Emergency Surgery: Evidence-Based Practice

Emergency Surgery: Evidence-Based Practice

Edited by Amy Walker

AMERICAN
MEDICAL PUBLISHERS
www.americanmedicalpublishers.com

American Medical Publishers,
41 Flatbush Avenue,
1st Floor, New York,
NY 11217, USA

Visit us on the World Wide Web at:
www.americanmedicalpublishers.com

ISBN: 978-1-63927-489-5

Cataloging-in-Publication Data

Emergency surgery : evidence-based practice / edited by Amy Walker.
p. cm.
Includes bibliographical references and index.
ISBN 978-1-63927-489-5
1. Surgical emergencies. 2. Evidence-based medicine. 3. Medical emergencies.
4. Surgery. I. Walker, Amy.

RD93 .E44 2022
617.026--dc23

Table of Contents

Preface IX

Chapter 1 **Management of spontaneous isolated dissection of the superior mesenteric artery** 1
Morihiro Katsura, Hidemitsu Mototake, Hiroaki Takara and Kazuhide Matsushima

Chapter 2 **Patient delay is the main cause of treatment delay in acute limb ischemia: an investigation of pre- and in-hospital time delay** 7
Louise S Londero, Birgitte Nørgaard and Kim Houlind

Chapter 3 **Extensive colonic necrosis following cardiac arrest and successful cardiopulmonary resuscitation** 13
Iraklis E Katsoulis, Alexia Balanika, Maria Sakalidou, Ioanna Gogoulou, Athanasios Stathoulopoulos and Michael K Digalakis

Chapter 4 **Correlation of the oxygen radical activity and antioxidants and severity in critically ill surgical patients** 17
Hongjin Shim, Ji Young Jang, Seung Hwan Lee and Jae Gil Lee

Chapter 5 **Isolated dissection of the superior mesenteric artery treated using open emergency surgery** 20
Markus Udo Wagenhäuser, Tolga Atilla Sagban, Mareike Witte, Mansur Duran, Hubert Schelzig and Alexander Oberhuber

Chapter 6 **An Observational Study of the Etiology, clinical presentation and outcomes associated with peritonitis in Lilongwe, Malawi** 26
Jonathan C Samuel, Javeria S Qureshi, Gift Mulima, Carol G Shores, Bruce A Cairns and Anthony G Charles

Chapter 7 **Acute cholecystitis: WSES position statement** 31
Fabio Cesare Campanile, Michele Pisano, Federico Coccolini, Fausto Catena, Ferdinando Agresta and Luca Ansaloni

Chapter 8 **Management of war-related vascular injuries: experience from the second gulf war** 37
Ali Jawas, Alaa K Abbas, Munier Nazzal, Marzoog Albader and Fikri M Abu-Zidan

Chapter 9 **Iatrogenic ureteric injuries following abdomino-pelvic operations: a 10-year tertiary care hospital experience** 42
Phillipo L Chalya, Anthony N Massinde, Albert Kihunrwa and Samson Simbila

Chapter 10 **Routine ultrasound examination by OB/GYN residents increase the accuracy of diagnosis for emergency surgery in gynecology**......50
Flavie Toret-Labeeuw, Cyrille Huchon, Thomas Popowski, Anne A Chantry, Alexandre Dumont and Arnaud Fauconnier

Chapter 11 **A technical modification for percutaneous tracheostomy: prospective case series study on one hundred patients**......57
Joao B Rezende-Neto, Argenil J Oliveira, Mario P Neto, Fernando A Botoni and Sandro B Rizoli

Chapter 12 **Acute appendicitis: proposal of a new comprehensive grading system based on clinical, imaging and laparoscopic findings**......64
Carlos Augusto Gomes, Massimo Sartelli, Salomone Di Saverio, Luca Ansaloni, Fausto Catena, Federico Coccolini, Kenji Inaba, Demetrios Demetriades, Felipe Couto Gomes and Camila Couto Gomes

Chapter 13 **World society of emergency surgery study group initiative on Timing of Acute Care Surgery classification (TACS)**......70
Yoram Kluger, Offir Ben-Ishay, Massimo Sartelli, Luca Ansaloni, Ashraf E Abbas, Ferdinando Agresta, et al.

Chapter 14 **Ten-year experiences with Tracheostomy at a University teaching hospital in Northwestern Tanzania: A retrospective review of 214 cases**......76
Japhet M Gilyoma, Darius D Balumuka and Phillipo L Chalya

Chapter 15 **Impact of high prevalence of pseudomonas and polymicrobial gram-negative infections in major sub-/total traumatic amputations on empiric antimicrobial therapy**......82
Moritz T Giesecke, Philipp Schwabe, Florian Wichlas, Andrej Trampuz and Christian Kleber

Chapter 16 **Proposal for a recovery prediction method for patients affected by acute mediastinitis**......91
Sławomir Jabłoński and Marcin Kozakiewicz

Chapter 17 **Splenic artery embolization: technically feasible but not necessarily advantageous**......103
F. Van der Cruyssen and A. Manzelli

Chapter 18 **Knowledge, awareness, and attitude towards infection prevention and management among surgeons: identifying the surgeon champion**......117
Massimo Sartelli, Yoram Kluger, Luca Ansaloni, Federico Coccolini, Gian Luca Baiocchi, Timothy C. Hardcastle, et al.

Chapter 19 **Acute mesenteric ischemia: guidelines of the World Society of Emergency Surgery**......123
Miklosh Bala, Jeffry Kashuk, Ernest E. Moore, Yoram Kluger, Walter Biffl, Carlos Augusto Gomes, Offir Ben-Ishay, Chen Rubinstein, Zsolt J. Balogh, Ian Civil, Federico Coccolini, Ari Leppaniemi, Andrew Peitzman, Luca Ansaloni, Michael Sugrue, Massimo Sartelli, Salomone Di Saverio, Gustavo P. Fraga and Fausto Catena

Chapter 20 **2017 WSES guidelines for the management of iatrogenic colonoscopy perforation 134**
Nicola de'Angelis, Salomone Di Saverio, Osvaldo Chiara, Massimo Sartelli, Aleix Martínez-Pérez, Franca Patrizi, et al.

Chapter 21 **Bologna guidelines for diagnosis and management of adhesive small bowel obstruction (ASBO): 2017 update of the evidence-based guidelines from the world society of emergency surgery ASBO working group 154**
Richard P. G. ten Broek, Pepijn Krielen, Salomone Di Saverio, Federico Coccolini, Walter L. Biffl, Luca Ansaloni, et al.

Chapter 22 **The *Global Alliance for Infections in Surgery*: defining a model for antimicrobial stewardship 167**
Massimo Sartelli, Francesco M. Labricciosa, Pamela Barbadoro, Leonardo Pagani, Luca Ansaloni, Adrian J. Brink, et al.

Chapter 23 **Resuscitative endovascular balloon occlusion of the aorta deployed by acute care surgeons in patients with morbidly adherent placenta 178**
Ramiro Manzano-Nunez, Maria F. Escobar-Vidarte, Claudia P. Orlas, Juan P. Herrera-Escobar, Samuel M. Galvagno, Juan J. Melendez, Natalia Padilla, Justin C. McCarty, Albaro J. Nieto and Carlos A. Ordoñez

Chapter 24 **Raising concerns about the Sepsis-3 definitions 184**
Massimo Sartelli, Yoram Kluger, Luca Ansaloni, Timothy C. Hardcastle, Jordi Rello, Richard R. Watkins, et al.

Chapter 25 **Predictors of Change in Functional Outcome at six months and twelve months after Severe Injury 193**
Aidan Lyanzhiang Tan, Yi Chiong, Nivedita Nadkarni, Jolene Yu Xuan Cheng, Ming Terk Chiu and Ting Hway Wong

Chapter 26 **Resuscitative Endovascular Balloon Occlusion of the Aorta in trauma 201**
Emiliano Gamberini, Federico Coccolini, Beatrice Tamagnini, Costanza Martino, Vittorio Albarello, Marco Benni, Marcello Bisulli, Nicola Fabbri, Tal Martin Hörer, Luca Ansaloni, Carlo Coniglio, Marco Barozzi and Vanni Agnoletti

Chapter 27 **Emergency abdominal surgery after solid organ transplantation 209**
Nicola de'Angelis, Francesco Esposito, Riccardo Memeo, Vincenzo Lizzi, Aleix Martìnez-Pérez, Filippo Landi, Pietro Genova, Fausto Catena, Francesco Brunetti and Daniel Azoulay

Permissions

List of Contributors

Index

Preface

Every book is a source of knowledge and this one is no exception. The idea that led to the conceptualization of this book was the fact that the world is advancing rapidly; which makes it crucial to document the progress in every field. I am aware that a lot of data is already available, yet, there is a lot more to learn. Hence, I accepted the responsibility of editing this book and contributing my knowledge to the community.

The purpose of emergency surgery is to deal with life-threatening conditions. It involves the stabilization and resuscitation of the patient, preparation of the patient for surgery as well as post- operative and recovery procedures. Conducting diagnostic tests, such as CT and MRI scans, X-rays, EKG and lab work are performed to determine the underlying condition and the severity of the problem. Certain medical conditions which require emergency surgery are acute respiratory failure, severe trauma to the chest, head, abdomen or other extremities, cardiac events (cardiac shocks, cardiac arrhythmia, heart attack), neurological or brain conditions, aneurysms, and abdominal emergencies including appendicitis, choecystitis, perforated ulcer and bowel blockage. After surgery, medication to control pain and prevent infections is prescribed. The time of recovery depends on the condition of the patients and in certain cases, rehabilitation therapy may be necessary. This book aims to shed light on some of the unexplored aspects of emergency surgery and the recent researches in this domain. It aims to give a general view of the various procedures, practices and complication management strategies that are crucial for the management of clinical emergencies. This book, with its detailed analyses and data, will prove immensely beneficial to professionals and students involved in this area at various levels.

While editing this book, I had multiple visions for it. Then I finally narrowed down to make every chapter a sole standing text explaining a particular topic, so that they can be used independently. However, the umbrella subject sinews them into a common theme. This makes the book a unique platform of knowledge.

I would like to give the major credit of this book to the experts from every corner of the world, who took the time to share their expertise with us. Also, I owe the completion of this book to the never-ending support of my family, who supported me throughout the project.

Editor

1

Management of spontaneous isolated dissection of the superior mesenteric artery

Morihiro Katsura[1*], Hidemitsu Mototake[2], Hiroaki Takara[3] and Kazuhide Matsushima[4]

Abstract

Background and method: The aim of this study was to assess retrospectively the clinical presentation, management and outcome of three patients with isolated SMA dissection encountered at Okinawa Prefectural Chubu Hospital, Japan from 2005 to 2006, along with a review of the literature. We follow up the patient's clinical symptoms and the image by using enhanced dynamic CT at 1 week, 1 or 2 months, 6 months, and yearly after onset.

Case presentation: We present three patients with acute abdominal pain due to spontaneous dissection of the superior mesenteric artery (SMA), who were treated by surgical revascularization or conservative management. Two patients underwent surgery because of signs or symptoms of intestinal ischemia and one patient elected conservative management. The SMA was repaired by bypass graft in two cases, and in one of these, the graft was occluded because of prominent native flow from the SMA. All patients were symptom free and there was no evidence of disease recurrence after a median follow-up of 4.3 years.

Conclusion: Although the indications for surgery are still controversial, we should proceed with exploratory laparotomy if the patient has acute symptoms with suspicion of mesenteric ischemia. A non-operative approach for SMA dissection requires close follow-up abdominal CT, with a focus on the clinical signs of mesenteric ischemia and the vascular supply of the SMA, including collateral flow from the celiac artery and inferior mesenteric artery.

Background

Spontaneous dissection of the superior mesenteric artery (SMA) is not associated with aortic dissection, and is a rare but potentially fatal disease. It is now being reported more often, which is a reflection of the increased use of imaging techniques, such as multidetector row computed tomography (MDCT), multiplanar (MPR) imaging, reconstruction imaging, and CT angiography (CTA) [1-4]. Three different therapeutic approaches are possible: conservative management [5-7], surgical revascularization [8-11], or endovascular therapy [12-18]. However, there is no consensus on the best treatment and its pathogenesis is unclear.

* Correspondence: morihiro@bj8.so-net.ne.jp
[1]Department of General Surgery, Okinawa Prefectural Hokubu Hospital, 2-12-3 Onaka, Nago, Okinawa 905-8512, Japan

Case presentation

Case 1

A 50-year-old man with an 8-day history of epigastric pain of acute onset was admitted. No associated symptoms of fever, nausea, constipation or diarrhea were present. He was previously healthy and had no remarkable medical history and trauma except for hypertension and appendectomy. On physical examination, mild tenderness and rebound tenderness over the epigastrium was observed, and no bruit was audible. Laboratory tests showed slightly elevated serum amylase and bilirubin. Therefore, we initially presumed that the patient had acute pancreatitis, but contrast-enhanced CT revealed isolated dissection of the SMA, in which the false lumen was thrombosed (figure 1a), and the dissecting portion began 6 cm from the origin of the SMA and extended to the distal branch. Bowel ischemia was suspected because of long-term continuous abdominal pain for 8 days and rebound tenderness, even though imaging

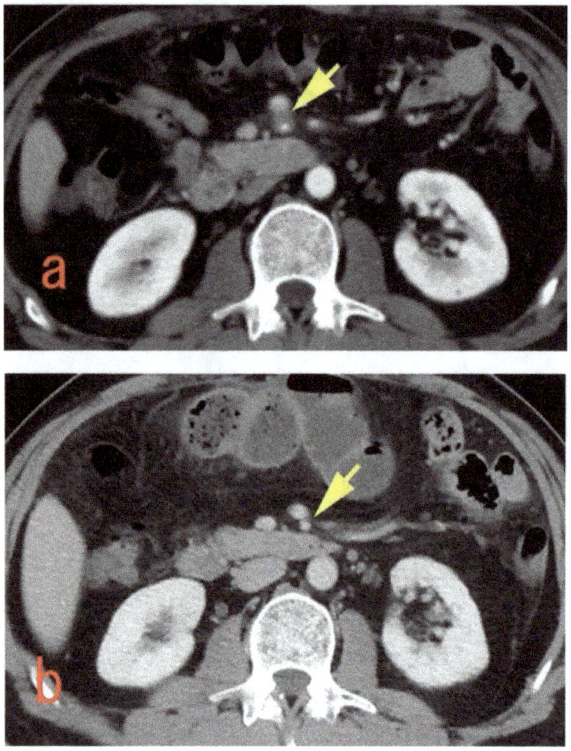

Figure 1 Sakamoto's type IV dissection of the SMA. (a) preoperative abdominal enhanced CT scan show isolated dissection of the SMA in which the false lumen was thrombosed without ulcer like projection(ULP). (b) postoperative 1 year abdominal enhanced CT scan show a thrombosed false lumen completely resolved with narrow true lumen.

showed no signs of ischemia. Exploratory laparotomy was performed and revealed a pale and pulseless small bowel without necrosis. We proceeded with a bypass operation between the distal portion of the SMA and the right common iliac artery, using the saphenous vein as a free graft. The postoperative course was uneventful without anticoagulation therapy, and follow-up CT showed good general vascularization of the bowel and full patency of the graft. The patient was discharge on postoperative day 14 and was symptom free 4 years after surgery with no recurrent symptoms or disease progression. One year after surgery, a thrombosed false lumen completely resolved with narrow true lumen on follow up CT(figure 1b).

Case 2

A 46-year-old woman presented to the emergency department with acute abdominal pain, back pain and vomiting. She had a history of hyperthyroidism but did not have any cardiovascular risk factors or recent trauma. On physical examination, mild periumbilical tenderness without signs of peritonitis was observed. Laboratory tests and abdominal radiography were unremarkable. Contrast-enhanced CT of the SMA showed abnormal wall thickness and irregular diameter, with a double lumen. Isolated dissection of the SMA began from just after the orifice of the SMA and separated the SMA into two distinct lumina for 3 cm from the origin of the artery; the distal portion of the SMA showed signs of thrombosis and stenosis, with the true lumen being compressed by the false lumen (figure 2a).

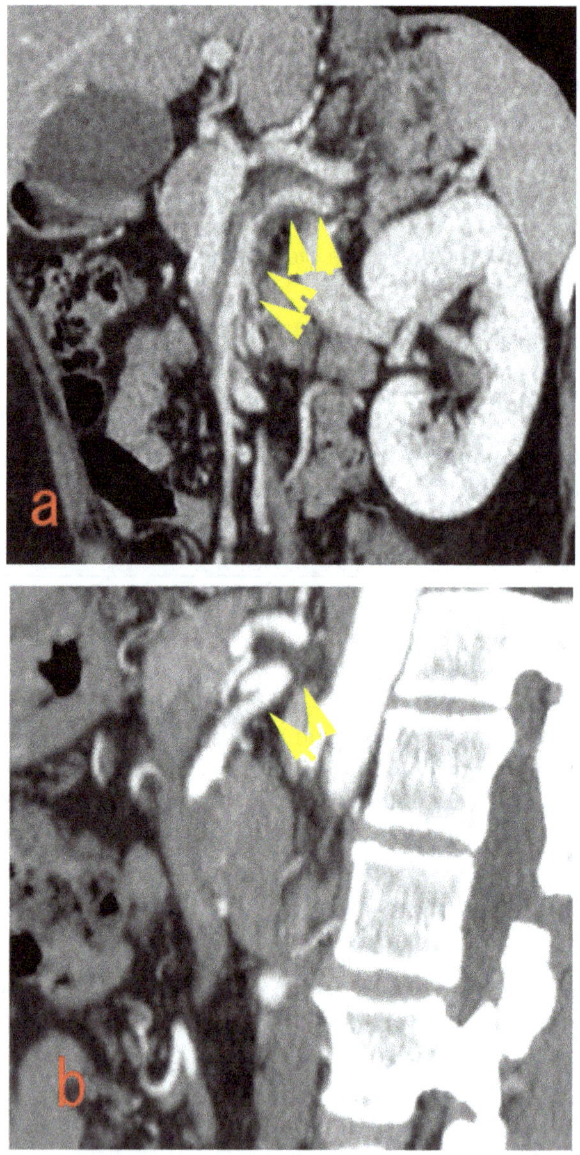

Figure 2 Sakamoto's type III dissection of the SMA. (a) preoperative MPR image of an abdominal enhanced CT scan show isolated dissection of the SMA began just after the orifice of the SMA and extended to the distal portion, with ULP and the narrow true lumen being compressed by the thrombosed false lumen. (b) postoperative 3 year abdominal enhanced CT scan show a thrombosed false lumen completely resolved without progressive dilation of ULP.

There were no signs of bowel ischemia, such as bowel thickening, abnormal contrast enhancement, or ascites. We proceeded with emergency laparotomy because of continuous severe abdominal pain, but no evidence of ischemia was found throughout the entire bowel with intraoperative duplex scanning. We performed a bypass operation between the distal portion of the SMA and the right common iliac artery, using the saphenous vein as a free graft, to prevent progression of SMA dissection. The postoperative course was uneventful without anticoagulation therapy, but follow-up CT showed thrombotic graft occlusion. We suppose that graft was occluded because of strong native flow from the SMA, that is, flow competition. The patient was discharge on postoperative day 8 and was symptom free 5 years after surgery, with no recurrent symptoms and disease progression. 3 year after surgery, a thrombosed false lumen completely resolved with ulcer like projection (ULP) on follow up CT(figure 2b).

Case 3

A 47-year-old man with a 5-day history of acute epigastric pain with radiation to the back was admitted. No associated symptoms of fever, nausea, constipation or diarrhea were present. He was previously healthy and had no cardiovascular risk factors and recent trauma. On physical examination, mild tenderness over the epigastrium without signs of peritonitis sign was observed, and no bruit was audible. Laboratory tests and abdominal radiography were unremarkable. Contrast-enhanced CT revealed a thin flap of the SMA, which began from just after the orifice of the SMA and separated the SMA into two distinct lumina; the resulting false lumen was thrombosed in the mid to distal portion of the SMA. Three-dimensionally reconstructed images demonstrated severe stenosis of the SMA, but no sign of bowel ischemia caused by prominent collateral flow from the celiac artery and inferior mesenteric artery (figure 3a). We chose conservative treatment without anticoagulation therapy. The abdominal pain completely disappeared on day 2 and he was discharged on day 4. The patient was symptom free 4 years after discharge with no recurrent symptoms and disease progression. One year after surgery, a thrombosed false lumen completely resolved with ULP on follow up CT (figure 3b).

Discussion and review of the literature

Spontaneous dissection of the SMA is a rare condition and is not associated with aortic dissection. It was first described by Bauerfield in 1947 [19]. In previously reported cases before 1972, the prognosis was very poor [19,20]. However, the prognosis has improved significantly since 1975 as a result of advancements in surgical techniques and imaging modalities [1-4].

The etiology of the disease has not yet been established, but atherosclerosis, cystic medial necrosis, and fibromuscular dysplasia have been implicated, often associated with untreated hypertension [3]. Solis et al. [21] have hypothesized that dissection usually begins 1.5-3 cm from the orifice of the SMA, thus sparing the origin of the artery. This segment of the SMA corresponds with the exit of the artery from the pancreas and is exposed to shearing force because this area forms the border zone between the fixed retropancreatic portion and the more distal mobile mesenteric portion. In two

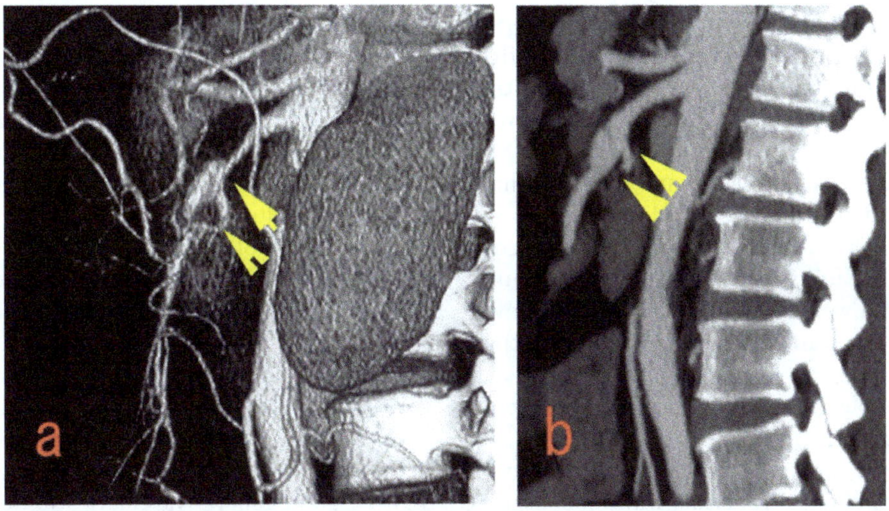

Figure 3 Sakamoto's type III dissection of the SMA. (a) preoperative three-dimensionally reconstructed images showing severe stenosis of the SMA with ULP, and the collateral flow from the celiac artery and inferior mesenteric artery. (b) postoperative 1 year abdominal enhanced CT scan show a thrombosed false lumen completely resolved without progressive dilation of ULP.

of the three present cases, dissection began from just after the orifice of the SMA, and in the other, dissection began 6 cm from the orifice. Our findings were not consistent with the hypothesis of Solis et al., but we suppose that the dissection plane can extend not only distally but also proximally.

The natural history of the disease is also unclear and depends on each case. Most patients present with acute epigastric pain, which is considered to be caused by the dissection itself or intestinal ischemia. Other common symptoms are nausea, vomiting, melena, and abdominal distention. These patients present acutely with symptom duration of <4 weeks [22]. Laboratory tests and abdominal radiography are usually unremarkable. Therefore, we often initially presume that the patient has enterocolitis and gastritis. Sometimes, laboratory tests show slightly elevated serum amylase, such as in our case 1, which might be caused by occlusion of the duodeno-pancreatic arcade [10].

Diagnosis in the acute stage has become possible as a result of advances and increased use of imaging techniques such as MDCT, leading to MPR and reconstruction imaging, and CTA [1-4]. Dynamic enhanced CT shows that the separated true lumen and false lumen can be identified by the presence of an intimal flap. Plain CT shows areas of high intensity if there is an acute clot in the false lumen. Sakamoto et al. [23] have categorized SMA dissection into four types based on contrast-enhanced CT scanning. Recently, Yun et al. [24] have added total thrombotic occlusion of the SMA trunk to Sakamoto's classification, and have devised a new classification of three types based on angiographic findings: type I: patent true and false lumina that show entry and re-entry sites; type II: patent true lumen but no re-entry flow from the false lumen; type IIa: visible false lumen but no visible re-entry site (blind pouch of false lumen); type IIb: no visible false luminal flow (thrombosed false lumen), which usually causes true luminal narrowing; and type III: SMA dissection with occlusion of SMA.

However, neither Sakamoto et al. nor Yun et al. have found a clear relationship between radiological appearance and clinical course. Abdominal color Doppler echo is also effective for following hemodynamic changes within the SMA, bowel movement, and signs of bowel ischemia, such as wall thickening and intestinal dilatation.

Some treatment algorithms for management of spontaneous SMA dissection have been reported [22,25,26]. At present, however, there is no established opinion on the indications for surgical revascularization, conservative medical management, or endovascular therapy. Some cases have been successfully treated by conservative therapy, such as anticoagulation [5,6]. Karacagi et al have reported that immediate anticoagulation therapy achieved prevention of clot formation in the true lumen in patients with spontaneous dissection of the carotid artery[27]. Nagai et al insisted that the disease pattern of SMA dissection seems similar with internal carotid artery and emphasized anticoagulation therapy is necessary for SMA dissection[5]. On the other hand, Sparks et al. [28] have reported a case in which the patient developed recurrent symptoms and disease progression 1 year later, which was a failure of the non-operative approach. This case indicates that a non-operative approach with anticoagulation of the isolated SMA dissection requires close follow-up, but it does not prevent disease progression. At that time, there is no consensus on the best drugs to be administered and administration period, so we didn't give anticoagulant for our case No.3. But we now suppose that anticoagulation therapy is valid for this disease when we chose conservative treatment.

Sparks et al. have suggested that indications for surgery are increasing size of the aneurysmal dilatation of the SMA, luminal thrombosis, or persistent symptoms despite anticoagulation. Various procedures for surgical intervention have been reported [8-11], including aorto-mesenteric or iliomesenteric bypass, thrombectomy, intimectomy with or without patch angioplasty, ligation, and resection. These surgical procedures have been performed with good short-term results.

Recent minimally invasive techniques, such as percutaneous endovascular stent placement and intralesional thrombolytic therapy, could be useful in certain cases, especially in patients at high risk for surgery [12-18]. However, it is usually difficult to find the site at which tearing of the artery wall started during dissection of the SMA, and the dissection often extends to the distal portion of the SMA, as in our present cases. There are still many problems with stent placement itself, such as risk of re-occlusion of a stented SMA and possible obstruction of side branches of the stented segment. Although we think that endovascular stent placement is feasible in patients without peritonitis or mesenteric ischemia, the long-term results should continue to be evaluated. Intralesional thrombolytic therapy with urokinase have also been reported, but some cases later underwent stenting [13] and laparotomy [29,30] because of clinical deterioration.

Table 1 summarizes the clinical characteristics of our three cases. In the patient whose small intestine we revascularized using an iliac-mesenteric bypass, because of bowel ischemia, postoperative follow-up CT showed good general vascularization of the bowel and full graft patency. On the other hand, in the patient whose small intestine we revascularized to prevent disease progression, although there was no sign of bowel

Table 1 Clinical characteristics of patients with SMA dissection

Case No.	Age/Sex	Dissection portion	Sakamoto's classification	Treatment	intestinal ischemia on surgery	Follow up CT
1	50/M	6 cm from the orifice of the SMA	type IV	Surgery	Yes	Graft patent ULP (-)
2	46/F	just after the orifice of the SMA	type III	Surgery	None	Graft occlusion ULP (+)
3	47/M	just after the orifice of the SMA	type III	Conservative	-	resolved false lumen ULP (+)

ULP: ulcer like projection

ischemia, postoperative follow-up CT showed thrombotic graft occlusion. We suppose that graft was occluded because of prominent native flow of the SMA, that is, flow competition. Our colleague Matsushima also has reported a case of SMA dissection [31]. In that case, emergency laparotomy was undertaken because the patient had signs that were suspicious of mesenteric ischemia. However, at the time of surgery, no evidence of ischemia was found throughout the entire bowel using intraoperative duplex scanning, which detected adequate blood flow to the peripheral branches, therefore, vascular reconstruction was not performed. Postoperatively, anticoagulants were administered and the patient was free of abdominal symptoms a few days later. We now suppose that it is not necessary to perform vascular reconstruction to prevent disease progression. Conservative management should have been indicated for our case No.2. If a initial CT demonstrated ULP, which was seen in the case like Sakamoto's classification type long term follow up are necessary for recognition of progressive dilation of ULP and aneurismal formation.

Conclusions

There is no consensus on the best treatment of spontaneous isolated dissection of the SMA. Although the indications for surgery are still controversial, we should proceed with exploratory laparotomy if the patient has acute symptoms with suspicion of mesenteric ischemia. A non-operative approach for SMA dissection requires close follow-up abdominal CT, with a focus on the clinical signs of mesenteric ischemia and the vascular supply of the SMA, including collateral flow from the celiac artery and inferior mesenteric artery.

Acknowledgements
The authors would like to thank all the surgical attending physicians and radiologists and residents at Okinawa Prefectural Chubu Hospital for their dedication and hard work in managing this study.

Consent
Written informed consent was obtained from the patients for publication of this case report and any accompanying images. A copy of the written consent is available for review by the Editor-in-Chief of this journal

Author details
[1]Department of General Surgery, Okinawa Prefectural Hokubu Hospital, 2-12-3 Onaka, Nago, Okinawa 905-8512, Japan. [2]Department of Cardiovascular Surgery, Okinawa Prefectural Chubu Hospital, Okinawa, Japan. [3]Department of Radiology, Okinawa Prefectural Chubu Hospital, Okinawa, Japan. [4]Department of Surgery, Penn State Milton S. Hershey Medical Center, PA, USA.

Authors' contributions
All authors except HT were involved in the preoperative and postoperative care of the patient. MK is the primary author and reviewed the case and the literature. HM and KM participated in the surgeries and provided editorial commentary. HT performed the angiography treatment. All authors conceived of the study, and participated in its design and coordination and helped to draft the manuscript. All authors have read and approved the final manuscript.

Competing interests
The authors declare that they have no competing interests.

References

1. Suzuki S, Furui S, Kohtake H, Sakamoto T, Yamasaki M, Furukawa A, Murata K, Takei R: **Isolated dissection of the superior mesenteric artery: CT findings in six cases.** *Abdom Imaging* 2004, **29**:153-157.
2. Hyodoh H, Hyodoh K, Takahashi K, Yamagata M, Kanazawa K: **Three-dimensional CT imaging of an isolated dissecting aneurysm of the superior mesenteric artery.** *Abdom Imaging* 1996, **21**:515-516.
3. Sheldon PJ, Esther JB, Sheldon EL, Sparks SR, Brophy DP, Oglevie SB: **Spontaneous dissection of the superior mesenteric artery.** *Cardiovasc Intervent Radiol* 2001, **24**:329-331.
4. Furukawa H, Moriyama N: **Spontaneous dissection of the superior mesenteric artery diagnosed on multidetector helical CT.** *J Comput Tomogr* 2002, **26**:143-144.
5. Nagai T, Torishima R, Uchida A, Nakashima H, Takahashi K, Okawara H, Oga M, Suzuki K, Miyamoto S, Sato R, Murakami K, Fujioka T: **Spontaneous dissection of the superior mesenteric artery in four cases treated with anticoagulation therapy.** *Intern Med* 2004, **43**:473-478.
6. Takayama H, Takeda S, Saitoh SK, Hayashi H, Takano T, Tanaka K: **Spontaneous isolated dissection of the superior mesenteric artery.** *Intern Med* 2002, **41**:713-716.
7. Cho YP, Ko GY, Kim HK, Moon KM, Kwon TW: **Conservative management of symptomatic spontaneous isolated dissection of the superior mesenteric artery.** *Br J Surg* 2009, **96**:720-723.
8. Kochi K, Orihashi K, Murakami Y, Sueda T: **Revascularization using arterial conduits for abdominal angina due to isolated and spontaneous dissection of the superior mesenteric artery.** *Ann Vasc Surg* 2005, **19**:418-420.
9. Tsuji Y, Hino Y, Sugimoto K, Matsuda H, Okita Y: **Surgical intervention for isolated dissecting aneurysm of the superior mesenteric artery: A case report.** *Vasc Endovasc Surg* 2004, **38**:469-472.
10. Picquet J, Abilez O, Pénard J, Jousset Y, Rousselet MC, Enon B: **Superficial femoral artery transposition repaire for isolated superior mesenteric artery dissection.** *J Vasc Surg* 2005, **42**:788-791.

11. Cormier F, Ferry J, Artru B, Wechsler B, Cormier JM: **Dissecting aneurysms of the main trunk of the superior mesenteric artery.** *J Vasc Surg* 1992, **15**:424-30.
12. Leung DA, Schneiber E, Kubik-Huch R, Marineck B, Pfammatter T: **Acute mesenteric ischemia caused by spontaneous isolated dissection of the superior mesenteric artery: treatment by percutaneous stent placement.** *Eur Radiol* 2000, **10**:1916-1919.
13. Yoon YW, Choi D, Cho SY, Lee DY: **Successful treatment of isolated spontaneous superior mesenteric artery dissection with stent placement.** *Cardiovasc Intervent Radiol* 2003, **26**:475-478.
14. Froment P, Alerci M, Vandoni RE, Bogen M, Gertsch P, Galeazzi G: **Stenting of a spontaneous dissection of the superior mesenteric artery:a new therapeutic approach?** *Cardiovasc Intervent Radiol* 2004, **27**:529-532.
15. Kim JH, Roh BS, Lee YH, Choi SS, So BJ: **Isolated spontaneous dissection of the superior mesenteric artery: percutaneous stent placement in two patients.** *Korean J Radiol* 2004, **5**:134-138.
16. Miyamoto N, Sakurai Y, Hirokami M, Takahashi K, Nishimori H, Tsuji K, Kang JH, Maguchi H: **Endovascular stent placement for isolated spontaneous dissection of the superior mesenteric artery: Report of a case.** *Radiat Med* 2005, **23**:520-524.
17. Casella IB, Bosch MA, Sousa WO Jr: **Isolated spontaneous dissection of the superior mesenteric artery treated by percutaneous stent placement: case report.** *J Vasc Surg* 2008, **47**:197-200.
18. Gobble RM, Brill ER, Rockman CB, Hecht EM, Lamparello PJ, Jacobowitz GR, Maldonado TS: **Endovascular treatment of spontaneous dissections of the superior mesenteric artery.** *J Vasc Surg* 2009, **50**:1326-1332.
19. Bauerfield SR: **Dissecting aneurysm of the aorta:a presentation of fifteen cases and a review of the recent literature.** *Ann Intern Med* 1947, **26**:873-889.
20. Hirai S, Hamanaka Y, Mitsui N, Isaka M, Kobayashi T: **Spontaneous dissection of the main trunk of the superior mesenteric artery.** *Ann Thorac Cardiovasc Surg* 2002, **8**:236-240.
21. Solis MM, Ranval TJ, McFarland DR, Eidt JF: **Surgical Treatment of superior mesenteric artery dissection aneurysm and simultaneous celiac artery compression.** *Ann Vasc Surg* 1993, **7**:457-462.
22. Subhas G, Gupta A, Nawalany M, Oppat WF: **Spontaneous isolated superior mesenteric artery dissection: a case report and literature review with management algorithm.** *Ann Vasc Surg* 2009, **23**:788-798.
23. Sakamoto I, Ogawa Y, Sueyoshi E, Fukui K, Murakami T, Uetani M: **Imaging appearances and management of isolated spontaneous dissection of the superior mesenteric artery.** *Eur J Radiol* 2007, **64**:103-110.
24. Yun WS, Kim YW, Park KB, Cho SK, Do YS, Lee KB, Kim DI, Kim DK: **Clinical and angiographic follow-up of spontaneous isolated superior mesenteric artery dissection.** *Eur J Vasc Endovasc Surg* 2009, **37**:572-577.
25. Morris JT, Guerriero J, Sage JG, Mansour MA: **Three isolated superior mesenteric artery dissections: update of previous case reports, diagnostics, and treatment options.** *J Vasc Surg* 2008, **47**:649-653.
26. Zerbib P, Perot C, Lambert M, Seblini M, Pruvot FR, Chambon JP: **Management of isolated spontaneous dissection of superior mesenteric artery.** *Langenbecks Arch Surg* 2010, **395**:437-443.
27. Karacagil S, Hardemark HG, Bergqvist D: **Spontaneous internal carotid artery dissection.** *Int Angiol* 1996, **15**:291-294.
28. Sparks SR, Vasquez JC, Bergan JJ, Owens EL: **Failure of nonoperative management of isolated superior mesenteric artery dissection.** *Ann Vasc Surg* 2000, **14**:105-109.
29. Javerliat I, Becquemin JP, d'Audiffret A: **Spontaneous isolated dissection of the superior mesenteric artery.** *Eur J Vasc Endovasc Surg* 2003, **25**:180-184.
30. Hwang CK, Wang JY, Chaikof EL: **Spontaneous dissection of the superior mesenteric artery.** *Ann Vasc Surg* 2010, **24**:254.e1-5.
31. Matsushima K: **Spontaneous isolated dissection of the superior mesenteric artery.** *Am Coll Surg* 2006, **203**:970-971.

2

Patient delay is the main cause of treatment delay in acute limb ischemia: an investigation of pre- and in-hospital time delay

Louise S Londero[1*], Birgitte Nørgaard[2] and Kim Houlind[3]

Abstract

Background: The prognosis of acute limb ischemia is severe, with amputation rates of up to 25% and in-hospital mortality of 9-15%. Delay in treatment increases the risk of major amputation and may be present at different stages, including patient delay, doctors´ delay and waiting time in the emergency department. It is important to identify existing problems in order to reduce time delay.
The aim of this study was to collect data for patients with acute limb ischemia and to evaluate the time delay between the different events from onset of symptoms to specialist evaluation and further treatment with focus on pre-hospital and in-hospital time delays.

Methods: We conducted a prospective cross-sectional cohort study including all patients suspected with acute limb ischemia who were admitted to the emergency department of a community hospital in a six months period. Temporal delay in the different phases between the time of occurrence of symptoms and completion of treatment was recorded prospectively. All patients who underwent intervention had a 30 days follow-up with regard to major amputation of the leg and survival.

Results: A total of 42 patients (21 men and 21 women) age 73 (20–95) years (median (range)) was identified. From onset of symptoms to first contact with a doctor the time for all patients were 24 (0–1200) hours. Thirty patients needed immediate intervention. In the group of fourteen patients who had immediate operation, the median time from vascular evaluation to revascularization was 324.5 (122–873) minutes and in the group of eight patients that went through an imaging procedure before an operation the median delay was 822 (494–1185) minutes from specialist assessment to revascularization. The median time for revascularization among four patients, who were treated with arterial thrombolysis was 5621 (1686–8376) minutes.
At 30 days follow up, six patients had had the ischemic limb amputated above the ankle and four patients had died.

Conclusions: We found that the largest time delay was between onset of symptoms and first contact to a medical doctor. A greater public awareness is needed, so as to facilitate urgent revascularisation and improve outcomes.

Keywords: Acute limb ischemia, ALI, Treatment delay, Fast track department, Diagnostic packages, Patient delay

* Correspondence: Louise.Skovgaard.Londero@rsyd.dk
[1]Department of Cardiothoracic- and Vascular Surgery, University Hospital of Odense, Sdr. Boulevard 29, 5000 Odense C, Denmark
Full list of author information is available at the end of the article

Background

Acute limb ischemia (ALI) is a sudden decrease in limb perfusion causing a potential threat to the limb viability [1]. The event may be caused by thrombosis, embolism, peripheral aneurysm with embolus/thrombosis, acute graft occlusion, iatrogenic intervention or by trauma. The prognosis is severe, with reported amputation rates of up to 25% and in-hospital mortality of 9-15% [1-3]. Delay in treatment of acute lower limb ischemia increases the risk of amputation [4-7].

The delay may be present at different stages, including patient delay, delay caused by the referring medical doctor, waiting time in the emergency department, waiting time for diagnostic imaging, or time for preparation at the operating theatre, including anaesthesia. Before creating strategies for reducing treatment delay, existing problems need to be identified.

It has been shown that implementation of ED fast track systems reduces ED waiting time and overcrowding [8-10]. In Denmark, the fast track organisation of Emergency Departments (ED's) has established length of stay time targets [11,12] similar to those known in the UK and Australia [13,14]. This has been done to ensure a punctual evaluation, examination and initiation of treatment of the patient including specialist examination within 30 minutes from arrival and a diagnosis within four hours. To optimize the patient flow 36 diagnostic packages have been prepared. These are based on main symptom with respect for triaging and time sensitive diagnosis. One of the packages is "Pain in extremity" and includes ALI [11]. The implementation in our hospital was done in September 2012. It is, however, unknown whether other causes for time delay are equally or more important for patients suspected with ALI.

The aim of this study was to collect data for patients with ALI and evaluate the time delay between the different events from onset of symptoms to specialist evaluation and further treatment with focus on pre-hospital and in-hospital time delays.

Methods

Design

We conducted a prospective cross-sectional cohort study. The study was approved by the Danish Data Protection Agency. Data collection took place from 01.10.12 to 31.03.13, at Kolding Hospital, a community hospital with a department for vascular surgery with a catchments area covering both suburban and rural districts.

Settings

The patients´ first contact with the medical care system is with a non-vascular specialist outside the hospital. When ALI is suspected, the non-vascular specialist consults a specialist in vascular surgery and the patients are admitted to the hospital. The ED fast track unit is notified by the vascular surgeon. All patients suspected with ALI are admitted to the fast track area in the ED.

The fast track unit is separated from the rest of the ED. It is open 24 hours a day and has its own nurses and staff station. There are two senior doctors, one specialist in internal medicine and one specialist in surgery, in the department from 08.00 am to 12.00 pm and at night they are on call. Also there are a number of junior doctors associated with unit.

The vascular specialist is summoned to the ED when the patient suspected with ALI arrives and will be the first doctor to see the patient within the ED fast track area.

Data collection

For each patient admitted, the specialist vascular surgeon on call started the data collection of the particular patient. A registration form was filled in with information about gender, age and earlier vascular procedures. Furthermore, onset of symptoms, first contact with a medical doctor (a non-vascular specialist), time for referral to the vascular department, time for arrival and time for vascular evaluation were registered. All patients were scored according to the classification suggested by Rutherford, where the severity of ALI is divided into four categories [6]. In class 1 the limb is not immediately threatened and is considered as subacute ischemia, while in class 2A and 2B the limb is threatened and needs immediate revascularization. Patients with class 3 ischemia have irreversible damage and there is no indication to improve the blood supply.

If the patient was not judged to have ALI the registration was stopped after the vascular examination. If they had ALI and needed further intervention, time was registered for the beginning and end of the procedure. Further interventions were computed tomography (CT) or magnetic resonance (MR)-imaging, operation, endovascular procedure or amputation.

When the patient arrived to the ED, examination of the leg was used to define the severity of the ischemia. ALI was classified into one of four categories based on clinical findings and Doppler measurements.

All patients who underwent intervention had a 30 days follow-up with regard to major amputation of the limb and death.

Analyses

For each patient the time between the registrations, in a chronological order, was measured. Descriptive statistics were performed using Microsoft Excel Version 7.0. To compare patient related time delay in patient with and without prior vascular surgery we performed Wilcoxon rank sum test using Stata, (Version 13.1, StataCorp LP, College Station, Texas).

Results

A total of 42 patients (21 men and 21 women) ages 73 (20–95) years (median (range) were admitted on suspicion of ALI. Twenty-one patients (50%) had a prior history of vascular surgery for periphery arterial disease (PAD) in one or both legs. Twelve patients did either not have ALI or had ALI class 1, which did not need immediate intervention, and registration stopped after vascular examination. Of these patients three had deep venous thrombosis (DVT), one had neuropathic pain, seven had ALI class 1 and one had class 2A ischemia, but it was found that no immediate treatment was required. The distribution of patients according to levels of severity of acute limb ischemia is shown in Figure 1.

Time from onset to specialist assessment (n = 42)

For all patients the time from onset of symptoms to specialist assessment the median time was 27.25 (1.65 – 1202.5) hours. This time period was divided into smaller time periods as showed in Figure 2.

Median time from onset of symptoms to first contact with a medical doctor was 24 (0–1200) hours. For patients with a prior history of vascular surgery the median time was 22 (0–240) hours and for patients with no earlier history of vascular surgery the time was 26.35 (0.17- 1200) hours. The time difference between the two groups was not significant (p = 0.4).

The time from first contact to a doctor until the ED was notified was 1.25 (0–67.5) hours and transportation time to the ED was 1.7 (0–19.9) hours. Median time from arrival to the ED to evaluation by a vascular specialist was 0.33 (0–1.5) hours. A total of 26 patients (62%) were assessed by the vascular surgeon on call within 30 minutes after arrival, 9 (21%) within an hour, and 7 (17%) waited for more than one hour.

ALI classified patients (n = 30)

Thirty patients were classified with ALI and needed immediate intervention as seen in Figure 3. Fourteen patients needed operation immediately, 11 patients went through diagnostic imaging before further intervention, one patient went directly to diagnostic angiography and thrombolysis and for 3 patients the ischemia was so severe, that revascularization was not indicated; they went directly for an amputation of the limb. One patient was classified with severe ALI in both legs caused by an occlusion of the aorta in the setting of a major myocardial infarct and died before any action could be taken.

Among the 14 patients operated immediately, it was possible to restore blood flow to the limb in 12. Eight of the 11 patients who underwent imaging had an operation afterwards; each having successful revascularization, yet two patients had re-operation due to new occlusions. Three patients underwent thrombolysis and one had an endovascular procedure, all of them resulting in restored blood flow.

In the group of patients who had immediate operation, 10 had an embolectomy, two had a thrombendarterectomy and two had peripheral bypass operation. The median time from vascular evaluation to revascularization (defined as time to end of successful surgery) was 324.5

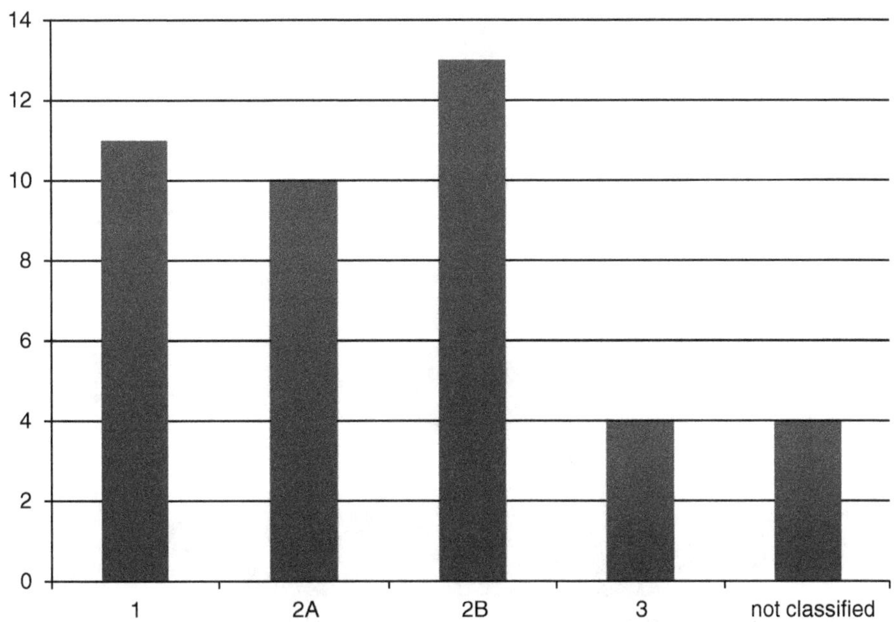

Figure 1 Distribution of patients. The distribution of patients (n = 42) according to levels of severity of acute limb ischemia.

Onset of symptoms –1. contact
24 hours [0-1200]
1. contact– ER notified
1.25 hours [0-67.5]
ER notified –arrival
1.7 hours [0-19.9]
Arrival – Specialist assessment
0.3 hours. [0-1.5]

Figure 2 Pre-hospital time delay. The time delay from onset of symptoms to specialist assessment (median time [range]) for all 42 patients suspected with ALI.

(122–873) minutes, whereas in the group of patients that went through an imaging procedure before operation the median delay was 822 (494–1185) minutes from vascular evaluation to revascularization. The median time for revascularization in the thrombolytic group was 5621 (1686–8376) minutes Figure 4.

30-days follow-up on amputation and death

At 30 days follow up, six patients had had the ischemic limb amputated above the ankle; four of these amputations were above the knee. Three of the patients were amputated without prior attempt of revascularization. In the amputation group (n = 6) the median time from onset of symptoms to arrival at the ER was 68.8 (24–1202) hours. The patient who did not arrive until 1202 hours (50 days) after onset of symptoms was an 83 years old man suffering from a neurodegenerative disease. He was referred acutely, without being able to tell for how long he had had symptoms. The hospital files showed that he had been seen in the emergency department 50 days earlier with complaints about pain in the leg. At that time, it was suspected to be muscle or join discomfort and he was released without seeing a vascular specialist. Fifty days later his family doctor was called to see him and he referred the patient to the hospital suspecting ALI.

Five out of the six patients who were amputated were assessed by a vascular specialist within 30 minutes after arrival; one waited 90 minutes. Three of these patients had an attempt of surgical revascularization. From vascular specialist assessment to revascularization it took 122, 365 and 620 minutes respectively. Two of the patients had an amputation above knee within 24 hours after attempt of revascularization and the last one had an amputation below knee after 9 days.

Four patients died within 30 days after referral to the vascular department, two had had a revascularization procedure that failed to restore blood flow, one had an amputation below the knee and the last one died of myocardial infarct shortly after arrival to the emergency department.

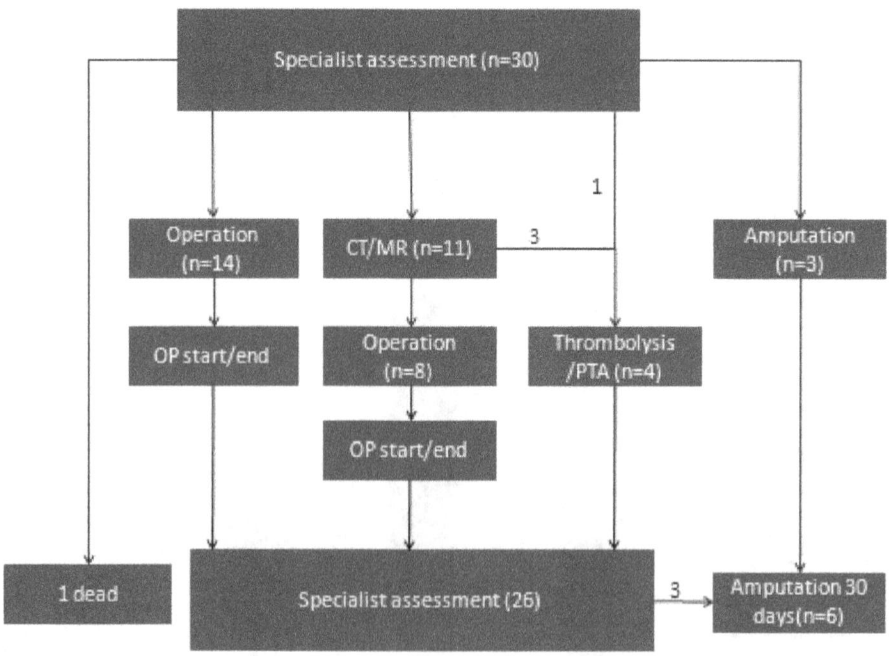

Figure 3 From specialist assessment to revascularization. The flowchart shows the distribution of the 30 patients, in need of acute intervention after specialist assessment.

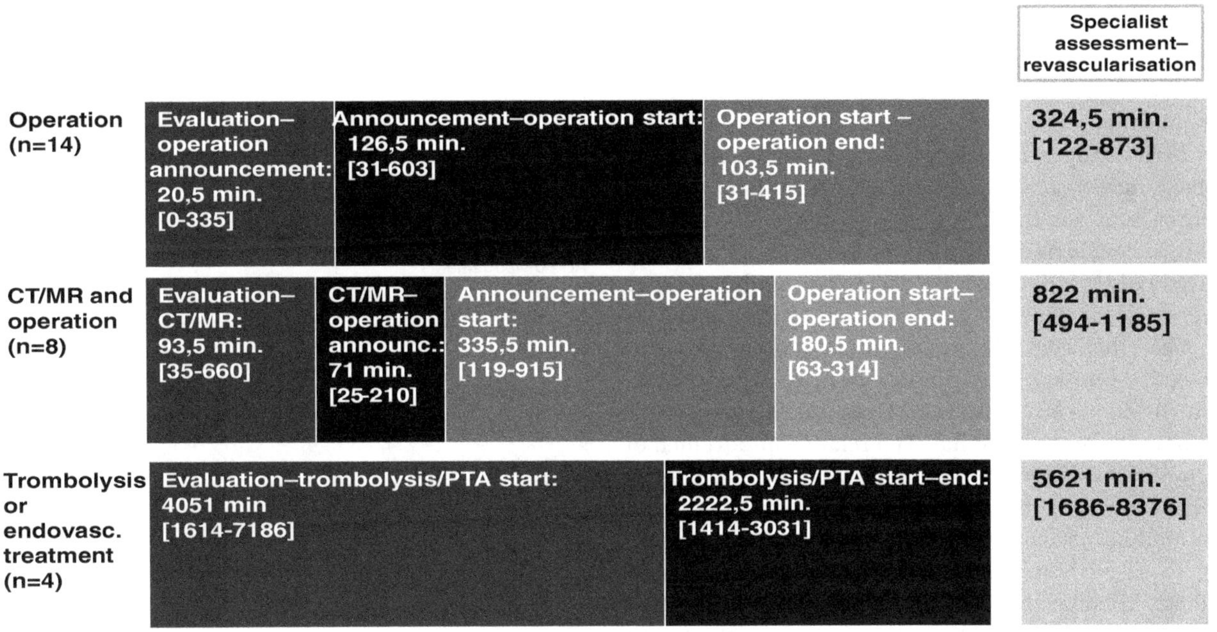

Figure 4 In-hospital time delay. The in-hospital time delay for all three groups with vascular intervention.

Discussion

Patients with acute limb ischemia have a poor prognosis with regard to major limb amputations and death. The rate of major amputations is reported to be up to 25%, including both non-salvageable limbs and limbs thought to be salvageable [1]. For patients with attempt of revascularization the amputation rate is 9-15% [1-3]. In our study six out of 30 (20%) patients found to have ALI underwent major amputation within the first 30 days, three of them had non-salvageable limbs at the time of vascular specialist assessment and no revascularization procedure was attempted.

Eliason and colleagues reported 9.3% in-hospital mortality for patients admitted with ALI [2], while Kuukasjärvi reported a 30 days mortality of 13% [15]. This is comparable to our findings where the 30 day's mortality rate was 13.3% (four out of 30).

There is a relationship between the delay from onset of symptoms to revascularisation and subsequent mortality or limb loss. As an example, Morris-Stiff and colleagues recently compared the results after peripheral arterial embolectomy from two different historical time periods in the same community hospital [16]. In both time periods, patients with an interval between symptoms and treatment of less than five hours had a more favourable outcome than those who suffered a longer delay. Therefore, it is of great importance that patients with suspected ALI are referred to a hospital with vascular specialists immediately.

In our study the largest pre-hospital time delay occurred between the onset of symptoms and the first contact to a doctor, this was the case for all patients, including the ones with irreversible ischemia. The median time was 24 hours, which is similar to findings in earlier studies [7,16]. Burgess and colleagues found that mean delay from onset of symptoms to first contact to a doctor was 29 hours and the main reason for delay was the patient. Also, Morris-Stiff and colleagues found that despite of advances in improvements in pre- and peri-operative management of ALI, the amputation rate was not significantly reduced and, therefore, concluded that the main reason was the fact that the patients still had a mean time from symptoms to revascularisation of 24 hours [16].

Patients with a prior history of vascular surgery for PAD tended to respond faster to symptoms than patients without prior history, suggesting that the first group is more aware of the importance of symptoms. This difference was, however, not statistically significant. Time delay between the first contact to a doctor and the arrival at the emergency department was reasonable taking into consideration that most patients were seen and examined by the non-vascular specialist outside the hospital before referral. To our knowledge, this is the first study evaluating the different time steps from onset of symptoms to revascularisation.

When looking at the in-hospital delay one of the main goals in the fast track program is to have the patients evaluated by a specialist within 30 minutes after arrival. In our study 62% of the patients were evaluated within 30 minutes, which leaves place for improvement. On the other hand, only 17% waited for more than one hour due to the fact that the surgeon was occupied with other acute tasks. Whether the fast track programme has shortened the in-hospital time delay is not certain, because our data collection started after the implementation.

A bit surprisingly we found that patients who went for imaging before further intervention had an almost 8.5 hours longer in-hospital delay than patients who needed immediately operation. This was mainly due to waiting time for the CT- or MR-imaging. Though imaging is considered a part of the fast track programme and should be done within the first four hours after arrival. Local changes have now been done in order to meet this goal of the fast track programme. We recognize limitations of the study, including especially a small sample size and also the fact that we only studied practice in one hospital. The relative importance of each of the different phases of in hospital delay cannot be expected to be the same in other locations, although the method used may be thought of as an inspiration for local analyses in other hospitals. However, the primary finding; that patient delay is the main reason for treatment delay in ALI, seems to be consistent with findings from other geographical areas and other time periods [7,16] and may be a finding of general interest.

Conclusions

In summary, we found that the main component of treatment delay is the time between onset of symptoms and the first contact to a doctor. Although we have not specifically asked the patients about the reasons for this delay, it seems safe to suggest that greater public awareness is needed, so as to facilitate urgent revascularisation and improve outcomes. Public campaigns, stressing the need for urgent treatment of ALI, might be a tool to improve results. In order to avoid misdiagnosing patients with ALI it may be helpful if all patients with acute pain in a leg, not caused by fractures or other obvious causes, are seen by a vascular specialist when referred to an emergency department according to the fast track organisation [11]. We recommend further studies including more centres and a larger number of patients in order to produce valid and generalizable results. We also recommend studies investigating the specific reasons for delay from onset of symptoms and the first contact to a doctor in order to minimize this delay and thereby improve outcomes for ALI patients.

Consent

According to Danish legislation and The National Committee on Health Research Ethics written consent from the patients is not required.

Competing interests

The authors declare that they have no competing interests.

Authors' contributions

LL and KH conceived the study and designed it with contribution from BN. LL designed the registration form and both LL and KH participated in the data collection. LL made the analysis and both BN and KH participated in the interpretation of data. LL drafted the manuscript and KH and BN contributed to critical revision and approved the final manuscript. LL had full access to all data in the study and takes responsibility for the integrity of the data and the accuracy of the data analysis. All authors read and approved the final manuscript.

Acknowledgements

We like to thank the vascular specialists at the department of vascular surgery at Kolding Hospital for the help with collecting the data.

Author details

[1]Department of Cardiothoracic- and Vascular Surgery, University Hospital of Odense, Sdr. Boulevard 29, 5000 Odense C, Denmark. [2]Institute of Public Health, University of Southern Denmark, Sdr. Boulevard 29, 5000 Odense C, Denmark. [3]Department of Vascular Surgery, Kolding Hospital, Skovvangen 2, 6000 Kolding, Denmark.

References

1. Norgren L, Hiatt WR, Dormandy JA, Nehler MR, Harris KA, Fowkes FG, Group TIW, Bell K, Caporusso J, Durand-Zaleski I, Komori K, Lammer J, Liapis C, Novo S, Razavi M, Robbs J, Schaper N, Shigematsu H, Sapoval M, White C, White J, Clement D, Creager M, Jaff M, Mohler E 3rd, Rutherford RB, Sheehan P, Sillesen H, Rosenfield K: **Inter-Society Consensus for the Management of Peripheral Arterial Disease (TASC II).** *Eur J Vasc Endovasc Surg: Off J Eur J Vasc Endovasc Surg* 2007, **33**(Suppl 1):S1–75.
2. Eliason JL, Wainess RM, Proctor MC, Dimick JB, Cowan JA Jr, Upchurch GR Jr, Stanley JC, Henke PK: **A national and single institutional experience in the contemporary treatment of acute lower extremity ischemia.** *AnnSurg* 2003, **238**(3):382–389.
3. Ouriel K, Veith FJ: **Acute lower limb ischemia: determinants of outcome.** *Surgery* 1998, **124**(2):336–341.
4. Rutherford RB, Baker JD, Ernst C, Johnston KW, Porter JM, Ahn S, Jones DN: **Recommended standards for reports dealing with lower extremity ischemia: revised version.** *J Vasc Surg* 1997, **26**(3):517–538.
5. Campbell WB, Ridler BM, Szymanska TH: **Current management of acute leg ischaemia: results of an audit by the Vascular Surgical Society of Great Britain and Ireland.** *British J Surg* 1998, **85**(11):1498–1503.
6. Karapolat S, Dag O, Abanoz M, Aslan M: **Arterial embolectomy: a retrospective evaluation of 730 cases over 20 years.** *Surg Today* 2006, **36**(5):416–419.
7. Burgess NA, Scriven MW, Lewis MH: **An 11-year experience of arterial embolectomy in a district general hospital.** *J R Coll Surg Edinb* 1994, **39**(2):93–96.
8. Ieraci S, Digiusto E, Sonntag P, Dann L, Fox D: **Streaming by case complexity: evaluation of a model for emergency department Fast Track.** *Emerg Med Australas* 2008, **20**(3):241–249.
9. Nash K, Zachariah B, Nitschmann J, Psencik B: **Evaluation of the fast track unit of a university emergency department.** *J Emerg Nurs* 2007, **33**(1):14–20.
10. Sanchez M, Smally AJ, Grant RJ, Jacobs LM: **Effects of a fast-track area on emergency department performance.** *J Emerg Med* 2006, **31**(1):117–120.
11. Region S: **Rapport Vedrørende Akutpakker til de Fælles AkutModtagelser [Report on Fast Track Packages in the Emergency Departments in the Region of Southern Denmark].** [www.fremtidenssygehuse.dk/dwn247348]
12. Region S: **Rapport om Fælles AkutModtagelser (FAM) i Region Syddanmark [Report on Emergency Departmenst in the Region of Southern Denmark].** [www.regionsyddanmark.dk/dwn105467]
13. Australian G: *A National Health and Hospitals Network:Further Investments in Australia's Health.* Canberra, Australia: Department of Health and Ageing; 2010 [http://www.health.gov.au/internet/main/publishing.nsf/Content/nhhnreport-2/$File/NHHN%20Report%20two.pdf]

3

Extensive colonic necrosis following cardiac arrest and successful cardiopulmonary resuscitation

Iraklis E Katsoulis[1*], Alexia Balanika[2], Maria Sakalidou[2], Ioanna Gogoulou[1], Athanasios Stathoulopoulos[1] and Michael K Digalakis[1]

Abstract

Non-occlusive colonic ischaemia is a recognized albeit rare entity related to low blood flow within the visceral circulation and in most reported cases the right colon was affected. This is the second case report in the literature of extensive colonic necrosis following cardiac arrest and cardiopulmonary resuscitation (CPR). A 83-year-old Caucasian woman was admitted to our hospital due to a low energy hip fracture. On her way to the radiology department she sustained a cardiac arrest. CPR started immediately and was successful. A few hours later, the patient developed increasing abdominal distension and severe metabolic acidocis. An abdominal multidetector computed tomography (MDCT) scan was suggestive of intestinal ischaemia. At laparotomy, the terminal ileum was ischaemic and extensive colonic necrosis was found, sparing only the proximal third of the transverse colon. The rectum was also spared. The terminal ileum and the entire colon were resected and an end ileostomy was fashioned. Although the patient exhibited a transient improvement during the immediate postoperative period, she eventually died 24h later from multiple organ failure. Histology showed transmural colonic necrosis with no evidence of a thromboembolic process or vasculitis. Therefore, this entity was attributed to a low flow state within the intestinal circulation secondary to the cardiac arrest.

Keywords: *Colonic necrosis, Non-occlusive ischaemia, CPR*

Introduction

Non-occlusive colonic ischaemia is a recognized albeit rare entity related to low blood flow within the visceral circulation. Post-traumatic shock-associated colonic ischaemia has been previously reported in young, healthy patients and has involved primarily the right colon in most instances [1-5]. Only a few cases of extensive non-occlusive colonic gangrene have been reported [6-10]. This is the second case report of colonic necrosis secondary to cardiac arrest followed by successful CPR.

Case presentation

A 83-year-old Caucasian woman was admitted to our hospital due to a low energy fracture of her left hip. The initial assessment in the Emergency Department revealed pallor, tachycardia and a systolic blood pressure of 110 mmHg. Her past medical history included coronary artery disease, arterial hypertension and depression for which the patient was under medication over the last three years. On her way to the radiology department the patient sustained a cardiac arrest. Cardiopulmonary resuscitation (CPR) started immediately and she was intubated. CPR was successful and the patient was subsequently transferred to the Intensive Care Unit (ICU). During her stay in the ICU, the vasoconstricting agent noradrenaline had to be installed in order to support her circulation and after a few hours she developed increasing abdominal distension and severe metabolic acidocis (PH = 7.14 with a Standard Base Excess = – 13.6 mEq/L). The patient underwent a multidetector computed tomography (MDCT) examination from the dome of the diaphragm to the symphysis pubis with a 6-row multidetector CT (Philips, Brilliance 6); using biphasic CT protocol for the abdomen without oral contrast administration. A 120 ml non-ionic contrast

* Correspondence: hrkats@yahoo.co.uk
[1]1st Surgical Department, Asklepieio General Hospital, Voula, Greece

medium (350mg/ml iobitridol) and 50 ml of normal saline flush were administered intravenously with a power injector at a flow rate 3mls/s, with scan delay for starting arterial and portal-venous phases at 10s and 100s, respectively. Image acquisitions parameters were: 5 mm slice thickness, slice collimation of 1.5 mm, pitch 1, 140 kV and 120mAs.

In the arterial phase, MDCT showed at least two focal areas of high attenuation (> 90 HU) within the lumen of the ascending colon and caecum suggestive of active bleeding [11]. Axial CT images at the level of the upper and the middle abdomen demonstrated thickened caecal and ascending colon wall (up to 11.5 mm) [12,13] with increased density due to intravenous contrast enhancement, pericaecal fat stranding and low-attenuation areas of intraperitoneal fluid at the root of the mesentery, at the perihepatic and Morrison's spaces (Figures 1–2). No endoluminal defect of mesenteric arteries and veins was noted.

The above CT findings were suggestive of intestinal ischaemia and in association with the patient's deterioration an exploratory laparotomy was undertaken which revealed ischaemia of the terminal ileum and extensive colonic necrosis sparing only the proximal third of the transverse colon. The rectum was also spared. The terminal ileum and the entire colon were resected and an end ileostomy was fashioned through the right abdominal rectus muscle sheath. The rectal stump was closed and left in the pelvis (Hartmann's pouch). Although the patient exhibited a transient improvement during the immediate postoperative period, she eventually died 24h later from multiple organ failure. Histology showed transmural colonic necrosis without evidence of a thromboembolic process or vasculitis. Therefore, the aetiology was felt to be a low flow state within the intestinal circulation most likely secondary to the cardiac arrest.

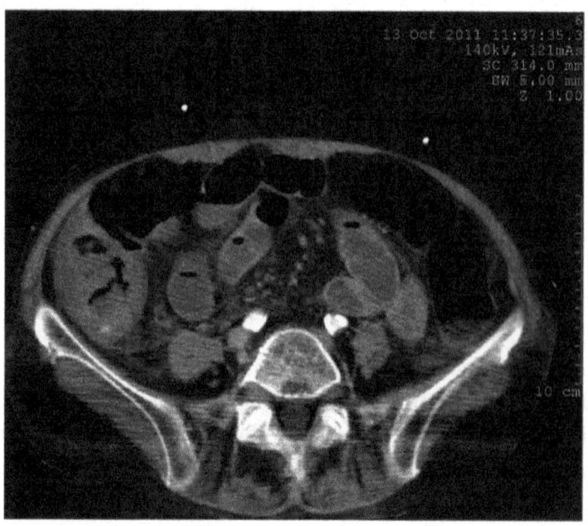

Figure 1 Axial CT image at arterial phase demonstrates a thickened caecal wall. A focal area of high attenuation suggesting active bleeding is seen in the lumen of the caecum.

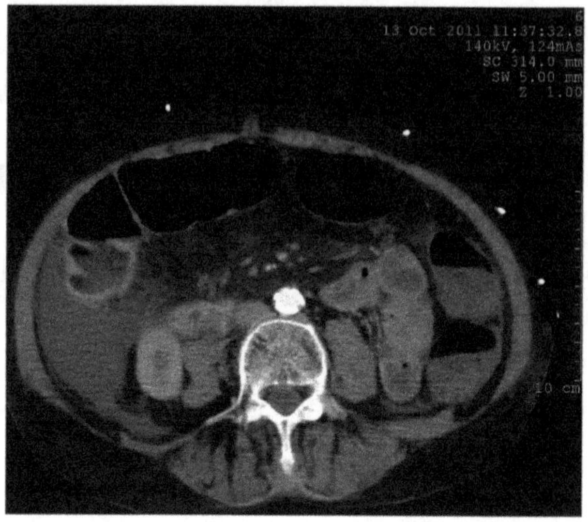

Figure 2 Axial CT image at venous phase shows intraperitoneal fluid and pericaecal fat stranding.

Discussion

The colon presents weak points on blood supply and poor autoregulation of blood flow that constitute the main predisposing factors for splachnic vasoconstriction and non-occlusive ischaemia [1]. Following experiments on flow characteristics within the mesenteric circulation when subjected to changing haemodynamics, Nikas D *et al.* found that the colon has the greatest sensitivity to hypotension [14].

An experimental model has also been used involving cardiogenic shock produced by pericardial tamponade [15]. This was associated with marked reductions in the intestinal blood flow. More recently Toung *et al.* [16], in another experimental model, involved variable degrees of hypovolaemic shock produced by graded levels of haemorrhage, from 12.5 to 50% of the calculated blood volume. This was associated with disproportional mesenteric ischaemia due to mesenteric vasoconstriction. They concluded that like cardiogenic shock, haemorrhagic shock generates selective mesenteric ischaemia by producing a disproportionate mesenteric vasospasm that, which is mediated primarily by the renin-angiotensin axis.

Both haemorrhagic and cardiogenic shocks can result in decreased perfusion pressure, prompting selective vasoconstriction of the mesenteric arterioles to maintain perfusion pressure of the vital organs, at the selective expense of the mesenteric organs. The response to any of these conditions can, variably and unpredictably, cause haemorrhagic gastric stress erosions, non-occlusive mesenteric ischaemia of the small bowel, ischaemic colitis, ischaemic hepatitis, acalculous cholecystitis, and ischaemic pancreatitis. Injury to the mesenteric organs can also initiate the systemic inflammatory response syndrome and, consequently, multiple organ failure [17,18].

Post-traumatic shock-associated colonic ischaemia has been previously reported in young, healthy patients and has involved primarily the right colon in most instances [1-5]. Only a few cases of extensive non-occlusive colonic necrosis have been reported [6-10] (Table 1). In all cases this entity has been attributed to decreased colonic perfusion but other factors could also have been involved, such as inadequate collateral circulation and increased plasma viscosity [8].

In the case presented here, the most plausible explanation of extensive colonic necrosis was cardiac arrest and a period of low cardiac output despite successful CPR. This is the second report in the literature of such a combination of events. In the previous report, however, the authors speculated that the complication might have been associated with the administration of vasopressin during CPR, leading to an exaggerated visceral vasoconstrictive response [10]. Although vasopressin was not used in the present case, non-occlusive necrosis of the colon still occurred. As mentioned above, in low flow states the result of selective vasoconstriction of the mesenteric arterioles may be variable and unpredictable and non-occlusive ischaemia of the colon is one of the possible complications.

Although angiography is the gold standard imaging method for the diagnosis of acute large bowel ischaemia, MDCT with increased spatial resolution and multiplanar reformatted images has become the imaging examination of choice for the evaluation of this condition [19]. The administration of contrast intravenously allows the rapid imaging of arterial and venous phases of the mesenteric circulation. MDCT findings such as abnormalities in the bowel wall and mesentery and intraluminal haemorrhage may help in the identification of the location and the severity of acute large bowel ischaemia. Prominent bowel wall thickness, hyperdensity due to mucosal hyperaemia, inhomogeneous enhancement and intraluminal haemorrhage are findings suggesting alterations in arterial circulation [20]. Active extravasation of contrast material is defined as a hyperdense focal area (> 90 HU) within the bowel lumen in arterial phase CT images [11,21]. In alteration from impaired venous drainage, submucosal hypodensity due to oedema, pericolic streakiness and peritoneal fluid are demonstrated [20]. Intramural gas, free peritoneal air and absence of bowel wall enhancement are findings of the late stage of the disease and represent irreversible infarction and necrosis [20]. Aschoff *et al.* reported MDCT sensitivity of 93% and specificity of 100% for diagnosing mesenteric ischaemia [22].

In patients with acute abdomen and evidence of intestinal ischaemia an emergency laparotomy is warranted. The extent of bowel resection depends on the length of the necrotic bowel. Most of these patients are critically ill and anastomosis of the stumps is contraindicated particularly in cases of non-occlusive necrosis. Rapid surgery and return to the ICU are of foremost importance. In all the reported cases of extensive colonic necrosis, including the case presented here, a subtotal colectomy with end ileostomy was performed [6-10] (Table 1).

Table 1 Characteristics of reported cases of non-occlusive extensive colonic necrosis

Author	Patient No	Age	Sex	Associated condition
Renton (1967)	1	18	M	Trauma/haemorrhagic shock
Wilson (1980)	2	20	M	Trauma/haemorrhagic shock
Welch (1986)	3	50	F	Cardiac Failure/hypotension
	4	77	F	Hypotension/multiple myeloma
Levandoski (1987)	5	12	F	Trauma/haemorrhagic shock
	6	19	M	Trauma/haemorrhagic shock
	7	32	F	Tricyclic overdose/ hypotension
Stockman (2006)	8	38	F	Cardiac arrest/CPR
Katsoulis (2012)	9	83	F	Cardiac arrest/CPR

Conclusion

Extensive ischaemia and even necrosis of the colon can occur following a period of low perfusion due to cardiogenic or hypovolaemic shock.

Competing interests
The authors declare that they have no competing interests.

Authors' contributions
IEK, who was the attending surgeon, designed the study and drafted the manuscript. AB helped to draft the manuscript. MS and IG performed the literature search using the PubMEd database. AS critically revised the manuscript. MKD coordinated the study. All authors read and approved the final version.

Author details
[1]1st Surgical Department, Asklepieio General Hospital, Voula, Greece.
[2]Computed Tomography Department, Asklepieio General Hospital, Voula, Greece.

References

1. Ludwig KA, Quebbeman EJ, Bergstein JM, Wallace JR, Wittmann DH, Aprahamian C: **Shock-associated right colon ischemia and necrosis.** *J Trauma* 1995, **39**(6):1171–1174.
2. Flynn TC, Rowlands BJ, Gilliland M, Ward RE, Fischer RP: **Hypotension-induced post-traumatic necrosis of the right colon.** *Am J Surg* 1983, **146**(6):715–718.
3. Byrd RL, Cunningham MW, Goldman LI: **Nonocclusive ischemic colitis secondary to hemorrhagic shock.** *Dis Colon Rectum* 1987, **30**(2):116–118.

4. Parry MMW, Nieuwouldt JHM, Stein C: **Gangrene of the right colon: a rare complication of trauma related systemic hypotension.** *Br J Surg* 1987, **74**:149.
5. Landreneau RJ, Fry WJ: **The Right Colon as a Target Organ of Non-occlusive Mesenteric Ischemia. Case report and review of the literature.** *Arch Surg* 1990, **125**(5):591–594.
6. Renton CJC: **Massive intestinal infarction following multiple injury.** *Br J Surg* 1967, **54**:399–402.
7. Wilson EA: **Extensive gangrene of the bowel after haemorrhagic shock: a case report.** *S Afr Med J* 1980, **57**(10):377–378.
8. Welch GH, Shearer MG, Imrie CW, Anderson JR, Gilmour DG: **Total colonic ischemia.** *Dis Colon Rectum* 1986, **29**(6):410–412.
9. Levandoski G, Deitrick JE, Brotman S: **Necrosis of the colon as a complication of shock.** *Am Surg* 1988, **54**(10):621–626.
10. Stockman W, De Keyser J, Brabant S, Spoelders K, Vuylsteke P, Beeusaert R, Coppe E: **Colon ischaemia and necrosis as a complication of prolonged but successful CPR.** *Resuscitation* 2006, **71**:260–262.
11. Jaeckle T, Stuber G, Hoffmann MHK, Freund W, Schmitz BL, Aschoff AJ: **Acute gastrointestinal bleeding: Value of MDCT.** *Abdom Imaging* 2008, **33**:285–293.
12. Wiesner W, Khurana B, Ji H, Ros PR: **CT of acute bowel ischemia.** *Radiology* 2003, **226**:635–650.
13. Horton KM, Fishman EK: **Multidetector CT angiography in the diagnosis of mesenteric ischemia.** *Radiol Clin North Am* 2007, **45**:275–288.
14. Nikas D, Ahn Y, Fielding LP: **Sensitivity of colon blood flow to changing haemorrhagic events.** *Curr Surg* 1985, **42**:20–23.
15. Bailey RW, Bulkley GB, Hamilton SR, Morris JB, Smith GW: **Pathogenesis of non-occlusive ischemic colitis.** *Ann Surg* 1986, **203**(6):590–599.
16. Toung T, Reilly PM, Fuh KC, Ferris R, Bulkley GB: **Mesenteric vasoconstriction in response to hemorrhagic shock.** *Shock* 2000, **13**(4):267–273.
17. Reilly PM, Wilkins KB, Fuh KC, Haglund U, Bulkley GB: **The mesenteric hemodynamic response to circulatory shock: an overview.** *Shock* 2001, **15**(5):329–343.
18. Ceppa EP, Fuh KC, Bulkley GB: **Mesenteric hemodynamic response to circulatory shock.** *Curr Opin Crit Care* 2003, **9**(2):127–132.
19. Chou CK: **CT manifestations of bowel ischaemia.** *AJR* 2002, **178**:87–91.
20. Romano S, Romano L, Grassi R: **Multidetector row computed tomography findings from ischaemia to infarction of large bowel.** *Eur J Radiol* 2007, **61**(30):433–441.
21. Suo BJ, Zhou LY, Ding SG, Guo CJ, Gu F, Zheng YA: **Analysis of etiological and related factors responsible for acute gastrointestinal hemorrhage.** *Zhonghua Yi Xue Za Zhi* 2011, **91**(25):1757–1761.
22. Aschoff AJ, Stuber G, Becker BW, Hoffmann MHK, Schmitz BL, Schelzig H, Jaeckle T: **Evaluation of acute mesenteric ischemia: accuracy of biphasic mesenteric multi-detector CT angiography.** *Abdom Imaging* 2009, **34**:345–357.

4

Correlation of the oxygen radical activity and antioxidants and severity in critically ill surgical patients

Hongjin Shim[1], Ji Young Jang[2], Seung Hwan Lee[2] and Jae Gil Lee[2*]

Abstract

Background: Surgical patients who require an emergent operation commonly have severe sepsis or septic shock, followed by high morbidity and mortality rates.

Despite advances in treatment however, no predictable markers are available. In severe sepsis, many pathophysiologic mechanisms are involved in progression to organ failure, and oxygen free radical and antioxidants are known to contribute to this process. Oxygen free radical and antioxidants contribute to progression of organ failure in severe sepsis. In fact, oxygen radical activity has been reported to be correlated with disease severity and prognosis in patients with severe sepsis or septic shock. Accordingly, we aim to assess the usefulness of oxygen free radical and antioxidant concentrations to predict the disease severity and mortality in a cohort of critically ill surgical patients.

Methods/Design: This is a prospective observation study including patient demographic characteristics, clinical information, blood sampling/serum oxygen radical activity, serum antioxidant activity, serum antioxidant concentrations (zinc, selenium and glutamate), disease severity scores, outcomes, lengths of stay in intensive care unit, hospital 30-day mortality.

Keywords: Oxygen radical activity, Antioxidant activity, Sepsis, Critically ill patient, Zinc, Selenium, Glutamate

Background

Critically ill surgical patients usually have a septic status combined with severe systemic inflammation and shock. Sepsis is commonly caused by a gastrointestinal tract perforation, bowel ischemia, or postoperative complications, such as, pneumonia, intra-abdominal infection, or anastomotic leakage. Severe systemic inflammation and sepsis can cause organ failure with high risk of mortality (4 ~ 15% vs. 1%). Sepsis affects about 18 million people annually, with a mortality rate of 25% for uncomplicated cases and 80% in patients developing multi-organ failure syndrome [1].

Prognostic markers like natriuretic peptide (NP), B-type natriuretic peptide (BNP), or pro-BNP are used to predict postoperative cardiac complications after cardiac or non-cardiac surgery, while procalcitonin is commonly used as prognostic marker and indicator of mortality and antibiotics usage in septic patients. In addition, lactate clearance was recently reported to be a useful indicator of resuscitation and prognosis in severe sepsis [2,3]. Furthermore, some scoring systems, such as, the acute physiologic and chronic health evaluation (APACHE) II, the sequential organ failure assessment (SOFA), and multiple organ dysfunction score (MODS) systems, are also used to evaluate critically ill patient's condition. However, no clinically adaptable markers, except lactate clearance and procalcitonin, are available for determining the outcomes of critically ill surgical patients with severe sepsis. Inflammatory processes after infection are known to involve cells, inflammatory mediators, cytokines, pro-inflammatory substances, nitric oxide, arachidonic acid metabolites, and oxygen free radicals. These mediate and induce organ injury leading to organ failure [4-10]. Recently, many reports have been issued on the roles of oxygen free radicals and antioxidants, such as, glutamine, zinc, and selenium, which act as cofactors of

* Correspondence: jakii@yuhs.ac
[2]Department of Surgery, Yonsei University College of Medicine, 50 Yonsei-ro, Seodaemun-gu, Seoul 120-752, Korea

glutathione peroxidase [11,12]. Oxygen free radicals (OFR) cause oxidative damage in cells, which lead to DNA damage and mitochondrial dysfunction culminates in cell death [13-15]. There is evidence that oxidative stress caused by reactive oxygen species(ROS) in sepsis is characterized by tissue ischemia reperfusion injury and intense systemic inflammatory response [16-19]. Furthermore, oxidative stress and OFR impair the microcirculation, which induce acute renal failure, and have been correlated with sepsis severity and sepsis-induced morbidity. In sepsis, the protective role of antioxidants against oxidative stress has been known for more than 15 years [20-22]. Supplementation with antioxidants, such as, glutamine, zinc, and selenium may decrease oxidative stress and increase antioxidant activity, but apparently, do not affect mortality [23-28]. Early recognition of oxidative damage in sepsis by assessment of oxidative stress biomarkers is an actual topic for future research [29,30].

Methods

Aim

The purpose of the study is to assess the usefulness of the concentration of the oxygen free radical and antioxidants to predict the severity and mortality of the critically ill surgical patients.

Study population

This prospective study will be performed over 2-year periods (May 2012 ~ April 2014) in single institution. About 50 patients having severe sepsis or septic shock requiring emergency operation due to the bowel perforation or strangulation will be included.

Study design

This study will not change or modify the clinical practices of the participitating physicians. Patients are enrolled after acquisition of the informed consent approved by a Severance hospital institutional review board (Approval No. of IRB: 4-2012-0188).

Blood sample is drawn at 1st day, 3rd day, and 7th day after admitting to intensive care unit (ICU) regardless of the disposition of the patients after discharge from the ICU.

The primary endpoint of this study is to evaluate the correlation of the level of oxygen radical activity and severity of the patients. And secondary endpoints are (1) correlation of the level of oxygen radical activity and outcome, i.e., LOS in ICU and hospital, 30 day mortality, in-hospital mortality; (2) correlation of the level of antioxidant and severity and outcome of the patients; (3) relationship of the level of the oxygen radical activity and antioxidants.

Data collection

Investigators have collected the data including the followings: (1) patient characteristics, i.e., demographic data, severity of sepsis (severe sepsis or septic shock), presence of shock; (2) severity score for 7 days in ICU, i.e., APACHE II score, SOFA score, MODS; (3) clinical progress, i.e., vital signs, daily intake and output; (4) clinical outcomes, i.e., duration of shock, use of mechanical ventilation (MV), duration of MV, length of stay (LOS) in ICU, LOS in hospital, 30 day mortality, in-hospital mortality, complications. Blood samples are drawn to check the level of oxygen radical activity, antioxidation activity, level of the antioxidant (zinc, selenium, and glutamate) (Table 1).

Oxygen radical activity and antioxidation activity are assessed using CR3000® (Callegari 1930, Italy). Free oxygen radicals test (FORT) kit check the serum H2O2 level directly as oxygen radical. Free oxygen radicals detection (FORD) kit assess the antioxidation activity that check the reactivity with vitamic C, Trolox, albumin, and glutathione to free radical – chromogen.

The levels of the zinc, selenium and glutamate are assessed in the laboratory.

Table 1 Collection of dataset of the enrolled patients

Day of ICU* admission	APACHE II** score	Severity scoring (MODS†, SOFA‡)	Clinical courses (Vasopressors, Shock, MV§, Complications)	Oxygen radical activity and antioxidation activity	Antioxidants (Zn‖, Se¶, Glutamate)
1st day	O	O	O	O	O
2nd day			O		
3rd day		O	O	O	O
4th day			O		
5th day			O		
6th day			O		
7th day		O	O	O	O

*ICU intensive care unit, **APACHE II acute physiology and chronic health evaluation II, †MODS multi-organ dysfunction score, ‡SOFA sequential organ failure assessment, §MV mechanical ventilation, ‖Zn zinc, ¶Se selenium.

Statistical analysis

The results will be expressed as standard statistical metrics: median (range), mean ± standard deviation for continuous variables.

The primary endpoint of this study is to evaluate the correlation of the level of oxygen radical activity and severity of the patients.

And secondary endpoints are (1) correlation of the level of oxygen radical activity and outcome, i.e., LOS in ICU and hospital, 30 day mortality, in-hospital mortality; (2) correlation of the level of antioxidant and severity and outcome of the patients; (3) relationship of the level of the oxygen radical activity and antioxidants.

Comparison will be performed using the Student's t-test and chi-test for the relationship of the oxygen radical activity and severity, and Student's t-test and logistic regression test for the relationship of the oxygen radical activity and antioxidants, and outcomes. Statistical significance will be defined as a *p*-value less than 0.05 ($p<0.05$).

Inclusion criteria

Patients with severe sepsis or septic shock undergoing emergency surgery due to bowel perforation or strangulation will be screened to enroll the study. And patients requiring ICU care due to postoperative septic complications, such as pneumonia, bacteremia or peritoneal abscess or leakage. After acquesition of the informed consent, they will be assigned as to study.

Exclusion criteria

The patients are excluded followings; (1) age < 20 years or > 80 years old; (2) other type shock except sepsis; (3) immune compromised patients, i.e., post-transplant status requiring immunosuppressant, patients using steroid due to immune disorders or other disease, patients having chemotherapeutic agents due to advanced malignancy; (4) patients who not agree the informed consent.

Competing interests

This research is supported by Basic Science Research Program through the National Research Foundation of Korea (NRF) funded by the Ministry of Education, Science, and Technology (Grant No. 2012R1A1A2007915).

Authors' contributions

LJG designed and wrote the manuscript. And SH, JJY and LSH will have performed the analyses of antioxidant and oxygen radical activity, and collecting the data. All authors read and approved the final manuscript.

Author details

[1]Department of Surgery, Yonsei University Wonju College of Medicine, Wonju, Korea. [2]Department of Surgery, Yonsei University College of Medicine, 50 Yonsei-ro, Seodaemun-gu, Seoul 120-752, Korea.

References

1. Galley H: **Bench-to-bedside review: targeting antioxidants to mitochondria in sepsis.** *Crit Care* 2010, **14**:230.
2. Noveanu M, Mebazaa A, Mueller C: **Cardiovascular biomarkers in the ICU.** *Curr Opin Crit Care* 2009, **15**:377–383.
3. Piechota M, Banach M, Irzmanski R, Barylski M, Piechota-Urbanska M, Kowalski J, *et al*: **Plasma endothelin-1 levels in septic patients.** *J Intensive Care Med* 2007, **22**:232–239.
4. Kotsovolis G, Kallaras K: **The role of endothelium and endogenous vasoactive substances in sepsis.** *Hippokratia* 2010, **14**:88–93.
5. Kumar A, Brar R, Wang P, Dee L, Skorupa G, Khadour F, *et al*: **Role of nitric oxide and cGMP in human septic serum-induced depression of cardiac myocyte contractility.** *Am J Physiol* 1999, **276**:R265–R276.
6. van der Poll T, van Zoelen MA, Wiersinga WJ: **Regulation of pro-and anti-inflammatory host responses.** *Contrib Microbiol* 2011, **17**:125–136.
7. Gustot T: **Multiple organ failure in sepsis: prognosis and role of systemic inflammatory response.** *Curr Opin Crit Care* 2011, **17**:153–159.
8. Galley HF: **Oxidative stress and mitochondrial dysfunction in sepsis.** *Br J Anaesth* 2011, **107**:57–64.
9. Aksu U, Demirci C, Ince C: **The pathogenesis of acute kidney injury and the toxic triangle of oxygen, reactive oxygen species and nitri oxide.** *Contrib Nephrol* 2011, **174**:119–128.
10. Schulte J, Struck J, Kohrle J, Muller B: **Circulating levels of peroxiredoxin 4 as a novel biomarker of oxidative stress in patients with sepsis.** *Shock* 2011, **35**:460–465.
11. Berger M, Chiolero R: **Antioxidant supplementation in sepsis and systemic inflammatory response syndrome.** *Crit Care Med* 2007, **35**:S584–S590.
12. Birben E, Sahiner UM, Sackesen C, Erzurum S, Kalayci O: **Oxidative stress and antioxidant defense.** *World Allergy Organ J* 2012, **5**:9–19.
13. Dare A, Phillips A, Hickey A, Mittal A, Loveday B, Thompson N, *et al*: **A systematic review of experimental treatments for mitochondrial dysfunction in sepsis and multiple organ dysfunction syndrome.** *Free Radic Bio Med* 2009, **47**:1517–1525.
14. Rocha M, Herance R, Rovira S, Hernandez-Mijares A, Victor VM: **Mitochondrial dysfunction and antioxidant therapy in sepsis.** *Infect Disord Drug Targets* 2012, **12**:161–178.
15. Hatwalne MS: **Free radical scavengers in anaesthesiology and critical care.** *Indian J Anaesth* 2012, **56**:227–233.
16. Crimi E, Sica V, Williams-Ignarro S, Zhang H, Slutsky AS, Ignarro LJ, *et al*: **The role of oxidative stress in adult critical care.** *Free Radic Biol Med* 2006, **40**:398–406.
17. Abiles J, de la Cruz AP, Castano J, Rodriquez-Elvira M, Aquavo E, Moreno-Torres R, *et al*: **Oxidative stress is increased in critically ill patients according to antioxidant vitamins intake, independent of severity: a cohort study.** *Crit Care* 2006, **10**:R146.
18. Huet O, Dupic L, Harrois A, Duranteau J: **Oxidative stress and endothelial dysfunction during sepsis.** *Front Biosci* 2011, **16**:1986–1995.
19. Kumar Y, Singh G, Davidson B: **Free radical and antioxidant levels in patients with secondary peritonitis and their prognostic significance.** *Dig Surg* 2007, **24**:331–337.
20. Oldham KM, Bowen PE: **Oxidative stress in critical care: is antioxidant supplementation beneficial?** *J Am Diet Assoc* 1998, **98**:1001–1008.
21. Cadenas S, Cadenas A: **Fighting the stranger-antioxidant protection against endotoxin toxicity.** *Toxicology* 2002, **180**:45–63.
22. Nathens A, Neff M, Jurkovich G: **Randomized, prospective trial of antioxidant supplementation in critically ill surgical patients.** *Ann Surg* 2002, **236**:814–822.
23. Oliveira GP, Dias CM, Pelosi P, Rocco PR: **Understanding the mechanisms of glutamine action in critically ill patients.** *An Acad Bras Cienc* 2010, **82**:417–430.
24. Andrews PJ, Avenell A, Noble DW, Campbell MK, Croal BL, Simpson WG, *et al*: **Randomised trial of glutamine, selenium, or both, to supplement parenteral nutrition for critically ill patients.** *BMJ* 2011, **342**:d1542.
25. Linko R, Karlsson S, Pettilä V, Varpula T, Okkonen M, Lund V, *et al*: **Serum zinc in critically ill adult patients with acute respiratory failure.** *Acta Anaesthesiol Scand* 2011, **55**:615–621.
26. Cander B, Dundar ZD, Gul M, Girisgin S: **Prognostic value of serum zinc levels in critically ill patients.** *J Crit Care* 2011, **26**:42–46.
27. Valenta J, Brodska H, Drabek T, Hendl J, Kazda A: **High dose selenium substitution in sepsis: a prospective randomized clinical trial.** *Intensive Care Med* 2001, **37**:808–815.
28. Giladi AM, Dossett LA, Fleming SB, Abumrad NN, Cotton BA: **High-dose antioxidant administration is associated with a reduction in post-injury complications in critically ill trauma patients.** *Injury* 2011, **42**:78–82.

Isolated dissection of the superior mesenteric artery treated using open emergency surgery

Markus Udo Wagenhäuser*, Tolga Atilla Sagban, Mareike Witte, Mansur Duran, Hubert Schelzig and Alexander Oberhuber

Abstract

Background: Isolated dissection of the superior mesenteric artery (IDSMA) remains a rare diagnosis. However, new diagnostic means such as computed tomography makes it possible to detect even asymptomatic patients. If patients present symptomatic on admission, the risk of bowel infarction makes immediate therapy necessary. Today, endovascular techniques are often successfully used; however, open surgery remains important for special indications. In this paper, we present two cases with IDSMA and show why open surgical repair is still important in current treatment concepts.

Methods: Two cases with ISDMA that presented in our department from January 1, 2014 to June 1, 2014 are described. Data collection was performed retrospectively. Additionally, a review of articles which reported small cases series on patients with IDSMA within the past five years is provided.

Results: Both patients underwent open surgical repair following interdisciplinary consultation. Both patients were transferred to the intensive care unit after surgical repair and needed bowel rest, nasogastric suction and intravenous fluid therapy. CT scans were performed within the first week after operation. Platelet aggregation inhibitors were used in both cases as postoperative medication. Both patients survived and are able to participate in everyday activities.

Conclusion: Open surgical repair remains important in cases of anatomic variants of visceral arteries and suspected bowel infarction. Therefore, it is important that knowledge about open surgical techniques still be taught and trained.

Keywords: Superior mesenteric artery, Dissection, Bowel infarction, Open surgery, Aorta

Introduction

Isolated dissection of the superior mesenteric artery (IDSMA) remains a rare diagnosis; however, following the implementation of CT-scans in clinical routines, an increasing number of reports concerning patients with IDSMA can be observed [1]. The first description of IDSMA in the literature occurred in 1947 [2]. The superior mesenteric artery (SMA) is involved in over 60% of all spontaneous visceral dissections; however, its isolated dissection remains uncommon [3]. The successive course of the dissection starts with progressive thrombosis of the false lumen and continues with progressive dissection to distal branches, finally resulting in either rupture through the adventitia or the expansion of the false lumen [4,5]. A review of the literature recently reported that about 88% of all cases published to date concern men at an mean age of 54 years [6]. As abdominal pain is the most frequent sign of symptomatic IDSMA, it has been classified into grade I (peritonitis absent) and grade II (peritonitis present) [7]. The clinical course is individually different and difficult to predict. Radiological results show that angiographic follow-up findings may vary from complete remodeling to aneurysmal changes of the false lumen [8]. It can be shown that the length of the dissection correlates with the severity of abdominal pain; however, it remains uncertain whether bowel ischemia or the distention of periarterial nerve fibers is responsible for pain as a leading symptom [9]. The etiology of IDSMA is still uncertain. Cystic medial

* Correspondence: markus.wagenhaeuser@med.uni-duesseldorf.de
Department of Vascular and Endovascular Surgery, University Hospital

necrosis, fibromuscular dysplasia and atherosclerosis have been identified as associated with this rare disease [10]. The entry of the dissection is mostly located at the beginning of the superior mesenteric artery (SMA), i.e., about 15 mm to 30 mm of its origin, as in this area, differential forces as a result of the transition of the fixed to the mobile segment of the artery are the highest [7,10]. The latest reports show that conservative management and endovascular therapy are common therapeutic options for patients with an IDSMA today [11-13]. Open surgery is only considered if complications occur during the clinical course. In this paper, we present two cases where initial open surgery had to be performed due to abnormal vascular anatomy and a complete occlusion of the dissected SMA. The suspicion of bowel infarction prevented less invasive endovascular approaches.

Methods

Data collection was performed retrospectively in both cases. The patients were treated in the Department of Vascular and Endovascular Surgery, Heinrich Heine University, Düsseldorf. Oral and written consent concerning the publication of medical histories and radiological findings was obtained from both patients.

Additionally, we performed a literature search to outline the increasing number of reports about patients with IDSMA during the past five years. Here, a PubMed search was performed using the keyword "superior mesenteric artery" in conjunction with the term "dissection". We only included peer-reviewed studies that had been published between January 1, 2009 and June 1, 2014. The patient cohort of the studies had to include at least 10 patients. Results were summarized in a table and cases were subdivided based on medical treatment into "medical management", "endovascular therapy" and "open surgery" to show the distribution of therapeutic strategies of the past five years.

Results and discussion

Results

Case 1

Our report concerns a 51-year-old Caucasian man who was admitted to our clinic with severe abdominal pain. Two weeks prior, he had undergone an emergency operation in another hospital due to an IDSMA. Colleagues resected the dissection membrane and the SMA was reconstructed with a Dacron® patch. According to their medical history, the patient suffered from hypertension and non-insulin dependent diabetes mellitus (NIDDM). The patient was discharged free of symptoms two weeks prior to presentation in our department. Following admission to our emergency room, an immediate CT-scan and a blood test were performed, as the patient showed signs of an initiating peritonitis.

The CT scan showed an isolated re-dissection in the proximal part of the SMA with embolization of a distal branch causing an almost complete decline of right hand side intestinal perfusion. Aggravating, the right hepatic artery originated from the proximal part of the SMA as an anatomical variant. The origin was located directly in the region of the dissection entry. Figure 1 shows the major findings of the CT scan on admission. As endovascular therapy had a high risk of post interventional liver failure, the decision for open surgery was taken at an interdisciplinary level. Blood test results showed a normal serum lactate level, while C-reactive protein (CRP) and leukocytes (WBC) were raised. Thus, the patient had to be transferred urgently to the operating theatre.

We resected the dissection membrane from the origin of the SMA and a selective embolectomy of the arcade arteries was performed. The SMA was re-constructed using a venous interponate. Thus, for the interposition the saphenous vein from the right upper leg was used. The patient was admitted to the intensive care unit (ICU) with an abdomen apertum. As hypercoagulability occurred during the operation and we suspected a heparin induced thrombopenia (HIT), anticoagulation was managed using Argatroban with an activated partial thromboplastin time (aPTT) of 50-70 seconds. This suspicion was later confirmed due to a Heparin-induced Thrombocytopenia Platelet Factor 4 Antibody Test. Figure 1 demonstrates the representative findings of a CT-scan control five days after the operation. As a further course, negative wound pressure therapy was performed with wound dressing changes at intervals of two days and conducted within in the operating theatre (four times). In this context, the small intestinum was carefully inspected. We could not find any signs of hypoperfusion lesions. As the patient described persistent abdominal pain, performing a colonoscopy six days after the operation meant that ischemic colitis could be ruled out.

A secondary closure of the abdomen apertum could eventually be performed using a mesh graft transplant as coverage. Anticoagulation was managed using Fondaparinux at a therapeutic dose. After closure of the abdomen, dual platelet inhibition with clopidogrel and acetylsalicylic acid was used as a long-term medication.

Following the operation, the patient needed a bowel rest, nasogastric suction and intravenous fluid therapy. Diet was resumed after complete resolution of abdominal pain and nutritional support was required in the interval. The patient needed prokinetic medication at the outset, but during their hospital stay, a normal ingestion and defection frequency without any medical

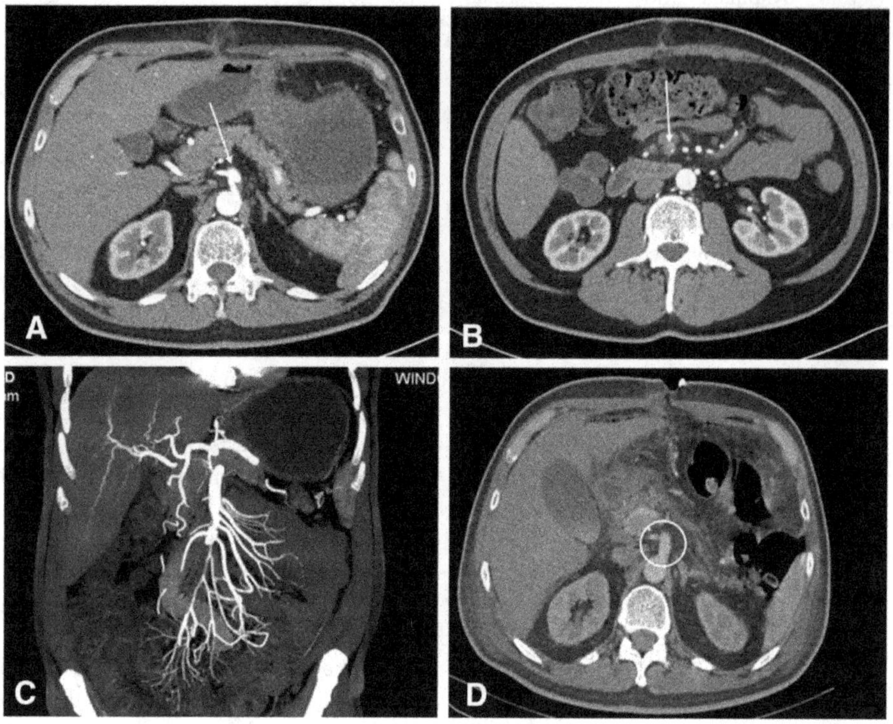

Figure 1 Representative CT scan findings. A: shown is the entry of the dissection at the proximal SMA. An abnormal origin of the right hepatic artery from the proximal SMA can be seen as an anatomical variant. **B**: An embolism of a distal branch of the SMA is shown. **C**: Reconstruction of the CT scan after admission. Almost complete decline of intestinal perfusion of the right abdominal side could be observed. **D**: findings of the control CT scan 5 days after operation. No residual membrane could be observed, normal perfusion of the SMA and the right hepatic artery.

support was achieved. The patient could be mobilized and will undergo postdischarge rehabilitation.

Case 2

The second case concerns a 50-year-old Caucasian man who was admitted to our clinic after a CT scan in an external hospital indicated suspicion of an acute occlusion of the SMA. Primary CT scan findings are shown in Figure 2. The patient presented with severe abdominal pain and vomiting. On reviewing the patient's medical history, it was discovered that he had a colitis ulcerosa, first diagnosed one year previously. In September 2013, the patient underwent a sigma-resection with the creation of a descendostoma resulting from a covered perforated sigma diverticulitis. At that time, thrombosis of the inferior mesenteric vein and a branch of the portal vein could be seen and as a result, anticoagulation with Rivaroxaban was initiated and has been maintained ever since.

Initial blood tests showed elevated CRP and leukocytes, whereas serum lactate level was within normal range. Following admission to the emergency room, the

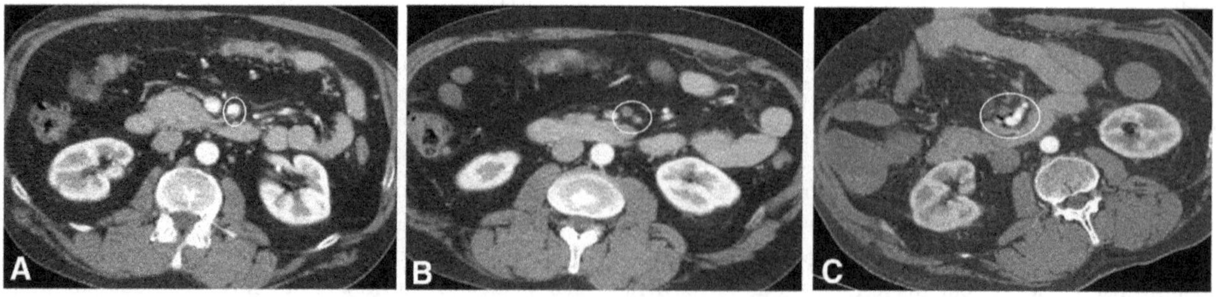

Figure 2 Representative CT scan findings. A: Dissection entry in the SMA at the typical location after passing behind the neck of the pancreas and the splenic vein. **B**: total occlusion of a branch of the SMA distal to the dissection entry. **C**: findings of the CT control 1 day after operation are shown. No residual membrane could be observed, normal perfusion of the SMA and the obstructed branch.

interdisciplinary decision was made to transfer the patient immediately to the operation theater, as clinical symptoms made a bowel infarction likely. We resected the dissection membrane from proximal SMA to the first arcade artery. Reconstruction was done using a saphenous vein patch. Macroscopic observation showed no signs of intestinal infarction; thus, intestinal resection was not necessary. Postoperative, the patient was admitted to the ICU with an abdomen apertum. Anticoagulation was managed using intravenous heparin and an aPTT of 50-70 seconds. In due course, medication was changed to platelet inhibition with acetylsalicylic acid.

A control CT scan was performed on the first day following the operation. Adequate intestinal perfusion could be seen with no signs of bowel infarction, as was verified by a second look laparotomy. Figure 2 shows the representative findings of the control CT scan. A colonoscopy five days after the operation was able to exclude intramural ischemic lesions and abdominal pain was already absent at this time. In due course, negative wound pressure therapy was performed with wound dressing changes at intervals of four days. It was possible to cover the abdomen and to bridge the fascia defect using a Vicryl mesh; thereafter, a definite closure could be performed.

Following the operation the patient needed a bowel rest, nasogastric suction and intravenous fluid therapy. We were able to initiate a light diet after the complete resolution of abdominal pain and eventually return the patient to a normal diet. The bridging of nutritional support was required. The patient could be mobilized and will perform postdischarge rehabilitation.

Discussion

IDSMA remains a rare condition, with postmortem investigations showing an incidence of about 0.06% [14]. However, to date, an agreement on the standardized treatment for this condition has not been reached. Within the past five years, reports featuring a small series of cases of patients with IDSMA can be found in the literature; prior to this period, only case reports are predominantly available. Based on a PubMed search, we identified 14 studies that fulfill the search criteria, which consisted of 323 cases altogether. Table 1 provides an overview of these publications.

Medical treatment seems to be effective in IDSMA. During a follow-up of 18 months a reduction of occlusion in the true lumen could be seen in up to 89% and progressive resolution of false lumen thrombosis in all patients [15]. Nevertheless, a fail rate of roughly 34% among conservative therapy approaches that includes the administration of effective anticoagulation through intravenous heparin makes such an approach appear questionable [27-29].

Endovascular therapy offers safe and quick therapy for patients with IDSMA. The first description of this approach by Leung et al. was followed by multiple reports of successful treatments by several authors describing complete resolution of the pain in most cases [30-33]. In a follow-up of 6 months stent patency could be found in 100%, a false lumen patency in 22% and new development of dissection in the SMA distal to the stent in 4% of all cases [19]. Other authors reported a fail rate of endovascular interventions of up to 50% and one author even described stent misplacement in the false lumen [7,22].

Table 1 Summary of small case series on patients with IDSMA

Year of publication	Author	Total number of cases	Medical treatment	Open surgery	Endovascular therapy
2014	Kim HK et al. [15]	27	27	-	-
2014	Ahn HY et al. [16]	13	12	1	0
2014	Li DL et al. [17]	42	24	7	11
2013	Dong Z et al. [7]	14	4	1	9
2013	Jia ZZ et al. [18]	17	14	0	3
2013	Li N et al. [19]	24	0	0	24
2013	Luan JY et al. [20]	18	7	0	11
2013	Choi JY et al. [21]	12	10	0	2
2012	Pang P [22]	12	3	0	9
2012	Zhang X [23]	10	6	2	2
2011	Min SI et al. [24]	14	7	1	6
2011	Park YJ et al. [25]	58	53	4	1
2011	Cho BS [26]	30	23	1	6
2009	Yun WS [9]	32	28	3	1
Sum		323	218	20	85

The investigation period was from January 1, 2009 to June 1, 2014. Cases are subdivided due to treatment strategies.

Open surgery is restricted to special indications. According to the literature available validity is limited as there are little reports up to now. It seems that if open surgery is performed the risk of operative revision is up to 28.6% and mortality rate is significantly elevated compared to other therapeutic options [17]. Thus, open surgery continues to be a choice of treatment with poor prognosis for patients.

In summary, most of cases emphasize that the clinical presentation of the patient on admission should have the strongest impact on the decision-making process. Preliminary algorithms derived from this small series of cases have been introduced. Dong et al. introduced an algorithm based on a study of 14 patients. They divided the patients into symptomatic (signs of peritonitis) and asymptomatic (no signs of peritonitis) groups and suggested an intervention or emergency operation only for symptomatic manifestations. Thus, asymptomatic patients should be treated conservatively [7]. The controversial discussion concerning whether asymptomatic patients should be treated to prevent a potential intestinal infarction remains unresolved [28,30,34,35]. Another algorithm was published by Garrett Jr. et al. [6]. In this instance, operative or interventional treatment is again suggested for symptomatic patients and the procedure should depend on the morphology and location of the dissection.

Both cases presented symptomatic on admission and we suspected an intestinal infarction due to clinical presentation. Generally, we followed the above- mentioned algorithms in general; however, the first case showed the anatomic variant of an abnormal origin of the right hepatic artery, while the second case was initially suspected to be an acute embolism with signs of intestinal infarction. Therefore, both cases needed open surgical intervention and demonstrated that open surgery should still be considered as a therapeutic option if endovascular therapy is not feasible. In this instance, we agree with Katsura et al., who described three cases of IDSMA and emphasized the necessity for open surgery in the management of this disease [36]. Considering the outcome (both patients survived), bowel resection was not necessary and after rehabilitation, they could participate in normal everyday activities.

The majority of reports about IDSMA have originated from Asia. This may reflect a genetic predisposition to SMA dissection in the Asian population [8]. However, different diet habits or viral infections in the Asian population might be causal, too. None of our patients had been to Asia prior to clinical presentation.

Suzuki et al. described characteristic CT findings concerning patients with IDSMA, which included a thrombosis of the false lumen, an intimal flap, an enlarged SMA diameter, an increased attenuation of the fat around the SMA and a hematoma in the mesentery with hemorrhagic ascites [37]. A residual intimal flap could be identified in the first case, whereas the second case only showed a complete thrombosis of the lumen in the absence of any additional radiological signs. Therefore, the second case outlines that one should also consider IDSMA as a diagnosis, even though clinical and radiological signs led to the conclusion of an acute embolism as a working diagnosis.

We performed a colonoscopy to exclude an ischemic lesion in both cases within the first week following operative treatment. We believe that endoscopic endoluminal control of the intestinal mucosa provides additional patient security. We suggest considering this approach to be standardized in the postoperative therapy of patients with IDSMA, even if patients present as asymptomatic.

Both patients received effective anticoagulation during direct postoperative therapy. In due course, this was changed to antiplatelet drugs. We intend to continue this medication for at least six months, after which the patients will be seen in our outpatient department and will undergo a follow-up CT scan. This regime has been described in a retrospective analysis by Li et al. and we consider it to be reasonable [17].

Conclusion

IDSMA remains a severe disease. Current therapeutic options suggest conservative management in asymptomatic patients, despite knowing that a failure rate of over 30% has been evidenced in such an approach [17,32]. Endovascular therapy should be the first therapeutic choice, as a hospital stay is shorter and mortality rate is lower compared to open surgery. Indications for open surgery are suspected bowel infarction or a rupture of the SMA [17]. In this paper, we presented two further cases where open surgery was performed. An anatomical variant and the suspicion of an acute embolism with bowel infarction made open surgery necessary.

Abbreviations

IDSMA: Isolated dissection of the superior mesenteric artery; CT: Computed tomography; SMA: Superior mesenteric artery; NIDDM: Non-insulin dependent diabetes mellitus; aPTT: Activated partial thromboplastin time; ICU: Intensive care unit; CRP: C-reactive protein; HIT: Heparin induced thrombopenia.

Competing interests

The authors declare that they have no competing interests.

Authors' contributions

MUW contributed substantially to the conception and design of the manuscript. He drafted the article, analyzed the data and revised them critically. TAS helped to concept the manuscript and contributed in data acquisition and interpretation. MW helped to write the article and contributed to its design. She participated in essential data interpretation. MD helped to improve the quality of the discussion as he revised this part critically. HS and AO helped to draft the manuscript. They participated in conceiving and designing the manuscript. All authors approved the final version of the manuscript.

References

1. Sartelet H, Fedaoui-Delalou D, Capovilla M, Marmonier MJ, Pinteaux A, Lallement PY: **Fatal hemorrhage due to an isolated dissection of the superior mesenteric artery.** *Intensive Care Med* 2003, **29:**505–506.
2. Bauersfeld SR: **Dissecting aneurysm of the aorta; a presentation of 15 cases and a review of the recent literature.** *Ann Intern Med* 1947, **26:**873–889.
3. Carter R, O'Keeffe S, Minion DJ, Sorial EE, Endean ED, Xenos ES: **Spontaneous superior mesenteric artery dissection: report of 2 patients and review of management recommendations.** *Vasc Endovascular Surg* 2011, **45:**295–298.
4. Subhas G, Gupta A, Nawalany M, Oppat WF: **Spontaneous isolated superior mesenteric artery dissection: a case report and literature review with management algorithm.** *Ann Vasc Surg* 2009, **23:**788–798.
5. Yasuhara H, Shigematsu H, Muto T: **Self-limited spontaneous dissection of the main trunk of the superior mesenteric artery.** *J Vasc Surg* 1998, **27:**776–779.
6. Garrett HE Jr: **Options for treatment of spontaneous mesenteric artery dissection.** *J Vasc Surg* 2014, **1433-9:**e1–e2.
7. Dong Z, Fu W, Chen B, Guo D, Xu X, Wang Y: **Treatment of symptomatic isolated dissection of superior mesenteric artery.** *J Vasc Surg* 2013, **57:**69S–76S.
8. Park UJ, Kim HT, Cho WH, Kim YH, Miyata T: **Clinical course and angiographic changes of spontaneous isolated superior mesenteric artery dissection after conservative treatment.** *Surg Today* 2014, [Epub ahead of print]. doi:10.1007/s00595-014-0849-9.
9. Yun WS, Kim YW, Park KB, Cho SK, Do YS, Lee KB, Kim DI, Kim DK: **Clinical and angiographic follow-up of spontaneous isolated superior mesenteric artery dissection.** *Eur J Vasc Endovasc Surg* 2009, **37:**572–577.
10. Solis MM, Ranval TJ, McFarland DR, Eidt JF: **Surgical treatment of superior mesenteric artery dissecting aneurysm and simultaneous celiac artery compression.** *Ann Vasc Surg* 1993, **7:**457–462.
11. Lim EH, Jung SW, Lee SH, Kwon BS, Park JY, Koo JS, Yim HJ, Lee SW, Choi JH: **Endovascular management for isolated spontaneous dissection of the superior mesenteric artery: report of two cases and literature review.** *J Vasc Interv Radiol* 2011, **22:**1206–1211.
12. van Uden DJ, Verhulst F, Robers-Brouwer H, Reijnen MM: **Images in vascular medicine: endovascular intervention for a spontaneous isolated superior mesenteric artery dissection.** *Vasc Med* 2011, **16:**79–80.
13. Jibiki M, Inoue Y, Kudo T: **Conservative treatment for isolated superior mesenteric artery dissection.** *Surg Today* 2013, **43:**260–263.
14. Foord AG, Lewis RD: **Primary dissecting aneurysms of peripheral and pulmonary arteries: dissecting hemorrhage of media.** *Arch Pathol* 1959, **68:**553–577.
15. Kim HK, Jung HK, Cho J, Lee JM, Huh S: **Clinical and radiologic course of symptomatic spontaneous isolated dissection of the superior mesenteric artery treated with conservative management.** *J Vasc Surg* 2014, **59:**465–472.
16. Ahn HY, Cho BS, Mun YS, Jang JH, Kim CN, Lee MS, Kang YJ: **Treatment results for spontaneous isolated superior mesenteric artery dissection according to our previous guidelines and collective literature review.** *Ann Vasc Surg* 2014, [Epub ahead of print]. doi:10.1016/j.avsg.2014.04.007.
17. Li DL, He YY, Alkalei AM, Chen XD, Jin W, Li M, Zhang HK, Liang TB: **Management strategy for spontaneous isolated dissection of the superior mesenteric artery based on morphologic classification.** *J Vasc Surg* 2014, **59:**165–172.
18. Jia ZZ, Zhao JW, Tian F, Li SQ, Wang K, Wang Y, Jiang LQ, Jiang GM: **Initial and middle-term results of treatment for symptomatic spontaneous isolated dissection of superior mesenteric artery.** *Eur J Vasc Endovasc Surg* 2013, **45:**502–508.
19. Li N, Lu QS, Zhou J, Bao JM, Zhao ZQ, Jing ZP: **Endovascular stent placement for treatment of spontaneous isolated dissection of the superior mesenteric artery.** *Ann Vasc Surg* 2014, **28:**445–451.
20. Luan JY, Li X, Li TR, Zhai GJ, Han JT: **Vasodilator and endovascular therapy for isolated superior mesenteric artery dissection.** *J Vasc Surg* 2013, **57:**1612–1620.
21. Choi JY, Kwon OJ: **Approaches to the management of spontaneous isolated visceral artery dissection.** *Ann Vasc Surg* 2013, **27:**750–757.
22. Pang P, Jiang Z, Huang M, Zhou B, Zhu K, Shan H: **Value of endovascular stent placement for symptomatic spontaneous isolated superior mesenteric artery dissection.** *Eur J Radiol* 2013, **82:**490–496.
23. Zhang X, Sun Y, Chen Z, Li X: **Therapeutic regimen options for isolated superior mesenteric artery dissection.** *Vasc Endovascular Surg* 2012, **46:**277–282.
24. Min SI, Yoon KC, Min SK, Ahn SH, Jae HJ, Chung JW, Ha J, Kim SJ: **Current strategy for the treatment of symptomatic spontaneous isolated dissection of superior mesenteric artery.** *J Vasc Surg* 2011, **54:**461–466.
25. Park YJ, Park KB, Kim DI, Do YS, Kim DK, Kim YW: **Natural history of spontaneous isolated superior mesenteric artery dissection derived from follow-up after conservative treatment.** *J Vasc Surg* 2011, **54:**1727–1733.
26. Cho BS, Lee MS, Lee MK, Choi YJ, Kim CN, Kang YJ, Park JS, Ahn HY: **Treatment guidelines for isolated dissection of the superior mesenteric artery based on follow-up CT findings.** *Eur J Vasc Endovasc Surg* 2011, **41:**780–785.
27. Nagai T, Torishima R, Uchida A, Nakashima H, Takahashi K, Okawara H, Oga M, Suzuki K, Miyamoto S, Sato R, Murakami K, Fujioka T: **Spontaneous dissection of the superior mesenteric artery in four cases treated with anticoagulation therapy.** *Intern Med* 2004, **43:**473–478.
28. Cho YP, Ko GY, Kim HK, Moon KM, Kwon TW: **Conservative management of symptomatic spontaneous isolated dissection of the superior mesenteric artery.** *Br J Surg* 2009, **96:**720–723.
29. Gobble RM, Brill ER, Rockman CB, Hecht EM, Lamparello PJ, Jacobowitz GR, Maldonado TS: **Endovascular treatment of spontaneous dissections of the superior mesenteric artery.** *J Vasc Surg* 2009, **50:**1326–1332.
30. Leung DA, Schneider E, Kubik-Huch R, Marincek B, Pfammatter T: **Acute mesenteric ischemia caused by spontaneous isolated dissection of the superior mesenteric artery: treatment by percutaneous stent placement.** *Eur Radiol* 2000, **10:**1916–1919.
31. Tsai HY, Yang TL, Wann SR, Yen MY, Chang HT: **Successful angiographic stent-graft treatment for spontaneously dissecting broad-base pseudoaneurysm of the superior mesenteric artery.** *J Chin Med Assoc* 2005, **68:**397–400.
32. Yoon YW, Choi D, Cho SY, Lee DY: **Successful treatment of isolated spontaneous superior mesenteric artery dissection with stent placement.** *Cardiovasc Intervent Radiol* 2003, **26:**475–478.
33. Wu XM, Wang TD, Chen MF: **Percutaneous endovascular treatment for isolated spontaneous superior mesenteric artery dissection: report of two cases and literature review.** *Catheter Cardiovasc Interv* 2009, **73:**145–151.
34. Woolard JD, Ammar AD: **Spontaneous dissection of the celiac artery: a case report.** *J Vasc Surg* 2007, **45:**1256–1258.
35. Zhang WW, Killeen JD, Chiriano J, Bianchi C, Teruya TH, Abou-Zamzam AM: **Management of symptomatic spontaneous isolated visceral artery dissection: is emergent intervention mandatory?** *Ann Vasc Surg* 2009, **23:**90–94.
36. Katsura M, Mototake H, Takara H, Matsushima K: **Management of spontaneous isolated dissection of the superior mesenteric artery: case report and literature review.** *World J Emerg Surg* 2011, **6:**16.
37. Suzuki S, Furui S, Kohtake H, Sakamoto T, Yamasaki M, Furukawa A, Murata K, Takei R: **Isolated dissection of the superior mesenteric artery: CT findings in six cases.** *Abdom Imaging* 2004, **29:**153–157.

6

An Observational Study of the Etiology, clinical presentation and outcomes associated with peritonitis in Lilongwe, Malawi

Jonathan C Samuel[1,2*], Javeria S Qureshi[1,2], Gift Mulima[1], Carol G Shores[3,4], Bruce A Cairns[2,5] and Anthony G Charles[2]

Abstract

Introduction: Peritonitis is a life-threatening condition with a multitude of etiologies that can vary with geographic location. The aims of this study were to elucidate the etiology, clinical presentation and outcomes associated with peritonitis in Lilongwe, Malawi.

Methods: All patients admitted to Kamuzu Central Hospital (KCH) who underwent an operation for treatment of peritonitis during the calendar year 2008 were eligible. Peritonitis was defined as abdominal rigidity, rebound tenderness, and/or guarding in one or more abdominal quadrants. Subjects were identified from a review of the medical records for all patients admitted to the adult general surgical ward and the operative log book. Those who met the definition of peritonitis and underwent celiotomy were included.

Results: 190 subjects were identified. The most common etiologies were appendicitis (22%), intestinal volvulus (17%), perforated peptic ulcer (11%) and small bowel perforation (11%). The overall mortality rate associated with peritonitis was 15%, with the highest mortality rates observed in solid organ rupture (35%), perforated peptic ulcer (33%), primary/idiopathic peritonitis (27%), tubo-ovarian abscess (20%) and small bowel perforation (15%). Factors associated with death included abdominal rigidity, generalized (versus localized) peritonitis, hypotension, tachycardia and anemia ($p < 0.05$). Age, gender, symptoms (obstipation, vomiting) and symptom duration, tachypnea, abnormal temperature, leukocytosis, hemoconcentration, thrombocytopenia and thrombocytosis were not associated with mortality (p = NS).

Conclusions: There are several signs and laboratory findings predictive of poor outcome in Malawian patients with peritonitis. Tachycardia, hypotension, anemia, abdominal rigidity and generalized peritonitis are the most predictive of death ($P < 0.05$ for each). Similar to studies from other African countries, in our population the most common cause of peritonitis was appendicitis, and the overall mortality rate among all patients with peritonitis was 15%. Identified geographical differences included intestinal volvulus, rare in the US but the 2nd most common cause of peritonitis in Malawi and gallbladder disease, common in Ethiopia but not observed in Malawi. Future research should investigate whether correction of factors associated with mortality might improve outcomes.

Introduction

Peritonitis is a common surgical emergency with a high mortality rate ranging from 10-60% depending on the study [1]. Though there are several distinct causes of peritonitis, prompt recognition and surgical treatment has been the mainstay of therapy since Kirschner first reported improved outcomes with surgical intervention [2]. This treatment approach requires both a knowledge of the signs and symptoms of peritonitis to aid diagnosis and an understanding of common causes to assist the surgeon in appropriate surgical care.

Despite a high prevalence of peritonitis reported in several African countries [3-5], little is known about the presentation, causes, and outcome of peritonitis in the

* Correspondence: jsamuel@unch.unc.edu
[1]Department of Surgery, Kamuzu Central Hospital, PO Box 149, Lilongwe, Malawi

south eastern African country of Malawi. Local environmental factors combined with genetic predispositions lead to marked variation in disease cause and presentation, and defining this can lead to improved local care and better overall understanding of the disease process. Like many resource-poor settings, acutely ill patients in Malawi often present late in the disease process and there is frequently limited time for diagnostic studies prior to definitive therapy. This knowledge gap, high morbidity and mortality, and delayed presentation illustrates a problem that has potential for improvement in care through a better ability to recognize and treat peritonitis. Therefore, the goals of this study were to better elucidate the etiology, presentation (history, physical, laboratory and ultrasound findings) and outcomes associated with peritonitis at a single large referral hospital in Lilongwe, Malawi.

Methods

Study Setting

This study was conducted at Kamuzu Central Hospital (KCH) in Lilongwe, the capital of Malawi, during the calendar year 2008. KCH is the 830-bed referral hospital for the central region of Malawi, serving a population of around 5 million people. The hospital has a 24-h casualty department, 4-bed intensive care unit, 4-bed high dependency unit, several open wards each with capacity for around 50 surgical patients, radiology department with plain radiography and limited ultrasound capabilities, and four operating rooms. The hospital lacked pathology capabilities in 2008 and hospital laboratory testing is limited to complete blood count, with more extensive testing available in only limited circumstances through off-site private laboratories. An onsite blood bank supplies whole blood and packed red blood cells, with occasional availability of plasma or platelets.

Subject Identification and Data Acquisition

All patients admitted to KCH who underwent an operation for treatment of peritonitis during the calendar year 2008 were eligible. Peritonitis was defined as abdominal rigidity, rebound tenderness, and/or guarding in one or more abdominal quadrants. Subjects were identified retrospectively through a review of all medical records of patients cared for in 2008 on the adult general surgical wards (approximately 5000) and from the operative log book. Data was collected from the medical record and included: gender, age, date of admission, date of surgery, date of discharge or death, surgical procedure and operative diagnosis, date of onset and type of symptoms, presence of guarding, rebound, or rigidity and abdominal quadrant(s) affected, vital signs on presentation including temperature, heart rate, blood pressure, and respiratory rate, date and results of initial complete blood count if performed, and results of abdominal ultrasound if performed. Data was collected and entered into a Microsoft Excel spreadsheet (Office 2007) and analyzed using Stata (version 11).

Analysis of Data

Descriptive statistics were calculated for the following: operative diagnosis; overall and diagnosis-specific mortality rates; age and gender distributions; time (in days) from symptom onset, presentation, and outcome (death versus discharge); presence of rigidity; localized versus generalized peritonitis; presenting vital signs including systolic blood pressure (< 90, ≥ 90), respiratory rate (< 30, ≥ 30), heart rate (< 100, ≥ 100), and temperature (< 35.5, 35.5-38.4, > 38.4); Complete blood count results including total leukocyte count (< 4, 4-11, > 11) hematocrit (< 31.6, 31.6-47.9, > 47.9), and platelet count (< 100, 100-399, ≥400); and ultrasound findings if performed (presence or absence of free fluid, abscess, and/or appendicitis).

Correlations between outcome (death during hospitalization versus discharge) and clinical data (age, gender, type of symptoms and symptom duration, examination findings, vital signs, and laboratory values) were calculated using chi-squared analyses. In comparison to operative diagnosis the sensitivity and specificity of ultrasound in diagnosing appendicitis and free fluid/abscess was reported.

Results

We identified 190 subjects meeting the definition of peritonitis who underwent celiotomy. Sixty-nine percent were male. The average age was 35 (median 32, range 10-84). The youngest subject was 10, and 10 subjects were under the age of 18. The most common etiologies were appendicitis (22%), intestinal volvulus (17%), perforated peptic ulcer (11%) and small bowel perforation (11%) (table 1). The overall mortality rate associated with peritonitis was 15%, with the highest mortality rates observed in solid organ rupture (35%), perforated peptic ulcer (33%), primary/idiopathic peritonitis (27%), tubo-ovarian abscess (20%) and small bowel perforation (15%) (table 1). Factors associated with increased mortality include abdominal rigidity, generalized peritonitis (versus localized peritonitis), hypotension, tachycardia and anemia ($p < 0.05$); age, gender, symptoms (obstipation, vomiting) and symptom duration, tachypnea, abnormal temperature, hemoconcentration, thrombocytopenia and thrombocytosis were not associated with increased mortality (p = NS) (table 2).

Preoperative ultrasound was performed in 51 of the 190 cases of peritonitis. Of the 51 ultrasounds, 22 were performed to evaluate for appendicitis and 23 were

Table 1 Etiology of peritonitis in relation to gender, age, and in-hospital mortality.

Diagnosis	Number	Male	Female	Mortality
Appendicitis	42 (22%)	30 (71%)	12 (29%)	2.4% (1/42)
Intestinal Volvulus*	32 (17%)	30 (94%)	2 (6.3%)	9.4% (3/32)
Perforated Peptic Ulcer†	21 (11%)	19 (90%)	2 (9.5%)	33% (7/21)
Small Bowel Perforation	20 (11%)	15 (75%)	3 (15%)	15% (3/20)
Solid Organ Rupture	17 (8.9%)	9 (53%)	8 (47%)	35% (6/17)
Primary/Idiopathic	15 (7.9%)	8 (53%)	7 (47%)	27% (4/15)
Ischemic Bowel‡	12 (6.3%)	5 (42%)	7 (58%)	8.3% (1/12)
Intussusception	8 (4.2%)	5 (63%)	3 (38%)	0% (0/8)
Tubo-Ovarian Abscess	5 (2.6%)	na	5 (100%)	20% (1/5)
Bowel Obstruction	5 (2.6%)	1 (20%)	4 (80%)	0% (0/5)
All Other§	13 (6.8%)	9 (69%)	4 (31%)	15% (2/13)
Total	190 (100%)	131 (69%)	57 (30%)	15% (28/ 190)

*Sigmoid volvulus (23), Mid-gut Volvulus (9)
†Duodenal (14), Gastric (7)
‡ischemic bowel not otherwise due to bowel obstruction or volvulus
§Colorectal (3), Postoperative (3), Small Bowel Cancer (2), hernia (2), TB (1), Pancreatitis (1), Traumatic Gastric Perforation (1)

performed to evaluate for fluid and/or abscesses. A comparison between ultrasound results and intra-operative findings revealed a sensitivity and specificity for appendicitis was 0.5 and 1.0, and for fluid and/or abscess 0.82 and 0.83, respectively (table 3).

Discussion

This study outlines the etiology, associated presenting signs and symptoms, and outcomes of surgically managed peritonitis in a tertiary care center in central Malawi. The most common etiologies of peritonitis were appendicitis and volvulus. Abdominal rigidity, generalized peritonitis (versus localized), hypotension, tachycardia and anemia were significantly associated with mortality. The overall mortality rate was 15%. Ultrasound was specific but not sensitive in diagnosing appendicitis.

There are several similarities between our findings and those from other African countries. Appendicitis was the most common cause of peritonitis in our series (21%) and in studies on acute abdomen from Ghana (43.1%), Nigeria (40.3%) and Ethiopia (24.5%)[3,5,6]. One important distinction is that our study included patients with peritonitis defined as rigidity, guarding, or rebound tenderness, while these other studies included all patients with acute abdomen. Nega (2009) was the only investigator to report specific symptoms and reported guarding in only 39% of his patients, and though tenderness was present in 78% this was not specifically peritoneal tenderness.

Table 2 Association between presentation and outcome.

Presenting Factor		Death	Discharge	p value (χ^2)
Age	< 50	21	133	
	≥50	7	27	0.303
Gender	Male	18	113	
	Female	10	47	0.501
Symptom Duration	< 4 days	12	79	
	≥4 days	10	75	0.776
Obstipation	Yes	8	63	
	No	16	93	0.511
Vomiting	Yes	7	69	
	No	17	87	0.164
Rigidity	Yes	10	36	
	No	13	122	0.033
Peritonitis	Localized	0	34	
	Generalized	23	124	0.014
Blood Pressure	≥90	24	152	
	< 90	3	2	0.004
Respiratory Rate	< 30	4	62	
	≥30	4	17	0.073
Heart Rate	< 100	3	60	
	≥100	24	93	0.005
Temperature	35.5-38.4	6	48	
	< 35.5 or > 38.4	2	10	0.593
Leukocytosis	4-11	6	60	
(WBC*10^4/μL)	< 4 or > 11	12	44	0.056
Anemia	> 31.5	9	84	
(Hematocrit, %)	≤31.5	9	20	0.005
Hemoconcentration	< 48	14	84	
(Hematocrit, %)	≥48	4	20	0.768
Thrombocytopenia	≥100	14	96	
(Platelets*10^4/μL)	< 100	4	8	0.056
Thrombocytosis	< 400	16	96	
(Platelets*10^4/μL)	≥400	2	8	0.625

Our mortality rate (15%) was similar to reported rates from Ethiopia (4.9-15.3%)[5,7]. A report from the 1960s in England also had a similar mortality rate of 20%, though this study included only patients with generalized peritonitis [8]. Interestingly, we found no correlation between the duration of symptoms and mortality, while Kotiso *et al.* noted 7.6% mortality rate in patients with symptoms of 2 days or less, compared with 25% among those with symptoms over 2 days in duration [7]. Though it is unclear why we did not observe a similar trend, one hypothesis is that our population had

Table 3 Comparison between ultrasound results and intra-operative findings.

Ultrasound for Appendicitis		Intraoperative Finding	
		Appendicitis	**No Appendicitis**
Ultrasound Finding	Appendicitis	9	0
	No Appendicitis	9	4
Ultrasound for Fluid/Abscess		Intraoperative Finding	
		Fluid/Abscess	No Fluid/Abscess
Ultrasound Finding	Fluid/Abscess	14	1
	No Fluid/Abscess	3	5

more "survivor bias" with the sickest dying prior to presentation; this bias is noted in a variety of epidemiologic studies from developing countries [9-11].

We found a significant correlation between outcome and several presenting signs and laboratory values. Generalized peritonitis (versus localized) was correlated with mortality. This is likely because localized peritonitis was most commonly seen in appendicitis which had a low mortality rate, whereas all cases of perforated peptic ulcer (with a high mortality rate) had generalized peritonitis (data not shown). We also found that hypotension, tachycardia, and anemia were associated with increased mortality. Several of these factors are also predictive of mortality in other surgical emergencies including traumatic injuries and necrotizing soft tissue infections [12,13]. Triage and care of patients with peritonitis might therefore be improved by using predictive tools similar to those applied to other acute surgical conditions such as trauma and necrotizing soft tissue infections.

Surgical diseases leading to peritonitis have a geographic variability. For example, in developed countries diverticulitis is a common cause of peritonitis, while we did not observe any cases of diverticulitis in our series [8]. Additionally, we noted variation even within Africa, as several studies from Ethiopia report gallbladder pathology including gangrenous cholecystitis and gallbladder empyema whereas in our study there was no gallbladder pathology [7,14].

The specificity of ultrasound (1.0) among those suspected of having appendicitis was similar to a that reported in a meta-analysis of ultrasound for appendicitis in adults (0.93), however our calculated sensitivity was considerably lower than the meta-analysis (0.50 versus 0.83) [15]. One potential explanation of why we observed a lower than expected sensitivity is the selection bias in our study related to including only patients with peritonitis, as it may be that appendicitis is more difficult to diagnose when peritonitis is present due to patient intolerance of the examination or less reliable ultrasound findings late in the disease process. An alternative explanation is that the test is operator-dependent and the ultrasonographers are not experienced or adequately trained to diagnose appendicitis. Regardless inability to diagnose appendicitis by ultrasound in patients with peritonitis did not sway the clinician away from surgical intervention. In this study, the sensitivity and specificity of ultrasound to detect free fluid and/or abscess was 0.82 and 0.83. Interpretation of this is limited without intra-operative quantification of fluid volume, as prior studies suggest a minimum of 100 mL to over 500 mL of fluid is necessary for an ultrasound to reveal fluid [16].

This retrospective study was not able to examine the utility of plain films in the management of peritonitis because patients often keep their radiographs upon discharge. Our analysis also showed association between preoperative factors and outcome, but this observational study does not prove causality. Future research should aim to determine if correction of factors associated with mortality (such as fluid resuscitation to correct tachycardia and/or hypotension) might improve outcomes. The generalizability of this study is also limited to adult patients at a tertiary care setting, as we did not include patients admitted to the pediatric ward or patients managed in district hospitals or health centers. Lastly, the definition of peritonitis, though standardized, assumes that all health care providers are adept at assessing the abdominal exam for guarding, rebound tenderness, and rigidity.

Conclusions

In our setting peritonitis is associated with an overall mortality rate of 15%. The most common causes are appendicitis and volvulus, and factors associated with death include abdominal rigidity, generalized (versus localized) peritonitis, hypotension, tachycardia and anemia. Future research should investigate whether preoperative correction of these factors improves survival.

Acknowledgements

We thank the UNC Project in Lilongwe, Malawi, and the UNC Division of Infectious Diseases for administrative assistance. Funding was provided by the NC Jaycee Burn Center at the University of North Carolina; the University of North Carolina Center for AIDS Research Developmental Award (P30 AI50410); and by the National Institutes of Health Office of the Director, Fogarty International Center, Office of AIDS Research, National Cancer Center, National Eye Institute, National Heart, Blood, and Lung Institute, National Institute of Dental & Craniofacial Research, National Institute On Drug Abuse, National Institute of Mental Health, National Institute of Allergy and Infectious Diseases Health, and National Institutes of Health Office of Women's Health and Research through the International Clinical Research Fellows Program at Vanderbilt University (R24 TW007988).

Author details

[1]Department of Surgery, Kamuzu Central Hospital, PO Box 149, Lilongwe, Malawi. [2]Department of Surgery, University of North Carolina, 4001 Burnett Womack Bldg, CB 7050, Chapel Hill, NC, 27599 USA. [3]Lineberger Comprehensive Cancer Center, University of North Carolina, CB 7295, Chapel Hill, NC, 27599 USA. [4]Department of Otolaryngology/Head & Neck Surgery, University of North Carolina, 170 Manning Drive, CB 7070, Physician's Office Bldg G-190, Chapel Hill, NC, 27599 USA. [5]NC Jaycee Burn Center, University of North Carolina, 101 Manning Drive, CB 7600, Chapel Hill, NC, 27599 USA.

Authors' contributions

Author contributions were as follows: Conception and design (JS); acquisition of data (JS, GM); analysis and interpretation of data (JS); drafting of the manuscript (JS, JQ, GM); critical revision of the manuscript (CS, BC, AC). All authors read and approved the final manuscript.

Competing interests

The authors declare that they have no competing interests.

References

1. Farthmann EH, Schoffel U: **Principles and limitations of operative management of intraabdominal infections.** *World J Surg* 1990, **14**:210-217.
2. Kirschner M: **Die Behandlung der akuten eitrigen freien Bauchfellentzundung.** *Arch Klin Chir* 1926, **142**:253-267.
3. Ohene-Yeboah M: **Causes of acute peritonitis in 1188 consecutive adult patients in Ghana.** *Tropical Doctor* 2005, **35**:84-85.
4. Savoie PH, Peycru T, Mingoutaud L, Sow A, Biance N, Pauleau G, Garcia L, Farthouat P: **[Primary peritonitis in Sub-Saharian Africa: a 15 case series].** *Med Trop (Mars)* 2007, **67**:154-158.
5. Nega B: **Pattern of acute abdomen and variables associated with adverse outcome in a rural primary hospital setting.** *Ethiopian Medical Journal* 2009, **47**:143-151.
6. Ajao OG: **Abdominal emergencies in a tropical African population.** *Br J Surg* 1981, **68**:345-347.
7. Kotiso B, Abdurahman Z: **Pattern of acute abdomen in adult patients in Tikur Anbessa Teaching Hospital, Addis Ababa, Ethiopia.** *East and Central African Journal of Surgery* 2007, **12**:47-52.
8. Dawson JL: **A study of some factors affecting the mortality rate in diffuse peritonitis.** *Gut* 1963, **4**:368-372.
9. Boerma JT, Sommerfelt AE, Bicego GT: **Child anthropometry in cross-sectional surveys in developing countries: an assessment of the survivor bias.** *Am J Epidemiol* 1992, **135**:438-449.
10. Depoortere E, Checchi F, Broillet F, Gerstl S, Minetti A, Gayraud O, Briet V, Pahl J, Defourny I, Tatay M, Brown V: **Violence and mortality in West Darfur, Sudan (2003-04): epidemiological evidence from four surveys.** *Lancet* 2004, **364**:1315-1320.
11. Hill K, Choi Y: **Neonatal mortality in the developing world.** *Demographic Research* 2006, **14**:429-452.
12. Champion H, Copes W, Sacco W, Lawnick M, Keast S, Bain L, Flanagan M, Frey C: **The major trauma outcome study: Establishing national norms for trauma care.** *The Journal of Trauma* 1990, **30**:1356-1365.
13. Wong CH, Khin LW, Heng KS, Tan KC, Low CO: **The LRINEC (Laboratory Risk Indicator for Necrotizing Fasciitis) score: a tool for distinguishing necrotizing fasciitis from other soft tissue infections.** *Crit Care Med* 2004, **32**:1535-1541.
14. Tsegaye S, Osman M, Bekele A: **Surgically treated acute abdomen at Gondar University Hospital, Ethiopia.** *East and Central African Journal of Surgery* 2007, **12**:53-57.
15. Doria AS, Moineddin R, Kellenberger CJ, Epelman M, Beyene J, Schuh S, Babyn PS, Dick PT: **US or CT for Diagnosis of Appendicitis in Children and Adults? A Meta-Analysis.** *Radiology* 2006, **241**:83-94.
16. Patel NY, Riherd JM: **Focused assessment with sonography for trauma: methods, accuracy, and indications.** *Surg Clin North Am* 2011, **91**:195-207.

7

Acute cholecystitis: WSES position statement

Fabio Cesare Campanile[1*], Michele Pisano[2], Federico Coccolini[2], Fausto Catena[3], Ferdinando Agresta[4] and Luca Ansaloni[2]

Abstract

Background: The management of acute calculous cholecystitis still offers room for debate in terms of diagnosis, severity scores, treatment options and timing for surgery.

Material and methods: A systematic review about the treatment of acute cholecystitis has been completed. The recommendations of recent guidelines have also been examined taking into account the results of the review.

Results: The evidence available in the literature supports the recommendation about laparoscopic cholecystectomy as treatment of choice for acute cholecystitis. Surgery should be performed as soon as possible after the diagnosis because early treatment reduces total hospital stay and does not increase complication or conversion rates. The antibiotics can play different roles and attention should be posed to the risk of emerging resistance. A surgical or percutaneous drainage of the gallbladder is advocated by some authors in the advanced forms of inflammation or patients with severe co-morbidities; however, the available evidence does not support it, and further studies are necessary to clarify its role.

Introduction

The literature about the treatment of acute calculous cholecystitis has been recently examined in more than one Consensus Conference [1-3]. The disease could present with a picture ranging from mild, self-limiting, to a potentially life-threatening illness, and the severity of inflammation and its life-threatening potential is also strongly determined by the general condition of the patient. The degree of inflammation of the gallbladder and the conditions of patients with their co-morbidities contribute to indicate the best therapeutic option for every single patient. However, such heterogeneity makes very difficult to standardize a therapeutic protocol for this condition.

The optimal surgical treatment for acute cholecystitis should be examined according to its severity; however, no uniform grading system is yet available, and the need for practical patient-related operative guidelines has been stressed elsewhere [4].

Even the evidences about the outcome of the therapeutic procedures adopted are difficult to evaluate in this heterogeneous context; studies available have not generally examined the optimal treatment for acute cholecystitis according to its severity. A systematic review of the literature must take into consideration this aspect.

The literature review has been presented to the 2nd World Society for Emergency Surgery held in Bergamo in July 2013. This position paper follows the indication emerged in that meeting.

Review of literature

The results of the systematic literature review performed for the EAES Consensus Conference about the laparoscopic approach to the acute abdomen, published in 2012 were entirely considered for this analysis; the literature search strategy adopted has been detailed in that paper [1].

An additional literature search was done from 2010 through February 2013 with the following limits and filters: adult, clinical trial, review and english language. The PICO (population, intervention, comparison, outcome) system was applied for the MeSH (Medical Subject Headings) search whenever possible. Analogous search has covered the Cochrane Collaboration database and the Google Scholar in order to gather all the remaining evidence, synopses and guidelines on the topic.

The following search string was used:

("cholecystitis, acute"[MeSH Terms] OR ("cholecystitis" [All Fields] AND "acute"[All Fields]) OR "acute cholecystitis" [All Fields] OR ("acute"[All Fields] AND "cholecystitis"[All

* Correspondence: campanile@surgical.net
[1]Division of Surgery, Ospedale San Giovanni Decollato - Andosilla, Civita Castellana, VT, Italy
Full list of author information is available at the end of the article

Fields]))) AND ((Clinical Trial [ptyp] OR Review [ptyp]) AND ("2010/01/01"[PDAT]: "2013/12/31"[PDAT]) AND "humans"[MeSH Terms] AND English [lang]).

A total of 79 citations was identified.

A search without the limits "clinical trial" and "review" was then carried out, obtaining 392 additional papers whose abstracts were examined for relevance. Two authors (FCC and MP) collected data independently.

After exclusion of duplicates, publications with no abstract and of low interest in the specific topics and key questions, 77 publications were taken into consideration: The papers have been classified for evidence strength following the Oxford CEBM 2011 scheme. In the rest of this paper, the level of evidence obtained has been specified after every relevant reference citation as evidence level (EL) 1–5.

The literature obtained has also been used to update the results of the above cited Consensus Conference. This update has been presented at the 32nd "Congresso Nazionale ACOI" held in Florence (Italy) in May 2013. For the purpose of publication, the search was extended to April 2014.

Timing of surgery

The issue of early versus delayed laparoscopic cholecystectomy for acute cholecystitis is examined in seven randomized controlled trials [5-11] and 5 meta-analyses (EL1) [12-17]. The studies show that an early treatment reduces total hospital stay and does not increase complication or conversion rates. In particular, the rate of bile duct injury has been shown to be higher in the delayed treated patients, but the difference was not statistically significant due to the small numbers analyzed in the trials.

The optimal delay for surgery after the onset of symptoms it is not completely clarified in the above mentioned studies and deserves a more precise definition. One of the systematic reviews examined above [10,12] performed a subgroup analysis and could not demonstrate a statistically significant difference between the patients treated less than four days from the onset of symptoms and those of the studies also including patients with a longer delay. One large population-based studies, mentioned above, examined the risk-adjusted association between outcomes and preoperative length of hospital stay (used as a proxy for the onset of symptoms). There was no significant association between preoperative length of stay and 30-day postoperative mortality or overall morbidity. However, patients hospitalized for two or more days preoperatively sustained longer operative times and were significantly more likely to require open cholecystectomy compared with patients who received operation on the day of admission [18]. The above mentioned evidence supported the EAES Consensus Conference to recommend early cholecystectomy for acute cholecystitis, and to state that surgery should be performed as soon as possible after the onset of symptoms.

On the contrary, the authors of the Tokyo guidelines maintain that, despite the demonstration that early cholecystectomy is indicated for acute cholecystitis in an unselected population, still it could be possible to improve the overall outcome of this condition tailoring the treatment according to the severity of the condition and to the patient status. They suggest a staging system based upon severity assessment criteria such as degree of local inflammation and patient conditions. According to their classification acute cholecystitis is defined as "severe (grade III)" if associated with organ dysfunction, "moderate (grade II)" if the completion of a cholecystectomy is likely to be difficult due to local inflammation ("criteria predicting when conditions might be unfavorable for cholecystectomy in the acute phase"), and "mild (grade I)" if it does not meet the criteria for grade II or III [19-21].

Based on that scheme, the Tokyo guidelines suggest early laparoscopic cholecystectomy only in the mild forms of the disease (grade I), in which a laparoscopic cholecystectomy is likely to be easy. In the moderate cases, medical therapy with or without early gallbladder drainage (surgical or percutaneous) followed by delayed cholecystectomy is indicated, except in "experienced" centers. The "severe" grade (with organ dysfunction) is trusted to cholecystostomy.

However, several reports show that early cholecystectomy is safe even in the severe forms of the disease [22-24] or in the elderly population [25-27]. In particular, a recent review of prospective and retrospective series (EL3) [28] did not show an increase in local postoperative complications in severe cholecystitis and confirmed that laparoscopic cholecystectomy is to be considered an acceptable indication for it, despite a demonstrated threefold conversion rate.

Laparoscopic vs open cholecystectomy

There are two randomized trials (EL2) [29,30], a population-based outcome research (EL3) [31] and numerous comparative studies demonstrating that laparoscopic cholecystectomy is associated with faster recovery and shorter hospital stay than open cholecystectomy; the population-based outcome research showed also lower morbidity and mortality [31]. This evidence supported the EAES Consensus Conference recommendation that laparoscopic cholecystectomy be the treatment of choice for acute cholecystitis.

The preference for laparoscopic cholecystectomy is also expressed in the Tokyo guidelines [3]; however, the "severity" tailored approach suggested in those guidelines limits the indication for surgery only to the mildest forms of acute cholecystitis and takes in consideration the above evidence only in part (EL5). One of the trials mentioned above, specifically included gangrenous cholecystitis (to be classified in the "moderate" form according to the Tokyo guidelines) [29] and a recent meta-analysis shows that straight laparoscopic cholecystectomy is indicated in severe (gangrenous, empyematous) cholecystitis (EL3) [28].

Advanced age also does not preclude the indication for laparoscopic cholecystectomy (EL3) [32-35].

Antibiotic treatment

Different antibiotic regimens can be employed in acute cholecystitis; the choice must be based on the most common pathogens, community acquired or health care associated infections, pharmacodynamics and pharmacokinetics of the antibiotic and evolution of sepsis. Moreover, the antibiotics can be administered with different intent: as an ancillary role for early surgery or cholecystostomy or as the unique treatment for acute episode in the non-operative setting and delayed surgery.

The most accredited guidelines arise from TG 2013 and the WSES: the last one is the most updated and take into consideration also "new drugs" such a Tigecycline (see Table 1) [36,37].

Percutaneous cholecystostomy (PC)

Percutaneous tube cholecystostomy (followed or not by surgery) is reported in the literature as an alternative for the emergency treatment in septic high-risk patients. In particular, as mentioned above, the Tokyo guidelines consider the percutaneous (or surgical) drainage as mandatory in the severe grade of acute cholecystitis and also suggest its use in the moderate grade, in order to overcoming the technical difficulties of an inflamed gallbladder. However, gallbladder drainage has never been proven to be an effective alternative to early surgery; the evidence on its role is still poor. The panel of the Tokyo Guidelines states that it is known to be an effective option in critically ill patients, especially in elderly patients and patients with complications; however, no evidence is provided to support the statement, and it is recognized that there have been no randomized controlled trials on the issue.

As a matter of fact, a Cochrane systematic review included two trials, and none of them addressed the comparison of early cholecystectomy vs. percutaneous cholecystostomy [38].

A recent review performed a particularly detailed examination of 53 papers about cholecystostomy as an option in acute cholecystitis (EL3). It found no evidence to support the recommendation of percutaneous drainage rather than straight early emergency cholecystectomy even in critically ill patients. Actually, it suggested that cholecystectomy seems to be a better option for treating acute cholecystitis in the elderly and/or critically ill population [39]. Even if the results obtained from the studies reviewed are non-homogeneous, the mortality rate after PC (15.4%) is significantly higher than reported after early cholecystectomy (4.5%) in published series of similar patients. Of course, the reports analyzed in the PC group take into account also patients who could not have tolerated any surgery, and this limitation has to be considered.

After their review, about 27 further observational studies have been published, confirming that the groups considered in the studies, their inclusion criteria, the results and even the conclusions reached by different authors are largely non-homogeneous. With these limitations in mind, the reported in-hospital mortality for cholecystostomy varies between 4 and 50% (vs. 4.5% reported for cholecystectomy) and its morbidity ranges between 8.2 and 62%.

The role of percutaneous drainage of the gallbladder is difficult to investigate also because different definitions are used to identify "high-risk patients".

At the present time, percutaneous cholecystostomy cannot be recommended as part of a routine protocol for treatment of acute cholecystitis, but only considered as a possible alternative to reduce anesthesiology risk in a small subset of patients unfit for emergency surgery due to their severe co-morbidities. A randomized controlled trial (CHOCOLATE Trial) has been planned to attempt to clarify the largely conflicting evidence [40].

Recommendations

We recommend that laparoscopic cholecystectomy be considered the treatment of choice for acute cholecystitis and that surgery be performed as soon as possible after the diagnosis.

The role of antibiotics is relevant both in conservative therapy of the inflammation or as support to invasive

Table 1 Recommendation for antibiotic strategy in acute cholecystitis (modified from WSES 2013)

Community acquired		Healt care associated	
Infectious situation	**Drug**	**Infectious situation**	**Drug**
No Severe Sepsis ESBL -	*Amox-Clav*	*No Severe Sepsis*	*Pipera-Tazo + Tigecycline + −Fluconazole*
No Severe Sepsis ESBL +	*Tigecycline*		
Severe Sepsis ESBL -	*Pipera-Tazo*	*Severe Sepsis*	*Pipera-Tazo + Tigecicline + Echinocandin or Carbap Antibiotics + Teicoplanin + Echinocandin*
Severe Sepsis ESBL +	*Pipera-Tazo + Tigecycline + −Fluconazole*		

procedures. A frequent assessment of the therapeutic protocol is necessary to deal with bacterial resistance. We recommend the use of the 2013 WSES guidelines because they take into account several new drugs compared to TG13.

At present, we do not recommend that cholecystostomy (surgical or percutaneous) be included in routine protocols for treatment of acute cholecystitis, and we suggest that it be considered, only in those patient clearly unfit for emergency surgery, until better evidence are available.

Discussion

The above reported literature review clarifies the advantages of early laparoscopic cholecystectomy in an unselected population. It has to be stressed, however, that acute cholecystitis is a very heterogeneous disease as far as general and local factors are concerned. The severity of inflammation and its life-threatening potential is strongly determined by the general status of the patient, and the choice of surgical treatment cannot disregard this aspect [4]. Also, the general principles expressed in the literature have to be applied taking into account the environment, the socio-economic context in which such an emergency develops and the related logistics.

The Tokyo guidelines attempted to address such heterogeneity with the above described classification, that takes into account both local and general factors, and a therapeutic protocol based on such scheme.

Such a tailored approach, however, has not been validated by studies showing an improved outcome after its introduction, and a retrospective series did not find any significant benefit [41]. It ends up in a large use of delayed cholecystectomy, despite several meta-analysis of RCTs establish that early laparoscopic cholecystectomy is to be considered the gold standard. It also disregards the examined literature about the safety of early laparoscopic cholecystectomy in the severe forms of the disease. Furthermore, the role of percutaneous cholecystostomy is far from being established as discussed above: its therapeutic potential needs to be confirmed by the literature evidence and integrated in an evidence-based algorithm.

The risk of early surgery for acute cholecystitis should be evaluated against a well-established risk score in order to identifying the patients with reduced functional reserve who should undergo a treatment alternative to surgery. However, none of the available clinical scores for the evaluation of surgical risk for acute conditions [42,43] has been validated for this disease. Further investigations could help in validating a clinical score useful for clinical and therapeutic decision making for acute cholecystitis.

In addition, it has to be stressed that the general principles expressed in the evidence based recommendations have to be adapted to the technical, environmental and social conditions of the different areas of the world. The indications suggested by the Tokyo Guidelines, too limited for most of the Western countries, still have been shown to increase the adoption of early laparoscopic cholecystectomy in a Japanese context, as reported by Asai [44].

In many developing areas complex technology is not readily available, the diffusion of laparoscopy is still extremely sparse [45] and percutaneous drainage is not available. It is still debated if the introduction of minimally invasive surgery is proper in many developing countries where safe performance cannot always be assured [46] and economic resources could be better employed on more essential health programs [47]. The interpretation of our recommendations in those environments has to take into account that the value of early cholecystectomy for acute cholecystitis is supported by a level of evidence stronger than the laparoscopic approach. Therefore, in those areas where laparoscopy is not readily available, an early laparotomic operation may be preferred to a long transfer to a far away facility, taking into consideration the local situation, the logistics and the patient conditions.

Competing interests
The authors declare that they do not have any competing interests.

Authors' contributions
FCC collected and reviewed the literature, prepared the evidence report, presented the results at the congress, drafted the final manuscript. MP collected the literature and reviewed the manuscript. LA reviewed the manuscript and drafted the antibiotic treatment paragraph. FC, FC and FA reviewed the manuscript. All authors read and approved the final manuscript.

Author details
[1]Division of Surgery, Ospedale San Giovanni Decollato - Andosilla, Civita Castellana, VT, Italy. [2]General Surgery Department, Papa Giovanni XXIII hospital, Bergamo, Italy. [3]Department of Emergency Surgery, Maggiore Parma Hospital, Parma, Italy. [4]Department of General Surgery, ULSS19 del Veneto, Adria, RO, Italy.

References

1. Agresta F, Ansaloni L, Baiocchi GL, Bergamini C, Campanile FC, Carlucci M, Cocorullo G, Corradi A, Franzato B, Lupo M, Mandalà V, Mirabella A, Pernazza G, Piccoli M, Staudacher C, Vettoretto N, Zago M, Lettieri E, Levati A, Pietrini D, Scaglione M, De Masi S, De Placido G, Francucci M, Rasi M, Fingerhut A, Uranüs S, Garattini S: **Laparoscopic approach to acute abdomen from the Consensus Development Conference of the Società Italiana di Chirurgia Endoscopica e nuove tecnologie (SICE), Associazione Chirurghi Ospedalieri Italiani (ACOI), Società Italiana di Chirurgia (SIC), Società Italiana di Chirurgia d'Urgenza e del Trauma (SICUT), Società Italiana di Chirurgia nell'Ospedalità Privata (SICOP), and the European Association for Endoscopic Surgery (EAES).** *Surg Endosc* 2012, **26:**2134–2164.
2. Yamashita Y, Takada T, Kawarada Y, Nimura Y, Hirota M, Miura F, Mayumi T, Yoshida M, Strasberg S, Pitt HA, de Santibanes E, Belghiti J, Büchler MW, Gouma DJ, Fan ST, Hilvano SC, Lau JW, Kim SW, Belli G, Windsor JA, Liau KH, Sachakul V: **Surgical treatment of patients with acute cholecystitis: Tokyo guidelines.** *J Hepatobiliary Pancreat Surg* 2007, **14:**91–97.

3. Yamashita Y, Takada T, Strasberg SM, Pitt HA, Gouma DJ, Garden OJ, Büchler MW, Gomi H, Dervenis C, Windsor JA, Kim S-W, de Santibanes E, Padbury R, Chen X-P, Chan ACW, Fan S-T, Jagannath P, Mayumi T, Yoshida M, Miura F, Tsuyuguchi T, Itoi T, Supe AN: **TG13 surgical management of acute cholecystitis.** *J Hepatobiliary Pancreat Sci* 2013, **20:**89–96.
4. Campanile FC, Catena F, Coccolini F, Lotti M, Piazzalunga D, Pisano M, Ansaloni L: **The need for new "patient-related" guidelines for the treatment of acute cholecystitis.** *World J Emerg Surg* 2011, **6:**44.
5. Lai PB, Kwong KH, Leung KL, Kwok SP, Chan AC, Chung SC, Lau WY: **Randomized trial of early versus delayed laparoscopic cholecystectomy for acute cholecystitis.** *Br J Surg* 1998, **85:**764–767.
6. Lo CM, Liu CL, Fan ST, Lai EC, Wong J: **Prospective randomized study of early versus delayed laparoscopic cholecystectomy for acute cholecystitis.** *Ann Surg* 1998, **227:**461–467.
7. Dàvila D, Manzanares C, Pichò ML, Albors P, Càrdenas F, Fuster E: **Experience in the treatment (early vs delayed) of acute cholecystitis via laparoscopy.** *Cir Esp* 1999, **66**(suppl 1):233.
8. Chandler CF, Lane JS, Ferguson P, Thompson JE, Ashley SW: **Prospective evaluation of early versus delayed laparoscopic cholecystectomy for treatment of acute cholecystitis.** *Am Surg* 2000, **66:**896–900.
9. Johansson M, Thune A, Blomqvist A, Nelvin L, Lundell L: **Management of acute cholecystitis in the laparoscopic era: results of a prospective, randomized clinical trial.** *J Gastrointest Surg* 2003, **7:**642–645.
10. Kolla SB, Aggarwal S, Kumar A, Kumar R, Chumber S, Parshad R, Seenu V: **Early versus delayed laparoscopic cholecystectomy for acute cholecystitis: a prospective randomized trial.** *Surg Endosc* 2004, **18:**1323–1327.
11. Yadav RP, Adhikary S, Agrawal CS, Bhattarai B, Gupta RK, Ghimire A: **A comparative study of early vs. delayed laparoscopic cholecystectomy in acute cholecystitis.** *Kathmandu Univ Med J (KUMJ)* 2009, **7**(25):16. 20.
12. Papi C, Catarci M, D'Ambrosio L, Gili L, Koch M, Grassi GB, Capurso L: **Timing of cholecystectomy for acute calculous cholecystitis: a meta-analysis.** *Am J Gastroenterol* 2004, **99:**147–155.
13. Shikata S, Noguchi Y, Fukui T: **Early versus delayed cholecystectomy for acute cholecystitis: a meta-analysis of randomized controlled trials.** *Surg Today* 2005, **35:**553–560.
14. Lau H, Lo CY, Patil NG, Yuen WK: **Early versus delayed-interval laparoscopic cholecystectomy for acute cholecystitis: a metaanalysis.** *Surg Endosc* 2006, **20:**82–87.
15. Gurusamy KS, Davidson C, Gluud C, Davidson BR: **Early versus delayed laparoscopic cholecystectomy for people with acute cholecystitis.** *Cochrane Database Syst Rev* 2013, **6:**CD005440. doi:10.1002/14651858.CD005440.pub3.
16. Siddiqui T, MacDonald A, Chong PS, Jenkins JT: **Early versus delayed laparoscopic cholecystectomy for acute cholecystitis: a meta-analysis of randomized clinical trials.** *Am J Surg* 2008, 195:40–47.
17. Gurusamy K, Samraj K, Gluud C, Wilson E, Davidson BR: **Meta-analysis of randomized controlled trials on the safety and effectiveness of early versus delayed laparoscopic cholecystectomy for acute cholecystitis.** *Br J Surg* 2010, **97:**141–150.
18. Banz V, Gsponer T, Candinas D, Güller U: **Population-based analysis of 4113 patients with acute cholecystitis: defining the optimal time-point for laparoscopic cholecystectomy.** *Ann Surg* 2011, **254:**964–970.
19. Hirota M, Takada T, Kawarada Y, Nimura Y, Miura F, Hirata K, Mayumi T, Yoshida M, Strasberg S, Pitt H, Gadacz TR, Santibanes E d, Gouma DJ, Solomkin JS, Belghiti J, Neuhaus H, Büchler MW, Fan S-T, Ker C-G, Padbury RT, Liau K-H, Hilvano SC, Belli G, Windsor JA, Dervenis C: **Diagnostic criteria and severity assessment of acute cholecystitis: Tokyo Guidelines.** *J Hepatobiliary Pancreat Surg* 2007, **14:**78–82.
20. Mayumi T, Takada T, Kawarada Y, Nimura Y, Yoshida M, Sekimoto M, Miura F, Wada K, Hirota M, Yamashita Y, Nagino M, Tsuyuguchi T, Tanaka A, Gomi H, Pitt HA: **Results of the Tokyo Consensus Meeting Tokyo Guidelines.** *J Hepatobiliary Pancreat Surg* 2007, **14:**114–121.
21. Yokoe M, Takada T, Strasberg SM, Solomkin JS, Mayumi T, Gomi H, Pitt HA, Gouma DJ, Garden OJ, Büchler MW, Kiriyama S, Kimura Y, Tsuyuguchi T, Itoi T, Yoshida M, Miura F, Yamashita Y, Okamoto K, Gabata T, Hata J, Higuchi R, Windsor JA, Bornman PC, Fan S-T, Singh H, de Santibanes E, Kusachi S, Murata A, Chen X-P, Jagannath P, *et al*: **New diagnostic criteria and severity assessment of acute cholecystitis in revised Tokyo Guidelines.** *J Hepatobiliary Pancreat Sci* 2012, **19:**578–585.
22. Choi SB, Han HJ, Kim CY, Kim WB, Song T-J, Suh SO, Kim YC, Choi SY: **Early laparoscopic cholecystectomy is the appropriate management for acute gangrenous cholecystitis.** *Am Surg* 2011, **77:**401–406.
23. Lo H-C, Wang Y-C, Su L-T, Hsieh C-H: **Can early laparoscopic cholecystectomy be the optimal management of cholecystitis with gallbladder perforation? A single institute experience of 74 cases.** *Surg Endosc* 2012, **26:**3301–3306.
24. Nikfarjam M, Niumsawatt V, Sethu A, Fink MA, Muralidharan V, Starkey G, Jones RM, Christophi C: **Outcomes of contemporary management of gangrenous and non-gangrenous acute cholecystitis.** *HPB (Oxford)* 2011, **13:**551–558.
25. Riall TS, Zhang D, Townsend CM Jr, Kuo YF, Goodwin JS: **Failure to perform cholecystectomy for acute cholecystitis in elderly patients is associated with increased morbidity, mortality, and cost.** *J Am Coll Surg* 2010, **210**(5):668–679.
26. Sánchez Beorlegui J, Lagunas Lostao E, Lamata Hernández F, Monsalve Laguna EC: **Tratamiento de la colecistitis aguda en en el anciano: cirugía urgente frente a terapia médica y cirugía diferida.** *Rev Gastroenterol Peru* 2009, **29**(4):332–340.
27. Lupinacci RM, Nadal LR, Rego RE, Dias AR, Marcari RS, Lupinacci RA, Farah JFM: **Surgical management of gallbladder disease in the very elderly: are we operating them at the right time?** *Eur J Gastroenterol Hepatol* 2013, **25:**380–384. doi:10.1097/MEG.0b013e32835b7124.
28. Borzellino G, Sauerland S, Minicozzi AM, Verlato G, Di Pietrantonj C, de Manzoni G, Cordiano C: **Laparoscopic cholecystectomy for severe acute cholecystitis. A meta-analysis of results.** *Surg Endosc* 2008, **22:**8–15.
29. Kiviluoto T, Siren J, Luukkonen P, Kivilaakso E: **Randomised trial of laparoscopic versus open cholecystectomy for acute and gangrenous cholecystitis.** *Lancet* 1998, **351:**321–325.
30. Johansson M, Thune A, Nelvin L, Stiernstam M, Westman B, Lundell L: **Randomized clinical trial of open versus laparoscopic cholecystectomy in the treatment of acute cholecystitis.** *Br J Surg* 2005, **92:**44–49.
31. Csikesz N, Ricciardi R, Tseng JF, Shah SA: **Current status of surgical management of acute cholecystitis in the United States.** *World J Surg* 2008, **32**(10):2230–2236.
32. Pessaux P, Regenet N, Tuech JJ, Rouge C, Bergamaschi R, Arnaud JP: **Laparoscopic versus open cholecystectomy: A prospective comparative study in the elderly with acute cholecystitis.** *Surg Laparosc Endosc Percutan Tech* 2001, **11**(4):252–255.
33. Lujan JA, Sanchez-Bueno F, Parrilla P, Robles R, Torralba JA, Gonzalez-Costea R: **Laparoscopic vs. open cholecystectomy in patients aged 65 and older.** *Laparosc Endosc Percutan Tech* 1998, **8**(3):208–210.
34. Chau CH, Tang CN, Siu WT, Ha JP, Li MK: **Laparoscopic cholecystectomy versus open cholecystectomy in elderly patients with acute cholecystitis: retrospective study.** *Hong Kong Med* 2002, **J8:**394–399.
35. Massie MT, Massie LB, Marrangoni AG, D'Amico FJ, Sell HW: **Advantages of laparoscopic cholecystectomy in the elderly and in patients with high ASA classifications.** *J Laparoendosc Surg* 1993, **3:**467–476.
36. Gomi H, Solomkin JS, Takada T, Strasberg SM, Pitt HA, Yoshida M, Kusachi S, Mayumi T, Miura F, Kiriyama S, Yokoe M, Kimura Y, Higuchi R, Windsor JA, Dervenis C, Liau K-H, Kim M-H: **Tokyo Guideline Revision Committee: TG13 antimicrobial therapy for acute cholangitis and cholecystitis.** *J Hepatobiliary Pancreat Sci* 2013, **20:**60–70. doi:10.1007/s00534-012-0572-0.
37. Sartelli M, Viale P, Catena F, Ansaloni L, Moore E, Malangoni M, Moore FA, Velmahos G, Coimbra R, Ivatury R, Peitzman A, Koike K, Leppaniemi A, Biffl W, Burlew CC, Balogh ZJ, Boffard K, Bendinelli C, Gupta S, Kluger Y, Agresta F, Di Saverio S, Wani I, Escalona A, Ordonez C, Fraga GP, Junior GAP, Bala M, Cui Y, Marwah S, *et al*: **2013 WSES guidelines for management of intra-abdominal infections.** *World J Emerg Surg* 2013, **8:**3. doi:10.1186/1749-7922-8-3.
38. Gurusamy KS, Rossi M, Davidson BR: **Percutaneous cholecystostomy for high-risk surgical patients with acute calculous cholecystitis.** *Cochrane Database Syst Rev* 2013, **8:**CD007088. doi:10.1002/14651858.CD007088.pub2.
39. Winbladh A, Gullstrand P, Svanvik J, Sandström P: **Systematic review of cholecystostomy as a treatment option in acute cholecystitis.** *HPB (Oxford)* 2009, **11**(3):183–193.
40. Kortram K, van Ramshorst B, Bollen TL, Besselink MGH, Gouma DJ, Karsten T, Kruyt PM, Nieuwenhuijzen GAP, Kelder JC, Tromp E, Boerma D: **Acute cholecystitis in high risk surgical patients: percutaneous cholecystostomy versus laparoscopic cholecystectomy (CHOCOLATE trial): study protocol for a randomized controlled trial.** *Trials* 2012, 13:7.
41. Lee S-W, Yang S-S, Chang C-S, Yeh H-J: **Impact of the Tokyo guidelines on the management of patients with acute calculous cholecystitis.** *J Gastroenterol Hepatol* 2009, **24:**1857–1861.
42. Rix TE, Bates T: **Pre-operative risk scores for the prediction of outcome in elderly people who require emergency surgery.** *World J Emerg Surg* 2007, **2:**16. doi:10.1186/1749-7922-2-16.

43. Vaid S, Bell T, Grim R, Ahuja V: **Predicting risk of death in general surgery patients on the basis of preoperative variables using American College of Surgeons National Surgical Quality Improvement Program data.** *Perm J* 2012, **16:**10–17.
44. Asai K, Watanabe M, Kusachi S, Matsukiyo H, Saito T, Kodama H, Dotai K, Hagiwara O, Enomoto T, Nakamura Y, Okamoto Y, Saida Y, Nagao J: **Changes in the therapeutic strategy for acute cholecystitis after the Tokyo guidelines were published.** *J Hepatobiliary Pancreat Sci* 2013, **20:**348–355. doi:10.1007/s00534-012-0536-4.
45. Afuwape OO, Akute OO: **The challenges and solutions of laparoscopic surgical practice in the developing countries.** *Niger Postgrad Med J* 2011, **18:**197–199.
46. Manning RG, Aziz AQ: **Should laparoscopic cholecystectomy be practiced in the developing world?: the experience of the first training program in Afghanistan.** *Ann Surg* 2009, **249:**794–798. doi:10.1097/SLA.0b013e3181a3eaa9.
47. Teerawattananon Y, Mugford M: : **Is it worth offering a routine laparoscopic cholecystectomy in developing countries? A Thailand case study.** *Cost Eff Resour Alloc* 2005, **3:**10. doi:10.1186/1478-7547-3-10.

8

Management of war-related vascular injuries: experience from the second gulf war

Ali Jawas[1], Alaa K Abbas[1], Munier Nazzal[2,3], Marzoog Albader[2] and Fikri M Abu-Zidan[1,2*]

Abstract

Aim: To study the biomechanism, pattern of injury, management, and outcome of major vascular injuries treated at Mubarak Al-Kabeer Teaching Hospital, Kuwait during the Second Gulf War.

Methods: This is a descriptive retrospective study. War-related injured patients who had major vascular injuries and were treated at Mubarak Al-Kabeer Teaching Hospital from August 1990 to September 1991 were studied. Studied variables included age, gender, anatomical site of vascular injury, mechanism of injury, associated injuries, type of vascular repair, and clinical outcome.

Results: 36 patients having a mean (SD) age of 29.8 (10.2) years were studied. 32 (89%) were males and 21 (58%) were civilians. Majority of injuries were caused by bullets (47.2%) and blast injuries (47.2%). Eight patients (22%) presented with shock.

There were 31 arterial injuries, common and superficial femoral artery injuries were most common (10/31). Arterial repair included interposition saphenous vein graft in seven patients, thrombectomy with end-to-end / lateral repair in twelve patients, vein patch in two patients, and arterial ligation in four patients. Six patients had arterial ligation as part of primary amputation. 3/21 (14.3%) patients had secondary amputation after attempted arterial vascular repair of an extremity. There were a total of 17 venous injuries, 13 managed by lateral suture repair and 4 by ligation. The median (range) hospital stay was 8 (1–76) days. 5 patients died (14%).

Conclusions: Major vascular injuries occurred in 10% of hospitalized war-related injured patients. Our secondary amputation rate of extremities was 14%. The presence of a vascular surgeon within a military surgical team is highly recommended. Basic principles and techniques of vascular repair remain an essential part of training general surgeons because it may be needed in unexpected wars.

Keywords: Injury, Management, Trauma, Vascular, War

Background

War is a type of collective violence which is defined as an instrumental use of violence by members of a group against another in order to achieve political, economic or social objectives [1]. The highest rates of war-related deaths are in the WHO African Region followed by parts of the WHO Eastern Mediterranean region. More than half a million people died during the first Gulf War (1980–1988) between Iraq and Iran [1].

* Correspondence: fabuzidan@uaeu.ac.ae
[1]Department of Surgery, College of Medicine and Health Sciences, United Arab Emirates University, PO Box 17666, Al-Ain, United Arab Emirates
[2]Department of Surgery, Mubarak Al-Kabeer Teaching Hospital, Jabriya, Kuwait

Explosive weapons are designed to increase the number and energy of casing fragments leading to multiple penetrating wounds [2]. This is why vascular injuries are often associated with multiple trauma leading to high mortality unless prompt and appropriate surgical management is made. The evacuation time, climate, and availability of medical resources will impact the outcome of surgical management of war-injured patients [3]. Shortening the evacuation time in the prehospital setting reduced the war-related mortality [4-6], while prolonged evacuation resulted in high mortality [7].

Ideally, war injuries should be treated by surgeons having military surgery experience. In fact, civilian surgeons may find themselves trapped in wars practicing military surgery without prior training or experience in this field [4].

The mechanism and pattern of vascular injury will vary in the same community in war and peace. The commonest mechanism of injury in civilian practice in most parts of the world is road traffic collisions. We have found in a prospective cohort study that vascular injuries constituted 1.2% of all hospitalized motor vehicle collision trauma patients in a civilian setting [8]. However in countries with armed conflicts penetrating trauma causes most of the vascular injuries [9]. Interestingly, effects of war on vascular injuries extend after the war. Asfar et al. have shown that penetrating vascular injuries increased in civilian surgical practice after the Second Gulf War reflecting the aftermath of the Gulf War on Kuwait [10].

Mubarak Al-Kabeer Teaching Hospital is a 400 bed hospital located in the centre of Kuwait City. During the Second Gulf War, fighting occurred close to the hospital leading to a short evacuation time. This gave us a unique opportunity for treating vascular injuries in multiply severe injured patients similar to a front line field hospital. [4]. We aimed to study the biomechanism, pattern of injury, magnitude, and outcome of vascular injuries treated at Mubarak Al-Kabeer Teaching Hospital, Kuwait during the Second Gulf War and to highlight lessons learned from that period.

Patients and methods

All war-related injured patients who had vascular injury and were treated at Mubarak Al-Kabeer Teaching Hospital from August 1990 to September 1991 were studied. During the study period Mubarak Al-Kabeer Teaching Hospital received more than 1100 war-injured patients out of whom 361 patients were admitted. Data were retrieved from the Gulf War Injury Database which was retrospectively collected. A special form was designed to collect the data. Data were coded and an Access Program was used to design the database.

Studied variables included age, gender, site of vascular injury, mechanism of injury, associated trauma, type of vascular repairs, and clinical outcome. Comminuted/complicated open fractures were primarily managed by external fixators. Data were analyzed with the PASW Statistics 18, SPSS Inc, USA. Data were presented as mean (SD), median (range) or numbers (%) as appropriate.

Results

There were a total of 36 patients with major vascular injuries during the study period. This constituted 10% (36/361) of all war-related hospitalized patients while 32 (89%) were males. Their mean (SD) age was 29.8 (10.2) years. 21 (58%) were civilian and 15 (42%) were soldiers.

Majority of injuries were caused by bullets (47.2%) and blast injuries (47.2%) (Table 1). Thirteen patients were Iraqi (36%), 11 were Kuwaiti (31%) and 12 were from other nationalities. Eight patients (22%) presented with shock on arrival to the hospital.

Table 2 shows the anatomical distribution of injuries. Majority of patients had head and neck injuries beside the extremity injuries. Only 2.8% had chest trauma.

Type of arterial injury and their operative management are shown in Table 3. Injuries to the common femoral and superficial femoral arteries were most common (32%) followed by injuries to the popliteal arteries (19.4%) and brachial arteries (16.1%). Arterial repair included interposition saphenous vein graft in seven patients, thrombectomy with end-to-end / lateral repair in twelve patients, vein patch in two patients, and arterial ligation in four patients. Six patients had arterial ligation as part of a primary amputation. No prosthetic grafts were used in these patients. Types of venous injuries and their management are shown in Table 4. There were a total of 17 venous injuries. 13 were managed by lateral suture repair and 4 by ligation.

Amputation was performed in nine patients. Six patients underwent primary amputation for mangled extremities. These included, above knee amputation in two patients, below knee amputation in two patients and below elbow amputation in two patients.

All primary repairs, except two, were performed on the same day of injury. The exact time between vascular injury and surgery was unknown in majority of the cases. Three patients had secondary amputation after attempted vascular repair for 21 limbs (14.3%). One patient had a gunshot injury to the knee with multiple fractures, and popliteal artery, vein and nerve injuries. He underwent primary repair of the popliteal artery with end-to-end anastomosis and fasciotomy 24 hours after the injury. The patient subsequently developed thrombosis of the graft and limb ischemia which required above knee amputation. A 7-year-old boy was involved with a blast injury and transferred to our hospital from Iraq, underwent delayed primary repair of the femoral artery seven days after the injury. He had thrombectomy and end-to-end anastomosis but this ended with a below knee amputation because of delayed ischaemia. Another patient had a blast injury, underwent popliteal artery repair with interposition saphenous vein graft within six hours of injury. This was complicated by deep soft tissue infection and graft

Table 1 Mechanism of vascular injuries

Cause of injury	Number	%
Bullet injury	17	47.2
Blast injury	17	47.2
Stab wound	2	5.6
Total	36	100%

Table 2 Distribution of injuries of patients having vascular war-related injuries, n = 36, August 1990 to September 1991, Mubarak Hospital, Kuwait

Region	Number	%
Head and neck	7	19.4%
Chest	1	2.8%
Abdomen and pelvis	3	8.3%
Upper limbs	8	22%
Lower limbs	21	58%

thrombosis that needed above knee amputation. The median (range) hospital stay of our patients was 8 (1–76) days. 5 patients died (14%).

Discussion

Blast and bullet injuries caused majority of vascular injuries in our study. Most occurred in extremities and head and neck. The rarity of chest vascular injuries in our study is possibly related to early death of chest injury patients at the field before arrival to the hospital.

Common femoral, superficial femoral, and brachial arteries were the most common injured arteries in our study. This is similar to other reports. In Vietnam Vascular Registry, the superficial femoral and brachial arteries were the most common injured arteries [5]. Similarly, Fox et al. reported involvement of superficial femoral and brachial arteries in 44% of their cases [7]. Among 6808 reported vascular injuries in the literature, femoral artery injury was the most common (35%) followed by the brachial (31%) and then popliteal artery injuries (19.5%) [11]. Balad Vascular Registry from Iraq war included 90 femoral arteries and 44 popliteal arteries [12]. That is different from blunt vascular injuries caused by road traffic collisions in civilian practice, in which brachial artery is the most common injured vessel [8].

Table 3 Types and operative management of arterial injuries

Artery	Vein graft	Vein patch	Primary repair	Ligation	Total
Common femoral	3	1	2	1	7
Popliteal	1		3	2	6
Brachial		1	2	2	5
Superficial femoral	2	-	1		3
Tibial	-	-		2	2
Radial	-	-	1	1	2
Carotid	-	-	2	-	2
Subclavian	1	-	-	-	1
Ulnar	-	-	-	1	1
Epigastric	-	-	-	1	1
Iliac	-	-	1	-	1
Total	7	2	12	10	31

Table 4 Types and operative management of venous injuries

Vein	Primary repair	Ligation	Total
Popliteal	2	1	3
Internal jugular	1	1	2
Femoral	2	-	2
Subclavian	2	-	2
Superficial femoral	2	-	2
Inferior vena cava	2	-	2
Iliac	1	-	1
Pulmonary	1	-	1
Brachial	-	1	1
Tibial	-	1	1
Total	13	4	17

Arterial primary repair was the most common method of repair in our study (12/31). Only seven patients have their arterial repair performed with reversed saphenous vein graft. In contrast, most studies recommended using the interposition vein graft [7,13]. Experienced vascular and transplant surgeons were available through the whole war period in our hospital explaining the variation of techniques used in our study. Management of arterial repair with autologous vein graft remains the most durable and effective means of vascular repair [7,13]. Arterial injuries usually have a segmental arterial loss preventing tensionless primary anastomosis. Ligation of arterial injuries is a good strategy only in selected vessels. In our study, ligation of the radial, ulnar and tibial arteries did not cause ischaemia of the involved limbs. Examination of extremities after ligation is important to confirm limb viability. Prosthetic grafts were not used in any of our patients. Using prosthetic grafts remains a controversial issue because they are associated with increased risk of infection and consequently poor outcome [5,14].

Ligation of injured veins was commonly used during war [5,15]. However, in our series only four out of 17 venous injuries had ligation. This can be also explained by the presence of experienced vascular surgeons in our hospital. Venous repair remains a controversial issue in patients with vascular injuries. However, most would agree that venous repair by means, other than simple lateral suturing and end-to-end anastomosis, is a time-consuming process with uncertain benefits especially in multiply injured patients [5]. In our series most patients with venous injury underwent simple lateral repair or ligation if the first option was not possible.

Primary amputation was performed mainly because of mangled extremity with massive tissue loss, and bone injury, while secondary amputation was related to delayed presentation and infectious complications. Wani et al. treated 360 war-related arterial injuries over 13 years in Kashmir [16]. Their annual proximal peripheral arterial injuries were similar to ours. Nevertheless, their extremity amputation rate (less than 5%) was much less than ours (14%).

The decision for limb amputation is more difficult than it seems. We tried at the early period of the war to save as much limbs as we could but we learned later that this cannot be achieved all the time. Sometimes, early amputation can be the best option for some patients that saves their lives. Amputation rate depends on many factors including the severity of limb injury, mechanism of injury, ischaemia time, presence of associated injuries, and disaster situations when treating mass causalities [17].

It is a major principle in management of war-injured patients that saving a life comes before saving a limb. Mine injuries of the lower limbs are specifically more notorious and cause internal limb damage more than what appears on the skin. The blast injury of the mine causes high pressure that is transmitted proximally between the muscles causing major damage to the tissues.

We did not cover the vascular graft of the popliteal region with healthy viable tissue in two patients because of loss of all superficial tissues. We learned that this is a major problem that can lead to limb loss even with a successful graft because the graft has to be covered by viable tissue to prevent dehydration and infection. A rotational gastrocnemius flap if used to cover the popliteal vessels [18] could have possibly saved two secondarily amputated limbs having popliteal injuries in our series.

Limitations of the study

The data of the present study is a historical data of our Gulf War Registry. Nevertheless, we think that it is very important to share this information with others. Civilian surgeons suddenly practicing war surgery without previous experience in this field tend to repeat the same old mistakes that surgeons learned from previous wars.

We could not define the exact time between vascular injury and surgery in majority of the cases. Nevertheless, we think that majority were operated within 6 hours of injury because fighting occurred very close to our hospital and the evacuation time was less than one hour [4]. There were no extensive diagnostic radiological procedures and wounds were explored in the operating theatre as soon as possible depending mainly on the clinical findings.

There have been many technical developments in the last two decade including principles of damage control surgery, use of portable ultrasound machines, and endovascular techniques. Despite that, we have recently noticed in the recent war conflicts in our region that most of these advanced techniques are not affordable except damage control surgery. Basic principles of using the least expensive surgical methods that help the maximum number of patients is still the major principle.

We did not use temporary vascular shunts for peripheral vascular injuries. Simple damage control surgery methods can reduce the operating time in mass casualty situations [19,20]. Rasmussen *et al.,* have used temporary vascular shunts in 30 extremities as a damage control adjunct in the Iraq war, especially for major proximal vascular injuries [21]. There were no shunt related complications, 86% were patent and only 7% needed early amputation [21]. This simple technique was useful to stabilize and then transport patients.

Ultrasound technology has dramatically evolved during the last two decades. New portable hand held ultrasound machines with excellent images and doppler color facility can be used in the battle field [22]. Duplex ultrasound has been successfully used to diagnose vascular injuries during the recent Iraq Conflict [17].

Angiography / Endovascular means was not used in our series. Therefore, it is possible that occult vascular injuries have been possibly missed and those usually present later [23]. The value of endovascular approach for both diagnosis and treatment of vascular injury in civilian and war practice is well studied [7,24,25] Fox et al. reported their experience of managing 107 soldiers with vascular injuries during the Iraq/Afghanistan wars [7]. They found that endovascular interventions resulted in lower morbidity and mortality in multiply injured patients.

Conclusions

Major vascular injuries occurred in 10% of hospitalized war injured patients. The presence of vascular surgeons within a military surgical team is highly recommended. Basic principles and techniques of vascular repair remain an essential part of training general surgeons as it may be needed in unexpected wars.

Competing interests

The authors declare that they have no competing interests.

Authors' contributions

AJ helped in the idea and design of the study, analyzed the data and wrote the manuscript. AA helped in the idea and analysis of the data and approved its final version. MN helped in the idea, drafting the first version of manuscript, and critically reading it. MA helped in the idea, and edited the manuscript. FAZ had the idea, designed the study protocol, collected and assessed the quality of the data, helped in writing the first draft of the paper, and repeatedly critically edited it. All authors have read and approved the final version of the manuscript.

Author details

[1]Department of Surgery, College of Medicine and Health Sciences, United Arab Emirates University, PO Box 17666, Al-Ain, United Arab Emirates. [2]Department of Surgery, Mubarak Al-Kabeer Teaching Hospital, Jabriya, Kuwait. [3]Division of Vascular and Endovascular Surgery, University of Toledo Medical Center, Toledo, Ohio, USA.

References

1. Zwi AB, Garfield R, Loretti A: **Collective Violence**. In *World report on violence and health*. Edited by Krug EG, Dahlberg LL, Mercy JA, Zwi AB, Lozano R. World Health Organization; 2002:215–240. Available on http://whqlibdoc.who.int/publications/2002/9241545615_chap8_eng.pdf [Accessed on March 20, 2013].
2. Champion HR, Holcomb JB, Young LA: **Injuries from explosions: Physics, biophysics, pathology, and required research focus.** *J Trauma* 2009, **66:**1468–1477.
3. Rautio J, Paavolainen P: **Afghan war wounded; experience with 200 cases.** *J Trauma* 1988, **28:**523–525.
4. Behbehani A, Abu Zidan F, Hasaniya N, Merei J: **War Injuries in the Gulf war: experience of a teaching hospital in Kuwait.** *Ann R Coll Surg Engl* 1994, **76:**407–411.
5. Hafez HM, Woolgar J, Robbs JV: **Lower extremity arterial injury: Results of 550 cases and review of risk factors associated with limb loss.** *J Vasc Surg* 2001, **33:**1212–1219.
6. Fosse E, Husum H, Giannou C: **The siege of Tripoli 1983. War surgery of Lebanon.** *J Trauma* 1988, **28:**660–663.
7. Fox C, Gillespie D, O'Donnell S, Rasmussen T, Goff J, Johnson C, Galgon R, Sarac T, Rich N: **Contemporary management of wartime vascular trauma.** *J Vasc Surg* 2005, **41:**638–644.
8. Jawas A, Hammad F, Eid H, Abu Zidan F: **Vascular injuries following road traffic collisions: a population- based study.** *World J Emerg Surg* 2010, **5:**13.
9. Rich NM, Hughes CW: **Vietnam vascular registry: a preliminary report.** *Surgery* 1969, **65:**218–226.
10. Asfar S, Al-Ali J, Safar H, Al-Bader M, Farid E, Ali A, Kansou J: **155 vascular injuries: A retrospective study in Kuwait. 1992–2000.** *Eur J Surg* 2002, **168:**626–630.
11. Frykberg ER, Schinco MA: **Peripheral vascular injury**. In *Trauma*. 5th edition. Edited by Moore EE, Feliciano DV, Mattox KL. NewYork: McGraw-Hill; 2004:969–1004.
12. Woodward EB, Clouse WD, Eliason JL, Peck MA, Bowser AN, Cox MW, Jones WT, Rasmussen TE: **Penetrating femoropopliteal injury during modern warfare: Experience of the Balad Vascular Registry.** *J Vasc Surg* 2008, **47:**1259–1264.
13. Rich NM, Rhee P: **An historical tour of vascular injury management: from its inception to the new millennium.** *Surg Clin North Am* 2001, **81:**1199–1215.
14. Scott R: **British military surgery.** *J Trauma* 1988, **28:**S83–S85.
15. Yelon JA, Scalea TM: **Venous injuries of the lower extremities and pelvis: repair versus ligation.** *J Trauma* 1992, **33:**532–536.
16. Wani ML, Ahangar AG, Lone GN, Hakeem ZA, Dar AM, Lone RA, Bhat MA, Singh S, Irshad I: **Profile of missile-induced cardiovascular injuries in Kashmir, India.** *J Emerg Trauma Shock* 2011, **4:**173–177.
17. Starnes BW, Beekley AC, Sebesta JA, Andersen CA, Rush RM Jr: **Extremity vascular injuries on the battlefield: Tips for surgeons deploying to war.** *J Trauma* 2006, **60:**432–442.
18. Coupland RM: **The role of reconstructive surgery in the management of war wounds.** *Ann R Coll Surg Engl* 1991, **73:**21–25.
19. Olofsson P, Vikström T, Nagelkerke N, Wang J, Abu-Zidan FM: **Multiple small bowel ligation compared to conventional primary repair after abdominal gunshot wound with haemorrhagic shock.** *Scand J Surg* 2009, **98:**41–47.
20. Blackbourne LH: **Combat damage control surgery.** *Crit Care Med* 2008, **36:**S304–S310.
21. Rasmussen TE, Clouse WD, Jenkins DH, Peck MA, Eliason JL, Smith DL: **The use of temporary vascular shunts as a damage control adjunct in the management of wartime vascular injury.** *J Trauma* 2006, **61:**8–15.
22. Abu-Zidan FM: **Point-of-care ultrasound in critically ill patients: Where do we stand?** *J Emerg Trauma Shock* 2012, **5:**70–71.
23. Yilmaz AT, Arslan M, Demirkiliç U, Ozal E, Kuralay E, Tatar H, Oztürk OY: **Missed arterial injuries in military patients.** *Am J Surg* 1997, **173:**110–114.
24. Rosa P, O'Donnell SD, Goff JM, Gillespie DL, Starnes B: **Endovascular management of a peroneal artery injury due to a military fragment wound.** *Ann Vasc Surg* 2003, **17:**678–681.
25. McArthur CS, Martin ML: **Endovascular therapy for the treatment of arterial trauma.** *Mt Sinai J Med* 2004, **71:**4–11.

Iatrogenic ureteric injuries following abdomino-pelvic operations: a 10-year tertiary care hospital experience in Tanzania

Phillipo L Chalya[1*], Anthony N Massinde[2], Albert Kihunrwa[2] and Samson Simbila[3]

Abstract

Background: Iatrogenic ureteric injuries are rare complications of abdomino-pelvic surgery but associated with high morbidity and even mortality. There is paucity of data regarding iatrogenic ureteric injuries in Tanzania and Bugando Medical Centre in particular. This study describes our experience in the management and outcome of ureteric injuries following abdomino-pelvic operations outlining the causes, clinical presentation and outcome of management of this condition in our local setting.

Methods: This was a retrospective descriptive study of patients with iatrogenic ureteric injuries following abdomino-pelvic operations that were managed in Bugando Medical Centre between July 2004 and June 2014.

Results: A total of 164 patients (M: F = 1: 1.6) were studied. Of these, 154 (93.9%) were referred to Bugando Medical Centre having had their initial surgeries performed at other hospitals, whereas 10 (6.1%) patients sustained ureteric injuries during abdomino-pelvic surgery at Bugando Medical Centre. The median age at presentation was 36 years. The most common cause of iatrogenic ureteric injuries was total abdominal hysterectomy occurring in 69.2% of cases. The distal ureter was more frequently injured in 75.6% of cases. Suture ligation was the commonest type of injury accounting for 36.6% of patients. One hundred and sixteen (70.7%) patients had delayed diagnosis but underwent immediate repair. Ureteroneocystostomy was the most frequent reconstructive surgery performed in 58.0% of cases. Of the 164 patients, 152 (92.7%) were treated successfully. Twelve (7.3%) patients died in hospital. The main predictors of deaths were delayed presentation, deranged renal function tests on admission, missed ureteric injuries and surgical site infections ($P < 0.001$). The overall median length of hospital stay was 12 days. Follow up of patients was generally poor as more than half of patients were lost to follow up.

Conclusion: Total abdominal hysterectomy still accounts for most cases of iatrogenic ureteric injuries in our environment. Meticulous surgical technique as well as identification of the course of the ureter and associated anatomic locations where injury is most likely to occur is important to decrease the risk of ureteric injury. Timely recognition of ureteric injury and its management is associated with good outcome.

Keywords: Ureteric injuries, Iatrogenic, Abdomino-pelvic operations, Management, Outcome, Tanzania

* Correspondence: drphillipoleo@yahoo.com
[1]Department of Surgery, Catholic University of Health and Allied Sciences-Bugando, Mwanza, Tanzania
Full list of author information is available at the end of the article

Background

Injury to the ureter is one of the most serious complications of any abdominal or pelvic procedure whether from gynaecological, urological or general surgical disease and the medico-legal implication has always been a major area of concern [1]. These complications can result in high morbidity and even mortality for the patients, which can create anxiety and psychosocial concerns for the patients and their spouses [2]. The morbidity arising from ureteric injury includes increased hospital stay, secondary invasive interventions, reoperation, potential loss of renal function and deterioration patient's quality of life [3].

The incidence of iatrogenic ureteric injuries varies from 0.5–10% in different studies [4-6]. It can occur following any abdomino-pelvic surgery. Obstetric and gynaecological surgery, vascular surgery, general surgical procedures especially colorectal surgery and urological procedures are commonly responsible for ureteric injuries [6]. Endo-urological procedures also account for many ureteric injuries [6,7]. Traditionally, gynaecological procedures have been reported to account for between 50 and 75% of iatrogenic ureteric injuries since the ureter lies very near the female reproductive organs throughout its course from the pelvic brim to the bladder [8-10]. While recent reports from developed countries have however indicated a change in the pattern of these iatrogenic injuries with urological endoscopy being the major source, recent literature from the sub-Saharan Africa is relatively sparse, with the few ones available also indicating a change in pattern however of a different variety with a high incidence of injuries arising from gynaecological causes [11-14]. Intra-operative injury to the ureter is possible not only during complicated surgical procedures but also during uncomplicated procedures [10]. Such complication can occur even in the hands of experienced surgeons [10,15].

The risk factors for iatrogenic ureteric injury include nature and indication of the abdominal or pelvic surgery, patient related factors such as: pelvic adhesions from previous surgeries, history of pelvic radiation, enlarged uterus, pelvic malignancy, pelvic endometriosis, and anatomical abnormalities [16,17]. Experience of the operating surgeon may also be an important risk factor [18,19].

During abdomino-pelvic surgery, ureteric injury may be in the form of crush injury by a clamp, inadvertent diathermy injury, suture ligation, transaction, resection of a segment of ureter, kinking of ureter, and devascularization of a segment of ureter due to extensive dissection close to ureter. Patient may develop urinary fistula with adjacent organ or end up with non-functioning kidney later on [19,20].

The most important determinant of outcome of ureteric injuries is the interval between the injury and repair: the longer the interval, the worse the outcome [20]. Prompt intraoperative identification and appropriate correction decrease morbidity and eliminate mortality. However, most cases of ureteric injuries are recognized late [6,7,16,17,20]. Patients may present with flank pain, fever, prolonged ileus, ascites, urinary incontinence, anuria and azotemia with 5% patients present very late with hydronephrosis and non-functioning kidney [16,17].

The management of iatrogenic ureteric injuries in our environment poses major challenges to urologist practicing in developing countries such as Tanzania where most ureteric injuries after abdomino-pelvic surgeries are diagnosed late postoperatively with fever, loin pain, per-vaginal urine leak, prolonged ileus, oliguria, anuria and uraemic symptoms [21,22]. Some patients may remain asymptomatic and present years later with hydro-nephrotic, non-functioning kidney on investigations [21]. Lack of advanced diagnostic and therapeutic facilities is the hallmark of the disease in these countries. In addition to late presentation and lack of advanced diagnostic and therapeutic facilities, the majority of abdomino-pelvic operations in developing countries are performed by general practitioners and junior doctors who may have limited experiences in performing major abdomino-pelvic operations as well as prompt intraoperative identification and appropriate correction of ureteric injury [19,21,22],

There is a paucity of information regarding iatrogenic ureteric injuries in Tanzania and Bugando Medical Centre in particular. This is partly due to a paucity of published local data regarding this condition in this region. This study was designed to describe our experiences in the management and outcome of iatrogenic ureteric injuries, highlighting the causes, clinical presentation and treatment outcome of iatrogenic ureteric injuries in our local setting.

Methods

Study design and setting

This was a retrospective descriptive study of consecutive patients with iatrogenic ureteric injuries who were referred and managed in the department of urology of Bugando Medical Centre over a period of ten years from July 2004 to June 2014. Bugando Medical Centre is a tertiary and teaching hospital for the Catholic University of Health and Allied Sciences-Bugando (CUHAS-Bugando). It is located in Mwanza city and has a bed capacity of 1000.

Study population

The study included all patients who were referred to the urology department with a suspected diagnosis of iatrogenic ureteric injury. Patients with incomplete data were excluded from the study. The information was obtained from medical record database and from patients' files, operating theatre, surgical, urological and gynecological ward registries. Variables such as gender, age at the time of injury and side of injury were recorded as well as information about the indication for surgery, type of surgery performed, location of injury, when the injury was identified, method of repair and outcome of repair. The outcome of repair included post operative complications, length of hospital stay and mortality. A repair was deemed successful if there are no anastomotic related complications and the subsequent preservation of unilateral kidney function on follow up. Intravenous urography (IVU) was used to assess renal function and exclude strictures or hydronephrosis.

Definition of terms

Iatrogenic ureteric injury was defined as any inadvertent injury to the ureter which necessitates additional period of observation or intervention. The recognition time of injury was arbitrarily divided into: intraoperative, early (within seven days of the primary operation) and late (after seven day of primary operation). The primary disease referred to the disease condition that necessitated the abdomino-pelvic surgery (primary procedure).

Statistical data analysis

The statistical analysis was performed using the Statistical Package for Social Sciences (SPSS) version 17.0 for Windows (SPSS, Chicago, Illinois, United States). The median (and IQR) and ranges were calculated for continuous variables, whereas proportions and frequency tables were used to summarize categorical variables. The chi-square ($\chi2$) test was used to test for the significance of association between the independent (predictor) and dependent (outcome) variables in the categorical variables. The level of significance was considered as $P < 0.05$. Multivariate logistic regression analysis was used to determine predictor variables that predicted the outcome.

Ethical consideration

Ethical approval to conduct the study was obtained from the CUHAS-Bugando/BMC joint institutional ethic review committee before the commencement of the study.

Results

Out of 6424 patients who had abdomino-pelvic operations performed either at our centre or in the peripheral hospital and referred here for management of complications of abdomino-pelvic operations during the study period, 176 (2.7%) had iatrogenic ureteric injuries. Of these, 12 patients were excluded from the study due to incomplete data. Thus, a total of 164 patients were enrolled in the study. One hundred and fifty-four (93.9%) patients with ureteric injuries following abdomino-pelvic surgery were referred to Bugando Medical Centre having had their initial surgeries performed at other hospital, whereas only 10 (6.1%) patients sustained ureteric injuries during abdomino-pelvic surgery at Bugando Medical Centre. The age of patients at presentation ranged from 24 to 74 years with a median age of 36 years (interquartile range, 34 to 38 months). The peak age incidence was in the age group 31–40 years. Out of 164 patients, 62 (37.8%) were males and 102(62.2%) were females with a male to female ratio of 1: 1.6. The most common cause of iatrogenic ureteric injuries was obstetric and gynaecological procedures (55.5%) mainly total abdominal hysterectomy occurring in 69.2% of cases (Table 1). Gross pelvic adhesions from previous surgeries were reported in 6 (3.7%) patients. Previous history of pelvic inflammatory diseases was reported in 10 (6.1%) patients. Massive intraoperative bleeding during pelvic tumour surgeries was reported in 4 (2.4%) patients. No patient in this study had history of pelvic radiation or anatomical abnormalities. All patients who were referred from peripheral hospitals had their abdomino-pelvic surgeries performed by general practitioners who might have limited experience.

Out of 164 abdomino-pelvic surgeries, 72(43.9%) were elective and 92(56.1%) were emergency. Ninety-eighty (59.8%) patients had left sided ureteric injuries and (36.6%) had right sided ureteric injuries with a right-to-left ratio of 2.1: 1. Six (20.4%) patients had bilateral ureteric injuries. The distal ureter was more frequently injured in 75.6% of cases. Suture ligation was the commonest type of injury accounting for 36.6% of patients (Table 2). The diagnosis was made intra-operatively in 28 (17.1%) patients and it was characterized by urinary extravasations into the peritoneal cavity in 20 (12.2%) patients. In the remaining 136 (82.9%) patients the diagnosis was postoperative. Of these, the diagnosis was made early within seven days in 20 (12.2%) and in 116 (70.7%) patients the diagnosis was made

Table 1 Etiology of iatrogenic ureteric injuries

Etiology of iatrogenic ureteric injuries	Frequency	Percentages
Gynaecological/obstetric operations	**91**	**55.5**
• Total abdominal hysterectomy	63	69.2
• Caesarean section	14	15.4
• Excision of huge tubo-ovarian mass	12	13.2
• Vaginal operations	2	2.2
General surgical operations	**68**	**41.5**
• Large bowel resection (colectomy)	32	47.1
• Intraabdominal tumour excision	30	44.1
• Abdomino-perineal resection (APR)	4	5.9
• Pull through operation	2	2.9
Urological operations	**5**	**3.0**
• Endourological procedures	3	60.0
• Other urological operations	2	40.0

Table 2 Demographic data and injury characteristics

Study variable	Frequency	Percentages
Age		
• <40	71	43.3
• ≥40	93	56.7
Sex		
• Male	62	37.8
• Female	102	62.2
Nature of the primary surgery		
• Elective	72	43.9
• Emergency	92	56.1
Laterality		
• Left	98	59.8
• Right	60	36.6
• Bilateral	6	3.6
Site of injury		
• Upper (Proximal) third	12	7.3
• Middle third	28	17.1
• Lower (Distal) third	124	75.6
Type of injury		
• Suture ligation	60	36.6
• Ureteric transection	44	26.8
• Excision of ureteric segment	28	17.1
• Crush injury	16	9.8
• Uretero-vaginal fistula	12	7.3

late after 7 days. The time interval from injury to urological consultations ranged from 2 to 172 days with a median of 14 days ((interquartile range, 12 to 16 days). Missed ureteric injuries were reported in 8 (4.9%) patients who presented with prolonged ileus, fever, frank pain, anuria, haematuria and elevated serum creatinine. Of these, 6 (75.5%) were found to have non-functioning kidney. The presenting features are shown in Table 3.

Table 3 Postoperative clinical presentation (N = 136)

Clinical presentation	Frequency	Percentages
Leakage of urine per vagina or through the surgical wound	57	41.9
Loin pain/mass	30	22.1
Fever	23	16.9
Urinary incontinence	18	13.2
Abdominal pain	16	11.8
Haematuria	13	9.6
Peritonitism	10	7.4
Non-functioning kidney	9	6.6
Anuria	6	4.4

Pre-operative assessment included Ultrasound scan, Intravenous urography (IVU), Computed tomography (CT) scan, examination under anaesthesia, dye test and cystoscopy as indicated.

All patients except two who died before definitive surgery had surgical intervention. All the injuries were repaired as soon as possible after diagnosis was made and stabilization of their condition done. Ureteroneocystostomy was the most frequent reconstructive surgery performed in 58.0% of cases (Table 4).

A total of thirty-eight patients postoperative complications were recorded in 30 (18.5%) patients, the commonest being surgical site infections in 36.8% of patients (Table 5). A total of six patients required re-laparotomy for postoperative complications as follows; three patients for intra-abdominal abscess /peritonitis, two patients for wound dehiscence and one patient intra-abdominal bleeding after excision of huge intraabdominal tumor. One patient required ureteroscpy for postoperative ureteral stenosis. Other postoperative complications were treated successfully with good results.

The overall length of hospital stay (LOS) ranged from 1 day to 75 days with a median of 12 days. The LOS for non-survivors ranged from 1 day to 14 days (median 4 days). According to multivariate logistic regression analysis, patients who developed post-operative complications stayed longer in the hospital and this was significant ($P = 0.011$). Delayed diagnosis and treatment were also associated with longer hospital stay ($P < 0.001$).

Of the 164 patients, 152 (92.7%) were treated successfully and discharged home and the remaining twelve (7.3%) patients died in hospital. The causes of deaths were sepsis in six patients, renal failure in three patients and in the remaining patients the causes of death were not documented. According to multivariate logistic regression analysis, delayed presentation [OR = 3.8, 95% CI (2.4- 6.5), $p = 0.011$], deranged renal function tests on admission [OR = 2.9, 95%CI (1.7-8.6), $p = 0.001$], missed ureteric injuries [OR = 8.0, 95%CI (3.7-9.3), $p = 0.000$], and presence of postoperative complications mainly surgical site infections [OR = 5.3, 95% CI (3.5-11.5), $p = 0.001$] were the main predictors of mortality.

Patients were followed up for a period ranging between two and twelve months. At the end of follow up period only 65 (42.8%) of survivors were available for follow up and the remaining 87 (57.2%) were lost to follow up. Follow up evaluation mainly consisted of clinical evaluation and abdomino-pelvic ultrasound scan with IVU and cystoscopy when indicated.

Discussion

Iatrogenic Injury to the ureter is the most common complication of abdomino- pelvic surgery, ranging from less than 1 to 10 percent of procedures, depending on

Table 4 Surgical procedures for the Treatment of Ureteric Injuries (n = 162)

Surgical procedures	Frequency	Percentages
Ureteroneocystostomy	94	58.0
End to end uretero-ureterostomy	34	21.0
Psoas hitch + Ureteroneocystostomy	15	9.3
Psoas hitch + Boari flap + Ureteroneocystostomy	12	7.4
Nephrectomy	9	5.6
Percutanaous nephrostomy	7	4.3

Note: All patients with percutaneous nephrostomy underwent definitive surgery after stabilization of their condition.

the complexity of the procedure [4-6]. In this study, iatrogenic ureteric injuries were reported in 2.7% of all abdomino-pelvic operations, a figure which is comparable with what is reported in literature [4-6]. However, the figure of 2.7% in this study may actually be an underestimate and the magnitude of the problem may not be apparent because many cases may have been missed or excluded from the study due to missing data owning to the retrospective nature of the study.

The majority of patients in this study were referred to our centre having had their initial surgeries performed at other hospitals by general practitioners and only 6.1% of ureteric injuries were related to abdomino-pelvic surgeries performed at our centre mainly by junior doctors. Similar observation was reported by Tijani *et al.* [10] in Nigeria. High incidence of ureteric injuries among patients who had abdomino-pelvic operations performed in peripheral hospitals may be attributed to the fact that in this hospitals abdomino-pelvic surgeries were performed by general practitioners who might have limited experience.

In keeping with other studies [10,11,19], the peak age incidence of iatrogenic ureteric injuries in this study was found to be in the third decade of life indicating that this often befalls women during the reproductive periods.

In this study, females were more affected than males, an observation which is in accordance with the results of other workers [10,14,19]. The female predominance demonstrated in this study can be explained by the fact that the most common cause of iatrogenic ureteric injuries in this study was related to obstetric and gynaecological procedures in more than fifty-percent of patients.

In agreement with other studies [10,11,14,19,22], total abdominal hysterectomy (TAH) was the leading cause of ureteric injuries in this study contributing to 69.2% of cases. The ureter is most at risk for injury during gynecologic procedures (such as TAH) at the pelvic brim, beneath the infundibulopelvic ligaments, where it is crossed by the uterine artery, near the cervix [9,11]. In sub-Saharan Africa including Tanzania, with an endemic scarcity of gynaecologists, the practice of major gynaecological surgical procedures such as TAH is not limited to the specialists alone [12]. Ureteric injury may result from such practices and if not properly managed could lead to increase in morbidity and mortality [12]. Injuries may however be almost unavoidable in some situations, even in the hands of the most skilled and experienced gynaecologists. In this study, the majority of abdomino-pelvic operations including TAH were performed by general practitioners in peripheral hospitals who might have limited experience to perform major abdomino-pelvic operations such as TAH. The best defenses against ureteric injury are meticulous surgical technique as well as identification of the course of the ureter and the associated anatomic locations where injury is most likely to occur.

Patients at high risk of iatrogenic ureteric injuries include those with altered anatomy, fibrosis or direct extension of disease process, as in cases of chronic pelvic inflammatory disease, endometriosis, large fibroids (especially in the broad ligament), previous pelvic surgery, malignancy, previous irradiation and congenital abnormalities of the urogenital system [16,17]. Surgeon's experience is also an important risk factor [18-20]. In our series, gross pelvic adhesions from previous surgeries, previous history of pelvic inflammatory diseases and massive intra-operative bleeding during operations for large pelvic tumours were reported to be risk factors for iatrogenic ureteric injuries.

In the present study, more than half of patients were operated on emergency basis which is in keeping with Tijani et al. [10] in Nigeria, but at variance with other authors [19,21] who reported that majority of patients were operated electively. In emergency situations, the surgeon typically has inadequate time to prepare the patient and to perform meticulous surgery; in the process, the surgeon may clamp or even transect a vessel along with the ureter; moreover, at odd hours of the day, competent hands may not always be available.

Ureteric injuries have been found to be more common on the left side [9,10]. This was also observed in our series, where more than half of the ureteric injuries were

Table 5 Postoperative complications

Postoperative complications	Frequency	Percentages
Surgical site infection	14	36.8
Postoperative pyrexia	6	15.8
Urinary tract infections	3	7.9
Intraabdominal abscesses/peritonitis	3	7.9
Wound dehiscence	2	5.3
Intra-abdominal haemorrhage	2	5.3
Paralytic ileus	1	2.6
Ureteral stenosis	1	2.6

on the left side, but at variance with that of Oboro et al. [14] who reported that the right ureter was commonly injured. The left ureter has a greater proximity to the cervix compared to the right ureter, and is thus more liable to injury [9]. Bilateral ureteric injuries have been reported in literature to occur in 5–10% of patients [21]. In this study, bilateral injury was seen in 20.4%. These figures are comparable to that reported by other studies [6,10,22,23].

Most ureteric injuries occur in the distal most part of the ureter where it is closely related to the uterine vessels [9,11]. In the present study, more than three quarter of ureteric injuries occurred in the distal portion of the ureter, which is in agreement with other studies [10,11,22,24]. The distal portion of the ureter is not only embryologically related to the female genital organs but is also involved in diseases affecting them [9]. At the base of the cardinal ligament where it crosses the uterine artery, the ureter is just 12 mm from the vagina and as it moves towards the bladder it becomes even closer to the vagina, and this predisposes the ureter to injury during surgical procedures in the pelvis [9,11].

Ligation injury was the most common form of iatrogenic ureteric injuries reported in the operation notes by accounting for about 36.6% of cases. This is consistent with the findings of Chinakwana *et al.* [13] and most other reports in literature [10,25] but contrasts with the findings of Oboro *et al.* [14] who reported transection injury as the most common.

The management of ureteric injury depends on the time of diagnosis, patient's condition, nature and site of ureteric injury. If the injury is recognized intra-operatively then it must be managed immediately [10,26]. In this study, the diagnosis of ureteric injury was made intra-operatively in less than twenty percent (17.1%) of the patients. However, immediately intra-operatively management of ureteric injury was not performed in any of our patients due to the fact that the majority of primary abdomino-pelvic operations were performed by general practitioners in peripheral hospitals who might have limited experience in the immediate management of ureteric injury.

Many authors have suggested that early recognition and management of ureteric injuries is associated with better outcome [21,22]. In agreement with other studies performed in developing countries [10,11,14,19], the diagnosis of ureteric injury was usually delayed at the Bugando Medical Centre in more than seventy percent of patients as majority of them were referred from peripheral hospitals. Delayed diagnosis of ureteric injury is often associated with high morbidity, uretero-vaginal fistula and the potential loss of kidney function or even mortality. The risk of impairment or loss of kidney function is increased when ureteral injury is not recognized until the post-operative period when ureteral obstruction or urinary leakage is diagnosed in an expected uneventful convalescent period [10]. In this study, missed ureteric injuries were reported in 8 (4.9%) patients and more than three quarters were found to have non-functioning kidney which necessitated nephrectomy.

Imaging is essential for diagnosis especially in cases where bilateral lesions are suspected. Ultrasound may show the eventual hydronephrosis, but this may not be obvious initially. Repeated ultrasound examinations may be necessary. Intravenous pyelogram is indispensable in delineating the degree and level of ureteric obstruction [11]. Delayed function of the involved kidney, poor function on one side, hydronephrosis, extravasation of contrast, and the finding of a urinoma are late findings that all point to ureteral injury [25]. In this study, pre-operative assessment included Ultrasound scan, Intravenous urography (IVU), Computed tomography (CT) scan, examination under anaesthesia, dye test and cystoscopy as indicated.

The objectives of the surgery for repair of iatrogenic ureteric injuries include amongst others preservation of renal function on the affected side and restoration of anatomic continuity of the urinary tract. There is a general agreement that when inadvertent injury to the ureter is detected during surgery, immediate repair is the treatment of choice [10,26]. However, when the diagnosis is delayed the optimal time for definitive treatment is subject to some controversies. Some have advocated for immediate repair while many others still prefer a delayed repair usually preceded by a period of upper tract drainage [10,17,25]. However, recent studies have reported similar results after early and delayed repair [6,17,27,28]. Early repair is associated with shorter hospital stay compared to delayed repair. In a study by Al-Awadi *et al.* [6] mean hospital stay was 4.8 days after early repair; hospital stay was 10.1 days after delayed repair. In our study, all the patients with delayed diagnosis underwent open surgical repair soon after diagnosis and stabilization. This is comparable with other studies [10,11,19,21]. Percutaneous nephrostomy has been reported to be essential when ureteric injury and obstruction is associated with infection or if the patient is not stable for definitive surgery [10,11]. In some cases nephrostomy is essential in order to preserve renal function when scarring and fibrosis at site of ureteric injury prevents immediate repair. A nephrostomy can also permit ante grade contrast studies, ureteroscopy and or ante grade ureteric catheterization [11]. In the present study, percutaneous nephrostomy was performed in only 7 patients representing 4.3% of cases. However, nephrostomy tube in this study was used only to stabilize the patients and all of these patients required additional definitive procedures.

Various reconstructive surgical options include ureteroneocystostomy, Boari flap, Psoas hitch, end to end ureteroureterostomy and trans-ureteroureterostomy [6,22,27]. Other options include ileal segment replacement, appendix interposition and auto-transplantation [10,11]. In our study, fifty-eight percent of patients underwent ureteroneocystostomy which is consistent with other studies [10,14,19]. Ureteroneocystostomy with Boari flap and Psoas hitch was performed in 16.7% of cases. In our study, nephrectomy in patients who had non-functioning kidneys was carried out in 5.6% of cases; this is similar to that reported by other authors [10].

As reported by others [10,19], surgical site infection was the most common postoperative complication in our study. High rate of surgical site infection in the present study may be attributed to contamination of the laparotomy wound during the surgical procedure.

In this study, mortality rate was 7.3% which is higher than that reported by others. [10,11]. High mortality rate in this study is attributed to delayed presentation, deranged renal function tests on admission, missed ureteric injuries and presence of postoperative complications mainly surgical site infections.

The overall median length of hospital stay was 12 days, a figure which is higher than that reported by Al-Awadi *et al.* [6]. Our overall median length of hospital stay was significantly long in patients who developed complications postoperatively. Delayed diagnosis and treatment were also associated with longer hospital stay. Prolonged length of hospitalization results in consumption of large amounts of healthcare resources such as personnel, theatre space, medications, and hospital beds.

The outcome of our management was generally good, with a 92.7% success rate and no complications that were detected during the follow up period. This may be related to the fact that the all reconstructive procedures were performed by experienced urologists. However, the follow up of patients were generally poor as more than half of patients were lost to follow up.

The potential limitation of this study is the fact that information about some patients was incomplete in view of the retrospective nature of the study and this might have introduced some bias in our findings. However, despite this limitation, the study has provided local data that can help healthcare providers in the management of patients with iatrogenic ureteric injuries. The prevention of ureteric injuries during abdomino-pelvic operations is of utmost important. Surgeon must have adequate knowledge of abdominal and pelvic anatomy especially the close relation of ureter with adjacent structures. Urologist must be consulted in the preoperative period in patients at risk for ureteral injury such as those with pelvic adhesions, pelvic radiation, pelvic malignancy, extensive surgery etc. Appropriate imaging of the urinary tract may be required in the preoperative period.

Conclusion

Our experience in this study shows that iatrogenic ureteric injuries are still common in our environment and total abdominal hysterectomy accounts for most cases. The majority of injuries are a result of complications of abdomino-pelvic operations by general practitioners in the peripheral hospitals. Meticulous surgical technique as well as identification of the course of the ureter and associated anatomic locations where injury is most likely to occur is important to decrease the risk of ureteric injury. Early recognition and prompt repair of ureteric injuries is the key to a successful outcome. Treatment of these injuries by experienced team may minimize long-term consequences.

Competing interests

The authors declare that they have no competing interests.

Authors' contributions

PLC conceived the study and did the literature search, coordinated the write-up, editing and submission of the article. ANM, AK and SS participated in the writing of the manuscript and editing. All authors read and approved the final manuscript.

Acknowledgements

The authors are grateful to all who provided assistance during the preparation of this manuscript. Special thanks go to the staff members of the medical record department, theatre, obstetrics & gynaecological, urology and general surgical wards for their support during data collection.

Author details

[1]Department of Surgery, Catholic University of Health and Allied Sciences-Bugando, Mwanza, Tanzania. [2]Department of Obstetrics /Gynecology, Catholic University of Health and Allied Sciences-Bugando, Mwanza, Tanzania. [3]Department of Urology, Catholic University of Health and Allied Sciences-Bugando, Mwanza, Tanzania.

References

1. Preston JM. Iatrogenic ureteric injury: common medicolegal pitfalls. BJU Int. 2001;86:313–7.
2. Vakili B, Chesson RR, Kyle BL, Shobeiri SA, Echols KT, Gist R, et al. The incidence of urinary tract injury during hysterectomy: a prospective analysis based on universal cystoscopy. Am J Obstet Gynecol. 2005;192:1599–604.
3. Obarisiagbon EO, Olagbuji BN, Onuora VC, Oguike TC, Ande ABA. Iatrogenic urological injuries complicating obstetric and gynaecological procedures. Singapore Med J. 2011;52:738–41.
4. Carver BS, Bozeman CB, Venable DD. Ureteral injury due to penetrating trauma. South Med J. 2004;97:462–4.
5. Fraga GP, Borges GM, Mantovani M, Ferreira U, Laurito TL, Netto NR. Penetrating ureteral trauma. Int Braz J Urol. 2007;33:142–50.
6. Al-Awadi K, Kehinde EO, Al-Hunayan A, Al-Khayat A. Iatrogenic ureteric injuries: incidence, aetiological factors and the effect of early management on subsequent outcome. Int Urol Nephrol. 2005;37:235–41.
7. Geavlete P, Georgescu D, Niţă G, Mirciulescu V, Cauni V. Complications of 2735 retrograde semirigid ureteroscopy procedures: a single-center experience. J Endourol. 2006;20:179–85.
8. Liapis A, Bakas P, Giannopoulos V, Creatsas G. Ureteral injuries during gynecological surgery. Int Urogynecol J. 2001;12:391–4.
9. Fröber R. Surgical atlas, surgical anatomy of the ureter. BJU Int. 2007;100:949–65.
10. Tijani KH, Onwuzurigbo KI, Ojewola RW, Afolabi BB, Akanmu NO. Iatrogenic ureteric injuries in a Nigerian teaching hospital: experience in the last decade. East Afr Med J. 2011;88:304–9.

11. Mteta KA, Mbwambo J, Mvungi M. Iatrogenic ureteric and bladder injuries in obstetric and gynaecological surgeries. East Afr Med J. 2006;83:79–85.
12. Williams G, Broughton S, Worku H, Tekle H. Five years' experience of ureterovaginal fistulae following obstetric or gynaecological intervention in Ethiopia. Afr J Urol. 2010;16:17–9.
13. Chinakwana GU, Okafor PI, Ikechebelu JI. Urology injuries following gynaecological operation – our experience in a teaching hospital in Nigeria. West Afr J Med. 2006;25:153–6.
14. Oboro V, Dare FO, Fadiora SO, Aderounmu AOA, Adeoti ML, Ajadi AM. Ureteric injury following pelvic operations. East Afr Med J. 2002;79:611–3.
15. Aronson MP, Bose TM. Urinary tract injury in pelvic surgery. Clin Obstet Gynaecol. 2002;45:428–38.
16. Chou MT, Wang CJ, Lien RC. Prophylactic ureteral catheterization in gynaecologic surgery: a 12-year randomized trial in a community hospital. Int Urogynecol J Pelvic Floor Dysfunct. 2009;20:689–93.
17. Kim J-H, Moore C, Jones JS, Rackley R, Daneshgari F, Goldman H, et al. Management of ureteral injuries associated with vaginal surgery for pelvic organ prolapse. Int Urogynecol J. 2006;17:531–5.
18. Hammad FT, Alqaiwani KM, Shirodkar SS. The role of urologists in the management of urological injuries during obstetric and gynaecologic surgery. Int Urogynecol J Pelvic Floor Dysfunct. 2010;21:1237–41.
19. Durrani SN, Rehman A, Khan S, Ullah H, Khan MK, Ullah A. Ureteral trauma during open surgery: etiology, presentation and management. J Ayub Med Coll Abbottabad. 2013;25:86–9.
20. Schimpf MO, Gottenger EE, Wagner JR. Universal ureteral stent placement at hysterectomy to identify ureteral injury: a decision analysis. BJOG. 2008;115:1151–8.
21. Rafique M, Arif MH. Management of iatrogenic ureteric injuries associated with gynaecological surgery. Int Urol Nephrol. 2002;34:31–5.
22. Anwar MS, Tariq M, Saeed K, Ghafoor T, Mustafa G. Causes of ureteric injuries and outcome of different surgical procedures for the repair of ureter. J Sheikh Zayed Med Coll. 2010;1:16–20.
23. Matani YS, Bani-Hani KE, Bani-Hani IH. Ureteric injuries during obstetric and gynecologic procedures. Saudi Med J. 2003;24:365–8.
24. Mahendran HA, Singam P, Ho C, Hee TG, Zainuddin ZM. Iatrogenic ureter injuries: eleven years experience in a tertiary hospital. Med J Malaysia. 2012;67:169–72.
25. Brandes S, Micheal C, Noel A, Jackmcaninch. Diagnosis and management of ureteric injury: an evidence-based analysis. BJU Int. 2004;94:277–89.
26. Visco AG, Taber KH, Weidner AC, Barber MD, Myers ER. Cost-effectiveness of universal cystoscopy to identify ureteral injury at hysterectomy. Obstet Gynecol. 2001;97:685–92.
27. Routh JC, Tollefson MK, Ashley RA, Husmann DA. Iatrogenic ureteral injury: can adult repair techniques be used on children? J Pediatr Urol. 2009;5:53–5.
28. Mensah J, Klufio G, Ahiaku F, Osafo C, Gepi-Attee S. Delayed recognition of bilateral ureteral injury after gynaecological surgery. Ghana Med J. 2008;42:133–6.

10

Routine ultrasound examination by OB/GYN residents increase the accuracy of diagnosis for emergency surgery in gynecology

Flavie Toret-Labeeuw[1], Cyrille Huchon[1,2*], Thomas Popowski[1], Anne A Chantry[3], Alexandre Dumont[4] and Arnaud Fauconnier[1,2]

Abstract

Introduction: Diagnostic accuracy of first-line sonographic evaluation by obstetrics/gynecology residents in determining the need for emergency surgery in women with acute pelvic pain is unknown. Aim of this study was to evaluate the diagnostic accuracy of routine ultrasound evaluation by obstetrics/gynecology residents, available 24 hours a day, in patients with acute pelvic pain.

Methods: A cross-sectional retrospective study included consecutive patients who underwent emergency laparoscopy for acute pelvic pain at a teaching hospital gynecologic emergency unit, between January 1, 2004, and December 31, 2006. The laparoscopic diagnosis was the reference standard. Gynecologic and nongynecologic conditions requiring immediate surgery to avoid severe morbidity or death were defined as *surgical emergencies*. In all patients, obstetrics/gynecology residents routinely performed clinical examination and standardized ultrasonography was routinely recorded. Sonograms were re-interpreted for the study, blinded to physical examination and laparoscopic findings, according to evidence-based predetermined criteria. Sensitivity, specificity, and likelihood ratios were computed for clinical data alone, sonographic data alone, and the combination of both.

Results: Emergency laparoscopy was performed in 234 patients, diagnosing 139 (59%) *surgical emergencies*. Clinical and sonographic examinations performed by the residents each independently predicted a need for emergency surgery. Combining both examinations was superior over each examination alone and had an acceptable false-negative rate of 1%.

Conclusions: First-line combined clinical and sonographic examination by obstetrics/gynecology residents is effective in ruling out *surgical emergencies* in patients with acute pelvic pain.

Keywords: Acute pelvic pain, Physical examination, Ultrasonography, Laparoscopy, Gynecologic emergency, Sensitivity, Specificity

Introduction

Acute pelvic pain accounts for up to 40% of visits to gynecologic emergency departments (EDs) [1] and may indicate a life-threatening emergency. A prompt diagnosis is crucial to prevent severe morbidity or death [2]. The physical examination is not fully reliable [2-5]. Extensive use of diagnostic laparoscopy has been suggested to avoid missing gynecologic or non gynecologic disorders requiring emergency surgical treatment [1,6]. However, laparoscopy is an invasive procedure associated with a number of complications [7], and its use as a diagnostic tool should therefore be avoided whenever possible [8].

Since the 1990s, transvaginal ultrasonography (TVUS) has become an essential diagnostic tool for gynecologic emergencies [9]. Nonetheless, the impact of around-the-clock access to TVUS in gynecologic EDs remains unclear. In most of the studies establishing the diagnostic

* Correspondence: cyrillehuchon@yahoo.fr
[1]Department of Gynecology & Obstetrics, Centre Hospitalier Intercommunal de Poissy – Saint-Germain, University of Versailles Saint-Quentin (UVSQ), 78103 Poissy, France
[2]EA7285, Risques cliniques et sécurité en santé des femmes et en santé périnatale, University of Versailles Saint-Quentin (UVSQ), Poissy, France

accuracy of TVUS in detecting gynecological emergencies, the examination was performed by board-certified radiologists or obstetricians/gynecologists. These specialized physicians are not available around-the-clock when resources are limited, as is increasingly the case in this era of patient care in the case of cost containment. It has been suggested that obstetrics/gynecology residents can perform reliable ultrasound scans in the ED to increase the rapidity and improve the quality of patient care in case of gynecologic emergencies [10].

In France, obstetrics/gynecology residents perform the initial evaluation of patients seen in gynecologic EDs, including bedside TVUS. In a previous study, we demonstrated that standardizing the gynecologic emergency ultrasonogram allowed scoring and quality control and also significantly improved the quality of ultrasonography in the gynecologic EDs [11].

The aim of this retrospective cross-sectional study was to evaluate and compare the diagnostic accuracy of first-line clinical and sonographic evaluation by obstetrics/gynecology residents available 24 hours a day in determining the need for emergency surgery in women with acute pelvic pain.

Materials and methods

This study was approved by the CEROG (French Ethics Committee for Research in Obstetrics and Gynecology).

Study design

We retrospectively reviewed the medical records of consecutive women who underwent laparoscopy for acute pelvic pain at the gynecologic ED of the Poissy-St Germain Hospital, France, a teaching hospital serving a large population. This historical cohort was studied between January 1, 2004, and December 31, 2006.

One resident and one senior gynecologist are available at the gynecologic ED around the clock. In France, women with acute pelvic pain are evaluated either in general EDs, in which case they are then referred to a gynecologic ED, or directly in gynecologic EDs, to which all women have free access. Thus, all patients with suspected gynecologic emergencies are seen in gynecologic EDs.

Study population

All patients seen at our gynecologic ED for acute pelvic pain of less than 7 days' duration and who underwent emergency laparoscopy were included. Exclusion criteria were hemodynamic shock, pregnancy of more than 13 gestational weeks, secondary laparoscopy for ectopic pregnancy initially managed with methotrexate, surgery within the last month, or virgin patients.

Among patients who did not undergo emergency laparoscopy, those who were pregnant were followed until a definitive diagnostic was made [12]. In nonpregnant patients, when the findings of all examinations were thought to be normal and the pain subsided with appropriate analgesia by the end of the visit or hospitalization, a diagnosis of idiopathic acute pelvic pain was made. After discharge, the patients were encouraged to return to our ED in case of pain recurrence.

Study protocol

In all patients, a nurse performed an initial assessment including measurement of vital signs (Heart rate, arterial pressure and temperature), a urine hCG test and a pain intensity measurement using a Numerical Rating Scale (NRS). Then, the obstetrics/gynecology resident on duty performed standardized physical and TVUS examinations. If needed, additional investigations were performed (laboratory tests, complete ultrasound examination by a certified obstetrician/gynecologist, computed tomography). Residents were between their third and eight semester of formation in gynecology and obstetrics and were non titular of ultrasound diploma.

The senior gynecologist decided whether to perform emergency laparoscopy based on all the available data. Criteria for emergency laparoscopy were suspected adnexal torsion [13], ectopic pregnancy with a contraindication to medical treatment according to French recommendations [14], suspected tubo-ovarian abscess or peritonitis due to pelvic inflammatory disease [15], suspected massive hemoperitoneum and persistence of severe pain. For patients who did not undergo laparoscopy and before discharge, a routine time of observation of about 24 hours is usually performed in the department of gynecology.

Data collection

The physical examination included palpation of the abdomen, speculum examination, and digital vaginal examination. The results were considered normal when there was no guarding, rebound, mass, or thickening on abdominal palpation [2 5 16] and no cervical motion tenderness, adnexal tenderness, or adnexal mass or thickening on vaginal examination [4,16]. If one of these features was present, the physical examination was considered abnormal.

TVUS was performed using a 3.5-5 MHz transabdominal probe and a 7 MHz transvaginal probe with a General Electric Voluson 730 Expert machine (GE Medical System Europe). The residents followed a standardized TVUS protocol including at least five images, and including a routinely recording of: (i) a longitudinal view of the uterus to visualize the midline stripe indicating an empty uterus, (ii) a transverse view of the uterus, (iii and iv) a view of each ovary with the transvaginal probe, and (v) a view of Morison's pouch with the transabdominal probe (Figure 1). One to three additional views could be obtained as dictated by the abnormal ultrasound findings (e.g., view of an

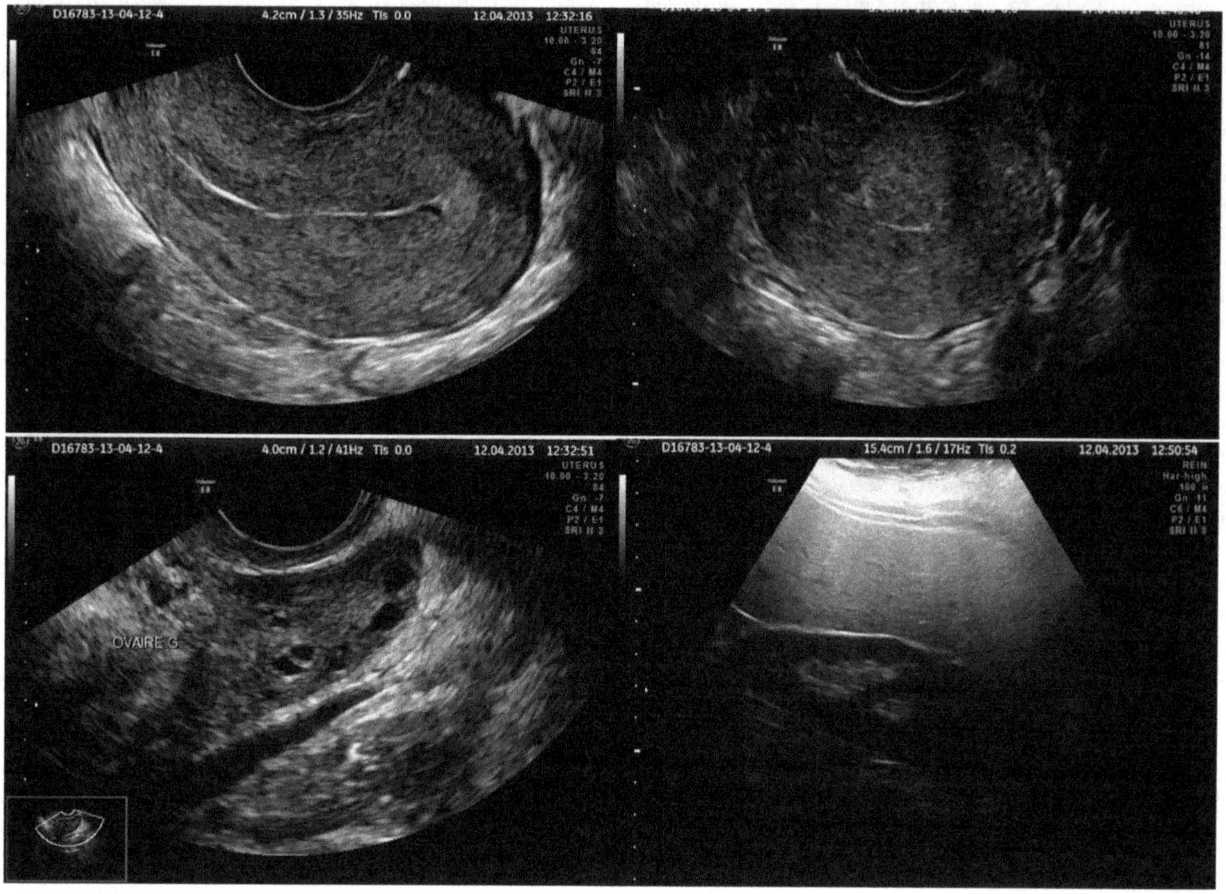

Figure 1 Standardized ultrasonography scans. (**i**) longitudinal view of the uterus, (**ii**) transverse view of the uterus, (**iii**) view of left ovary, and (**iv**) view of Morison's pouch.

ectopic gestational sac) [11]. Residents received a 1-hour class taught by a board-certified senior obstetrician/gynecologist with special expertise in gynecological ultrasonography available online (www.e-campus.uvsq.fr/claroline/course/index.php?cid=SAFE). This class covered image acquisition, normal and abnormal findings and image quality criteria. A copy of the written protocol for bedside emergency ultrasonography was also given to each resident.

For the present study, all sonograms were retrospectively re-interpreted by two authors: a board-certified obstetrician/gynecologist (FTL) with special expertise in gynecological ultrasonography and a research nurse (AC), who were blinded to the physical and laparoscopic findings. TVUS was considered abnormal if any of the following was seen: pelvic fluid reaching the uterine corpus or around the ovary [17], fluid in Morison's pouch [18], abnormal adnexal mass separate from the ovary [10,19], and ovary larger than 50 mm and containing a cyst [13].

Key outcome measures

The laparoscopy diagnosis was the reference standard. Patients were classified as having a *surgical emergency* or a *benign emergency. Surgical emergencies* were defined as gynecologic or nongynecologic disorders diagnosed by laparoscopy and associated with a high risk of complications likely to cause severe morbidity or death in the absence of appropriate emergency surgical treatment [2]. They included ectopic pregnancy with tubal rupture or active bleeding or cardiac activity or hemoperitoneum exceeding 300 mL [17]; pelvic inflammatory disease complicated by tubo-ovarian abscess or peritonitis; adnexal torsion; rupture of hemorrhagic ovarian cysts with hemoperitoneum exceeding 300 mL; appendicitis; and intestinal obstruction. *Benign emergencies*, as defined for this study, included acute conditions expected to resolve spontaneously or with appropriate medical treatment such as uncomplicated ectopic pregnancy, uncomplicated pelvic inflammatory disease, uncomplicated cyst, intra-cystic hemorrhage, myoma, endometriotic lesions, and pelvic adhesions.

Data analysis

The preoperative physical and TVUS examinations, recorded as normal or abnormal, were compared to the laparoscopy findings as indicating a *surgical emergency* or a *benign emergency*. We used multiple logistic regression to compute the crude and adjusted diagnostic odds ratios (DORs) of having a laparoscopically confirmed surgical emergency depending on the preoperative clinical and TVUS results. The parameter values of the model were estimated using the maximum likelihood ratio method. The adjusted diagnostic odds ratios (aDORs) and their confidence intervals (CIs) were computed from the model coefficients and their standard deviations. *P* values lower than 0.05 were considered significant.

To compare the performances of physical examination alone, TVUS alone, and both in combination for diagnosing a *surgical emergency*, we computed sensitivity (Se), specificity (Sp), and the positive and negative likelihood ratios (LR+ and LR-). In the strategy including both examinations in combination, the results were considered to suggest a *surgical emergency* if the physical examination OR the TVUS OR both showed abnormalities; this strategy reflected routine use of TVUS in first line, regardless of clinical findings as we perform at our ED.

To be clinically effective and safe, a first-line diagnostic strategy had to have a low false-negative rate (i.e., sensitivity of 95% or more), with sufficient sensitivity to produce an LR- lower than 0.25. The three different strategies were compared based on the 95% confidence intervals (95% CIs) for Se and Sp according to Taylor's formula [20]. If the point estimate of one value was not included within the 95% CI of the other, then they differed significantly with *P* smaller than 0.05. The analyses were first performed on the overall population of patients then separately in the pregnant and nonpregnant patients.

The required sample size was estimated as follows. The expected prevalence of surgical emergencies among patients who underwent laparoscopy was 50%. Using computation of the 95% CI with an unknown ratio estimator of the standard deviation, including 200 patients with laparoscopy would produce a lower limit of the 95% CI of 0.95 if the true false-negative rate is less than or equal to 2%. To take into account the occurrence of exclusion criteria and missing data in some patients, we planned to include 300 patients.

Results

Of the 300 patients who met the inclusion criteria between January 1, 2004, and December 31, 2006, 34 had one or more exclusion criteria (Figure 2). Among the 266 eligible patients, 32 had missing physical examination data or no recorded ultrasound images, leaving 234 patients for the analysis. The characteristics of the patients with missing data did not differ from those of the patients included in the analysis.

The main patient characteristics and laparoscopy diagnoses are shown in Table 1. Of the 234 patients, 139 (59%) had laparoscopically confirmed *surgical emergencies* and the remaining 95 (41%) patients had *benign emergencies* that did not require immediate surgery, including 7 (6.3%) entirely normal findings at laparoscopy.

Both the physical examination alone (DOR, 3.5; 95% CI, 1.8 to 6.9; $P<0.001$) and TVUS alone (DOR, 6.6; 95% CI, 2.8 to 15.6; $P<0.0001$) independently predicted a laparoscopy diagnosis of *surgical emergency*. However, when used alone, neither the physical examination nor TVUS performed sufficiently well to rule out a surgical emergency (Table 2). TVUS alone was better than the physical examination alone (false-negative rates, 5.8% and 13.0%,

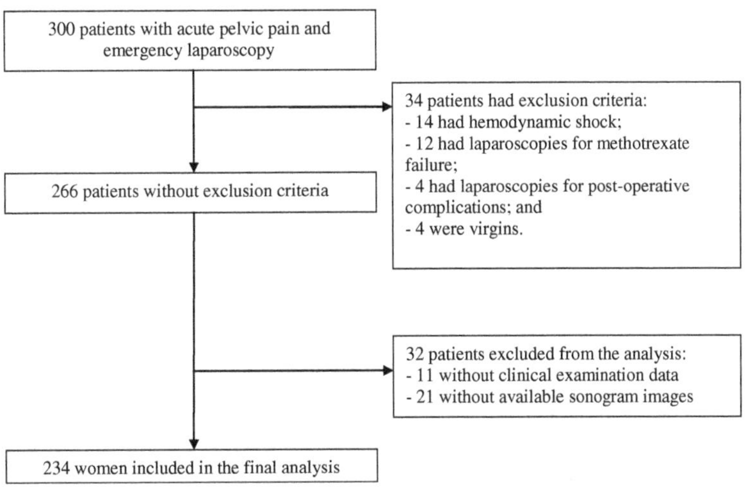

Figure 2 Flow chart of the study population.

Table 1 Characteristics of the study population and laparoscopy diagnoses

	Overall population N=234	*Surgical emergencies* N=139	*Benign emergencies* N=95
Age in years, mean±SD	31.3 ± 7.0	31.9 ± 6.9	30.5 ± 7.1
Gravidity, median [range]	2 [0–9]	2 [0–9]	1 [0–6]*
Parity, median [range]	1 [0–6]	1 [0–6]	0 [0–4]*
Contraception, n (%)	65 (27.9)	37 (26.8)	28 (29.5)
Pain NRS score at admission, mean±SD	6.7 ± 2.6	6.9 ± 2.6	6.4 ± 2.5
Positive hCG test, n (%)	150 (64.1)	97 (69.8)†	53 (55.8)†
Laparoscopy diagnosis			
Ectopic pregnancy, n (%)	136 (58.1)	91 (65.5)	45 (47.4)
Pelvic inflammatory disease, n (%)	31 (13.2)	25 (18.0)	6 (6.3)
Adnexal torsion, n (%)	15 (6.4)	15 (10.8)	NA
Appendicitis, n (%)	4 (1.7)	4 (2.9)	NA
Ruptured hemorrhagic cyst, n (%)	5 (3.0)	2 (1.4)	3 (5.3)
Other diagnosis, n (%)	36 (15.0)	2 (1.4)‡	34 (34.7)‡
Normal, n (%)	7 (2.6)	NA	7 (6.3)

Surgical emergencies were ectopic pregnancies with tubal rupture or active bleeding or cardiac activity or hemoperitoneum over 300 mL; pelvic inflammatory disease complicated with pyosalpinx, tubo-ovarian abscess, or pelvic peritonitis; adnexal torsion; hemorrhagic ovarian cyst rupture with hemoperitoneum exceeding 300 mL; appendicitis; and intestinal obstruction.
Benign emergencies were conditions expected to resolve spontaneously or with appropriate medical treatment.
NRS, numerical rating scale for pain severity; hCG, human chorionic gonadotropin; NA, not applicable; SD, standard deviation; NRS, Numerical rating scale; hCG, serum human chorionic gonadotrophin; NA, not applicable.
*$P<0.05$, Student's *t* test; †$P<0.05$, Chi-square; ‡ Intestinal obstruction; ‡ uncomplicated ovarian cysts or intracystic hemorrhage.

respectively). Table 3 lists the diagnoses of the false-negative results of the physical examination and TVUS.

The strategy combining physical examination and TVUS in first-line was better than the strategy including only physical examination according to our criteria in which surgical emergencies were suspected based on abnormal clinical OR TVUS findings. This strategy decreased the false-negative rate from 13% (physical examination alone) to less than 1% (Table 3). The strategy combining physical examination and TVUS was the one maximizing Se and decreased negative LR to an acceptable rate of 0.1. When pregnant and nonpregnant patients were analyzed separately, the results were unchanged (Table 2).

Discussion

According to our data, physical examination cannot be used alone to safely rule out a *surgical emergency* in a woman presenting with acute pelvic pain. Inversely when both the physical examination and TVUS are normal, the risk of a *surgical emergency* is less than 1%. This suggests the benefit of adding bedside standardized ultrasonography in the first-line diagnostic management of suspected gynecologic emergencies.

One of the strengths of our study is that TVUS findings are recorded routinely at our institution using a standardized protocol [11]. This standardized protocol, with a routine recording of standardized images, allows a reviewing of those scans, even a long time after. Recording pictures

Table 2 Diagnostic accuracy of physical examination, transvaginal ultrasonography, and both for diagnosing surgical emergencies

	Physical examination alone				TVUS alone				Strategy combining physical examination andTVUS†			
	Se% (n/N) [95% CI]	Sp% (n/N) [95% CI]	LR +	LR −	Se (n/N) [95% CI]	Sp (n/N) [95% CI]	LR +	LR −	Se (n/N) [95% CI]	Sp (n/N) [95% CI]	LR +	LR −
Overall population	87% (121/139) [82–93]	33% (31/95) [23–42]	1.3	0.4	94% (131/139) [90–98]	27% (26/95) [18–36]	1.3	0.2	99% (138/139) [98–100]	7% (7/95) [2–13]	1.1	0.1
Pregnant women	84% (81/97) [76–91]	42% (22/53) [28–55]	1.4	0.4	96% (93/97) [92–100]	13% (7/53) [4–22]	1.1	0.3	99% (96/97) [97–100]	6% (3/53) [0–12]	1.1	0.2
Non-pregnant women	95% (40/42) [89–100]	21% (9/42) [19–34]	1.2	0.2	91% (38/42) [82–99]	45% (19/42) [30–60]	1.6	0.2	100% (42/42) [92 – 100]	10% (4/42) [1–18]	1.1	0

Se, sensitivity; CI, confidence interval; Sp, specificity; LR, likelihood ratio.
†Corresponds to a strategy of routine TVUS regardless of the clinical findings, abnormal findings include abnormal examination OR abnormal TVUS.
TVUS, transvaginal ultrasonography; Se, sensitivity; Sp, specificity; LR+, positive likelihood ratio; LR-, negative likelihood ratio; 95%CI, 95 % confidence interval.

Table 3 Diagnoses in patients with a laparoscopy diagnosis of surgical emergency but had negative physical examination or negative transvaginal ultrasonography or negative with both examinations combined

	FN, physical examination, n (%)	FN, TVUS, n (%)	FN, physical examination combined with TVUS†, n (%)	Total number of patients with surgical emergencies, N
Ectopic pregnancy	14 (15%)	1 (1%)	0	91
Pelvic peritonitis	0	1 (4 %)	0	25
Adnexal torsion	3 (20%)	3 (20%)	1 (7%)	15
Appendicitis	0	1 (25%)	0	4
Intestinal obstruction	0	2 (100%)	0	2
Ruptured hemorrhagic cyst	1 (50%)	0	0	2
Total	18 (13%)	8 (6%)	1 (0.7%)	139

Percentages were computed by dividing the number of false negatives by the total number of surgical emergencies.
FN, False negatives; TVUS, transvaginal ultrasonography.
†Corresponds to a strategy of routine TVUS regardless of the clinical findings, abnormal findings include abnormal examination OR abnormal TVUS.

in the patient's chart may also decrease the need for subsequent repeat ultrasonography, thereby saving time and diminishing healthcare costs. Furthermore, we did not have to rely on a written description of the TVUS findings in the medical record. The TVUS findings were determined by blinded observers using objective criteria. These criteria are reliable and have been proven useful for diagnosing specific gynecologic emergencies [9,10,13,15,21].

It has been demonstrated that the availability of TVUS at the initial assessment of both pregnant and nonpregnant women decreased patient time management, unnecessary admissions, outpatient follow-up examinations and also modified treatment decisions [22,23]. Nonetheless, we did not find any published study showing clear-cut evidence that routine ultrasonography decreases unfavorable patient outcomes. We demonstrate that including around-the -clock TVUS as a first step investigation in addition to the physical examination is an effective strategy to rule out surgical emergencies at the gynecologic ED by reducing the risk of diagnostic errors.

In France, there is at least one resident on duty around the clock with unlimited access to TVUS in gynecological EDs, even when no radiologist or board-certified obstetrician/gynecologist is available. Another particularity in France is that ultrasonography for gynecologic emergencies are under the supervision of board-certified obstetricians/gynecologists instead of radiologists. In contrast, in most of the developed countries, emergency ultrasonography is performed at the request of ED physicians by radiologists or board-certified obstetricians/gynecologists [22,23]. Although, this strategy optimizes the quality of ultrasound examination, our results suggest that suspecting surgical emergencies based on the physical examination alone does not perform well for the diagnosis of gynecologic emergencies. Instead, the French strategy of first-line ultrasonography performed by non-specialized healthcare providers should be compared with the so-called "limited" sonogram in the 2nd/3rd trimester of pregnancy. These examinations do not replace a standard complete ultrasound examination but are performed to obtain an immediate answer to a specific clinical question [24], as FAST scanning in EDs. Bedside abdominal ultrasonography by a surgeon was also introduced several years ago as a routine examination for patients with acute abdominal pain and produced similar results, improving the rate of correct diagnoses [25].

The quality of bedside ultrasonography by obstetrics/gynecology residents is obviously not comparable to that obtained by board-certified specialists, as the quality of examination is highly variable [11]. Furthermore, experience is a key factor in the ability of transvaginal ultrasound to manage women with pelvic pain with accuracy [9]. Nonetheless, in our center, we made important efforts to implement a standardized ultrasonography protocol [11] to reduce the heterogeneity of the quality of ultrasonography performed by residents. This quality process probably increased the usefulness of bedside TVUS for the diagnosis of gynecologic emergency. One application of this process would that these scans could be performed by anyone involved in gynecologic emergencies management with appropriate training (ie ED physicians, Family Medical doctors, midwife or advanced nurse practitioners). This training should include rigorous implementation of standardized ultrasonography protocol in EDs, with quality control of ultrasonography by board-certified obstetricians/gynecologists or radiologists to obtain individual accreditation. Thus, this accreditation could decrease the heterogeneity of ultrasound examination and allow correct interpretation in order to make correct clinical decision regarding surgical emergencies.

Nonetheless, our study has several limitations. First, we were not able to have the physical examination and TVUS done by two different individuals, in contrast to another group [23]. The physical examination was performed before TVUS, and its results may therefore have influenced the recording of the images. However, calculating the conditional statistics of one examination according to the result of the other showed no differences with the main results (data not shown).

Second, our strategy of including only women who underwent laparoscopy may have led to verification bias. We chose to select patients with laparoscopy to ensure that the final diagnosis was established with certainty. However, the decision to perform laparoscopy was taken by a senior physician, based possibly on the result of the physical and TVUS findings by the resident, which may have artificially increased Se and decreased Sp of both examinations.

Third, our follow-up data on patients in whom emergency laparoscopy was deemed unnecessary may have been incomplete. We believe that the risk of missing a surgical emergency among patients who leave the ED without undergoing laparoscopy is low as pregnant women received very close follow-up after ED discharge until the hCG test became negative and patients discharged with undiagnosed surgical emergencies would eventually come back to our ED, which serves a vast geographic area.

Conclusions

Our findings indicate that combining routine bedside TVUS with the physical examination performed by gynecology/obstetrics residents on duty around-the-clock in gynecologic EDs is more effective than physical examination alone in ruling out potentially life-threatening emergencies in women with acute pelvic pain. The use of a standardized TVUS protocol and stringent objective criteria for interpreting the images may play a role in the beneficial effects of routine TVUS.

Consent

Written informed consent was obtained from the patient for publication of accompanying images.

Competing interests

The authors have no conflicts of interest.

Authors' contributions

AF and AD design the study; Acquisition of data were performed by FTL, TP an AC, Statistical analysis were performed by TP, CH and AF; Analysis and interpretation of data were performed by AC, AD, CH and AF; FTL, CH and AF draft the manuscript; AD and AF made critical revision of the manuscript for important intellectual content; AF and CH have full access to all of the data and take responsibility for the integrity of the data and the accuracy of the data analysis. All authors read and approved the final manuscript.

Author details

[1]Department of Gynecology & Obstetrics, Centre Hospitalier Intercommunal de Poissy – Saint-Germain, University of Versailles Saint-Quentin (UVSQ), 78103 Poissy, France. [2]EA7285, Risques cliniques et sécurité en santé des femmes et en santé périnatale, University of Versailles Saint-Quentin (UVSQ), Poissy, France. [3]INSERM, UMR S953, 75014 Paris, France. [4]Institut de recherche pour le développement (Research Institute for Development), UMR IRD 216, 75014 Paris, France.

References

1. Kontoravdis A, Chryssikopoulos A, Hassiakos D, Liapis A, Zourlas PA: **The diagnostic value of laparoscopy in 2365 patients with acute and chronic pelvic pain.** *International Journal of Gynaecology & Obstetrics* 1996, **52**:243–248.
2. Abbott J, Emmans LS, Lowenstein SR: **Ectopic pregnancy: ten common pitfalls in diagnosis.** *Am J Emerg Med* 1990, **8**(6):515–522.
3. Huchon C, Fauconnier A: **Adnexal torsion: a literature review.** *Eur J Obstet Gynecol Reprod Biol* 2010, **150**(1):8–12.
4. Kahn JG, Walker CK, Washington E, Landers DV, Sweet RL: **Diagnosing pelvic inflammatory disease: a comprehensive analysis and considerations for developing a new model.** *JAMA* 1991, **226**(18):2594–2604.
5. Mol BW, Hajenius PJ, Engelsbel S, Ankum WM, van der Veen F, Hemrika DJ, *et al*: **Should patients who are suspected of having an ectopic pregnancy undergo physical examination?** *Fertil Steril* 1999, **71**(1):155–157.
6. Mikkelsen AL, Felding C: **Laparoscopy and ultrasound examination in women with acute pelvic pain.** *Gynecol Obstet Invest* 1990, **30**:162–164.
7. Chapron C, Querleu D, Bruhat MA, Madelenat P, Fernandez H, Pierre F, *et al*: **Surgical complications of diagnostic and operative gynaecological laparoscopy: a series of 29,966 cases.** *Hum Reprod* 1998, **13**(4):867–872.
8. Morino M, Pellegrino L, Castagna E, Farinella E, Mao P: **Acute nonspecific abdominal pain: a randomized, controlled trial comparing early laparoscopy versus clinical observation.** *Ann Surg* 2006, **244**(6):881–886. discussion 86–8.
9. Okaro E, Condous G: **Diagnostic and therapeutic capabilities of ultrasound in the management of pelvic pain.** *Curr Opin Obstet Gynecol* 2005, **17**(6):611–617.
10. Timor-Tritsch IE, Lerner JP, Monteagudo A, Murphy KE, Heller DS: **Transvaginal sonographic markers of tubal inflammatory disease.** *Ultrasound Obstet Gynecol* 1998, **12**(1):56–66.
11. Salomon LJ, Nassar M, Bernard JP, Ville Y, Fauconnier A: **A score-based method to improve the quality of emergency gynaecological ultrasound examination.** *Eur J Obstet Gynecol Reprod Biol* 2009, **143**(2):116–120.
12. Barnhart KT, Fay CA, Suescum M, Sammel MD, Appleby D, Shaunik A, *et al*: **Clinical factors affecting the accuracy of ultrasonography in symptomatic first-trimester pregnancy.** *Obstet Gynecol* 2011, **117**(2 Pt 1):299–306.
13. Huchon C, Staraci S, Fauconnier A: **Adnexal torsion: a predictive score for pre-operative diagnosis.** *Hum Reprod* 2010, **25**(9):2276–2280.
14. CNGOF: **[Guidelines for clinical practice: Ectopic pregnancy management].** *J Gynecol Obstet Biol Reprod (Paris)* 2003, **32**(7 Suppl):3S6–3S112.
15. Varras M, Polyzos D, Perouli E, Noti P, Pantazis I, Akrivis C: **Tubo-ovarian abscesses: spectrum of sonographic findings with surgical and pathological correlations.** *Clin Exp Obstet Gynecol* 2003, **30**(2–3):117–121.
16. Dart RG, Kaplan B, Varaklis K: **Predictive value of history and physical examination in patients with suspected ectopic pregnancy.** *Ann Emerg Med* 1999, **33**(3):283–290.
17. Fauconnier A, Mabrouk A, Salomon LJ, Bernard JP, Ville Y: **Ultrasound assessment of haemoperitoneum in ectopic pregnancy: derivation of a prediction model.** *World J Emerg Surg* 2007, **2**:23.
18. Baque P, Iannelli A, Dausse F, de Peretti F, Bourgeon A: **A new method to approach exact hemoperitoneum volume in a splenic trauma model using ultrasonography.** *Surg Radiol Anat* 2005, **27**(3):249–253.
19. Condous GS: **Ultrasound diagnosis of ectopic pregnancy.** *Semin Reprod Med* 2007, **25**(2):85–91.
20. Simel DL, Samsa GP, Matchar DB: **Likelihood ratios for continuous test results–making the clinicians' job easier or harder?** *J Clin Epidemiol* 1993, **46**(1):85–93.
21. Popowski T, Huchon C, Toret-Labeeuw F, Chantry AA, Aegerter P, Fauconnier A: **Hemoperitoneum assessment in ectopic pregnancy.** *Int J Gynaecol Obstet* 2012, **116**(2):97–100.
22. Bignardi T, Burnet S, Alhamdan D, Lu C, Pardey J, Benzie R, *et al*: **Management of women referred to an acute gynecology unit: impact of an ultrasound-based model of care.** *Ultrasound Obstet Gynecol* 2010, **35**(3):344–348.

11

A technical modification for percutaneous tracheostomy: prospective case series study on one hundred patients

Joao B Rezende-Neto[1*], Argenil J Oliveira[2], Mario P Neto[2], Fernando A Botoni[1] and Sandro B Rizoli[3]

Abstract

The purpose of this study is to describe a technical modification of percutaneous tracheostomy that combines principles of the Percu Twist™ and the Griggs-Portex® methods in a reusable kit. One hundred patients underwent the procedure. There were no false passage, tube misplacement, or deaths related to the procedure. There were two minor bleedings managed conservatively. The technical modification described in this study is safe and simple to execute.

Keywords: Percutaneous tracheostomy, technique.

Introduction

Tracheostomy is one of the most frequently performed surgical procedures in intensive care unit (ICU) patients [1]. Percutaneous tracheostomy has gained widespread acceptance as an alternative to open surgical tracheostomy with the advantage of "bedside" performance and minimal morbidity [2-4]. Most percutaneous tracheostomy methods incorporate the Seldinger technique to gain initial access to the tracheal lumen. However, after that initial step, a number of variations have been described [2,4-10]. The method introduced by Ciaglia and colleagues in 1985, has become the most popular technique for percutaneous tracheostomy [2]. Different strategies to dilate the tracheal breach are utilized in the Percu Twist™technique (Rüsch, Kernen, Germany) and in the Griggs method (Portex® Smiths Medical International Ltd., Hythe, Kent, UK) [5,10-12]. In the Percu Twist™technique a tracheal stoma is created by a screwlike dilating device, whereas in the method introduced by Griggs a pair of forceps are used to dilate the tracheal breach [5,9-14]. Compression of the anterior tracheal wall is minimal in both methods potentially reducing injury to the posterior wall [12,13].

* Correspondence: jbrezende.ufmg@gmail.com
[1]Universidade Federal de Minas Gerais and Risoleta Tolentino Neves Hospital, Brazil

The aim of this study is to describe a technical modification of percutaneous tracheostomy that combines the principles of the Percu Twist™ and the Griggs-Portex® methods.

Materials and methods

This prospective case series study was approved by the Research Ethics Committee of the Universidade Federal de Minas Gerais, Belo Horizonte, Brazil (resolution number: ETIC 0392.0.203.000-10), in accordance with the WMA Declaration of Helsinki - Ethical Principles for Medical Research Involving Human Subjects. A family member responsible for the patient was contacted for informed consent prior to the procedure. Data were obtained prospectively (data collecting sheet) at the Risoleta Tolentino Neves University Hospital Trauma Center (affiliated to the Universidade Federal de Minas Gerais) from June 1, 2010 to March 31, 2011. Inclusion criteria were age 18 years or older and an indication for tracheostomy. All percutaneous tracheostomies, as well as, ultrasound and bronchoscopy were performed by the authors JBRN, AJO, MPN. General surgery residents of the Federal University of Minas Gerais performed the procedure under supervision. Data included demographics, indication for tracheostomy, body mass index (BMI), thyromental distance (measured from the thyroid notch to the inferior border of the mentum), tracheostomy tube size (internal diameter), and acute complications. Procedure time was recorded by a nurse with a digital stopwatch. It is our practice to correct the coagulation parameters of the patients prior to percutaneous tracheostomy. Therefore, we also reviewed the data pertaining to prothrombin time, activated partial prothrombin time, platelet count, and the international normalized ratio (INR).

Modified Percutaneous Tracheostomy Technique

The instruments used for percutaneous tracheostomy in this work were manufactured from stainless steel and are reusable (Figure 1). All mechanically ventilated patients are sedated (midazolan 1-2 mg and fentanyl 100-200 mcg), paralyzed (pancuronium 0.04-0.1 mg/Kg), and placed on 100% oxygen starting 5 minutes before and until 5 minutes after the completion of the procedure. Positive end expiratory pressure (PEEP) setting is not changed for the procedure. A pulse oximeter (Datex-Ohmeda Inc., Tewksbury, MA) is used to assess hemoglobin oxygen saturation. Trauma patients with cervical spine cleared by physical examination in addition to radiograph of the neck and/or computed tomography scan, have their neck slightly extended by a 10 cm high pillow placed underneath the shoulders. Otherwise, the patient's neck and the bed are maintained in neutral position. If the cervical collar has to be removed a head immobilization device is used to stabilize the cervical spine (HeadBed™ II, Laerdal do Brasil, Barueri, SP, Brazil).

The operative site is prepared with 10% povidone iodine solution and infiltrated with 2% lidocaine (Astra Zeneca, Sao Paulo, Brazil);10 mg/Kg maximum dose. Ultrasound of the neck is performed with an 8 MHz Ultrasound Vascular Probe (Toshiba Nemio XG, Toshiba America Medical Systems, Inc. Tustin, CA) to assess vascular anatomy of the anterior neck, the distance between the skin and the trachea in the midline, as well as, to identify the thyroid isthmus, the cricoid cartilage, and 1st to 3rd tracheal rings (Figure 2). The endotracheal tube is pulled back under ultrasound guidance until the cuff is at the level of the thyroid cartilage, thus avoiding puncture of the cuff. The cricoid cartilage is palpated, and a 1.5 cm vertical incision is made immediately below that point. The subcutaneous tissue is bluntly dissected with hemostats until the pretracheal fascia is exposed. The trachea is punctured between the first and second, or the second and the third tracheal rings with a 14 G intravenous catheter needle (Jelco®; Medex, Carlsbad, CA) attached to a fluid filled 10 cc syringe, under ultrasound guidance. As soon as aspiration of air into the syringe is confirmed, the intravenous catheter is advanced into the trachea and the needle is removed. A flexible guidewire is gently passed through the intravenous catheter into the trachea; the catheter is removed afterwards (Figure 3). Ultrasound is once again used to verify endotracheal positioning of the guidewire. A threaded dilator (6 mm internal diameter) is advanced into the trachea, over the guidewire, for approximately 1 cm by clockwise rotation; minimal pressure is exerted on the anterior tracheal wall (Figure 4). The threaded dilator is removed by counter clockwise rotation after air escape through the lumen is detected. A self-retaining retractor forceps, with a limiter ridge, is passed over the guidewire into the trachea in locked position. The retractor is opened to enlarge the tracheal breach laterally, and to maintain the

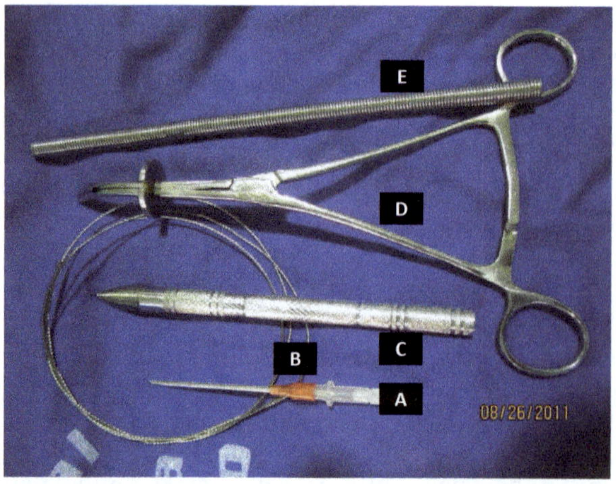

Figure 1 The instruments used for percutaneous tracheostomy. (A) The 14G intravenous catheter- Jelco®; (B) the guidewire; (C) the threaded tip dilator; (D) the self retaining retractor; (E) the spherical tip flexible introducer.

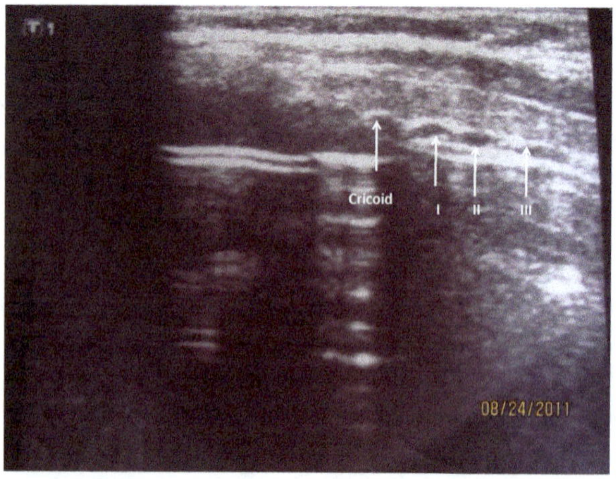

Figure 2 Ultrasound image of the trachea. Longitudinal view of the trachea shows the cricoid cartilage and the tracheal rings; important anatomical references to localize the site of puncture of the trachea. The endotracheal tube has been pulled back. I, II, III (first, second, and third tracheal rings); image obtained with an 8 MHz vascular probe.

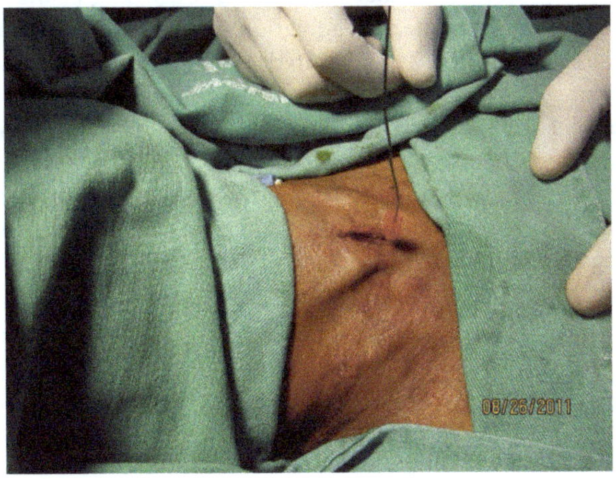

Figure 3 The guidewire in position. The guidewire is passed into the tracheal lumen through the 14 G intravenous catheter.

tracheal orifice open (Figure 5). A flexible, spherical tip introducer (6 mm internal diameter) is inserted into the airway under direct vision, facilitated by the retractor which is removed afterwards (Figure 6). A tracheostomy tube is placed inside the trachea passing over the guidewire and the flexible introducer (Figure 7). At this point the flexible introducer and the guidewire are removed, the cuff is inflated, and the patient is ventilated via the tracheostomy tube. The endotracheal tube is completely removed after adequate ventilation is confirmed by end-expiratory volume on the ventilator and auscultation of the patient. The tracheostomy cannula is secured in place with a neckband, and a chest radiograph is performed. Statistical analysis was performed using Graph Pad Prism (GraphPad Prism Software, Inc., San Diego, CA). Data are reported as the mean ± SEM and percentages.

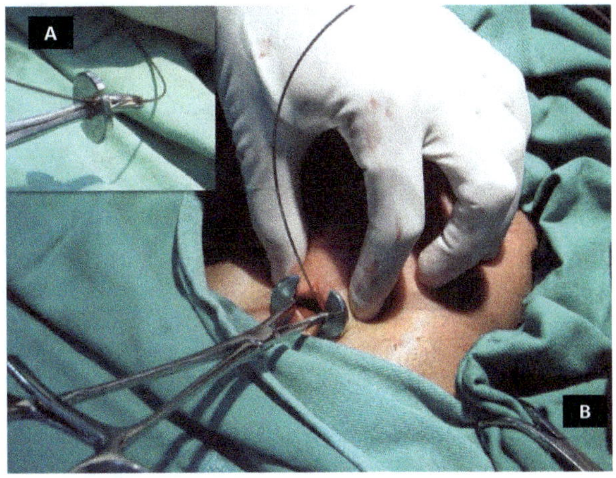

Figure 5 The self-retaining retractor. Insert (A) depicts how the self-retaining retractor is passed over the guidewire in locked position. Picture (B) shows how the retractor enables hands free lateral retraction of the pre-tracheal soft tissue, and the aperture on the anterior tracheal wall. The limiter ridge prevents insertion of the retractor too far into the trachea.

Results

During the study period, 100 patients underwent percutaneous tracheostomy by the modified technique described in this study. All percutaneous tracheostomies were performed on intubated patients at the bedside. Ninety patients (90%) underwent the procedure in the ICU. The remaining 10 patients were in another hospital location: 4 patients were in the hospital step-down unit, 3 in the trauma room, and 3 in the post-anesthesia

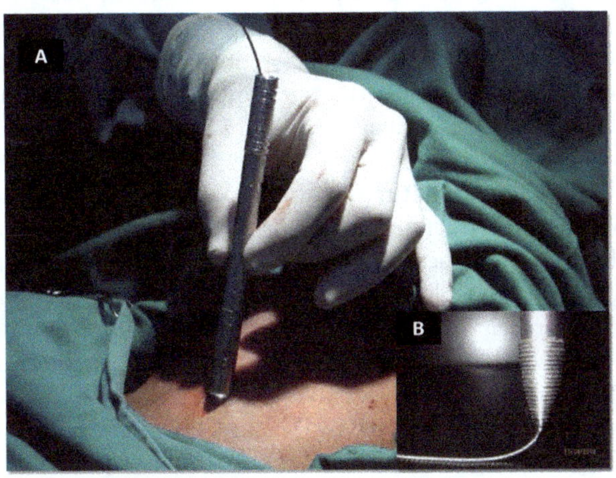

Figure 4 The threaded tip dilator. Picture (A) shows the threaded tip dilator in the incision. Insert (B) depicts how the guidewire, passing through the tip of the threaded dilator, prevents the threads from "catching" other structures.

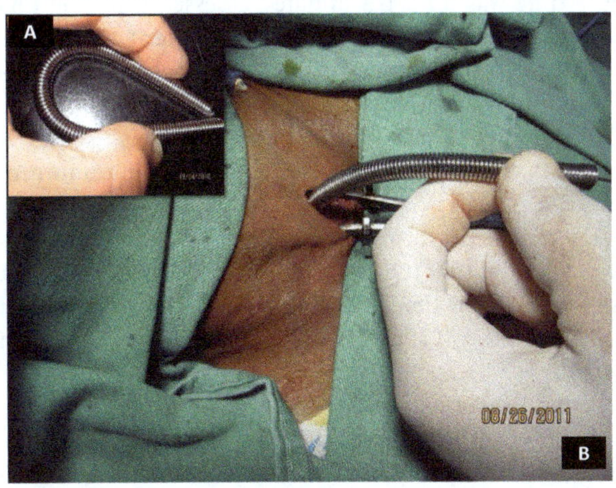

Figure 6 The spherical tip flexible introducer. Insert (A) depicts the elastic property of the introducer constructed with a circular helical spring. Picture (B) shows the flexible introducer positioned in the trachea facilitated by the self-retaining retractor.

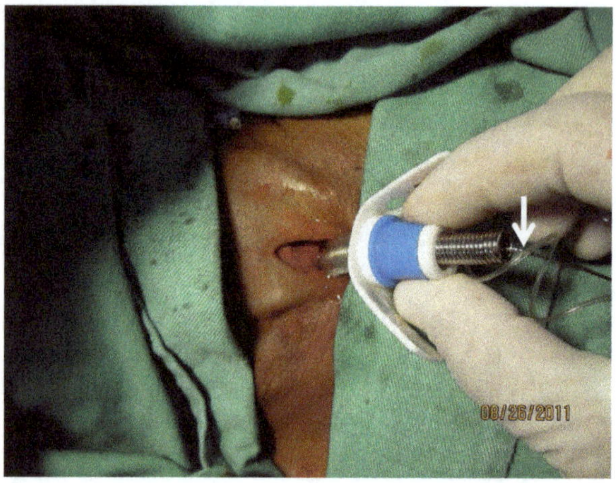

Figure 7 Insertion of the tracheostomy tube in the trachea. Picture shows the insertion of the tracheostomy tube in the trachea over the spherical tip flexible introducer. Arrow depicts the guidewire inside the introducer.

recovery room. Demographic data showed that the majority of the patients were men (68%) with a mean age of 49 ± 2.2 years. The mean BMI of the patients was 25.6 ± 2.1, and the thyromental distance was 6.2 ± 0.3 cm. The pretracheal tissue thickness was 1.5 ± 0.7 cm. Twenty five percent of the percutaneous tracheostomies were performed on trauma patients, and18% on acute care surgery non-trauma patients. The remaining patients were admitted to the hospital because of clinical (29%) or neurologic (28%) related diseases. The most common indication for percutaneous tracheostomy (95 patients) was the need for prolonged ventilatory support, with a mean intubation period of 9.5 ± 4.2 days. Five patients underwent the procedure because of severe maxillofacial trauma. Percutaneous tracheostomy procedure time was 5.1 ± 0.3 minutes, assessed from the time of skin incision to the time of placement of the tracheostomy tube inside the airway. A tracheostomy tube size 9.0 mm (internal diameter) was used in 70 patients (70%), a size 8.5 mm (internal diameter) was used in 20 patients, and a tube size 8.0 mm in the remaining patients.

The mean prothrombin time prior to the procedure was 80.9 ± 5.5% (Quick Value), the activated partial thromboplastin time was 30.6 ± 1.9 seconds, the mean INR was 1.2 ± 0.1, and platelet count was 216.3 ± 35.5 $x10^3$/uL.

Patients were followed for an average of 6.6 ± 2.2 days for complications. There were no inadvertent extubations, tracheostomy cannula misplacements and false passages, or oxygen desaturation below 95%, in the patients of the study. Furthermore, post-procedure chest radiograph showed no pneumothorax and no subcutaneous emphysema in the neck. There were two bleeding complications (2%) that resolved with dressing changes. Hemodialysis and anticoagulation shortly after the procedure could have contributed to the bleeding episode in one of the cases. There were no conversions to open surgical tracheostomy, and no deaths related to percutaneous tracheostomy in this study.

Bronchoscopy was performed in the first ten patients. In all cases, midline tracheal puncture, proper positioning of the thread tip dilator, as well as, integrity of the posterior wall of the tracheal were confirmed during the procedure.

Discussion

Percutaneous tracheostomy via the modified Seldinger technique was first described in 1969, and has gained several variants since then [2,5-17]. One of the main advantages of percutaneous tracheostomy is bedside performance, thus eliminating the expenses and logistics involved in operating room set-up usually required for open surgical tracheostomies. Furthermore, several investigators have reported shorter procedure times and lower complication rates with percutaneous tracheostomy compared to open surgical tracheostomy [4,11,14,15,18-22].

The percutaneous tracheostomy method described in this study combines technical principles common to other well consolidated techniques, particularly the Percu Twist™, and the Griggs-Portex® procedures; and to a lesser extent the Schachner method [2,4,5,7,10,23-25].

Our experience of 100 cases underscores three important features of the technical variation described herein. First is the capability to produce the initial breach on the trachea smoothly, with minimal compression, facilitated by the fine threads on the dilator. Additionally, the anterior tracheal wall is pulled away from the posterior wall as the dilator is threaded into the trachea, thus reducing posterior wall injury. Furthermore, passage of the guidewire through the tip of the dilator prevents the threads from "catching" the posterior wall, also reducing inadvertent injury (Figure 4).

The second feature is the capability to maintain hands-free retraction of the pre-tracheal soft tissue, and the tracheal aperture, with the self retaining retractor. The device enables controlled lateral dilation of the tracheal breach up to 2 cm maximum, thereby preventing excessive dilatation. Interestingly, a safety evaluation study in adult cadavers demonstrated that the mean force required to dilate the trachea 1.5 to 2 cm with a Griggs forceps, was two times that for therapeutic tracheal dilatation and three times the force required for tracheal disruption (31.6 N vs. 97.7 N), respectively [26]. The strategic location of the limiter ridge on the retractor (1.5 cm from the tip) is an additional safety feature to prevent insertion of the retractor too far into the trachea, and posterior wall injury.

The third feature relates to the flexible introducer which is constructed with a circular helical spring that confers elasticity, and enough rigidity to safely avoid false passage and tracheostomy tube misplacement. Tracheostomy tubes of 7 to 9.5 mm internal diameter can be passed over the introducer and placed inside the airway.

Even though the percutaneous tracheostomy procedure described in this study incorporates technical principles of at least two different methods the mean procedure time (5.1 minutes) was consistent with single dilator techniques reported by others [10,13,21,27].

Acute complications with the percutaneous tracheostomy method described by us were restricted to hemorrhage. The post-procedure bleeding rate of 2% in our study is comparable to other reports (1.6 - 4%) [3-5,10,11,15,18,19,23,24]. Even though comparison of the method described herein was not the purpose of this study, a contemporary analysis of 30 open surgical tracheostomies performed in our institution showed a 4% incidence of post-procedure bleeding, 50% of those cases required a surgical intervention to control the hemorrhage (unpublished data- Joao B. Rezende-Neto). On the contrary, none of the percutaneous tracheostomy patients who had a bleeding complication required a surgical intervention in the present study. Interestingly, prothrombin (Quick Value) time and INR were equivalent among the patients, respectively; 80.9 ± 5.5% in percutaneous tracheostomy vs. 87.2 ± 3.1% in open surgical tracheostomy patients (p = 0.27, Student's t-Test), and 1.2 ± 0.1 in percutaneous tracheostomy vs. 1.3 ± 0.15 in open surgical tracheostomy patients (p = 0.64, Student's t-Test). Furthermore, time to perform time to perform percutaneous tracheostomy was significantly shorter than that of open surgical tracheostomy (5.1 ± 0.3 minutes vs. 12.2 ± 1.4 minutes; $p < 0.001$, Student's t-Test)

Several studies highlight the importance of bronchoscopy to reduce complications during percutaneous tracheostomies, and most institutions routinely perform the procedure under bronchoscopic guidance [4,11,18,19,24,28-32]. Unfortunately, our institution did not have bronchoscopy routinely available during the study period.

Even though bronchoscopy is considered an important adjunct to percutaneous tracheostomy, that enables confirmation of midline puncture of the trachea, correct position of the guidewire and the tracheostomy tube, as well as, visualization of posterior tracheal wall injury, it is not without complications [4,31,33,34]. Studies have shown that bronchoscopy can cause hypoventilation that leads hypercarbia and respiratory acidosis during percutaneous tracheostomy [12,35,36]. Nonetheless, percutaneous tracheostomy without bronchoscopic guidance remains a controversial issue [4,12,19,29,31,34,37-40].

Investigators who forgo bronchoscopy during percutaneous tracheostomy usually implement additional measures to compensate for the lack of intraluminal visualization of the trachea [12,18,37-39,41-44]. For example, dissection of the subcutaneous tissue down to the pre-tracheal fascia prior to tracheal puncture, palpation of the trachea through the incision during endotracheal tube positioning and tracheal puncture, verification of free mobility of the guidewire throughout the procedure, and capnography assessed at the puncture site [12,18,37-39,41-44]. Additionally, ultrasound has become an increasingly used adjunct to percutaneous tracheostomy when bronchoscopy is not available, particularly in obese patients. Several studies have shown that sonography is helpful to delineate the anatomy of the neck prior to the procedure; particularly the thyroid gland, pre-tracheal vascular structures, the thyroid and cricoid cartilages, and the first three tracheal rings [18,24,45-48]. Real-time ultrasound guidance makes it possible to follow the needle path during tracheal puncture, and the final position of the tracheostomy tube [46,49-51]. Because of unavailability of bronchoscopy in our institution, real time ultrasound was the main adjunct to the percutaneous tracheostomy technique described in this study.

There are several limitations to this study. There is the possibility that the low complication rate with our technique could be linked to the favorable anatomic features of our patients, defined by a mean thyromental distance > 6 cm and a mean BMI of 25.6. Previous studies have shown that a short thyromental distance and a high BMI are useful predictors of difficult intubation and a challenging surgical airway [52-55]. Another point is the coagulation parameters of our patients. There is the possibility that the low incidence of bleeding complications with the technique would not have been obtained if patients with abnormal coagulation parameters were included in the study. Unfortunately we did not assess the patients for other risk factors, such as, pre-procedure positive end expiratory pressure > 10 cm H_2O or fraction of inspired oxygen > 50% [4]. Even though, the follow-up period in the study was sufficiently long for the determination of acute complications, it did not extend long enough for detection of long term complications, such as post-procedure tracheal stricture, associated with our method. That limitation is corroborated by previous reports that show late symptoms related to percutaneous tracheostomies in up to 20% of the patients followed for 39 months

[4,20,46,56]. Furthermore, only 10 patients in our study underwent bronchoscopic guided percutaneous tracheostomy, thus significantly limiting our capability to determine complications and the shortcomings of the technique. Even though the technique can be performed without bronchoscopic guidance, it should be used whenever available, particularly during the learning curve which is of approximately 20 patients for percutaneous dilatational tracheostomy [57]. Lastly, we did not compare our method to other percutaneous tracheostomy techniques; unfortunately, we do not have commercial tracheostomy kits readily available at our institution. Nonetheless, our results were in accordance with the data from other publications.

Conclusions

In our experience, percutaneous tracheostomy performed with the technical modification described in this study, is safe and simple to execute. However, long term follow-up for complications, is warranted. Additionally, reproducibility of results and a comparison to commercially available tracheostomy kits are required to further validate the method.

Abbreviations

ICU: Intensive Care Unit; BMI: Body Mass Index; and INR: International Normalized Ratio.

Acknowledgements

We thank Coordenacao de Aperfeicoamento de Pessoal de Nivel Superior (CAPES) - Brazil, and Fundacao de Amparo a Pesquisa do Estado de Minas Gerais - Brazil, for support in the decision to submit the manuscript for publication. We thank Emanuelle Savio - Trauma Case Manager, and the Respiratory Therapists of the Risoleta Tolentino Neves Hospital for their support.

Author details

[1]Universidade Federal de Minas Gerais and Risoleta Tolentino Neves Hospital, Brazil. [2]Risoleta Tolentino Neves Hospital, Brazil. [3]University of Toronto and Sunnybrook Hospital, Canada.

Authors' contributions

Conception of the technique, design of the study, acquisition and interpretation of data, and drafting of the manuscript (JBRN); acquisition and interpretation of data, and execution of bedside ultra-sound (AJO); acquisition and interpretation of data, and drafting of the manuscript (MPN); interpretation of data and drafting of the manuscript (FAB); drafting of the manuscript and revision for important intellectual content (SBR). All authors read and approved the final manuscript.

Authors' information

JBRN - Associate Professor Department of Surgery Universidade Federal de Minas Gerais, Brazil. Chief of Trauma and Acute Care Surgery Risoleta Tolentino Neves Hospital.

AJO - Intensivist Risoleta Tolentino Neves Hospital.

MPN - Trauma Surgeon Risoleta Tolentino Neves Hospital.

FAB - Assistant Professor of Internal Medicine Universidade Federal de Minas Gerais, Brazil. Chief of Critical Care Medicine Risoleta Tolentino Neves Hospital.

SBR - Associate Professor of Surgery and Critical Care Medicine University of Toronto and Sunnybrook Hospital, De Souza Trauma Research Chair.

Competing interests

The Universidade Federal de Minas Gerais (Dr. Joao B. Rezende-Neto) filed a patent application for the technique and the device described in this manuscript (Patent Pending Number 902833073 - INPI - Brazil). All other authors declare that they have no competing interests in relation to this manuscript.

References

1. Yu M: **Tracheostomy patients on the ward: multiple benefits from a multidisciplinary team.** *Critical Care* 2010, **14**:109.
2. Ciaglia P, Firsching R, Syniec C: **Elective percutaneous dilational tracheostomy: a new simple bedside procedure; preliminary report.** *Chest* 1985, **87**:715-719.
3. Petros S: **Percutaneous tracheostomy.** *Crit Care* 1999, **3**:R5-R10.
4. Kornblith LZ, Burlew CC, Moore EE, Haenel JB, Kashuk JL, Biffl WL, Barnett CC, Johnson JL: **One thousand bedside percutaneous tracheostomies in the surgical intensive care unit: time to change the gold standard.** *J Am Coll Surg* 2011, **2**:163-170.
5. Griggs WM, Worthley LIG, Gilligan JE, Thomas PD, Myburg JA: **A simple percutaneous tracheostomy technique.** *Surg Gynec Obstet* 1990, **170**:543-545.
6. Fantoni A, Ripamonti D: **A non-derivative, non-surgical tracheostomy: the trans-laryngeal method.** *Intensive Care Med* 1997, **23**:386-389.
7. Schachner A, Ovil Y, Sidi J, Rogev M, Heilbronn Y, Levy MJ: **Percutaneous tracheostomy - A new method.** *Crit Care Med* 1989, **17**:1052-1089.
8. Sheldon CH, Pudenz RH, Freshwater DB, Cure BL: **A new method for tracheostomy.** *J Neurosurg* 1995, **12**:428-431.
9. Toy FJ, Weinstein JD: **A percutaneous tracheostomy device.** *Surgery* 1969, **65**:384-389.
10. Westphal K, Maeser D, Scheifler G, Lischke V, Byhahn C: **PercuTwist: A new single-dilator technique for percutaneous tracheostomy.** *Anesth Analg* 2003, **96**:229-232.
11. Fernandez L, Norwood S, Roettger R, Gass D, Wilkins H: **Bedside percutaneous tracheostomy with bronchoscopic guidance in critically ill patients.** *Arch Surg* 1996, **131**:129-132.
12. Paran H, Butnaru G, Hass I, Afanasyv A, Gutman M: **Evaluation of a modified percutaneous tracheostomy technique without bronchoscopic guidance.** *Chest* 2004, **126**:868-871.
13. Sengupta N, Ang KL, Prakash D, George SJ: **Twenty months' routine use of a new percutaneous tracheostomy set using controlled rotation dilation.** *Anesth Analg* 2004, **99**:188-192.
14. Toye FJ, Weinstein JD: **Clinical experience with percutaneous tracheostomy and cricothyroidotomy in 100 trauma patients.** *J Trauma* 1986, **26**:1130-1140.
15. Bove MJ, Afifi MS: **Tracheotomy procedure.** In *Tracheostomies: the complete guide.* Edited by: Morris L, Afifi S. New York: Springer Publishing Company; 2010:17-40.
16. Toye FJ, Weinstein JD: **A percutaneous tracheostomy device.** *Surgery* 1969, **65**:384-389.
17. Ernest LW, Brink PRG: **The history of percutaneous tracheostomy.** *J Laryngol Otol* 1996, **110**:723-726.
18. Marx WH, Ciaglia P, Graniero KD: **Some important details in the technique of percutaneous dilatational tracheostomy via the modified Seldinger technique.** *Chest* 1996, **110**:762-766.
19. Marelli D, Paul A, Manolidis S, Walsh G, Odim JN, Burdon TA, Shennib H, Vestweber KH, Fleiszer DM, Mulder DS: **Endoscopic guided percutaneous tracheostomy: early results and consecutive trial.** *J Trauma* 1990, **30**:433-435.
20. van Heurn LW, Goei R, Ploeg I, Ramsay G, Brink PR: **Late complications of percutaneous dilatational tracheostomy.** *Chest* 1996, **110**:1572-1576.
21. Kost KM: **Percutaneous tracheostomy: comparison of Ciaglia and Griggs techniques.** *Crit Care* 2000, **4**:143-146.
22. Delaney A, Bagshaw SM, Nalos M: **Percutaneous dilatational tracheostomy surgical tracheostomy in critically ill patients: a systematic review and meta-analysis.** *Crit Care* 2006, **10**:R55.
23. Friedman Y, Mayer AD: **Bedside percutaneous tracheostomies in critically ill patients.** *Chest* 1993, **104**:532-535.

24. Hill BB, Zweng TN, Maley RH, Charash WE, Tourasarkissian B, Kearney PA: **Percutaneous dilational tracheostomy: report of 356 cases.** *J Trauma* 1996, **40**:238-243.
25. Brambrink A: **Percutaneous dilatation tracheostomy: which technique is the best for the critically ill patient, and how can we gather further scientific evidence?** *Crit Care* 2004, **8**:319-321.
26. Watters M, Thorne G, Cox C, Monk C: **Tracheal trauma from percutaneous tracheostomy using the Griggs method.** *Anaesthesia* 2002, **57**:249-252.
27. Montcriol A, Bordes J, Asencio Y, Prunet B, Lacroix G, Meaudre E: **Bedside percutaenous tracheostomy: a prospective randomised comparison of PercuTwist versus Griggs' forceps dilational tracheostomy.** *Anaesth Intensive Care* 2011, **39**:209-216.
28. Sarkar S, Kelly A, Townsend R: **Survey of percutaneous tracheostomy practice in UK intensive care units.** *JICS* 2009, **10**:138-140.
29. Hinerman R, Alvarez F, Keller CA: **Outcome of bedside percutaneous tracheostomy with bronchoscopic guidance.** *Intensive Care Med* 2000, **26**:1850-1856.
30. Kluge S, Baumann HJ, Maier C, Klose H, Meyer A, Nierhaus A, Kreymann G: **Tracheostomy in the intensive care unit: A nationwide survey.** *Anesth Analg* 2008, **107**:1639-1643.
31. Barba CA, Angood PB, Kauder DR, Latenser B, Martin K, McGonigal MD, Phillips GR, Rotondo MF, Schwab W: **Bronchoscopic guidance makes percutaneous tracheostomy a safe, cost-effective, and easy-to-teach procedure.** *Surgery* 1995, **118**:879-883.
32. Fikkers BG, van Veen JA, Kooloos JG, Pickkers P, van den Hoogan FJA, Hillen B, van der Hoeven JG: **Emphysema and pneumothorax after percutaneous tracheostomy: Case reports and an anatomic study.** *Chest* 2004, **125**:1805-1814.
33. Trottier SJ, Hazard PB, Sakabu SA, Levine JH, Troop BR, Thompson JA, McNary R: **Posterior tracheal wall perforation during percutaneous dilatational tracheostomy: An investigation into its mechanism and prevention.** *Chest* 1999, **115**:1383-1389.
34. Reilly PM, Shapiro MB, Malcynski JT: **Percutaneous dilatational tracheostomy under the microscope: justification for intra-procedural bronchoscopy?** *Intensive Care Med* 1999, **25**:3-4.
35. Reilly PM, Anderson HL III, Sing RF, Schwab W, Bartlett RH: **Occult hypercarbia: An unrecognized phenomenon during percutaneous endoscopic tracheostomy.** *Chest* 1995, **107**:760-763.
36. Reilly PM, Sing RF, Giberson FA, Anderson HL III, Rotondo MF, Tinkoff GH, Schwab CW: **Hypercarbia during tracheostomy: a comparison of percutaneous endoscopic, percutaneous Doppler, and standard surgical tracheostomy.** *Intensive Care Med* 1997, **23**:858-864.
37. Ahmed R, Rady SR, Siddique JIM, Iqbal M: **Percutaneous tracheostomy in critically ill patients: 24 months experience at a tertiary care hospital in the United Arab Emirates.** *Ann Thorac Med* 2010, **5**:26-29.
38. Veenith T, Ganeshamoorthy S, Standley T, Carter J, Young P: **Intensive care unit tracheostomy: a snapshot of UK practice.** *Int Arch Med* 2008, **1**:21-27.
39. Park SS, Goldenberg D: **Percutaneous tracheostomy: Griggs technique.** *Operative Techniques in Otolaryngology* 2007, **18**:95-98.
40. Grundling M, Pavlovic D, Kuhn SO, Feyerherd F: **Is the method of modified percutaneous tracheostomy without bronchoscopic guidance really simple and safe?** *Chest* 2005, **128**:3774-3775.
41. Dawood AA, Haddad S, Arabi Y, Dabbagh O, Cook DJ: **The safety of percutaneous tracheostomy in patients with coagulopathy of thrombocytopenia.** *MEJ Anesth* 2007, **19**:37-50.
42. Maddalli M, Pratap M, Fahr J, Zarroug AW: **Percutaneous tracheostomy by guidewire dilating forceps technique: is bronchoscopic guidance mandatory?** *Middle East J Anesthesiol* 2002, **16**:509-519.
43. Mallick A, Venkatanath D, Elliot SC, Hollins T, Kumar CGN: **A prospective randomised controlled trail of capnography vs. bronchoscopy for Blue Rhino™ percutaneous tracheostomy.** *Anaesthesia* 2003, **58**:864-868.
44. Atweh NA, Possenti PP, Caushaj PF, Burns G, Pineau MJ, Ivy M: **Dilatational percutaneous tracheostomy: Modification of technique.** *J Trauma* 1999, **47**:142-144.
45. Sustic A, Kovac D, Zgaljardic Z, Zupan Z, Krstulovic B: **Ultrasound-guided percutaneous dilatational tracheostomy: A safe method to avoid cranial misplacement of the tracheostomy tube.** *Intensive Care Med* 2000, **26**:1379-1381.
46. Kollig E, Heydenreich U, Roetman B, Hopf F, Muhr G: **Ultrasound and bronchoscopic controlled percutaneous tracheostomy on trauma ICU.** *Injury* 2000, **31**:663-668.
47. Hatfield A, Bodenham A: **Portable ultrasound scanning of the anterior neck before percutaneous dilatational tracheostomy.** *Anesthesia* 1999, **54**:660-663.
48. Brueggeney MK, Greif R, Ross S, Eichenberger U, Moriggl B, Arnold A, Luyet C: **Ultrasound-guided percutaneous tracheal puncture: A computer-tomographic controlled study in cadavers.** *Br J Anaesth* 2011, **106**:738-742.
49. Rajajee V, Fletcher JJ, Rochlen LR, Jacobs TL: **Real-time ultrasound-guided dilatational percutaneous tracheostomy: a feasibility study.** *Crit Care* 2011, **15**:R67.
50. Sustic A: **Role of ultrasound in the airway management of critically ill patients.** *Crit Care Med* 2007, **35(Suppl 5)**:137-177.
51. Szeto C, Kost K, Hanley JA, Roy A, Christou N: **A simple method to predict pretracheal tissue thickness to prevent accidental decannulation in the obese.** *Otolaryngol Head Neck Surg* 2010, **143**:223-229.
52. Baker PA, Depuydt A, Thompson JM: **Thyromental distance measurement: Fingers don't rule.** *Anaesthesia* 2009, **64**:878-882.
53. Aldawood AS, Arabi YM, Haddad S: **Safety of percutaneous tracheostomy in obese critically ill patients: A prospective cohort study.** *Anaesth Intensive Care* 2008, **36**:69-73.
54. Kim WH, Ahn HJ, Lee CJ, Shin BS, Ko JS, Choi SJ, Ryu SA: **Neck circumference to thyromental distance ratio: A new predictor of difficult intubation in obese patients.** *Br J Anaesth* 2011, **106**:743-748.
55. Connor CW, Segal S: **Accurate classification of difficult intubation by computerized facial analysis.** *Anesth Analg* 2011, **112**:84-93.
56. Rosenbower TJ, Morris JA Jr, Eddy VA, Ries WR: **The long term complications of percutaneous dilatational tracheostomy.** *Am Surg* 1998, **64**:82-86.
57. Massick DD, Powell DM, Price PD, Chang SL, Squires G, Forrest LA, Young DC: **Quantification of the learning curve for percutaneous dilatational tracheostomy.** *Laryngoscope* 2000, **110**:222-228.

12

Acute appendicitis: proposal of a new comprehensive grading system based on clinical, imaging and laparoscopic findings

Carlos Augusto Gomes[1*], Massimo Sartelli[2], Salomone Di Saverio[3], Luca Ansaloni[4], Fausto Catena[5], Federico Coccolini[4], Kenji Inaba[6], Demetrios Demetriades[6,7], Felipe Couto Gomes[8] and Camila Couto Gomes[9]

Abstract

Advances in the technology and improved access to imaging modalities such as Computed Tomography and laparoscopy have changed the contemporary diagnostic and management of acute appendicitis. Complicated appendicitis (phlegmon, abscess and/ or diffuse peritonitis), is now reliably distinguished from uncomplicated cases. Therefore, a new comprehensive grading system for acute appendicitis is necessary. The goal is review and update the laparoscopic grading system of acute appendicitis and to provide a new standardized classification system to allow more uniform patient stratification. During the last World Society of Emergency Surgery Congress in Israel (July, 2015), a panel involving Acute Appendicitis Experts and the author's discussed many current aspects about the acute appendicitis between then, it will be submitted a new comprehensive disease grading system. It was idealized based on three aspect of the disease (clinical and imaging presentation and laparoscopic findings). The new grading system may provide a standardized system to allow more uniform patient stratification for appendicitis research. In addition, may aid in determining optimal management according to grade. Lastly, what we want is to draw a multicenter observational study within the World Society of Emergency Surgery (WSES) based on this design.

Keywords: Appendicitis, Appendectomy, Laparoscopy, Treatment, Classification

Background

Appendicitis is the most common cause of an acute surgical abdomen, with an estimated lifetime prevalence of 7–8 %. Despite advances in diagnosis and treatment, it is still associated with significant morbidity (10 %) and mortality (1–5 %) [1]. The clinical history and physical examination represent the most important tools for early diagnosis of the disease. The overall accuracy for diagnosing acute appendicitis is approximately 90 %, with a false-negative appendectomy rate of 10 %. This is more frequent in atypical cases, especially in women of childbearing age, because the symptoms often overlap with others conditions [2, 3]. Recently 182 patients with suspicion of acute appendicitis were stratified to low, intermediate, and high probability of appendicitis by two different clinical scores (AIR / Alvarado) and by an experienced surgeon. The AIR score was especially good at identifying patients with high probability of appendicitis with a specificity of 0.97 for all appendicitis and 0.92 for advanced appendicitis, compared with 0.91 and 0.77, respectively, for the surgeon and Alvarado score. Therefore, in this series, the AIR score had both higher sensitivity and specificity than the Alvarado score and the experienced surgeon in the clinical diagnosis of the disease [4].

Imaging

The clinical scores represent an excellent and useful tool for pre-operative diagnosis of acute appendicitis, but regardless its accuracy it cannot be applied as a grading system for acute appendicitis, especially attempting to distinguish different complicated grades of the disease [5]. As we know, novel scoring systems are being described and introduced into clinical practice, based on clinical and imaging (CT and/or US). In addition, less

* Correspondence: caxiaogomes@gmail.com
[1]Surgery Department, Therezinha de Jesus University Hospital, Medical and Health Science School, Surgery Unit, Federal University of Juiz de Fora (UFJF), Rua Senador Salgado Filho 510 / 1002, Bairro Bom Pastor, Juiz de Fora, Minas Gerais 36021-660, Brasil
Full list of author information is available at the end of the article

invasive management options including percutaneous drainage, non-operative treatment and minimally invasive surgery are available [6].

Three imaging modalities are available in difficult cases of acute appendicitis: Ultrasound (US), Computed Tomography (CT), and Magnetic Resonance Imaging (MRI). Trans-abdominal ultrasound should be the first-line imaging test. Although there is a higher radiation burden, abdominal CT is superior to US and may be required in patients with an equivocal US or if perforation is suspected. Low-dose unenhanced CT is equivalent to standard-dose CT with intravenous contrast agents in the detection of the five signs of acute appendicitis (thickened appendiceal wall greater than 2 mm, cross-sectional diameter greater than 6 mm, increased pericolic fat density, abscess, and appendicolith) [7]. However, as pointed out by Saar, despite all available technologies, it remains very difficult to achieve a false negative appendectomy rates less than 10 % [8].

Operative versus non-operative treatment

Both open appendectomy and laparoscopic appendectomy are acceptable techniques and can be used interchangeably. The laparoscopic treatment of uncomplicated grades of acute appendicitis is well established and represent the approach of first choice some time ago. However, well-conducted trials to help guide the treatment for all complicated grades of acute appendicitis are limited, especially by the presence of bias and methodological flaws. However, the safety and efficacy of laparoscopy in the treatment of these cases is well established too [9–13].

A recent meta-analysis by Varadhan et al. 2015 [14] assessed four randomized controlled trials about safety and efficacy of antibiotics compared with appendectomy for treatment of uncomplicated acute appendicitis [15–18]. The primary outcome measure was the incidence of complications and secondary outcome was the efficacy of treatment. 900 patients (470 antibiotic treatment, 430 appendectomy) met the inclusion criteria. Antibiotic treatment was associated with a 63 % (277/438) success rate at 1 year. Meta-analysis of complications showed a relative risk reduction of 31 % for antibiotic treatment compared with appendectomy. The authors concluded that antibiotics are both effective and safe as primary treatment for patients with uncomplicated acute appendicitis. Initial antibiotic treatment deserves consideration as a primary treatment option for early-uncomplicated appendicitis.

Similarly, the study NOTA (Non Operative Treatment for Acute Appendicitis), assessed the safety and efficacy of antibiotic treatment for suspected acute uncomplicated appendicitis and monitored the long-term follow-up of non-operated patients. One hundred fifty-nine patients with suspected appendicitis were enrolled and underwent non-operative management with amoxicillin / clavulanate. The follow-up period was 2 years. Short-term (7 days) non-operative failure rate was 11.9 %. All patients with initial failures were operated within 7 days. At 15 days, no recurrences were recorded. After 2 years, the overall recurrence rate was 13.8 %. The authors concluded that antibiotics for suspected acute appendicitis are safe and effective and may avoid unnecessary appendectomy, reducing operation rate, surgical risks, and overall costs [19].

Although interesting and reducing the false negative appendectomy rate, both studies also contain methodological flaws, like the patients recruitment, surgery approach (laparotomy/laparoscopy), different antibiotics prescription and images diagnostic method criteria (CT scan / Ultrasound). In addition, the success rate of 63 % is very low and the relative risk of complication reduction very high. Therefore, the laparoscopic treatment of non-complicated acute appendicitis may show much less complication rates and represent the treatment of choice with acceptable false negative appendectomy rate about 10 % [11, 20].

Histologic diagnosis

As a rule, the acute appendicitis diagnosis was established according to the transmural appendix inflammation (neutrophilic infiltration of the mucosa, submucosa, and *muscularis propria*). The histologic assessment also defined the difference between endoappendicitis (neutrophils within mucosa and mucosal ulceration) and periappendicitis (inflammation restricted to serosa and sub-serosa) [21].

Why to propose a new acute appendicitis grading system?

The laparoscopic grading system of acute appendicitis proposed by Gomes et al. [20] is limited by its exclusive focus on just the intraoperative aspects (Table 1). Complicated grades (phlegmon, abscess and/or diffuse peritonitis), are now reliably distinguished from uncomplicated cases by clinical and imaging findings. Because the treatment options for these complicated cases of acute appendicitis includes non-operative modalities, a new comprehensive grading system for acute appendicitis is necessary (Table 2).

It was idealized a grading system for acute appendicitis that incorporates clinical presentation, imaging and laparoscopic findings. The goal of this new grading system is to provide a standardized classification to allow more uniform patient stratification for appendicitis research and to aid in determining optimal management according to grade (Table 2).

New acute appendicitis grading system

Grades

Grade- 0 (normal looking)

The grade 0 refers to the non-rare situation surgeon may faces, when the patient has a clinical diagnosis of acute appendicitis and laparoscopy shows a macroscopically

Table 1 Laparoscopic grading system of acute appendicitis

Grade	Laparoscopic findings
Grade 0	Normal looking appendix
Grade 1	Hyperemia and edema
Grade 2	Fibrinous exudate
Grade 3A	Segmental necrosis
Grade 3B	Base necrosis
Grade 4A	Abscess
Grade 4B	Regional Peritonitis
Grade 5	Difuse Peritonitis

Note: From Gomes et al. 2012 [13]

"normal looking appendix". In such case, if the appendix looks normal on laparoscopy but another disease is found to be the cause of the patient's symptom, then the appendix should be left in situ [22]. The 10-year follow-up by van Dalen et al. [23], demonstrated the safety of this approach in women. The situation is more complicated when the appendix shows no signs of inflammation and no other disease can be found (Fig. 1). Weighting the disadvantages of a negative appendectomy against the risk of overestimating a case of appendicitis is difficult. If symptoms and signs are typical for appendicitis, most surgeons still consider advised to perform an appendectomy, because in early appendicitis, the inflammation may be limited to intramural layers [11].

In surgical cases of pelvic endometriosis, surgeons need to preoperatively inform that appendix is found frequently involved, regardless the presence of concurrent symptoms or gross finding of the appendix. Furthermore, surgeons should take into account the possibility of performing an incidental appendectomy [24].

Table 2 Proposal of a new grading system of acute appendicitis based on clinical, imaging and laparoscopic findings (2015)

Non-Complicated Acute Appendicitis	
Grade 0 - Normal Looking Appendix (Endoappendicitis/Periappendicitis).	
Grade 1 - Inflamed Appendix (Hyperemia, edema ± fibrin without or little pericolic fluid).	
Complicated Acute Appendicitis	
Grade 2 – Necrosis	A - Segmental Necrosis. (without or little pericolic fluid).
	B - Base Necrosis. (without or little pericolic fluid).
Grade 3 - Inflammatory Tumor-	A Flegmom.
	B - Abscess less 5 cm without peritoneal free air.
	C - Abscess above 5 cm without peritoneal free air.
Grade 4 - Perforated - Diffuse Peritonitis with or without peritoneal free air.	

Note: Proposal for a new acute appendicitis grading system based on clinical, imaging and laparoscopic findings. (±) = Presence or absence of fibrinous exudate Gomes et al. (2015).

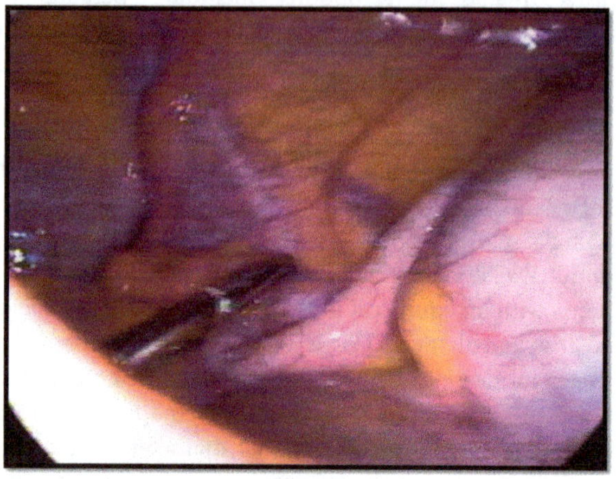

Fig. 1 "Normal looking appendix" without any other intra-abdominal disease and suggestive clinical set. The appendix was removed and the histopathological study shows intraluminal inflammation (Grade 0)

Grade-1 (inflamed)

Gomes et al. in 2012, published a series of 186 patients who underwent a laparoscopic appendectomy, according to the Laparoscopic Grading System for Acute Appendicitis (Table 1). This grading system has been developed to stratify the disease according to the inflammatory findings occurring within the appendix and the abdominal cavity. The impact of the grade on surgical site infection was also examined [20]. This score was externally validated in a cohort of 112 consecutive cases of complicated acute appendicitis patients by Di Saverio et al, where all patients had Gomes scores II–V and the scores were correlated with the outcomes [25]. Based on this series the safety and efficacy of laparoscopy compared to open appendectomy was also examined. The laparoscopic grading system was useful in stratify the disease; contributing and highlights some aspects, whose laparotomy could not be able to show at the same amplitude (Fig. 2) [20].

In addition, Gomes et al. documented an unusual situation. About 10 % of the patients where appendix presented with hyperemia, edema and fibrin exudates had a significant plasma exudation into the abdominal cavity. The study of the exudates diagnosed the presence of gram-negative bacteria in 10 % of the analyzed samples. These data could explain, at least partially, that acute appendicitis may get complicated with development of postoperative peritonitis and intra-abdominal abscesses after simple appendectomies, especially when antimicrobial prophylaxis was not administrated. Excessive plasma exudation in the absence of necrosis and/or perforation of resected appendices could be explained by bacterial translocation and plasma transudation [20].

Grade- 2A and 2B (necrosis)

Complicated appendicitis refers to gangrenous and/or perforated appendix, which may lead to abscess formation

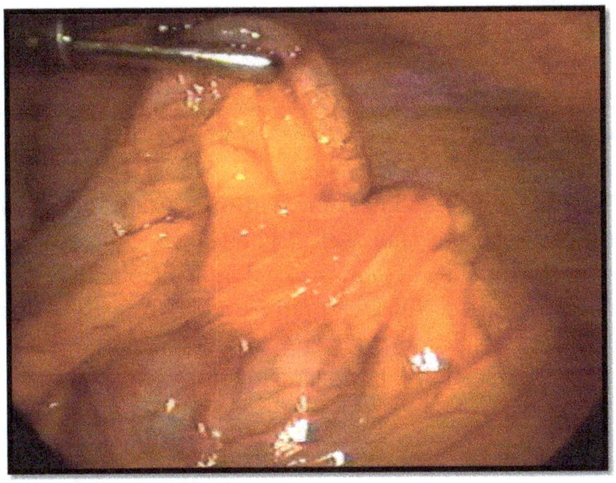

Fig. 2 The image shows hyperemia and edema of appendix, without fibrinous exudate (Grade-1)

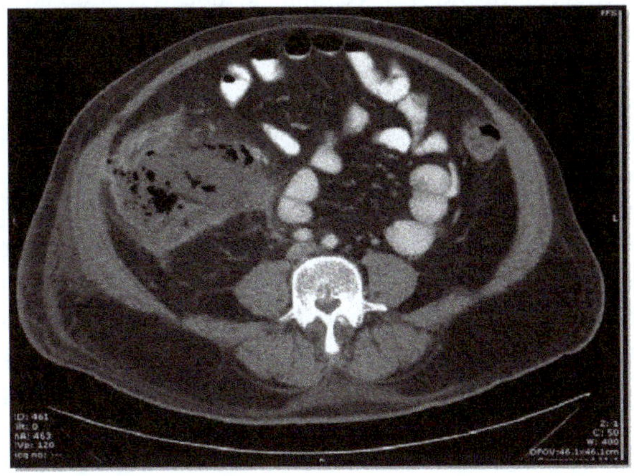

Fig. 4 The CT scan of abdomen showing an inflammatory tumor in the lower right quadrant. The patient was managed with antibiotics only; i. e non-operative treatment. (Grade 3A)

and degrees of peritonitis [26]. Therefore, these grades by definition are complicated cases of acute appendicitis. Nevertheless, the specific grade study, showed that in the grade 2A, the necrosis was an isolated phenomenon, restricted to the appendix, without or with minimal local exudation (Fig. 3). The majority of patients had an uneventful recovery and were discharged in the next post-operative day. More importantly, they had a clinical course similar to those with non-complicated appendicitis (grade 0, 1). They received short course antimicrobial therapy (3 to 5 days) and post-operative complication was a rare event. By the way, recent observational cohort study from van Rossem et al. showed that after appendectomy for complicated appendicitis, 3 days of antibiotic treatment is equally effective as 5 days in reducing postoperative infections [27].

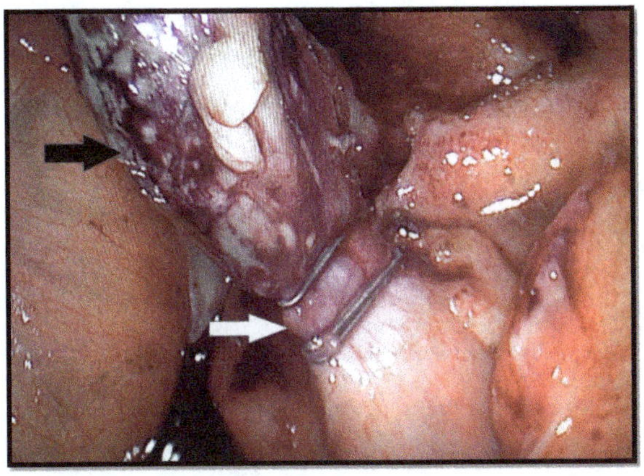

Fig. 3 Acute appendicitis with segmental necrosis (*black arrow*). Observe that the appendiceal base was not compromised by inflammatory and necrotic process, allowing appendicular stump closure by metallic clip (*white arrow*) In a healthy tissue (Grade 2A)

About 3.2 % there was presence of necrosis involving the appendicular base, at the level of its insertion on cecal wall (grade 2B). This condition makes the operation even more difficult and requires experience from the surgical team with intra-corporeal suturing, mainly when endostapler is not routinely used, justifying a new specific grade, which is rarely studied during laparoscopic appendectomy. Nowadays, this grade represents the most important situation, where the endostapler is used to closure the appendiceal stump in the Service. In the other grades the appendicular stump could be closure of different ways (endostapler, endoloop, metallic and polymeric clip and others one). We prefer its management by T-400 metallic endoclip, which is less expensive and have demonstrated safety and effectiveness in a prospective observational study [20]. In addition, it is oriented operating the patients under Day Hospital way. The study of Alvarez and Voitk [28], should be highlighted because, according the authors, in the ambulatory management of acute appendicitis (Day Hospital), the patients discharge is occurring less than 24 h after

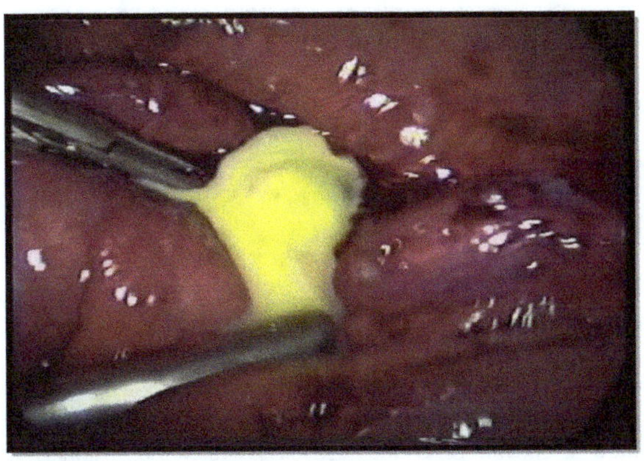

Fig. 5 Acute appendicitis complicated with inflammatory tumor and an abscess less than 5 cm, managed by laparoscopic approach (Grade 3B)

appendectomy and this recommendation was adopted for grades 0,1, 2 [28].

Grade- 3A - 3B - 3C (perforated - inflammatory tumor)

As it is already well known, sometimes the inflammation of the appendix may be enclosed by the patient's own defense mechanisms, by the formation of an inflammatory phlegmon or a circumscribed abscess of different diameter, often presenting some days after the onset of symptoms [29]. In fact, an inflammatory tumor in the right lower quadrant represents a spectrum, at least of three physiopathology stages of the acute appendicitis, very similar to what happens in the acute diverticulitis of sigmoid colon: phlegmon, inflammatory tumor with <5-cm abscesses and inflammatory tumor >5-cm abscess (Fig. 4). Thus, once again, such patients should not be considered as a whole, without distinction, since they have different aspects with regard to, physiopathology, treatment, complications, disease recurrence and prognosis. Moreover, according to Stefanidis et al 2008, acute abdominal pain lasting less than 7 days [30]. Therefore, assuming that we are evaluating patients with acute and subacute disease, since mostly patients classified within these grades, had the onset of symptoms occurring into seven or more days. These patients receive long course (5–10 days) antimicrobial therapy according their clinical post-operative recovery (Fig. 5).

Grade- 4 (perforate - diffuse peritonitis)

Controversy exists regarding the laparoscopic approach in the treatment of acute appendicitis complicated with diffuse peritonitis. The chance of potential surgical complications is high and consequently the outcomes are poorly documented. Our literature review found only two articles investigating the issue [31, 32]. Although the results seems to favor the use of laparoscopy, only a large multi-institutional study with appropriate design will be able to answer this question (Fig. 6).

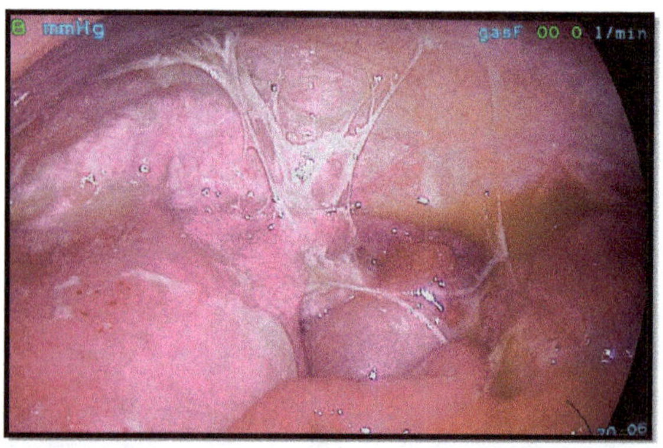

Fig. 6 Patient with perforated appendicitis and diffuse peritonitis operated on laparoscopy. He had an uneventful recovery in the postoperative day six. (Grade 4)

Summary

In summary, the new appendicitis grading system is based on three aspects of the disease. The clinical, imaging and laparoscopic findings and could be tested in multicenter observational study within the World Society of Emergency Surgery, in order to assess its actual practicality. It will enable the creation of homogeneous groups of patients with disease in the same well-defined stage. Ultimately, the goal of this grading system is to aid in determining optimal management according to grade, and to provide a standardized classification system to allow more uniform patient stratification for appendicitis research.

Competing interests

The authors have no conflicts of interest ties or financial funding source' to disclose.

Authors' contributions

CAG, MS, SDS: conception design and coordination and helped to draft the manuscript, acquisition of data, analysis and interpretation of data, entire manuscript reviewer. FC, FC, LA: Participated in the sequence alignment and revising it critically for important intellectual content; KI, DD: Participated in the sequence alignment, design and revising it critically for important intellectual content; FCG, CCG: have made substantial contributions in the graphic art and contribution in the manuscript conception and revision. All authors read and approved the final manuscript.

Acknowledgements

Manuscript produced at Surgery and Internal Medicine Unit. Monte Sinai Hospital, Juiz de Fora, Minas Gerais, Brazil.
*Presented in part at last World Society of Emergency Surgery (WSES) Congress, 2015 in Jerusalem - Israel.

Author details

[1]Surgery Department, Therezinha de Jesus University Hospital, Medical and Health Science School, Surgery Unit, Federal University of Juiz de Fora (UFJF), Rua Senador Salgado Filho 510 / 1002, Bairro Bom Pastor, Juiz de Fora, Minas Gerais 36021-660, Brasil. [2]Department of Surgery, Macerata Hospital, Macerata, Italy. [3]Trauma Surgery Unit, Maggiore Hospital, Bologna, Italy. [4]General Surgery I, Papa Giovanni XXIII Hospital, Bergamo, Italy. [5]Emergency Surgery Department, Maggiore Parma Hospital, Parma, Italy. [6]University of California, San Francisco, USA. [7]Department of Surgery (K.I.), Keck School of Medicine of University of Southern California, Los Angeles, CA, USA. [8]Internal Medicine Departament, Therezinha de Jesus University Hospital, Medical and Health Science School, Juiz de Fora, Brazil. [9]Internal Medicine Departament, Monte Sinai Hospital, Juiz de Fora, Minas Gerais, Brazil.

References

1. Prystowsky JB, Pugh CM, Nagle AP. Current problems in surgery. Appendicitis. Curr Probl Surg. 2005;42(10):688–742.
2. Andersson RE, Hugander A, Ravn H, Offenbartl K, Ghazil SH, Nyströn PO. Repeated clinical and laboratory examinations in patients with an equivocal diagnosis of appendicitis. World J Surg. 2000;24:479–85.
3. Birnbaun BA, Wilson SR. Appendicitis at the millennium. Radiology. 2000; 215:337–48.
4. Andersson RE. The magic of an appendicitis score. World J Surg. 2015; 39(1):110–1.
5. Atema JJ, van Rossem CC, Leeuwenburgh MM, Stoker J, Boermeester MA. Scoring system to distinguish uncomplicated from complicated acute appendicitis. Br J Surg. 2015;102:979–90 [Epub ahead of print].
6. Sartelli M, Moore FA, Ansaloni L, Di Saverio S, Coccolini F, Griffiths EA, et al. A proposal for a CT driven classification of left colon acute diverticulitis. World J Emerg Surg. 2015;10:3. Introduzido.

7. Karul M, Berliner C, Keller S, Tsui TY, Yamamura J. Imaging of appendicitis in adults. Röfo. 2014;186(6):551–8. Epub 2014 Apr 23.
8. Sarr M. Repeated clinical and laboratory examinations in patients with an equivocal diagnosis of appendicitis. World J Surg. 2000;(2):485. [Invited commented].
9. Korndorffer Jr JR, Fellinger E, Reed W. SAGES guideline for laparoscopic appendectomy. Surg Endosc. 2010;24(4):757–61.
10. Paterson HM, Qadan M, de Luca SM, Nixon SJ, Paterson- Brown S. Changing trends in surgery for acute appendicitis. Br J Surg. 2008;95(3):363–68.
11. Sauerland S, Agresta F, Bergamaschi R, Borzellino G, Budzynski A, Champault G, et al. Laparoscopy for abdominal emergencies: evidence-based guidelines of the European Association for Endoscopic Surgery. Surg Endosc. 2006;20(1):14–29.
12. Schick KS, Hüttl TP, Fertmann JM, Hornung HM, Jauch KW, Hoffmann JN. A critical analysis of laparoscopic appendectomy: how experience with 1,400 appendectomies allowed innovative treatment to become standard in a university hospital. World J Surg. 2008;32(7):1406–13.
13. Taguchi Y, Komatsu S, Sakamoto E, Norimizu S, Shingu Y, Hasegawa H. Laparoscopic versus open surgery for complicated appendicitis in adults: a randomized controlled trial. Surg Endosc. 2015 Aug 15. [Epub ahead of print]
14. Varadhan KK, Neal KR, Lobo DN. Safety and efficacy of antibiotics compared with appendicectomy for treatment of uncomplicated acute appendicitis: meta-analysis of randomized controlled trials. BMJ. 2012;344(5):e2156.
15. Hansson J, Korner U, Khorram-Manesh A, Solberg A, Lundholm K. Randomized clinical trial of antibiotic therapy versus appendicectomy as primary treatment of acute appendicitis in unselected patients. Br J Surg. 2009;96:473–81.
16. Vons C, Barry C, Maitre S, Pautrat K, Leconte M, Costaglioli B, et al. Amoxicillin plus clavulanic acid versus appendicectomy for treatment of acute uncomplicated appendicitis: an open-label, non-inferiority, randomised controlled trial. Lancet. 2011;377:1573–9.
17. Styrud J, Eriksson S, Nilsson I, Ahlberg G, Haapaniemi S, Neovius G, et al. Appendectomy versus antibiotic treatment in acute appendicitis. a prospective multicenter randomized controlled trial. World J Surg. 2006;30:1033–7.
18. Eriksson S, Granstrom L. Randomized controlled trial of appendicectomy versus antibiotic therapy for acute appendicitis. Br J Surg. 1995;82:166–69.
19. Di Saverio S, Sibilio A, Giorgini E, Biscardi A, Villani S, Coccolini F, et al. The NOTA Study (Non Operative Treatment for Acute Appendicitis): prospective study on the efficacy and safety of antibiotics (amoxicillin and clavulanic acid) for treating patients with right lower quadrant abdominal pain and long-term follow-up of conservatively treated suspected appendicitis. Ann Surg. 2014;260(1):109–17.
20. Gomes CA, Nunes TA, Fonseca Chebli JM, Junior CS, Gomes CC. Laparoscopy grading system of acute appendicitis: new insight for future trials. SurgLaparosc Endosc Percutan Tech. 2012;22(5):463–66.
21. Carr NJ. The pathology of acute appendicitis. Ann Diagn Pathol. 2000;4:46–58. 16.
22. van den Broek WT, Bijnen AB, de Ruiter P, Gouma DJ. A normal appendix found during diagnostic laparoscopy should not be removed. Br J Surg. 2001;88:251–4.
23. van Dalen R, Bagshaw PF, Dobbs BR, Robertson GM, Lynch AC, Frizelle FA. The utility of laparoscopy in the diagnosis of acute appendicitis in women of reproductive age. Surg Endosc. 2003;17:1311–3.
24. Wie HJ, Lee JH, Kyung MS, Jung US, Choi JS. Is incidental appendectomy necessary in women with ovarian endometrioma? Aust N Z J Obstet Gynaecol. 2008;48(1):107–11.
25. Di Saverio S, Mandrioli M, Sibilio A, Smerieri N, Lombardi R, Catena F, et al. A cost-effective technique for laparoscopic appendectomy: outcomes and costs of a case-control prospective single-operator study of 112 unselected consecutive cases of complicated acute appendicitis. J Am Coll Surg. 2014; 218(3):51–65.
26. Markides G, Subar D, Riyad K. Laparoscopic versus open appendectomy in adults with complicated appendicitis: systematic review and meta-analysis. World J Surg. 2010;34(9):2026–40.
27. van Rossem CC, Schreinemacher MH, Treskes K, van Hogezand RM, van Geloven AA. Duration of antibiotic treatment after appendicectomy for acute complicated appendicitis. Br J Surg. 2014;101(6):715–9.
28. Alvarez C, Voitk AJ. The road to ambulatory laparoscopic management of perforated appendicitis. Am J Surg. 2000;179(1):63–6.
29. Andersson RE. The Role of Antibiotic Therapy in the Management of Acute Appendicitis. Curr Infect Dis Rep. 2013;15(1):10–3.
30. Stefanidis D, Richardson WS, Chang L, Earle DB, Fanelli RD. The role of diagnostic laparoscopy for acute abdominal conditions: an evidence-based review. Surg Endosc. 2009;23(1):16–23.
31. Thereaux J, Veyrie N, Corigliano N, Servajean S, Czernichow S, Bouillot JL. Is laparoscopy a safe approach for diffuse appendicular peritonitis? Feasibility and determination of risk factors for post-operative intra-abdominal abscess. Surg Endosc. 2014;28(6):1908–13.
32. Quezada F, Quezada N, Mejia R, Brañes A, Padilla O, Jarufe N, et al. Laparoscopic versus open approach in the management of appendicitis complicated exclusively with peritonitis: a single center experience. Int J Surg. 2015;13:80–3.

13

World society of emergency surgery study group initiative on Timing of Acute Care Surgery classification (TACS)

Yoram Kluger[1*], Offir Ben-Ishay[2], Massimo Sartelli[2], Luca Ansaloni[3], Ashraf E Abbas[4], Ferdinando Agresta[5], Walter L Biffl[6], Luca Baiocchi[7], Miklosh Bala[8], Fausto Catena[9], Raul Coimbra[9], Yunfeng Cui[10], Salomone Di Saverio[11], Koray Das[12], Tamer El Zalabany[13], Gustavo P Fraga[14], Carlos Augusto Gomes[15], Ricardo Alessandro Teixeira Gonsaga[16], Jakub Kenig[17], Ari Leppäniemi[18], Sanjay Marwah[19], Gerson Alves Pereira Junior[20], Boris Sakakushev[21], Boonying Siribumrungwong[22], Norio Sato[23], Cristian Tranà[24], Nereo Vettoretto[25] and Ernest E Moore[26]

Abstract

Timing of surgical intervention is critical for outcomes of patients diagnosed with surgical emergencies. Facing the challenge of multiple patients requiring emergency surgery, or of limited resource availability, the acute care surgeon must triage patients according to their disease process and physiological state. Emergency operations from all surgical disciplines should be scheduled by an agreed time frame that is based on accumulated data of outcomes related to time elapsed from diagnosis to surgery. Although literature exists regarding the optimal timing of various surgical interventions, implementation of protocols for triage of surgical emergencies is lacking. For institutions of a repetitive triage mechanism, further discussion on optimal timing of surgery in diverse surgical emergencies should be encouraged. Standardizing timing of interventions in surgical emergencies will promote clinical investigation as well as a commitment by administrative authorities to proper operating theater provision for acute care surgery.

Introduction

Triage is the process of defining the priority of patients' management according to the severity of their disease process and clinical condition. This process is of paramount importance when resources are insufficient for patient demand and when medical team availability is lacking. Triage is also initiated to avoid resource exhaustion. The process ensures proper care in a timely manner for the sickest. The main principle is saving lives. The outcome and grading of patients is frequently the result of clinical assessment and physiological findings. Modern approaches to triage are scientific and systematic and some are algorithm-based. As triage concepts have become more sophisticated, software and hardware decision support products have evolved to guide caregivers in both hospitals and in the field. Triage is practiced in mass casualty incidents and its rationale is accepted worldwide. Such systems should also be implemented for the care of surgical emergencies other than injury related. In these cases, the concept of triage is especially important for managing multiple patients with diverse needs. Currently, timing emergency surgery is a matter of individual interpretation of the common adjectives used in the literature to express the degree that surgery is- emergent, prompt, early, urgent, expeditious and immediate. Further research on the proper timing of surgery will enable the translation of these adjectives to a more consistent time frame commitment. Evidence based data to support rigorous triage of non-traumatic surgical emergencies should be established and triage policies developed and implemented worldwide. Until this objective will evolve certain agreements on mechanism and principles of triage of emergency surgeries can be delineated.

* Correspondence: y_kluger@rambam.health.gov.il
[1]Department of Surgery, Rambam Health Care Center, Haifa, Israel
Full list of author information is available at the end of the article

This manuscript is an overview of the challenges of timing emergency, non- traumatic operations, with recommendations based on an international expert opinion survey (TACS study).

Review of literature and expert opinions

Acute care surgery requires punctual evaluation and early intervention, usually for diseases of short duration. The notion that expeditious management of acute surgical diseases is the appropriate strategy is based on the knowledge that delaying treatment may increase the risks of adverse outcomes. This study was approved by the ethical committee of the Rambam Health Care Center.

Most non-traumatized surgical patients present to the emergency department with one of three leading complaints: 1. abdominal or groin pain, 2. gastrointestinal bleeding 3. soft tissue infection. After thorough investigation, most of these clinical patterns evolve into unambiguous diagnoses. Some of the clinical patterns that represent acute surgical disease are managed by emergency surgery. Moreover, in certain situations, only surgery leads to proper diagnosis. Other situations require further nonsurgical investigation, and may be treated sufficiently by conservative management. Deferring surgery to daytime hours is appropriate in certain situations. On the other hand, inappropriate delaying of surgery may result in further contamination of the abdominal cavity (perforation of duodenal ulcer, perforated diverticulitis) or perforation of an inflamed organ (appendix) if left untreated. Soft tissue infections (perianal abscess, gluteal abscess) may progress to soft tissue gangrene if treatment is postponed, especially in patients who suffer co- morbidities, such as diabetes mellitus. Delaying treatment in a patient with mesenteric vascular insult may result in frank bowel necrosis or in extension of the ischemia, resulting in a protracted postoperative course and eventually death.

Papandria et al. found that delay to appendectomy is associated with increased perforation rates in children and adults [1]. This finding concurs with previous studies and with the conventional progressive pathophysiologic appendicitis model. On the other hand, Eko et al. found that timing of surgery for acute appendicitis did not affect the incidence of complications including perforation. However, in that study, delay in surgical consultation and treatment was associated with increased length of hospital stay and increased hospital costs. The investigators concluded that optimal timing of appendectomy for uncomplicated acute appendicitis appears to be within 18 hours of emergency department presentation [2]. In contrast, Abou Nukta et al. claimed that delaying appendectomy for 12–24 hours does not have a significant effect on perforation rate, operative time or length of hospital stay [3]. In an attempt to clarify the risk of surgical delay in acute appendicitis the ACS National Surgical Quality Improvement Program (ACS NSQIP) database was reviewed [4]. The primary outcomes were 30-day overall morbidity and 30-day serious morbidity and mortality. Patients who underwent appendectomy more than 12 hours after hospital admissions fared no worse than those who underwent surgery less than six hours from the time of admission. These data support the scheduling of appendectomies for the earliest, yet most suitable time for the surgeon and for proper hospital resource utilization and expenditure, which is usually in the morning. Several studies have addressed the optimal time for surgical intervention in acute cholecystitis [5] and diverticulitis [6]. Pakula et al. recently showed that delaying surgery in patients diagnosed with necrotizing fasciitis did not increase the risk of mortality [7]. Chao et al. [8] echoed Pakuals' observation indicating that timing of surgery (within 12 hours of admission) didn't impact outcome of patients admitted for Vibrio- vulnifics- related necrotizing fasciitis. Korkut et al. [9] on the contrary claim that the interval from the onset of clinical symptoms to the initial surgical intervention seems to be the most important prognostic factor with a significant impact on outcome of patients with Fournier's gangrene.

The objective of the management of acute surgical diseases is to save lives by controlling bleeding or contamination, or by improving organ perfusion. This objective obligates the need for strong commitment and effective mechanisms for prioritizing patient management according to physiological and clinical parameters. Resource availability along patient physiological and clinical parameters in the acute care arena justifies the development of triage tools and agreed criteria for proper timing of emergency operations. Most studies on timing of surgery have investigated delays in operations. This may reflect problems of resource availability, and indicate a need for all parties involved in surgical emergencies, both caregivers and their employers, to commit to high quality of care. Convenience for caregivers or administrators should not override patient safety. Investigations of the influence on patient outcomes of surgical delays due to constraints of resource utilization, must consider the availability of operating theaters at any given time.

Despite the widespread adoption of acute care surgery as a specialty among other surgical professions, the implementation, standardization and development of this discipline vary considerably among medical centers [10]. The World Society for Emergency Surgery (WSES) conducted an international expert opinion panel (TACS). Members of this panel were asked to fill a questionnaire that included information on their acute care service in regard to operating room availability for emergency cases, as well as hospital case load (Table 1). Of the 88 WSES expert panel members receiving the survey, 43 (48.6%) responded. Of the respondents, 79% indicated that a dedicated acute care surgery service operates in their hospital and 71.9% activate a dedicated operating theater (1–3, 72.9%). From this survey it appears that institutions around the world have adopted the concept of acute care services, and established appropriate use of their facilities. Nevertheless, only 51.2% of the respondents indicated that triage of surgical emergencies is performed by a surgeon.

In addition, 41.9% reported that an anesthesiologist is assigned as triage officer at their institution; 23.3% indicated that they already activate a triage system in their hospitals for general surgery emergencies, and 88.6% agreed to the need for such arrangement (Table 1).

When an injured patient presents to the Emergency Department with hemodynamic instability due to a traumatized bleeding spleen, the need for immediate surgery is apparent, and the healthcare team prepares in an almost routine fashion to deliver care and surgical intervention without delay. This is well-accepted, taught and practiced worldwide, and is the result of long standing efforts in education and proper trauma system organization. The simultaneous presentation of many injured patients in need of surgery prompts initiation of triage criteria. After establishing patent airway and ensuring normal breathing mechanism, hemodynamic instability is assigned first priority [11]. Triage criteria for the management of the injured are based on extensive experience gained during war times, and on research, knowledge acquisition and observations by surgeons who dedicated their career to the management of the wounded.

Table 1 International survey on ACS systems

	n- 43(%)
Number of Hospital Beds	
< 250	2 (4.8)
250–500	9 (21.4)
500–750	10 (23.8)
750–1000	10 (23.8)
> 1000	11 (26.2)
Number of General Surgery Cases	
< 1000	27 (62.8)
1000–2000	8 (18.6)
2000–3000	4 (9.3)
> 3000	3 [7]
Dedicated Acute Care Service	34 (79.1)
Dedicated OR for Emergency cases	34 (79.1)
Activated OR for Emergency Cases	
1–3	31 (72.9)
3–6	8 (18.6)
7–10	4 (9.3)
Triage system for Emergency Cases	10 (23.3)
Does Color Coding is Suitable for Triage of Emergency Cases	31 (88.6)
Who is Your Triage Officer	
General Surgeon	20 (46.5)
Anesthesiologists	18 (41.9)
Acute Care Surgeon	2 (4.7)
Anesthesiologist + General Surgeon	1 (2.3)
Casualty Medical Officer	1 (2.3)
None	1 (2.3)

OR – Operating Room

In the management of mass casualty incident, patients are triaged using a color coding system [12]. Prioritizing care of injured patients in need of surgical interventions is based on the same color coding system. This system was developed from the experience of military and civilian mass casualty incidents. Preparedness is crucial for successful treatment of the medical aspect of mass casualty incidents [13].

Hospital color codes alert staff to various emergencies. They convey common and repetitive language and are essential for the distribution of rapid, comprehensible and well-accepted information. We propose that the use of a color coding system to triage emergency surgery cases may help to reduce information loss and time spent on conferring with other caregivers regarding scheduling of emergency operations. Color coding will enable the use of common and standardized language among the members of the surgical team, and other acute care surgical disciplines and will allow proper documentation and improved quality of care.

Treating surgical emergency non- traumatized patients involves the same principles used in the management of the traumatized. Team availability and preparedness, prompt effort at diagnosis and early initiation of management protocols are the hallmarks of the acute care surgery approach for the most severely ill. Immediate availability of resources is essential. Triage concepts and color coding should therefore be adopted in the management of surgical emergencies as well.

In a busy Emergency Department with an influx of patients in need for early intervention, assigning patients to surgery in a "timely manner" is mastery. Triage criteria based on data and knowledge of disease processes need to be set forward for non- traumatic surgical emergencies. Setting proper time frames will promote the establishment of international standards, the initiation of worldwide research and the development of acute care services by national authorities and hospital management administrations. Triage criteria for acute surgical diseases should include simple hemodynamic and clinical data. These criteria would direct the acute surgical teams to properly tag each patient to the timing of surgery. While committing to the time frame set forward for managing patients with surgical emergencies, appropriate steps should be undertaken for optimizing patient physiological status alongside antibiotics administration and pain control during the wait for surgery. Acute Care Surgeons must decide on a proper time frame for the management of their patients, and to commit the medical system to such time frame. This commitment is essential especially in busy medical centers where the Emergency Department is crowded with patients in need of surgery, yet lacking availability of operating theaters.

Classification system

Considering the above (TACS study and current literature), the following categories could be incorporated into a triage system of acute care surgery cases as follows:

Immediate- implies an extreme or markedly decompensated physiological state, usually resulting from bleeding. This is rare in non- traumatic surgical emergencies, and for most bleeding patients initial resuscitative measures will enable further evaluation, diagnosis and even non-operative treatment. Active intra peritoneal bleeding due to a ruptured visceral aneurysm, a ruptured spleen due to hematological disorder with bleeding are examples of a condition that requires immediate surgery. In this category, life or tissue loss is imminent.

Within an hour from diagnosis- implies signs and symptoms of vascular compromise: incarcerated hernia with bowel entrapment, mesenteric vascular occlusion, or limb ischemia. Diffuse peritonitis due to uncontained hollow viscus perforation is another example of a condition that requires surgery "within an hour" as is the presence of necrotizing fasciitis with sepsis. Patients diagnosed with these pathologies need to be adequately resuscitated and managed while undergoing further diagnoses and other steps toward safe surgery. Physiologically, patients may have signs of sepsis or mild to moderate organ dysfunction requiring rapid resuscitation without delaying surgical intervention. In most cases, tissue loss is imminent.

Within 6 hours from diagnosis- implies localized peritonitis or soft tissue infection in need of surgery, but not a physiological state that entails spreading or progression of the disease process. These pathologies have the potential to evolve to more serious conditions if surgery is delayed. Antibiotic treatment and fluid administration should be initiated immediately upon diagnosis and repeat examination carried out while waiting for surgery.

Within 12 hours from diagnosis- implies a need of surgery, though evidence- based knowledge indicates that postponing surgery while under medical treatment does not lead to clinical deterioration. As an example, delay in treatment of acute appendicitis has been shown to have no deleterious effect on outcomes.

Within 24 or 48 hour from diagnosis- Suggests that intervention is indicated and the process may progress and worsen the morbidity of the operation. Examples include cholecystitis and thoracic empyema. The classification also applies to patients who were operated under emergency, and re-laparotomy was decided upon during the index procedure for peritoneal cavity rinsing or for assessment of bowel perfusion and viability. These principals need to be adopted, understood and appreciated by all personnel involved in the treatment of patients with surgical emergencies.

Timing of surgical intervention

Prompt, early, urgent, expeditious, immediate, and emergency are common adjectives used in the medical literature to describe the need for surgery "in a timely manner". The literature lacks evidence based data on proper timing of emergency surgery. Definitions of Time To Surgery (TTS), Ideal Time To Surgery (iTTS) and Actual Time To Surgery (aTTS) should therefore evolve and be standard for further discussions. Launching a triage system for non- trauma surgical emergencies will ensure that time to surgery (TTS) develops into a quality improvement tool. Actual TTS (aTTS, real time waiting for surgery) can be compared to the time assigned for each pathology by expert opinion, consistent with data from current literature (ideal time to surgery, iTTS). The ratio aTTS/iTTS will reflect efficiency and should be used for quality assessment. A ratio of ≤ 1 indicates compliance with standards for timing of surgery and a ratio >1 indicates that surgery was delayed. Delaying surgery from the time set by the acute surgical care team and determined by the triage system will be a matter for further quality improvement measures.

A reproducible tagging mechanism for acute surgical emergencies will clarify the vague adjectives commonly used to describe the urgency of "emergent" surgery. This will enable definitions of worldwide criteria for the timing of emergency surgery. When dealing with surgical emergencies, descriptive words for "timely surgery" should be substituted with unambiguous and reproducible time frames. This needs to be scrutinized, tested and validated on a worldwide scale.

In an effort to understand current occurrence in acute care of surgical emergencies and common practices of emergency surgery scheduling, WSES panel experts were asked to assign iTTS to a number of common surgical emergencies - acute appendicitis, incarcerated inguinal hernia, mesenteric ischemia, perforated duodenal ulcer and peri- anal abscess. The results are summarized in Table 2. The TACS study identified high agreement among responders regarding the time frame presented

Table 2 Expert opinion on timing of surgery in common surgical emergencies

	n-43(%)
Immediate Surgery	
Mesenteric Event	37 (86)
Evisceration	27 (62.8)
Hemodynamic Instability due to bleeding	42 (97.7)
Surgery Within an Hour	
Incarcerated Hernia	35 (83.3)
Perforated Viscus	35 (83.3)
*Necrotizing Fasciitis**	34 (79.1)
Surgery Within 6 Hours	
Soft Tissue Infection (Abscess)	37 (86)
*Appendicitis**	36 (83.7)
*Cholecystitis**	29 (67.4)
Surgery Within 24–48 Hours	
Second Look Laparotomy	41 (95.3)

*expert opinion not in aptness with current literature.

for common surgical emergencies. Although the data presented in the table does not concur with current views in the literature regarding some of the clinical entities surveyed, this may reflect availability of operating theaters in some of the institutions participating in the study. In most institutions, scheduling of unplanned is a matter of dialogue and negotiation where dedicated operating theaters are not assigned for surgical emergencies. The discrepancy revealed in iTTS assessment between TACS respondents and the current literature, e.g. timing of appendectomy [3] and cholecystectomy [5], indicate that further studies are needed to establish iTTS for surgical emergencies. Until this is accomplished a certain frame of iTTS can be proposed and implemented as an interim guideline for the timing of surgical interventions in surgical emergencies as proposed in Figure 1.

The National Confidential Enquiry into Patient Outcome and Death (NCEPOD) in the United Kingdom classifies interventions as immediate, urgent, expedited and elective [14]. For each of these categories, the respective target times to theatre from decision to operate is within minutes, hours, days or planned. There is general agreement that cases requiring immediate attention will be triaged before less urgent cases. Cases classified between these two groups raise the greatest debate in terms of patient priority. A standardized system for categorizing clinical urgency would be most beneficial to these types of surgical cases. It is clear from the TACS study and from other available guidelines [14] that iTTS is a matter of consensus among care providers based on clinical data.

iTTS needs further scrutinizing in regard to each and every surgical emergency and further investigation on the impact of actual time to surgery (aTTS) on outcomes. The goal is to establish evidence-based and feasible triage criteria for appropriate timing of operation in surgical emergencies.

Recommendations:

1. We recommend adopting a color-triage system for acute surgical emergencies.
2. We suggest that each medical institution should examine its aTTS and compare it to the iTTS proposed in this paper. This will facilitate the conduct and comparison of international research, and will ease adoption of triage protocols for surgical emergencies.

Timing- iTTS *from diagnosis*	*Possible Clinical Scenarios(TACS)*	*Color code*	*Note*
Immediate surgery	Bleeding emergencies		Immediate life saving surgical intervention, resuscitative laparotomy
Within an hour	Incarcerated hernia, perforated viscus, diffuse peritonitis, soft tissue infection accompanied with sepsis		Surgical Intervention as soon as possible but only after resuscitation (within 1 to 2 hours). administration of antibiotics upon diagnosis- no delay
Within 6 hours	Soft tissue infection (abscess) not accompanied with sepsis		Administration of antibiotics upon diagnosis- no delay
Within 12 hours	Appendicitis (local peritonitis), cholecystitis (optional)		Administration of antibiotics upon diagnosis- no delay
Within 24 or 48 hours	Second-look laparotomy		Schedule in advance. Intervention should occur during day time

Figure 1 Proposed Ideal Time to Surgery (iTTS) and color coding.

3. We recommend using the aTTS/iTTS ratio as a quality improvement tool and as an international index for comparison in future research.
4. We recommend that further studies on appropriate timing of emergency surgeries be initiated, and that the findings be implemented in more refined triage systems.

Conclusions

Accumulating evidence on the impact of delaying emergency surgical intervention on patient outcomes challenges common knowledge and intuitive paradigms held by acute care surgeons. The need for prospective multi-institutional studies on the appropriate timing of operations for surgical emergencies has become clear.

Competing interests

The authors declare that they have no competing interests.

Author details

[1]Department of Surgery, Rambam Health Care Center, Haifa, Israel. [2]Department of Surgery, Macerata Hospital, Macerata, Italy. [3]Department of General Surgery, Ospedali Riuniti, Italy. [4]Department of General Surgery, Mansoura University Hospital, Mansoura, Egypt. [5]Department of General Surgery, Department of Surgery, Adria Hospital, Adria, Italy. [6]Denver Health Medical Center, Denver, Colorado, USA. [7]Department of Medical and Surgical Sciences, Surgical Clinic, Brescia University, Brescia, Italy. [8]Department of General Surgery, Hadassah Medical Center, Jerusalem, Israel. [9]Department of Surgery, Division of Trauma, Surgical Critical Care, and Burns, University of California, San Diego Health System, San Diego, California, USA. [10]Department of Surgery, Tianjin Nankai Hospital, Nankai Clinical School of Medicine, Tianjin Medical University, Tianjin, China. [11]Department of Emergency and Trauma Surgery, Maggiore Hospital, Trauma Center, Bologna, Italy. [12]Department of General Surgery, Numune Training and Research Hospital, Adana, Turkey. [13]Department of General Surgery, Bahrain Defence Force Military Hospital, West Riffa, Bahrain. [14]Department of Surgery, University of Campinas, Campinas, São Paulo, Brazil. [15]Department of Surgery, Hospital Universitário, Universidade Federal de Juiz de Fora, Juiz de Fora, Minas Gerais, Brazil. [16]Department Chirurgia General e do Trauma, Catanduva, Brazil. [17]3rd Department of General Surgery, Jagiellonian Univeristy, Narutowicz Hospital, Krakow, Poland. [18]Department of Abdominal Surgery, University Hospital Meilahti, Helsinki, Finland. [19]Department of Surgery, Post-Graduate Institute of Medical Science, Rohatak, India. [20]Emergency Unit, Department of Surgery, Ribeirão Preto, Brazil. [21]First clinic of General Surgery, University Hospital Plovdiv, Plovdiv, Bulgaria. [22]Department of General Surgery, Thammsat University Hospital, Pathumthani, Thailand. [23]Department of Primary care and Emergency medicine, Kyoto University, Kyoto, Japan. [24]Department of Surgery, Ancona University, Ancona, Italy. [25]Department of Surgery, Mellini Hospital, Chiari, Italy. [26]Department of Surgery, Denver Health Medical Center, Denver, Colorado, USA.

References

1. Papandria D, Goldstein SD, Rhee D, Salazar JH, Arlikar J, Gorgy A, Ortega G, Zhang Y, Abdullah F: **Risk of perforation increases with delay in recognition and surgery for acute appendicitis.** *J Surg Res* 2012. doi:10.1016/j.jss.2012.12.008. [Epub ahead of print]. S0022-4804[12]01952-X.
2. Eko FN, Ryb GE, Drager L, Goldwater E, Wu JJ, Counihan TCN: **Ideal timing of surgery for acute uncomplicated appendicitis.** *Am J Med Sci. Jan;* 2013, **5**(1):22–7.
3. Abou- Nukta F, Bakhons C, Arroyo K, Martin J, Reinholds R, Ciadiello K: **Effect of delaying appendectomy for acute appendicitis for 12–24 hours.** *Arch Surg* 2006, **141**(5):504–6.
4. Ingraham AM, Choen ME, Bilimoria KY, Ko CY, Hall BL, *et al*: **Effect of delay to operation on outcomes in adults with acute appendicitis.** *Arch Sur* 2010, **145**:886–92.
5. Gurusamy KS, Samraj K, Fusai G, Davidson BR: **Early versus delayed laparoscopic cholecystectomy for biliary colic.** *Cochrane Database of Systematic Reviews* 2008, (4):CD007196. doi:10.1002/14651858.CD007196.pub2.
6. Stocchi L: **Current indications and role of surgery in the management of sigmoid diverticulitis.** *World J Gastroenterol* 2010, **16**(7):804–17.
7. Pakula AM, Kapadia R, Freeman B, Skinner RA: **A 3-year experience with necrotizing fasciitis: favorable outcomes despite operative delays in a busy acute care hospital.** *Am Surg* 2012, **78**(10):1059–62.
8. Chao WN, Tsai CF, Chang HR, Su KS, *et al*: **Impact of timing of surgery on outcome of Vibrio vulnificus- related necrotizing fasciitis.** *Am J Surg* 2013. Epub ahead of print.
9. Korkut M, Icoz G, Dayanac M, Akgun E, Yeniay L, *et al*: **Outcomes analysis in patients with Fournier's gangrene: report of 45 cases.** *Dis Colon Rectum* 2003, **46**(5):649–52.
10. Santry H, Pringle PL, Emhoff TA, Velmahos GC, *et al*: *Acute care surgery patterns in the current Era: results of a qualitative study.* http://escholarship.umassmed.edu/cgi/viewcontent.cgi?article.
11. Initial assessment and management , chapter 1: *Advanced trauma life support, student course manual.* 8th edition. Chicago, IL: American college of surgeons; 2008:1–19.
12. Kahn CA, Schultz CH, Miller KT, Anderson CL: **Does START triage work? An outcomes assessment after a disaster.** *Ann Emerg Med* 2009, **54**(3):424–30.
13. Kluger Y, Mayo A, Aladgem D, Halperin P: **Functions and principles in the management of bombing mass casualty incidents – lessons learned at the Tel-Aviv Sourasky medical center.** *Eur J Emerg Med* 2004, **11**:329–34.
14. *National confidential enquiry into patient outcome and death.* London: The NCEPOD classification of interventions [Online]; 2004. http://www.ncepod.org.uk/pdf/NCEPODClassification.pdf.

14

Ten-year experiences with Tracheostomy at a University teaching hospital in Northwestern Tanzania: A retrospective review of 214 cases

Japhet M Gilyoma†, Darius D Balumuka† and Phillipo L Chalya*

Abstract

Background: Tracheostomy remains a very important life saving surgical procedure worldwide and particularly in our environment where patients present late in upper airway obstruction. Little work has been done on this subject in our environment and therefore it was necessary to conduct this study to describe our own experiences with tracheostomy, outlining the common indications and outcome of tracheostomized patients in our setting and compare our results with those from other centers in the world.

Methods: This was a 10-year retrospective study which was conducted at Bugando Medical Centre from January 2001 to December 2010. Data were retrieved from patients' files kept in the Medical record department and analyzed using SPSS computer software version 15.0. Ethical approval to conduct the study was obtained from relevant authority before the commencement of the study.

Results: A total of 214 patients were studied. The male to female ratio was 3.1: 1. The majority of patients were in the 3rd decade of life. The most common indication for tracheostomy was upper airway obstruction secondary to traumatic causes in 55.1% of patients, followed by upper airway obstruction due to neoplastic causes in 39.3% of cases. The majority of tracheostomies (80.4%) were performed as an emergency. Transverse skin crease incision was employed in all the cases. Post-tracheostomy complication rate was 21.5%. Complication rate was significantly higher in emergency tracheostomy than in electives ($P < 0.001$). The duration of temporary tracheostomy ranged from 8 days to 46 months, with a median duration of 4 months. Tracheostomy decannulation was successively performed in 72.4% of patients who survived. Mortality rate was 13.6%. The mortality was due to their underlying illnesses, none had tracheostomy-related mortality.

Conclusion: Upper airway obstruction secondary to trauma and laryngeal tumors still remains the most common indication for tracheostomy in our centre and tracheostomy is still a life saving procedure in the surgical management of airway despite complications which are seen more commonly in paediatric patients. Most of tracheostomy related complications can be avoided by meticulous attention to the details of the technique and postoperative tracheostomy care by skilled and trained staff.

Keywords: Tracheostomy, Indications, Outcome, Tanzania

Background

Tracheostomy, an ancient surgical procedure originally described in the first century BC [1], is one of the more commonly performed surgical procedures in critically ill patients who require prolonged mechanical ventilation, and is predicted to become more common as demand for intensive care services increases [2,3]. Approximately 10% of mechanically ventilated critically ill patients receive a tracheostomy to facilitate prolonged airway and ventilatory support [4-7]. It is a life-saving procedure when performed with an appropriate indication and surgical technique [8,9]. Other methods of airway intervention include endotracheal intubation,

* Correspondence: drphillipoleo@yahoo.com
† Contributed equally
Department of Surgery, Weill-Bugando University Colleges of Health Sciences, Mwanza, Tanzania

cricothyroidotomy, and Percutaneous Dilatation Tracheostomy [10,11].

The most common indications for tracheostomy are relieve of upper airway obstruction, prolonged mechanical ventilation, airway protection in the comatose and facilitation of tracheo-bronchial toileting [11]. There is a changing trend in literature as regarding the indications and outcome of tracheostomy especially in children for the management of the airway [10-13]. In the past, short term tracheostomy for obstructive airway disease secondary to acute inflammatory infection was the most common indication [14] but in recent time trauma to the upper airway has become the commonest indication [10,11]. These have been attributed to the changes in the epidemiology of infectious diseases due to early diagnosis, adequate use of antibiotics and the improvement in the capabilities of medical technology [10,11,15].

Tracheostomy in the pediatric age group has been reported to be different from that in adults because in pediatric patients this procedure is challenging and technically more demanding and carries higher degree of morbidity and mortality when compared to the adult population [16].

The procedure of tracheostomy is associated with numerous complications which may occur anytime during the operative and postoperative periods [17,18]. These complications are more common in emergency tracheostomy than in elective ones [17]. Complication rates associated with tracheostomy have been reported in literature to range from 6 to 66 percent and the mortality rate related to tracheostomy is reported to be less then 2% [18]. Complications and mortality associated with tracheostomy are mostly avoidable if the procedure is carefully performed and the postoperative management strictly and conscientiously adhered to [19].

Despite the fact that tracheostomy is a common life saving procedure in the care of critically ill patients, there is paucity of information in our local setting regarding the subject. The aim of this retrospective study is to highlight our own experiences with tracheostomy outlining the common indications and outcome of patients with tracheostomy and compare our results with those from other centers in the world.

Methods

Study design and setting

A retrospective review of patients who had tracheotomies performed at Bugando Medical Centre during a ten-year period between January 2001 and December 2010 was carried out. Bugando Medical Centre is one of the four tertiary and referral hospitals in the country and has a bed capacity of 1000. It is also a teaching hospital for the Weill-Bugando University College of Health Sciences. The hospital has a 12-bed adult and 10-bed paediatric multi-disciplinary Intensive Care Unit (ICU) which is headed by a consultant anesthesiologist and run by trained ICU nurses.

Study subjects

The study included all patients who underwent tracheostomy at Bugando Medical Centre during the period under study. Patients who had incomplete or missed basic information were excluded from the study. Data were retrieved from patient registers kept in the Medical record departments, the surgical wards, and operating theatre and entered in a preformed questionnaire before analysis. Included in the questionnaire were; demographic profile (age, sex), primary diagnosis, indication for tracheotomy, surgical technique, duration of the tracheotomy before decannulation, hospital stay and outcome of management such as complications, death and cause of death. The primary diagnosis was classified based on the aetiology which is divided into trauma, infection/inflammation, Neoplasm, congenital and others. The indications for tracheostomy were divided into upper airway obstruction, respiratory insufficiency, bronchial toileting, adjunct to head and neck surgeries. Complications related to tracheostomy were classified as: immediate post-operative period (i.e. within the first 24 hours after surgery), early post-operative period (i.e. within the first week after surgery) and late post-operative period (i.e. beyond one week). Tracheostomies were performed in emergency and electively both under general as well as local anesthesia. The procedure was performed under general anaesthesia in the operating theatre and bedside tracheostomy was performed in the intensive care unit (ICU) under local anaesthesia. Transverse skin crease incision was employed in all the cases.

All the procedures were carried out by surgeons, residents or registrars, while trained ward staff carried out postoperative tracheostomy care. An electric suction machine was provided at bedside for suction as needed.

Tracheostomy decannulation was carried out depending upon the etiology and satisfactory maintenance of the airway. All of them were decannulated in the ward. They were kept under observation for 24 hours after decannulation and were sent home. Instruction was given to do air sealed dressing over the stoma, allowing healing by secondary intension. Patient and attendant were educated that if the patient develops respiratory distress he should be brought to the hospital immediately. First follow up was done after two weeks. When no complication was observed at home, then monthly check up for one year depending upon the condition of the patient.

Statistical analysis

The statistical analysis was performed using statistical package for social sciences (SPSS) version 15.0 for

Windows (SPSS, Chicago IL, USA). The mean ± standard deviation (SD), median and ranges were calculated for continuous variables whereas proportions and frequency tables were used to summarize categorical variables. Continuous variables were categorized. Chi-square ($\chi 2$) test were used to test for the significance of association between the independent (predictor) and dependent (outcome) variables in the categorical variables. The level of significance was considered as $P < 0.05$. Multivariate logistic regression analysis was used to determine predictor variables that predict the outcome.

Ethical consideration

Ethical approval to conduct the study was sought from the Weill-Bugando University College of Health Sciences/ Bugando Medical Centre joint institutional ethic review committee before the commencement of the study.

Results

Demographic profile

Two hundred and fourteen patients had tracheostomy within the study period. One hundred and sixty-two (75.7%) patients were males and females were fifty-two (24.3%) with a male to female ratio of 3.1: 1. Their ages ranged from 1 year to 76 years with the median and mean age of 36 and 38.34 ± 12.26 years respectively. The majority of patients were in the 3rd decade of life (36.7%).

Timing, purpose and indications of tracheostomy

One hundred and seventy-two tracheotomies (80.4%) were performed as an emergency while forty-two (19.6%) as elective procedures. Of the 214 tracheostomized patients, 184 (86.0%) had temporary tracheostomy and the remaining 30(14.0%) had permanent tracheostomy as part of their treatment.

The most common indication for tracheostomy was upper airway obstruction secondary to traumatic causes in 55.1% of patients, followed by upper airway obstruction due to neoplastic causes in 39.3% of cases (Table 1). High incidence of traumatic causes of upper airway obstruction was found between the third and fourth decades of life, while the 7-8th decades of life recorded high incidence of laryngeal and other head and neck

Table 1 Indications for Tracheostomy

Indications	Pathological causes	Frequency	Percentages
Upper airway obstruction		**178**	**83.2**
	Traumatic	***98***	***55.1***
	- Severe head injuries	69	70.4
	- Foreign body aspiration	13	13.3
	- Severe maxillofacial injuries	9	9.2
	- Cut throat	7	7.1
	Neoplastic	***70***	***39.3***
	- Laryngeal tumors	60	85.7
	- Thyroid cancer	4	5.7
	- Other neck tumors	6	8.6
	Infections	***18***	***10.1***
	- Tetanus	16	88.9
	- Retropharyngeal abscess	2	11.1
	Congenital lesions	***2***	***1.1***
	- Laryngeal web	1	50.0
	- Laryngeal stenosis	1	50.0
Mechanical ventilator support/ Tracheobronchial toileting		**26**	**9.3**
	Prolonged ventilation	24	92.3
	Diaphragmatic Injury	2	7.7
Adjunct to head and neck surgeries		**4**	**1.9**
	Anticipated difficult intubation	4	100.0
Others		**6**	**1.9**
	Post-thyroidectomy tracheomalacia	3	50.0
	? Gullein Barre syndrome	1	16.7
	Failed endotracheal intubation	1	16.7
	Cause not established	1	16.7

malignancies. Laryngeal papillomas causing upper airway obstruction were recorded as the most common indication for tracheostomy in the first decade of life.

In patients who had tracheostomy secondary to prolonged ventilation, the duration of intubation before tracheostomy was performed ranged from 4 to 62 days with a median duration of 26 days.

The vast majority of patients, 197 (92.1%) underwent tracheostomy under general anaesthesia in the operating theatre and the remaining 17 (7.9%) patients underwent bedside tracheostomy in the intensive care unit (ICU). Transverse skin crease incision was employed in all the cases.

Post-tracheostomy complications

Complications related to tracheostomy were seen in 46 patients giving a complication rate of 21.5%. Of these, 2 (4.3%) occurred in the immediate post-operative period (i.e. within the first 24 hours after surgery), 10 (21.7%) in the early post-operative period (i.e. within the first week after surgery) and 30 (65.2%) occurred in the late post-operative period (i.e. beyond one week). The period of post-operative complications was not recorded in 4 (8.7%). There were no intraoperative complications (Table 2). Post-tracheostomy complication rate was significantly higher in emergency tracheostomy than in elective one (73.9% versus 26.1%) ($P < 0.001$). Complication rate related to tracheostomy was also significantly higher in children aged 10 years and below than in adult patients ($P < 0.001$).

Outcome of tracheostomy

The duration of temporary tracheostomy depended on the primary pathology and ranged from 8 days to 46 months, with a median duration of 4 months. Tracheostomy decannulation was successively performed in 155 (72.4%) patients who survived. Of these, 102 (65.8%) patients were discharged home after decannulation and the remaining 53 (34.2%) were discharged home with their tracheotomies. In the group of patients who were discharged home with their tracheostomies, tracheostomy decannulation was accomplished successively in all patients during subsequent follow up visits. The median period of post-tracheostomy intensive care unit (ICU) stay was 18 days (range: 6-36 days) and median period of hospital stay was 26 days (range: 7-52 days). Thirty-two (14.0%) patients had permanent tracheostomy needed for either curative or palliative management. Twenty-nine patients died giving an overall mortality rate of 13.6%. The mortality was due to their underlying illnesses, none had tracheostomy-related mortality. Follow up of all patients after decannulation was uneventful.

Discussion

Since it was originally described in the first century B.C [1], tracheostomy remains a life-saving surgical procedure commonly performed in critically ill patients. In this review, the highest age incidence of the patients who had tracheostomy was in the third decade and males were more affected. Similar demographic profile was reported by other workers [10,11,18,20]. Male preponderance in this age group may be due to their increased susceptibility to trauma which necessitated prolonged intubation and assisted ventilation in some of them.

The indications of tracheostomy are diverse and changing. There has been a change in the' indications for tracheostomy over the past two decades [10-13]. In the past, infective conditions such as epiglottitis and laryngotracheobronchitis were major indications for tracheostomy but the better handling of infections with the use of intubation and conservative management in the intensive care unit has reduced the incidence of these indications [14,15]. The most common indication for tracheostomy in our series was upper airway obstruction secondary to traumatic causes followed by upper airway obstruction due to neoplastic causes, which is at variance with other reports which reported carcinoma of the larynx as the most common indication for

Table 2 Post-tracheostomy Complications (N = 46)

Period	Complications	Frequency	Percentage
Intraoperative	No complication	-	-
Immediate complications	Bleeding	1	2.2
	Subcutaneous emphysema	1	2.2
Early complications	Aspiration pneumonia	6	13.0
	Accidental decannulation	2	4.4
	Tracheal tube obstruction	2	4.4
Late complications	Suprastomal granulation tissue	17	37.0
	Stomal infection	11	23.9
	Tracheal stenosis	1	2.2
	Impacted tracheostomy tube	1	2.2

tracheostomy followed by prolonged ventilation and foreign body aspirations [10]. These variations between series might be due to different patient populations. The commonest indication recorded in the first decade of life in the present study was upper airway obstruction primarily from laryngeal papillomas, which necessitated emergency tracheostomy as these patients presented in respiratory distress as shown in other studies [16,21]. The high incidence of laryngeal papilloma could be because of mother to child transmission of the Human Papilloma virus (HPV) during delivery. Further research in our region is required to substantiate this. In agreement with other studies [11,22], upper airway obstruction secondary to laryngeal carcinoma and other neck malignancies were the main indications for tracheostomy in the 7th-8th decade of life. In our experience, all cases with laryngeal carcinoma and other neck malignancies present late in severe respiratory distress and so an emergency tracheostomy was always performed even before confirming the diagnosis. Higher incidence of laryngeal carcinoma in our series may also be that there is a possible increase in the incidence of laryngeal cancer in our society. Further study is needed in our setting to confirm this observation. Trauma to the head and neck was the leading indications in the 3rd decade of life in our series and interestingly the majority of these injuries were from road traffic crashes especially involving motorcycles which have become a major means of commuter transportation in Tanzania. This group represents the economically active age and portrays an economic loss both to the family and the nation and the reason for their high incidence of head and neck injuries reflects their high activity levels and participation in high-risk activities. The fact that the economically productive age-group were mostly involved calls for an urgent public policy response.

The surgical technique employed in all our patients was the transverse skin crease incision in the operating room. This is the method preferred by us whether it's an emergency or an elective tracheostomy because of the advantage of a better cosmetic result though, the vertical incision has the advantage of running in the line of the trachea and it is easy to perform and less vascular.

The presence of postoperative complications has an impact on the final outcome of tracheostomatized patients. The rate of postoperative complication in our study was 21.5%, which is higher than what was reported by others [10,20]. However, much higher complication rates have been reported from other centres in Nigeria [11,16,18,19]. In other studies, complication rates of between 6-66% have been quoted [20,23]. The reason for high rate of complications following tracheostomy in our study may be because the majority of tracheostomies in our patients were performed on emergency basis by non-otorhinolaryngologist junior doctors who may have little experiences in performing these procedures. It is therefore recommended that tracheostomy should be performed by an experienced surgeon with adequate facilities to reduce the potential complications. Post-tracheostomy complication rates were found to be significantly higher in emergency tracheostomy than in elective one, which is comparable to other studies done elsewhere [16,19]. This observation is at variance with one report which reported elective tracheostomy as the most frequent performed procedure [20]. Complication rates related to tracheostomy was also significantly higher in children aged 10 years and below than in adult patients which is in agreement with other studies [16,20]. High complication rate in patients who had emergency tracheostomy can be explained by the fact that the majority of patients with upper airway obstruction presented late to the Accident and Emergency department in severe respiratory obstruction and so emergency tracheostomy was always a rule. High rate of complication among children aged 10 years and below is attributed to the fact that tracheostomy in children is challenging and technically more difficult due to small caliber of their larynx and trachea and therefore carries higher postoperative complication rate when compared to the adult population. In the present study, suprastomal granulation tissue and stomal infection were found to be the most common complications of tracheostomy. Similar finding were also reported by Fasunla *et al* [24]. Complication rates associated with tracheostomy can be prevented by good surgical technique and meticulous postoperative care. Suprastomal granulation tissue is a notable late complication of tracheostomy that can be prevented with good surgical technique, sparing the cricoid cartilage during dissection. Stomal infection should be promptly treated and cuffed orotracheal intubation for more than a week in unconscious and tetanus patients should be avoided.

Tracheostomy decannulation in patients with temporary tracheostomy was successfully carried out in 72.4% of patients who survived, which is almost similar to the study done by Hussain *et al* [25] showing 74.1% decannulation accomplished successfully. The optimal timing of tracheostomy decannulation in patients with temporary tracheostomy depends mainly on the underlying disease and should be considered only if the original upper-airway obstruction is resolved, if airway secretions are controlled, and if mechanical ventilation is no longer needed [26].

The overall mortality recorded in our series was 13.6% and these were from underlying diseases. There was no mortality attributed to tracheostomy in this present review reflecting significant improvements not only in the skill of placing a tracheostomy but also in the post operative management of these patients in our hospital.

Our figures for the overall median duration of hospital stay in the present study was 26 days, which is higher compared to what is reported in other studies [10,11]. The reasons for the longer duration of hospital stay may be attributed to the underlying disease and presence of postoperative complications. Also, despite being a life-saving procedure, tracheostomy is not psychosocially acceptable to most patients because of the difficulty with phonation and the stigma associated with it by some uninformed people. Therefore, most patients with temporary tracheostomy desire decannulation before being discharged into the community from the hospital. This might have contributed to longer duration of hospital stay in this study. Due to the poor socio-economic conditions in our setting, the duration of inpatient stay for our patients may be longer than expected due to social reasons.

The potential limitation of this study is that it is retrospective from a single centre and the fact that information about some patients was incomplete in view of the retrospective nature of the study might have introduced some bias in our findings. A similar study in a prospective setting is highly recommended in order to describe our experiences of tracheostomies not only in our centre but also country-wide.

Conclusion

Upper airway obstruction secondary to trauma and laryngeal tumors still remains the most common indication for tracheostomy in our centre. Tracheostomy is still a life saving procedure in the surgical management of airway despite complications which are seen more commonly in paediatric patients. Most of complications related to tracheostomy can be avoidable by meticulous surgical technique and postoperative tracheostomy care by skilled and trained staff.

Acknowledgements

The authors thank all members of staff of Department of Surgery who participated in the preparation of this manuscript, and all those who were involved in the care of our tracheostomized patients. Special thanks go to members of the Medical record department for their assistance in the retrieval of patients' case notes.

Authors' contributions

JMG conceived the study and did the literature search, coordinated the write-up, editing. PLC participated in the literature search, writing of the manuscript, editing and submission of the article. All the authors read and approved the final manuscript

Authors' information

JMG: Senior Consultant General/ENT surgeon, Senior Lecturer and Head, Department of Surgery, Well Bugando University College of Health Sciences. PLC: Consultant general surgeon and Senior Lecturer, Department of Surgery, Well Bugando University College of Health Sciences.

Competing interests

The authors declare that they have no competing interests.

References

1. Walts PA, Murthy SC, DeCamp MM: **Techniques of surgical tracheostomy.** *Clin Chest Med* 2003, **24**:413-422.
2. Cox CE, Carson SS, Holmes GM, Howard A, Carey TS: **Increase in tracheostomy for prolonged mechanical ventilation in North Carolina, 1993-2002.** *Crit Care Med* 2004, **32**:2219-2226.
3. Needham DM, Bronskill SE, Calinawan JR, Sibbald WJ, Pronovost PJ, Laupacis A: **Projected incidence of mechanical ventilation in Ontario to 2026: Preparing for the aging baby boomers.** *Crit Care Med* 2005, **33**:574-579.
4. Esteban A, Anzueto A, Alía I, Gordo F, Apezteguía C, Pálizas F, Cide D, Goldwaser R, Soto L, Bugedo G, Rodrigo C, Pimentel J, Raimondi G, Tobin MJ: **How is mechanical ventilation employed in the intensive care unit? An international utilization review.** *Am J Respir Crit Care Med* 2000, **161**:1450-1458.
5. Frutos-Vivar F, Esteban A, Apezteguía C, Anzueto A, Nightingale P, González M, Soto L, Rodrigo C, Raad J, David CM, Matamis D, D' Empaire G, International Mechanical Ventilation Study Group: **Outcome of mechanically ventilated patients who require a tracheostomy.** *Crit Care Med* 2005, **33**:290-298.
6. Kollef MH, Ahrens TS, Shannon W: **Clinical predictors and outcomes for patients requiring tracheostomy in the intensive care unit.** *Crit Care Med* 1999, **27**:1714-1720.
7. Fischler L, Erhart S, Kleger GR, Frutiger A: **Prevalence of tracheostomy in ICU patients. A nation-wide survey in Switzerland.** *Intensive Care Med* 2000, **26**:1428-1433.
8. Ilce Z, Celayir S, Tekard GT, Murat NS, Ercogan E, Yeker D: **Tracheostomy in childhood: 20 years experience from a paediatric surgery clinic.** *Paediatr Int* 2002, **44**:306.
9. Wood DE: **Tracheostomy.** *Chest Surg Clin N Am* 1996, **6**:749.
10. Eziyi Josephine Adetinuola EJ, Bola AY, Olanrewaju MI, Oyedotun AA, Timothy OO, Alani AS, Adekunle A: **Tracheostomy in south western Nigeria: Any change in pattern?** *J Med Med Sci* 2011, **2(7)**:997-1002.
11. Amusa YB, Akinipelu VO, Fadiora SO, Agbakwuru EA: **Tracheostomy in surgical practice: Experience in a Nigerian Tertiary Hospital.** *West Afr J Med* 2004, **23(1)**:32-34.
12. Alladi A, Rao S, Das K, Charles AR, Cruz AJ: **Pediatric tracheostomy: a 13 year experience.** *Pediatr Surg Int* 2004, **20(9)**:695-8.
13. Primuharsa PSH, Wong CY, Hazim MY, Megat Shiraz MA, Goh BS: **Pediatric tracheostomy in Hospital University Kebangsaan Malaysia- a changing trend.** *Med J Malaysia* 2006, **61(2)**:209-13.
14. Parilla C, Scarano E, Guidi ML, Galli J, Paludetti G: **Current trends in pediatric tracheostomies.** *Int J Pediatr Otorhinolaryngol* 2007, **71(10)**:1563-7.
15. Kremer B, Botos-Kremer AI, Eckel HE, Schlorndoff G: **Indications, complications and surgical techniques for pediatric tracheostomies.** *J Pediatr Surg* 2002, **37(11)**:1556-62.
16. Adoga AA, Ma'an ND: **Indications and outcome of pediatric tracheostomy: results from a Nigerian tertiary hospital.** *BMC Surgery* 2010, **10**:2.
17. Hadi A, Ikram M: **Upper airway obstruction: Comparison of tracheostomy and endotracheal intubation.** *PJLO* 1995, **11**:25.
18. Asmatullah , Inayatullah , Rasool G, Billah M: **Complication of emergency tracheostomy.** *J Postgrad Med Inst* 2004, **18(2)**:225-9.
19. Onakoya PA, Nwaorgu OG, Adebusoye LA: **Complications of classical tracheostomy and management.** *Trop Doctor* 2003, **33**:148-150.
20. Khan FA, Ashrafi SK, Iqbal H, Sohail Z, Wadood : **Operative complications of tracheostomy.** *Pak J Surg* 2010, **26(4)**:308-310.
21. Adoga AA, Nimkur LT, Adoga AS: **Recurrent respiratory papillomatosis in Jos, Nigeria: clinical presentation, management and outcome.** *East Centr Afri J Surg* 2008, **13(2)**:105-8.
22. Okoye BCC: **Tracheostomy in Port Harcourt.** *Nig J Surg Sci* 2000, **10**:99-102.
23. Stock MC, Woodward CG, Shirpiro BA, Cane FD, Lewis V, Pecaro B: **Perioperative complications of elective tracheostomy in critically ill patients.** *Critical Care Medicine* 1986, , **14**: 861-3.
24. Fasunla JA, Aliyu A, Nwaorgu OGB, Ijaduola GTA: **Tracheostomy Decannulation: Suprastomal Granulation Tissue in Perspective.** *East Centr Afr J Surg* 2010, **15(1)**:81-85.

15

Impact of high prevalence of pseudomonas and polymicrobial gram-negative infections in major sub-/total traumatic amputations on empiric antimicrobial therapy

Moritz T Giesecke, Philipp Schwabe, Florian Wichlas, Andrej Trampuz and Christian Kleber*

Abstract

Introduction: Emergency treatment of major sub-/total traumatic amputations continue to represent a clinical challenge due to high infection rates and serious handicaps. Effective treatment is based on two columns: surgery and antimicrobial therapy. Detailed identification of pathogen spectrum and epidemiology associated with these injuries is of tremendous importance as it guides the initial empiric antibiotic regimen and prevents adverse septic effents.

Methods: In this retrospective study 51 patients with major traumatic amputations (n = 16) and subtotal amputations (n = 35) treated from 2001 to 2010 in our trauma center were investigated. All patients received emergency surgery, debridement with microbiological testing within 6 h after admission and empircic antimicrobial therapy. Additionally to baseline patient characteristics, the incidence of positive standardized microbiologic testing combined with clinical signs of infection, pathogen spectrum, administered antimicrobial agents and clinical complications were analyzed.

Results: 70.6% of the patients (n = 36) acquired wound infection. In 39% wounds were contaminated on day 1, whereas the mean length of duration until first pathogen detection was 9.1 ± 13.4 days after injury. In 37% polymicrobial colonization and 28% Pseudomonas were responsible for wound infections during hospitalization. In 45% the empirc antimicrobial therapy focussed on Gram positive strains did not cover the detected bacteria, according antimicrobial resistogram. It was significantly more often found in infections associated with Pseudomonas (p 0.02) or polymicrobial wound infections.

Conclusions: This epidemiologic study reveals a pathogen shift from Gram-positive to Gram-negative strains with high incidence of Pseudomonas and polymicrobial infections in sub-/total major traumatic amputations. Therefore, empiric antimicrobial treatment historically focussing on Gram-positive strains must be adjusted. We recommend the use of Piperacillin/Tazobactam for these injuries. As soon as possible antimicrobial treatment should be changed from empiric to goal directed therapy according to the microbiological tests and resistogram results.

Keywords: Trauma, Open fracture, Amputation, Infection, Pathogen, Pseudomonas, Antimicrobial therapy

* Correspondence: christian.kleber@charite.de
Center for Musculoskeletal Surgery, AG Polytrauma, Charité - Universitätsmedizin, Augustenburger Platz 1, 13353 Berlin, Germany

Background

The emergency treatment of subtotal and total traumatic amputations (type IIIC open fractures according to the Gustilo/Anderson and type IV according to Tscherne/Oestern classification) with extensive soft tissue injury represents a clinical challenge [1-3]. Although sub-/total traumatic amputations are rare injuries, the potential risk for individual detrimental consequences are serious, including limb loss, infections, osteomyelitis, delayed or non-union, bone segmental defects, soft tissue defects and sensomotor deficits, which in turn cause major socioeconomic costs [4-7].

The successful management of open fractures and traumatic amputations is limited due to high infection rate (<50%), poor soft tissue coverage, impaired fracture healing, non-union and secondary amputation. Traumatic amputations are known to be almost always contaminated with any sort of pathogen, predominately Gram-positive strains [8]. The infection rates are associated with the severity of soft tissue damage (muscle injury, wound contamination, blood supply, reperfusion injury), application of tourniquet in the field and need of fasciotomy in compartment syndrome [1,2,6,9-12]. In particular, sub-/total traumatic amputations with ischemia are more susceptible to infections. Moreover, following vascular repair and reperfusion, severe reperfusion edema and post-ischemic compartment syndrome are observed. Reperfusion syndrome additionally impairs the restored microcirculatory perfusion and local delivery of antibiotics due to endothelial leakage and pre-capillary shunting. Furthermore, traumatic coagulopathy and coagulation factor deficiency (e.g. factor XIII) are known to additionally impair wound healing and predispose towards wound infection [13].

The two cornerstones for successful sub-/total traumatic amputation treatment are emergency surgery with bleeding control, radical debridement, temporary stabilization and early, sufficient empiric antimicrobial therapy [7,14]. Despite high infection rates up to 66%, the most effective type or combination of empiric antimicrobial agent in open fractures and traumatic amputations are still a controversy [2,6,15-18]. In the last decades Staphylococcus aureus, Staphylococcus epidermidis and Gram-negative strains have been the predominate pathogens in these injuries [8]. Empiric antimicrobial therapy is focusing on epidemiologic data, plausible pathogens and patient's specific comorbidities (e.g. allergy, diabetes). But current epidemiologic data for sub-/total traumatic amputations are not available and microbiological spectrum and corresponding bacterial resistances are changing over the time.

Therefore, this study aimed to retrospectively analyze the characteristics, epidemiologic microbiological pathogen spectrum, incidence of multi-resistant pathogens, the efficiency of antimicrobial therapy, the incidence of multiple trauma and coagulopathy of all sub-/total traumatic amputations, treated in our center.

Methods

In this retrospective study we included 51 sub-/total traumatic amputations treated at the Campus Virchow Klinikum, Charité - Universitätsmedizin between 2001 and 2010. Due to the retrospective and observational character of the study no approval by our local ethic committee has been necessary.

Inclusion criteria

- Major sub-/total traumatic amputation (type IV Gustilo/Anderson Anderson and Tscherne/Oestern; n = 16) [2,3]
- Severe open fractures with vascular injury and large soft tissue injury (>5 cm defect or more than loss of 3/4 of circumference; type IIIC Gustilo/Anderson and type IV Tscherne/Oestern; n = 35) [2,3].

Exclusion criteria

- Type IIIc open fractures with <5 cm soft tissue defect or <3/4 of circumference [2]
- Minor traumatic amputations (finger, toe)
- Survival <24 hours or patients dying before obtaining microbiological test
- Lack of substantial information in medical record.

The baseline characteristics (gender, age, trauma mechanism, injury type, anatomical fracture location (AO classification) and following parameters were recorded:

- Abbreviated Injury Scale (AIS) and Injury Severity Score (ISS)
- Hanover Polytrauma Score (PTS)
- Clinical signs of wound infection (rubor, calor, dolor, wound secretion)
- Microbiological testing (swab, tissue, wound secretion)
- Pathogen type (Gram positive/negative)
- Laboratory findings (white blood count (WBC), C-reactive protein (CRP))
- Type and sufficiency of antimicobial therapy
- Risk factors for infection (diabetes, immune deficiency, compartment syndrome, arterial occlusive disease, nicotine/alcohol abuse)
- Length of hospital stay and critical care
- Type and number of surgical procedures, revisions and use of negative pressure wound therapy (NPWT/VAC)

- Late complications (osteomyelitis, removal of osteosynthesis materials due to infection, secondary amputation).

The leading injury was defined as the body region (head, face/neck, thorax, abdomen, extremities) with the highest AIS score. Polytrauma was classified according to ISS >15 and severe polytrauma ISS >25.

Traumatic coagulopathy on admission, negatively influencing wound healing, microcirculation and the clinical course of open fractures, was defined by INR >1.2 and/or platelet count <100 000/nl [13,19].

Microbiological assessment and definition of wound infections

All microbiological tests of the 51 patients were screened for pathogen type, number of simultaneous pathogens, resistance towards administered antimicrobial agent and time until positive pathogen proof.

Microbiological specimens (i.e. wound swabs, tissue samples, drain fluids) were obtained during surgery before debridement and administration of antibiotic therapy. Within operation at least 2 wound swabs (superficial and deep) were obtained. Based on surgeon's decision additionally tissue samples were obtain under sterile conditions. Drains were standardized removed within 2 days after surgery except high amount of wound secretion. Therefore, drain fluids were tested in case of persisting secretion >48 hours after surgery. Initial surgical debridement was performed within 2 hours after injury, followed by staged surgical debridement until conditioning of soft tissue or plastic surgery, depending on the clinical situation. Specimens were sent native (i.e. without transport media) and cultivated within 6 hours of sampling, except patient arrived at night, then samples were cultivated next morning. Samples were plated on sheep blood agar plates and incubated for 7 days under aerobic and anaerobic conditions at 37°C; an aliquot was in addition inoculated in thioglycolate broth. Identification and susceptibility testing of grown microorganisms were performed as standard microbiological methods. Wound cultures on day 1 refer to intraoperative microbiological samples collected before the first surgical debridement and antibiotic therapy, reflecting the incidence and spectrum of initial wound contamination.

Wound infection was defined as the proof of at least one pathogenic species in microbiological testing combined with clinical signs of infection (fever, pus, rubor, odor, macerated soft tissue) and elevated laboratory infectious parameter (WBC, CRP). A wound infection occurring within 14 days after trauma was defined as an early infection. Simultaneous detection of more than one pathogen species in the same sample was classified as polymicrobial wound infection. The initially applied antibiotic therapy was considered to be insufficient, if proven so by the microbiological resistance determination via antibiogram.

Surgical management

Our algorithm for limb salvage and surgical decision making was published in 2010 and performed with the help of the Mangled Extremity Severity Score ≥7, injury severity (polytrauma: "life before limb") and physiologic parameters (base deficit, lactate, blood pressure, and coagulopathy [6,20].

Out of 42 cases (82%) of limb salvage, revascularization was successfully performed in 37 cases (73%). In 18% primary (n = 9), 14% (n = 7) macro-replantation and 10% (n = 5) secondary amputation was performed.

Our soft tissue management is guided by the degree of open fracture, contusions, contamination and defect size. According to secondary swelling with progressive soft tissue necrosis and compartment syndrome primary wound closure in type III open fractures was an exception. In our protocol we performed open amputations in case of primary amputation. Criteria for stump formation were clean wean, no pathogen proof obtained in the microbiological test in the prior operation and no need for surgical debridement. We covered the soft tissue defects in type III open fractures with Epigard® + dry dressing in 44 patients, 5 open wound treatment with initial dry dressing and 1 primary NPWT. In 1 case primary wound closure was possible. The dressings were changed at least once every day. NPWT was used in 25 patients (49%) and were changed between 2–5 days according to wound conditions while surgery and results of microbiological testing.

Multiple trauma patients were treated according to their injury severity and hemodynamic constitution with life before limb principle for in extremis patients and damage control orthopedic surgery for hemodynamic unstable patients.

Statistic

Statistical analysis was conducted by use of PASW statistics 21.0 (IBM, USA; Mann–Whitney-/ Wilcoxon test). Continuous variables were described with standard variation (±) and p-values <0.05 were considered as statistically significant.

Results

Characteristics

51 patients were included in this study (male/female: n = 42/9; 82/18%, mean age: 37.5 ± 13.4 years, 62.7% coagulopathy at admission, 7.8% mortality rate). The length of hospitalization in non-survivors (mean 39 ± 42.4 days; range 16–103 days) compared to survivors (mean 39.5 ± 20.4 days;

range 7–103 days) showed no statistical significant difference. Therefore, non-survivors were not excluded from analysis.

The mean injury severity was 24.7 ± 13.0 points for ISS and 34.8 ± 20.7 points for PTS. 62% were polytraumatized (n = 31, ISS > 15 points) and 52.9% suffered a severe polytrauma (n = 27, ISS >25 points). The trauma mechanisms are shown in Table 1.

In polytraumatized patients the most common injury according to the AIS was extremity trauma (n = 39; 76.5%), followed by chest trauma (n = 9; 17.6%) and abdomen trauma (n = 3; 5.9%). The anatomic location of the open fractures are shown in Figure 1.

Risk factors for infection

Risk factors for wound infection were negligible (Table 2). We found no significant difference for the rate of wound infections in patient's with-/out risk factors or/and compartment syndrome.

Injuries

68.6% of the patients sustained subtotal (n = 35) and 31.4% total traumatic amputation (n = 16). No statistical significant differences was found for subtotal and total traumatic amputation referring injury severity, hospitalization (39.1 ± 22.4, range 7–103 days), ICU-days (11.9 ± 14.2, range 0–78 days), survival, acute (OF:51%/n = 18; amputation: 69%/n = 11) and total infection rate (OF:66%/n = 23; amputation: 81%/n = 13), type of infection, number and type of needed surgical interventions. Also no differences for the above listed parameters were detected for limb salvage (72.6%; n = 37), primary (17.6%; n = 9) and secondary amputation (9.8%; n = 5). But the mean ISS showed a trend to primary (27.9 ± 12.5 points) and secondary amputation (28.8 ± 15.1 points) compared to limb salvage group (23.3 ± 13 points). Severe polytrauma (ISS > 25) was more frequent in primary (67%) and secondary amputation (60%) compared to limb salvage group (49%).

The number of surgical interventions was 4.4 ± 3.6 for limb salvage, 4.3 ± 3.2 for primary amputation and 9.2 ± 4.4 for secondary amputations. We observed a higher number operations in the secondary compared to the primary amputation and limb salvage group (p 0.04).

The analysis of common laboratory testing (CRP, leucocyte count) revealed no association with the incidence and type of infection.

The traumatic coagulopathy was significantly associated with higher injury severity (PTS p 0.003, ISS p 0.008), severe polytrauma (p 0.02), increased number of surgical revisions (p 0.003) and most relevant, significantly higher infection rate (p 0.03).

In 47.1% (n = 24) late complications occurred (45.8% osteomyelitis, 25% early implant removal due to infection, 29.2% secondary amputation).

Microbiological findings

In total more than two thirds of the patients (70.6%, n = 36) acquired a wound infections during their hospitalization. The rate of polymicrobial wound infections and Pseudomonas infections in all patients (n = 51) during hospitalization were 37.3% (n = 19) and 27.5% (n = 14), respectively. 14 out of 36 patients with wound infections had a positive Pseudomonas wound swab (38.9%) during hospitalization, in which 50%/n = 7 were detected within 72 hours after admission. The distribution of 14 pseudomonas species have been: 9 P. aeruginosa, 2 P. putida and 1 P. oryzihabitans, P.fluorescens and Aeromonas hydrphilia, respectively.

First pathogen proof

In 38.9% (n = 14) the first microbiologic test, obtained under sterile conditions within 2 hours after trauma, was positive, indicating that nearly 40% are admitted with contaminated wounds. In contrast, the first positive pathogen proof within several surgical debridement was detected in mean 9.1 ± 13.4 days (range 1–61 days) after injury. Epidemiologic analyses of all pathogen revealed polymicrobial infections (25.5%/n = 13) and Pseudomonas (23.5%/n = 12) as the most frequently detected pathogen in the first positive microbiological testing. Polymicrobial infections assembled in 51.9% from gram-negative and positive strains, 25.9% more than one gram-negative strain and 7.4% more than one gram-positive strain.

Early infections

In 56.9% (n = 29) patients fulfilled the criteria of an early infection within 14 days after trauma. In 25.5% (n = 13)

Table 1 Trauma mechanism in sub-/total traumatic amputation

	Trauma mechanism							
Injury pattern	**Fall**	**Pedestrian vs. train**	**Motor-cyclist**	**Pedestrian vs. auto**	**Bicyclist**	**Vehicle occupant**	**Other**	**Total n**
Type IIIC open fracture	11	6	5	6	3	2	2	35
Amputation	1	6	5	2	1	1	0	16
Total	12	12	10	8	4	3	2	51

Distribution of injury pattern according to underlying trauma mechanism in type IIIC open fractures (subtotal amputations) and total traumatic amputations.

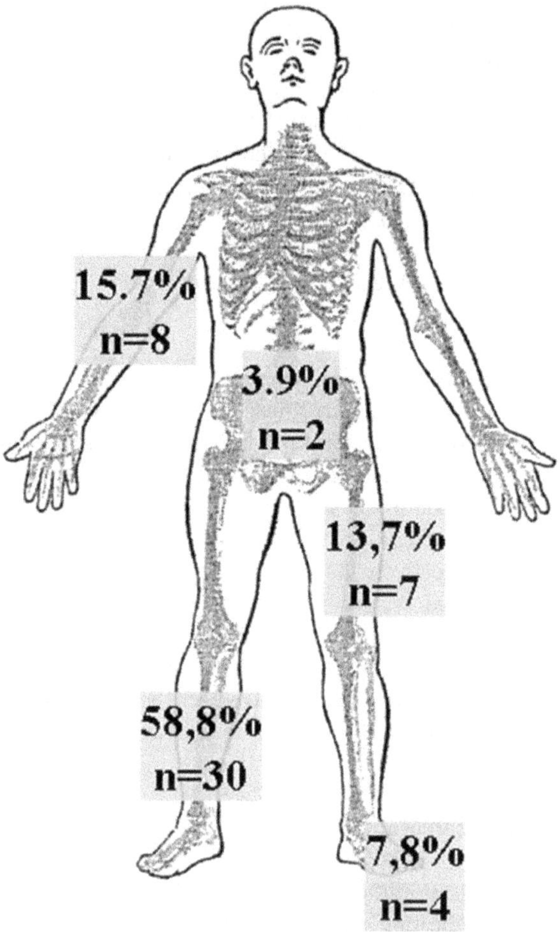

Figure 1 Anatomic location of sub-/total traumatic amputations. The lower leg was the predominate injured body region followed by the upper extremity.

Pseudomonas species and 23.5% polymicrobial infection (n = 12) were detected in the first positive microbiologic test within 14 days.

An overview of the epidemiology of pathogens in open fractures and amputations during hospitalization is shown in Table 3 and the temporal distribution of positive pathogen proof in Figure 2.

Table 2 Risk factors for infection

Risk factor	Incidence	
	n	Total %
Diabetes	1	2
Immune deficiency	0	0
Arterial occlusive disease	1	2
Smoker	3	5.9
Alcohol abuse	1	2
Compartment syndrome	8	15.7

Risk factors in 51 patients with type IIIC open fractures (subtotal-) and traumatic amputations to acquire infection.

Patients with acute Pseudomonas wound infections within 14 days after trauma (n = 13, NPWT 85%, p 0.01) and Pseudomonas wound infections while hospitalization (n = 14, NPWT 79%, p 0.03) were significantly more often treated with negative pressure wound therapy (NPWT) compared to no acute (n = 38, NPWT 37%) or no Pseudomonas wound infection (n = 37, NPWT 38%). We observed no methicillin-resistant Staphylococcus aureus (MRSA) but 13.7% (n = 7) carbapenem-resistant Gram-negative strains. The carbapenem-resistant Gram-negative pathogens were detected at mean 17 ± 10 days (Range 3-31days) after injury.

Neither the incidence of early wound infection nor the fact of completed sufficient initial antibiotic therapy did show a significant effect on the length of critical care treatment and hospitalization period. Also the number of revision surgeries conducted to reach wound closure, soft tissue coverage and skeletal reconstruction did also not significantly differ in patients with early wound infections compared to patients without wound infection. Furthermore, no relation was found between the injury severity and infection rate. Additionally, the injury severity according to ISS and PTS had no significant impact on the incidence of a Pseudomonas or polymicrobial wound infection. We found also no statistical significant differences referring the infection rate, acute infection, Pseudomonas infection, combined infections and appropriate antimicrobial treatment in polytrauma (ISS > 15 points) and severe polytrauma (ISS >25 points) compared to non polytraumatized patients.

Antimicrobial therapy

All 51 patients received empiric antibiotic therapy after admission. The most common antibiotic agents and frequency of application are shown in Table 4.

Initial antimicrobial mono-therapy (aminopenicillin plus a beta-lactamase inhibitor) was performed in 66.7% (n = 33) while 29.4% (n = 15) received a double antibiotic therapy. In 45.1% the empiric antibiotic therapy was insufficient according to the later reported microbiological findings and antibiogram. Additionally, the insufficient antibiotic therapy according antibiogram was significantly associated with an increase of Pseudomonas wound infection (<14 days p 0.05; during hospitalization p 0.02).

Discussion

Open fractures and major traumatic amputations are typically observed among high-energy velocity victims. Appropriate therapeutic management of these severe and rare injuries, including radical debridement, microsurgical revascularization and replantation belongs to the most advanced techniques in orthopedic surgery and requires enormous experience.

Table 3 Epidemiology of pathogens in sub-/total traumatic amputation

	Pathogen	1st wound culture n	Acute infection (<14d) n	Total n
Bacteria				
Aerobic				
Gram-positive	Staphylococcus aureus	4	2	7
	Bacillus cereus	6	5	6
	Enterococcus faecalis	2	2	5
	Staphylococcus epidermidis	2	2	4
	Enterococcus faecium	3	1	3
	Staphylococcus saprophyticus	1	1	1
	Staphylococcus capitis	0	1	1
	Streptococcus spp.	1	1	1
	Rothia mucilaginosa	1	1	1
	Lactobacillus spp.	1	1	1
Gram-negative	**Pseudomonas spp.**	**12**	**13**	**14**
	E.coli	3	3	5
	Enterobacter spp.	2	2	5
	Acinetobacter spp.	3	3	3
	Pantoea agglomerans	3	3	3
	Stenotrophomonas spp.	0	1	2
	Acromobacter spp.	0	1	2
	Klebsiella spp.	0	1	1
	Proteus spp.	0	0	1
	Chryseomonas luteola	1	1	1
	Acromonas hydrophila	1	1	1
Anaerobic				
	Bacteroides fragiles	1	1	1
	Fusobacterium spp.	1	1	1
	Anaerococcus prevotei	1	1	1
	Clostridium spp.	0	1	1
Fungi				
	Candida spp.	1	0	3
	Aspergillus spp.	1	1	2
	Paecilomyces ilacinus	0	0	1
	Seedosporium spp.	0	0	1
	Mucor spp.	1	1	1
	Fusarium spp.	1	1	1
	Combined pathogens (>1 species simultaneously)	**13**	**12**	**19**

Pathogen spectrum of 51 patients with type IIIC open fractures (subtotal-) and traumatic amputations; spp = species. Highest incidence of Pseudomonas spp. and combined pathogens (bolt letters).

Injuries and coagulopathy

The predominantly injured body region in our collective was the lower leg, which confirms the findings of various other studies [5,18,21-27]. Notably, most of the studies exclusively investigated open fractures (type I-III) of the lower leg, whereas our study includes all major traumatic amputations and only type IIIC open fracture within the study period [9,11,28-31]. More than half of the patients included in our study were severely polytraumatized (ISS >25 points). We could not find a significant relation

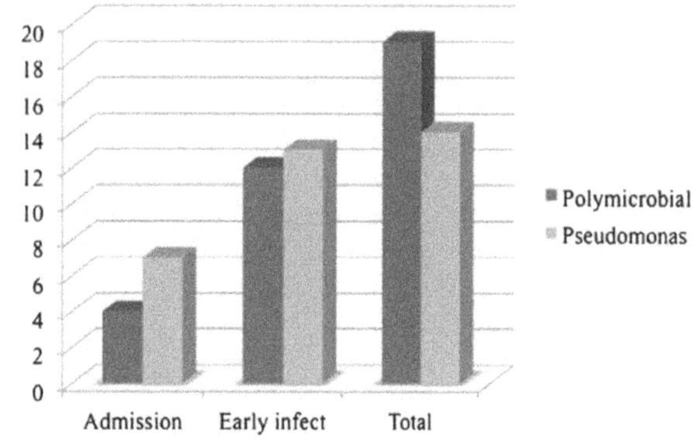

Figure 2 Temporal incidence of positive polymicrobial and Pseudomonas pathogen proof. Temporal distribution of positive polymicrobial and Pseudomonas pathogen proof in sub-/total traumatic amputations; y-axis: days after trauma; x-axis: admission: Specimen obtain within emergency surgery; early infect: positive pathogen proof within 14 days after trauma; total: incidence of positive pathogen proof within hospitalization period.

between injury severity and infection rate in our study, confirming previously published data for battlefield injuries [12]. We postulate that the individual posttraumatic immune response predispose for infection due to immune depression or pro-inflammatory reactions, not measurable by an anatomical injury severity score [32]. We definitely suggest a specific subgroup of polytrauma patients to be susceptible to acquire infection. Therefore, we need immunological tools to detect and characterize posttraumatic immune response and allocate an individual risk guiding decision-making in polytrauma [32]. In contrast, traumatic coagulopathy was significantly associated with higher infection rate and higher injury severity. Our data suggest that traumatic coagulopathy predisposes for wound infections underscoring the recent detected cross talk of complement system and coagulation factors [33]. We found no statistically significant differences for wound infections in subtotal traumatic amputation and primary major traumatic amputations. It is conceivable, that at this high level of severe soft tissue damage with ischemia in both injury types the already high risk of wound infection does not further increase. Comparison with previous publications is critical, because most studies include all types of open fractures and no traumatic amputation injuries [34-36].

Table 4 Antimicrobial therapy

Antibiotic agent	n	%
Ampicillin/Sulbactam	25	49.0
Ampicillin/Sulbactam + Clindamycin	5	9.8
Amoxycillin/Clavulanic acid	4	7.8
Cefuroxime	3	5.9
Cefuroxime + Clindamycin	2	3.9
Ceftriaxone + Clindamycin	2	3.9
Ciprofloxacin + Clindamycin	2	3.9
Clindamycin	2	3.9

Empiric antimicrobial therapy and frequency of application.

Microbiology

Due to exclusively type IIIc open fracture the rate of wound infections (70.6%) in our study exceeds the infection rates of previously published data (5-40%) supporting the fact, that the infection rate is strongly related to the extend of the soft tissue injury and vascularization [2,6,15,16,37].

The epidemiologic part of this study revealed a shift from Gram-positive to Gram-negative pathogens in subtotal and total traumatic amputation compared to literature [1,8]. We observed a high rate of Pseudomonas and polymicrobial wound infections already at admission to the hospital within emergency operation less then 2 hours after trauma and within hospitalization. This fact indicates the change of natural pathogen environment. Especially Pseudomonas was considered as a late hospitalization infection [12]. We detect a unique high Pseudomonas infection rate of 39% compared to the literature [8,11,34]. Furthermore, in our clinical experience we observe more and more primary Gram-negative contaminations or infections also in type II/IIIa/IIIb open fractures. For us, there is a clear trend towards Gram-negative strains in open fractures.

The use of NPWT is a controversy with positive and negative effects [31,38-40]. In our study we found a significant association between Pseudomonas wound infection and treatment with NPWT. A study revealed the NPWT foam as a hatchery for especially Pseudomonas. Therefore, NPWT has also disadvantages and should not be abused to delay or substitute plastic surgery in traumatic amputations [41]. Temporary soft tissue coverage with artificial skin coverage (Epigard®) or dry dressings can induce moistening and maceration of the wound. The humid wound atmosphere, fluid collections, bradytrophic tissue in an environment of Gram-positive focused empiric antimicrobial therapy might lead to a survival advantage and secondary selection of Gram-negative pathogens. Additionally the abuse of antimicrobial therapy combined with NPWT has the potential to select multiresistant pathogens, e.g. the carbapenem-resistant Gram-negative strains in our study. All multiple resistances were detected after hospitalization and under antimicrobial therapy at mean 10 days after trauma.

In contrast, the initial temporary vacuum-assisted wound coverage followed by early wound closure or plastic surgery has the potential to lower the secondary infection rates with Gram-negative rods, especially Pseudomonas, because of droughty effects on the wound side and removal of fluid collections predisposed for bacterial secondary colonization with hospitality pathogens in the future.

Antimicrobial therapy

The change of pathogen spectrum to Gram-negative strains has tremendous impact on the choice of empiric antimicrobial therapy and morbidity of our patients. Former empiric therapy focused on the reported epidemiologic data from 1990s with predominate Gram-positive strains. Therefore, we detect in 45% of our patients the empiric antibiotic regimen as insufficient and were significantly associated with Pseudomonas or polymicrobial wound infections. The data of this study clearly indicate the need to adjust the empiric antimicrobial therapy for type IIIc open fractures and traumatic amputations. However, remarkable controversy exists about the use of antibiotic therapy and guidelines similar to e.g. the 2013 WSES guidelines for intra-abdominal infections are absent [42,43].

Successful treatment of open fractures and traumatic amputations has two cornerstones, sufficient empiric antimicrobial therapy in combination with immediate radical surgical debridement [1,6,10,15,18,31]. We recommend the use of empiric antimicrobial therapy in sub-/total traumatic amputations with Piperacillin/Tazobactam (4.5 g i.v. 3 times per day) [44]. In case of penicillin allergy but no type I allergy (quincke edema, anaphylaxis) we use Cefepim (2 g i.v. 3 times per day). In type I penicillin allergy we use a combination of ether Vancomycin or Daptomycin in combination with Gentamicin or Ciprofloxacin. We always tried to preserve Ciprofloxacin as the only oral Pseudomonas active agent for ambulant long-term treatment of our patients. As soon as available we change from empiric to goal directed antimicrobial treatment according to the microbiological test and resistogram results.

Conclusions

This epidemiologic study reveals a pathogen shift from Gram-positive to Gram-negative strains with high incidence of Pseudomonas and combined pathogen infections in type IIIC open fractures and major traumatic amputations. Therefore, empiric antimicrobial treatment must be adjusted. We recommend the use of Piperacillin/Tazobactam in sub-/total traumatic amputations. As soon as available antimicrobial treatment must change from empiric to goal directed therapy according to the microbiological test and resistogram results.

Competing interests

There is no conflict of interest. The corresponding author affirms that he has no relationships with a company whose product is mentioned in the article or with one that sells a competitive product. The presentation is impartial and the content is independent of commercial influence.

Authors' contributions

MTG: conception and study design, data acquisition, manuscript drafting. PS: data acquisition, manuscript revision. FW: data analysis and interpretation, manuscript revision. AT: conception and study design, data analysis and interpretation, manuscript revision. CK: conception and study design, data analysis and interpretation, manuscript drafting. All authors read and approved the final manuscript.

Acknowledgements

Contributions of Dr. med. C. Kleber were made possible by DFG funding through the Berlin-Brandenburg School for Regenerative Therapies GSC 203.

References

1. Gustilo RB, Anderson JT: **Prevention of infection in the treatment of one thousand and twenty-five open fractures of long bones: retrospective and prospective analyses.** *J Bone Joint Surg Am* 1976, **58**(4):453–458.
2. Gustilo RB, Mendoza RM, Williams DN: **Problems in the management of type III (severe) open fractures: a new classification of type III open fractures.** *J Trauma* 1984, **24**(8):742–746.
3. Tscherne H, Oestern HJ: **[A new classification of soft-tissue damage in open and closed fractures (author's transl)].** *Unfallheilkunde* 1982, **85**(3):111–115.
4. Dillingham TR, Pezzin LE, MacKenzie EJ: **Incidence, acute care length of stay, and discharge to rehabilitation of traumatic amputee patients: an epidemiologic study.** *Arch Phys Med Rehabil* 1998, **79**(3):279–287.
5. Court-Brown CM, Rimmer S, Prakash U, McQueen MM: **The epidemiology of open long bone fractures.** *Injury* 1998, **29**(7):529–534.
6. Schwabe P, Haas NP, Schaser KD: **Fractures of the extremities with severe open soft tissue damage. Initial management and reconstructive treatment strategies.** *Unfallchirurg* 2010, **113**(8):647–670. quiz 671–642.
7. Kleber CHN: **Biologics in open fractures.** *Surg Orthop Traumatol* 2013, doi:10.1007/978-3-642-34746.7_199 Springer-Verlag Berlin Heidelberg 2013.
8. Robinson D, On E, Hadas N, Halperin N, Hofman S, Boldur I: **Microbiologic flora contaminating open fractures: its significance in the choice of primary antibiotic agents and the likelihood of deep wound infection.** *J Orthop Trauma* 1989, **3**(4):283–286.
9. Yokoyama K, Itoman M, Nakamura K, Uchino M, Nitta H, Kojima Y: **New scoring system predicting the occurrence of deep infection in open upper and lower extremity fractures: efficacy in retrospective re-scoring.** *Arch Orthop Trauma Surg* 2009, **129**(4):469–474.
10. Lenarz CJ, Watson JT, Moed BR, Israel H, Mullen JD, Macdonald JB: **Timing of wound closure in open fractures based on cultures obtained after debridement.** *J Bone Joint Surg Am* 2010, **92**(10):1921–1926.
11. Khatod M, Botte MJ, Hoyt DB, Meyer RS, Smith JM, Akeson WH: **Outcomes in open tibia fractures: relationship between delay in treatment and infection.** *J Trauma* 2003, **55**(5):949–954.
12. Brown KV, Murray CK, Clasper JC: **Infectious complications of combat-related mangled extremity injuries in the British military.** *J Trauma* 2010, **69**(Suppl 1):S109–S115.
13. Stutz CM, O'Rear LD, O'Neill KR, Tamborski ME, Crosby CG, Devin CJ, Schoenecker JG: **Coagulopathies in orthopaedics: links to inflammation and the potential of individualizing treatment strategies.** *J Orthop Trauma* 2013, **27**(4):236–241.
14. Gosselin RA, Roberts I, Gillespie WJ: **Antibiotics for preventing infection in open limb fractures.** *Cochrane Database Syst Rev* 2004, **1**:CD003764.
15. Patzakis MJ, Bains RS, Lee J, Shepherd L, Singer G, Ressler R, Harvey F, Holtom P: **Prospective, randomized, double-blind study comparing single-agent antibiotic therapy, ciprofloxacin, to combination antibiotic therapy in open fracture wounds.** *J Orthop Trauma* 2000, **14**(8):529–533.
16. Patzakis MJ, Wilkins J: **Factors influencing infection rate in open fracture wounds.** *Clin Orthop Relat Res* 1989, **243**:36–40.
17. Stannard JP, Volgas DA, Stewart R, McGwin G Jr, Alonso JE: **Negative pressure wound therapy after severe open fractures: a prospective randomized study.** *J Orthop Trauma* 2009, **23**(8):552–557.
18. Al-Arabi YB, Nader M, Hamidian-Jahromi AR, Woods DA: **The effect of the timing of antibiotics and surgical treatment on infection rates in open long-bone fractures: a 9-year prospective study from a district general hospital.** *Injury* 2007, **38**(8):900–905.
19. Richardson VR, Cordell P, Standeven KF, Carter AM: **Substrates of Factor XIII-A: roles in thrombosis and wound healing.** *Clin Sci (Lond)* 2013, **124**(3):123–137.

20. Helfet DL, Howey T, Sanders R, Johansen K: **Limb salvage versus amputation. Preliminary results of the mangled extremity severity score.** *Clin Orthop Relat Res* 1990, **256:**80–86.
21. Barmparas G, Inaba K, Teixeira PG, Dubose JJ, Criscuoli M, Talving P, Plurad D, Green D, Demetriades D: **Epidemiology of post-traumatic limb amputation: a national trauma databank analysis.** *Am Surg* 2010, **76**(11):1214–1222.
22. Dellinger EP, Miller SD, Wertz MJ, Grypma M, Droppert B, Anderson PA: **Risk of infection after open fracture of the arm or leg.** *Arch Surg* 1988, **123**(11):1320–1327.
23. DeLong WG Jr, Born CT, Wei SY, Petrik ME, Ponzio R, Schwab CW: **Aggressive treatment of 119 open fracture wounds.** *J Trauma* 1999, **46**(6):1049–1054.
24. Busse JW, Jacobs CL, Swiontkowski MF, Bosse MJ, Bhandari M: **Complex limb salvage or early amputation for severe lower-limb injury: a meta-analysis of observational studies.** *J Orthop Trauma* 2007, **21**(1):70–76.
25. Harley BJ, Beaupre LA, Jones CA, Dulai SK, Weber DW: **The effect of time to definitive treatment on the rate of nonunion and infection in open fractures.** *J Orthop Trauma* 2002, **16**(7):484–490.
26. Mirzayan R, Itamura JM, Vangsness CT Jr, Holtom PD, Sherman R, Patzakis MJ: **Management of chronic deep infection following rotator cuff repair.** *J Bone Joint Surg Am* 2000, **82-A**(8):1115–1121.
27. Seligson D, Ostermann PA, Henry SL, Wolley T: **The management of open fractures associated with arterial injury requiring vascular repair.** *J Trauma* 1994, **37**(6):938–940.
28. Seekamp A, Regel G, Ruffert S, Ziegler M, Tscherne H: **Amputation or reconstruction of IIIB and IIIC open tibial fracture. Decision criteria in the acute phase and late functional outcome.** *Unfallchirurg* 1998, **101**(5):360–369.
29. Sirkin M, Sanders R, DiPasquale T, Herscovici D Jr: **A staged protocol for soft tissue management in the treatment of complex pilon fractures.** *J Orthop Trauma* 2004, **18**(8 Suppl):S32–S38.
30. Cole JD, Ansel LJ, Schwartzberg R: **A sequential protocol for management of severe open tibial fractures.** *Clin Orthop Relat Res* 1995, **315:**84–103.
31. Melvin JS, Dombroski DG, Torbert JT, Kovach SJ, Esterhai JL, Mehta S: **Open tibial shaft fractures: I. Evaluation and initial wound management.** *J Am Acad Orthop Surg* 2010, **18**(1):10–19.
32. Kleber C, Becker CA, Schmidt-Bleek K, Schaser KD, Haas NP: **Are pentraxin 3 and transsignaling early markers for immunologic injury severity in polytrauma? a pilot study.** *Clin Orthop Relat Res* 2013, **471**(9):2822–2830. doi:10.1007/s11999-013-2922-x.
33. Amara U, Flierl MA, Rittirsch D, Klos A, Chen H, Acker B, Bruckner UB, Nilsson B, Gebhard F, Lambris JD, Huber-Lang M: **Molecular intercommunication between the complement and coagulation systems.** *J Immunol* 2010, **185**(9):5628–5636.
34. Akinyoola AL, Oginni LM, Adegbehingbe OO, Orimolade EA, Ogundele OJ: **Causes of limb amputations in Nigerian children.** *West Afr J Med* 2006, **25**(4):273–275.
35. McIntosh J, Earnshaw JJ: **Antibiotic prophylaxis for the prevention of infection after major limb amputation.** *Eur J Vasc Endovasc Surg* 2009, **37**(6):696–703.
36. Sadat U, Chaudhuri A, Hayes PD, Gaunt ME, Boyle JR, Varty K: **Five day antibiotic prophylaxis for major lower limb amputation reduces wound infection rates and the length of in-hospital stay.** *Eur J Vasc Endovasc Surg* 2008, **35**(1):75–78.
37. Stannard JP, Atkins BZ, O'Malley D, Singh H, Bernstein B, Fahey M, Masden D, Attinger CE: **Use of negative pressure therapy on closed surgical incisions: a case series.** *Ostomy Wound Manage* 2009, **55**(8):58–66.
38. Dedmond BT, Kortesis B, Punger K, Simpson J, Argenta J, Kulp B, Morykwas M, Webb LX: **The use of negative-pressure wound therapy (NPWT) in the temporary treatment of soft-tissue injuries associated with high-energy open tibial shaft fractures.** *J Orthop Trauma* 2007, **21**(1):11–17.
39. Herscovici D Jr, Sanders RW, Scaduto JM, Infante A, DiPasquale T: **Vacuum-assisted wound closure (VAC therapy) for the management of patients with high-energy soft tissue injuries.** *J Orthop Trauma* 2003, **17**(10):683–688.
40. Labler L, Trentz O: **The use of vacuum assisted closure (VAC) in soft tissue injuries after high energy pelvic trauma.** *Langenbecks Arch Surg* 2007, **392**(5):601–609.
41. Yusuf E, Jordan X, Clauss M, Borens O, Mader M, Trampuz A: **High bacterial load in negative pressure wound therapy (NPWT) foams used in the treatment of chronic wounds.** *Wound Repair Regen* 2013, **21**(5):677–681.
42. Hauser CJ, Adams CA Jr, Eachempati SR: **Surgical infection society guideline: prophylactic antibiotic use in open fractures: an evidence-based guideline.** *Surg Infect (Larchmt)* 2006, **7**(4):379–405.
43. Sartelli M, Viale P, Catena F, Ansaloni L, Moore E, Malangoni M, Moore FA, Velmahos G, Coimbra R, Ivatury R, Peitzman A, Koike K, Leppaniemi A, Biffl W, Burlew CC, Balogh ZJ, Boffard K, Bendinelli C, Gupta S, Kluger Y, Agresta F, Di Saverio S, Wani I, Escalona A, Ordonez C, Fraga GP, Junior GA, Bala M, Cui Y, Marwah S, *et al*: **2013 WSES guidelines for management of intra-abdominal infections.** *World J Emerg Surg* 2013, **8**(1):3.
44. Kleber CTA: **Antibiotic prophylaxis and therapy in orthopedic and traumatology surgery _ What, When and How long to administer?** *OP-Journal* 2014, **30:**8–10.

Proposal for a recovery prediction method for patients affected by acute mediastinitis

Sławomir Jabłoński[1*] and Marcin Kozakiewicz[2]

Abstract

Background: An attempt to find a prediction method of death risk in patients affected by acute mediastinitis. There is not such a tool described in available literature for that serious disease.

Methods: The study comprised 44 consecutive cases of acute mediastinitis. General anamnesis and biochemical data were included. Factor analysis was used to extract the risk characteristic for the patients. The most valuable results were obtained for 8 parameters which were selected for further statistical analysis (all collected during few hours after admission). Three factors reached Eigenvalue >1. Clinical explanations of these combined statistical factors are: Factor1 - proteinic status (serum total protein, albumin, and hemoglobin level), Factor2 - inflammatory status (white blood cells, CRP, procalcitonin), and Factor3 - general risk (age, number of coexisting diseases). Threshold values of prediction factors were estimated by means of statistical analysis (factor analysis, Statgraphics Centurion XVI).

Results: The final prediction result for the patients is constructed as simultaneous evaluation of all factor scores. High probability of death should be predicted if factor 1 value decreases with simultaneous increase of factors 2 and 3. The diagnostic power of the proposed method was revealed to be high [sensitivity =90%, specificity =64%], for Factor1 [SNC = 87%, SPC = 79%]; for Factor2 [SNC = 87%, SPC = 50%] and for Factor3 [SNC = 73%, SPC = 71%].

Conclusion: The proposed prediction method seems a useful emergency signal during acute mediastinitis control in affected patients.

Introduction

Severe sepsis is still a major cause of postoperative morbidity and mortality after surgery in patients with acute mediastinitis (AM). The disease is characterized by rapid and severe course and poor prognosis despite undertaken on time aggressive surgical management and supportive treatment in the intensive care conditions. The cause of the failure of the treatment is complex. Local anatomical conditions favor the infection spread in mediastinal anatomical loose tissues and the systemic reaction to infection [1]. An association is emphasized between the increase in mortality and the delay in surgical intervention [1-4]. The etiology of AM does not remain insignificant. The best chance of survival have the patients previously healthy without earlier mediastinal pathologies in whom infection develops as a result of injury or as a complication related to endoscopic diagnostic procedures [5-7]. If the disease develops in a patient with previous history of diseases, especially of carcinoma or as the result of complications related to thoracosurgical or cardiosurgical procedures, the death risk increases [8-10]. It should be expected that a number of factors can affect the final prognosis e.g. age, etiology, delay in diagnosis, the type of surgical procedure, the kind and number of coexisting diseases, the type of a pathogen, postoperative complications and others.

The management in this severe disease could facilitate categorizing patients into appropriate risk groups in order to undertake the most optimal treatment strategy for the developing severe sepsis. Working out a simple prognostic scale on the basis of the data obtained from the medical history, clinical examination, diagnostic imaging and preliminary biochemical investigations can be one of the useful solutions. Similar prognostic scales are applied in other diseases such as e.g. acute pancreatitis: the Acute Physiology and Chronic Health Evaluation

* Correspondence: jablonski_s@vp.pl
[1]Department of Thoracic Surgery, General and Oncological Surgery, Medical University of Lodz, 113 Żeromskiego St., 90-547, Łódź, Poland

(APACHE II) scale, Ranson criteria, the Atlanta Classification of Severe Acute Pancreatitis [11-13]. Scales trying to determine the prognosis for severely sick patients have also been created e.g.: Nutritional Risk Index (NRI) [14,15] and Prognostic Inflammatory and Nutritional Index(PINI) [16].

To date no method has been available for the evaluation of the probability of recovery if a patient is affected by acute mediastinitis.

Therefore, we attempt to find a clinically useful preoperative method of predicting the prognosis for patients with AM on the basis of clinical examination and simple laboratory investigations.

Material and methods

In the years 1998–2010, at the Department of Thoracic Surgery, General and Oncological Surgery of the Medical University of Lodz, there were treated 44 consecutive patients with AM. The study group comprised the patients fulfilling modified criteria of mediastinitis diagnosis worked out by Esterra et al. [17], which in the original version were related to descending necrotizing mediastinitis: (1) clinical manifestation of severe infection; (2) demonstration of AM etiological factors; (3) characteristic radiological picture of mediastanitis; (4) isolation of the pathogen in microbiological cultures from the mediastinal area; (5) intraoperative or postmortem documentation of mediastinitis. Exponents of sepsis in the form of: fever, tachycardia, hyperventilation and leucocytosis were observed in all patients.

The study was given an approval by the institutional Ethical Review Committee (ERC).

The age of the patients was from 19 to 83 years, mean age 52.5 years (median 54.5). There were 31 men, mean age 50,9 years (median 55) and 13 women, mean age 56.4 years (median 58). Majority of them were referred to our department after earlier treatment in other centers which had an impact on the delay in diagnosis and on appropriate surgical treatment.

The time of hospitalization was on the average about 3 weeks (23.84 ± 11.96 days, median 21.5). All patients were operated, 14 patients died. The total death rate was 31.82% (38.7% in male and 15.4% in female group).

The etiology of AM was extremely differentiated (Table 1). Iatrogenic complications were the most frequent cause of mediastinal infection. They were found in 19 patients (43.2%) and associated with esophageal and tracheal surgeries or with injuries to these organs during endoscopy or intubation. Non-iatrogenic esophageal and tracheal injuries were the cause of AM in 11 patients (25%). This group also included perforations caused by a foreign body. Descending AM was detected in 9 patients (20.4%). In 5 patients (11.4%) AM resulted from a spontaneous perforation of advanced esophageal cancer or

Table 1 Aetiology and surgical procedures in patients with acute mediastinitis

AETIOLOGY		Number	Procedure	Death
Iatrogenic (19)				
	Oesophageal endoscopy	4	PR-3E SPH-1	1
	Oesophagotomy	4	EX-2 PR-2	2
	Nissen operation	2	ESPH-1PR-1	1
	Post-intubation tracheal rupture	2	PR-2	0
	Complications of thyroid surgery	2	CRD + MDV-1 CRD + MDT-1	0
	Oesophageal rupture during intubation	1	PR-1	0
	Sternotomy complications in cardiac surgery	1	RVM-1	1
	Colonic perforation to retroperitoneal space	1	MDV-1	0
	Complications of neurosurgical procedures	1	CRD + MDV-1	0
	Complications of funnel chest surgery	1	RVM-1	0
Traumatic (11)				
	Oesophageal perforation	3	PR-3	0
	Tracheal rupture	2	PR-2	0
	Oesophageal rupture (foreign body)	3	PR-3	0
	Boerhaave syndrome	1	PR-1	1
	Burn of oesophagus with perforation	1	ESPH-1	0
	Foreign body in mediastinum (traffic accident)	1	MDS-1	0
Descending (9)				
	Dental abscess	4	DCUM- 2 CRD + MDT-2	1
	Retropharyngeal abscess	3	DCUM- 2 CRD + MDV- 1	1
	Peritonsillar abscess	2	CRD + MDT- 1 DCUM- 1	1
Neoplastic (4)				
	Esophageal spontaneous perforation after prosthesis/ stent implantation	2	EX + PN-1 EX-1	2
	Spontaneous oesophageal perforation in advanced cancer	3	PR-1 EX-1 TD-1	3

Legends of surgical procedures:
- EX: exclusion
- PR: primary repair
- ESPH: oesophagectomy
- MDT: mediastinal drainage by thoracotomy
- MDV: mediastinal drainage by videothoracoscopy
- MDS: mediastinal drainage by sternotomy
- TD: T-tube drainage
- CRD: cervical drainage
- PN: pneumonectomy
- DCUM: drainage of cervix and upper mediastinum
- RVM: revirage and mediastinal drainage

lung cancer with infiltration to the esophagus (neoplastic etiology).

All patients underwent surgery. The time from the establishment of the diagnosis of AM to the introduction of surgical treatment ranged from 2 h to 11 days, mean 1.62 days (±1.86), median (1.0). Surgical strategy was determined individually dependently on the etiology, delay from the diagnosis establishment, local conditions and the patient's general condition. The surgery, first of all, aimed at controlling the infection source and at limiting local inflammation by means of a wide cervical and/or mediastinal drainage through various surgical approaches. A detailed list of the performed surgical procedures and mortality rate of AM patients is presented in Table 1.

The following clinical risk features were evaluated: age, gender, etiology of coexisting diseases, delay in surgical treatment, isolated pathogens, type of surgical procedure, the number and type of postoperative complications. Then, the association between mortality rate and selected biochemical risk factors was investigated analyzing the following parameters: hemoglobin level, hematocrit, red blood cell count, leucocytosis, platelet count, serum sodium and potassium level, values of the inflammation markers: C-reactive protein (CRP) and procalcitonin (PCT) in preoperative period and on day 3 postoperatively. General and biochemical data were included (Table 2). The factors for which in statistical analysis no association was found with the prognosis were excluded from further studies.

Statistical analysis

Statistical method of the factor analysis was used to extract the risk aspects for the patients (Statgraphics Centurion XVI, StatPoint Technologies, Inc. Warrenton, USA). Then, the clinical value of the extracted factors was evaluated by ANOVA, where the treatment outcome was investigated. Variances were checked by Levene's test. As p value for this statistics was less than 0.05, Kruskal-Wallis Test was applied to check the significance.

Finally, the number of significant preoperative factors for the prognosis was reduced to 8 parameters which were grouped into 3 prognostic factors named respectively: proteinic status, inflammatory status and general status arranged dependently on their statistical power. All utilized parameters can be collected in a simple way during examination of the patient directly after admission to the ward and after laboratory investigations (within 2–3 hours).

The first factor explained as "proteinic status" informs about the initial state of protein metabolism. This parameter is composed of results of laboratory tests of blood: serum protein, albumin and hemoglobin (HGB) level.

The second factor "inflammatory status" allows to estimate the patient's septic state on the basis of three laboratory parameters determined prior to the treatment: white blood cell count (WBC_pre), CRP value (CRP_pre), PCT value (PCT_pre).

The third factor of the prediction schema "general risk" focuses on the evaluation of the patient's clinical state and includes only two important parameters: age (Age) and the number of coexisting diseases (Coex_disease).

Coefficients of sensitivity (SNC) and specificity (SPC) were calculated for the extracted factors to check the prediction power of the suggested method. The proposed method is designed for the prediction of recovery. Thus, the result of the test is positive (P) if the test predicts the recovery, and negative (N) if the test does not predict the recovery but i.e. "death". Respectively, the result of the test is true (T) if the test predicts recovery when the observed result is "recovery", and the result of the test is false (F) if the test does not predict the recovery. Therefore: TP-patient recovered and predicted as "recovery", TN-patient died and predicted as "death", FP-patient died but predicted as "recovery", and FN - patient recovered but predicted as "death". Basing on the above definitions, the suggested sensitivity and specificity coefficients equations are:

$$\text{Sensitivity coefficient: } SNC = \frac{TP}{TP+FN} \times 100\%$$

$$\text{Specificity coefficient: } SNC = \frac{TP}{TP+FN} \times 100\%$$

Results

Three factors have been extracted as statistically requested (Eigenvalue > 1), they are presented in Table 3. Together they account for over 69% of the variability in the original data. The initial communality estimates have been set to assume that all of the variability in the data is due to common factors (principal components method).

Table 2 Data included into this paper from treated patients affected with acute mediastinitis

	Age	Coex_diseas	HGB	WBC_pre	CRP_pre	PCT_pre	Proteins	Albumins
Average	52,5455	1,97727	11,5677	15,2432	202,891	2,93409	57,3864	31,6773
Standard deviation	13,7595	1,42223	2,14823	5,14417	50,1198	3,92167	7,35118	3,90652

Legend: Coex_diseas – coexisting diseases; HGB – level of hemoglobin in venous blood (g/dl) WBC_pre – white blood cell count in venous blood collected before surgical treatment immediately after department admission [x10^6/µl]; CRP_pre – C-reactive protein collected before surgical treatment immediately after department admission (mg/l); PCT_pre – procalcitonin in serum collected before surgical treatment immediately after department admission (ng/ml); Proteins – level of total serum proteins (g/l); Albumins – albumin level in serum (g/l).

Table 3 Factor Analysis – presentation of the factors

Factor Number	Eigenvalue	Percent of Variance	Cumulative Percentage	Initial Communality
1	3,31109	41,389	41,389	1,0
2	1,16325	14,541	55,929	1,0
3	1,04991	13,124	69,053	1,0
4	0,754858	9,436	78,489	1,0
5	0,682004	8,525	87,014	1,0
6	0,540662	6,758	93,772	1,0
7	0,358296	4,479	98,251	1,0
8	0,139929	1,749	100,000	1,0

Note: for 3 factors the Eigenvalue is >1.

Next, factor loading matrix was calculated. In order to simplify the clinical explanation of the factors, the rotation of the matrix was performed. Table 4 shows the parameters for equations, which estimate the common factors after rotation has been performed. Basing on those scores in the next statistical step, the factor (rotated) equations were constructed:

$$\begin{aligned} \text{Factor1} = {} & 0,712131\text{HGB} + 0,854481\text{Proteins} \\ & -0,131796\text{Coex}_{\text{diseas}} + 0,00534419\text{WBC}_{\text{pre}} \\ & -0,141942\text{Age} + 0,908303\text{Albumins} \\ & -0,651832\text{CRP}_{\text{pre}} - 0,560482\text{PCT}_{\text{pre}} \end{aligned}$$

$$\begin{aligned} \text{Factor2} = {} & 0,152337\text{HGB} - 0,0461529\text{Proteins} \\ & -0,0604516\text{Coex}_{\text{diseas}} + 0,914729\text{WBC}_{\text{pre}} \\ & +0,263779\text{Age} - 0,0949298\text{Albumins} \\ & +0,514794\text{CRP}_{\text{pre}} + 0,371643\text{PCT}_{\text{pre}} \end{aligned}$$

$$\begin{aligned} \text{Factor3} = {} & -0,243032\text{HGB} - 0,0418942\text{Proteins} \\ & +0,863627\text{Coex}_{\text{diseas}} + 0,108861\text{WBC}_{\text{pre}} \\ & +0,685527\text{Age} - 0,167625\text{Albumins} \\ & +0,0364827\text{CRP}_{\text{pre}} + 0,141625\text{PCT}_{\text{pre}} \end{aligned}$$

where the values of the variables (x) in the equations are standardized by subtracting their means (μ) and dividing by their standard deviations (σ). It also shows the estimated communalities, which can be interpreted as estimating the proportion of the variability in each variable attributable to the extracted factors.

Visual presentation of extracted factors is shown in Figure 1. Final factor scores calculated for all factors included into this study, together with easy explanation of their meanings are presented in Table 5.

There are three separate groups: HGB + Proteins + Albumim, WBC_pre + CRP_pre + PCT_pre, and Age + Coex_diseas.

According to the above, clinical meaning of the factors was established. Factor1 (F1) is "proteinic status" of the patient, Factor2 (F2) – "inflammatory status", and Factor3 (F3) – "general risk" understood as the composite of age and number of coexisting diseases. The statistics of these factors in the presented clinical series is shown in Table 6.

Finally, clinical verification was done by checking the extracted factors value in our series of patients concerning the outcome of the treatment as recovery or death (Table 7). ANOVA results are presented in Figure 2 for F1 ($F = 21.78$, $p < 0.0001$; Levene`s test = 4.0978, $p < 0.05$; Kruskal-Wallis test = 11.9168, $p < 0.001$), for F2 ($F = 8.45$, $p < 0.01$; Levene`s test = 8.9967, $p < 0.01$; Kruskal-Wallis test = 4.9168, $p < 0.05$), and for F3 ($F = 14.18$, $p < 0.001$; Levene`s test = 0.0001, $p = 0.9929$).

The final number of extracted factors was three. Furthermore, the coefficients of sensitivity and specificity were calculated for each factor (for F1: SNC = 87%, SPC = 79%; for F2: SNC = 87%, SPC = 50%; for F3: SNC = 73%, SPC = 71%), and next the prevalence test classification (TP, TN, FP, FN) was performed to establish the whole prognostic power of the method: SNC = 90%, SPC = 64%.

The schema of the proposed prediction method application is presented in Figure 3.

The probability of recovery increases when F1 is higher. In other words, when "proteinic status" is worse the risk of death is higher. As far as the "inflammatory status" (F2) is concerned, in our series, lower scores are observed in recovery outcome cases. The same trend is noticed in

Table 4 Factor loading matrix after varimax rotation

Parameter	Factor score coefficients			Estimated Communality	Specific Variance
	Factor1	Factor2	Factor3		
HGB	0,712131	0,152337	−0,243032	0,589401	0,410599
Proteins	0,854481	−0,0461529	−0,0418942	0,734023	0,265977
Coex_diseas	−0,131796	−0,0604516	0,863627	0,766875	0,233125
WBC_pre	0,00534419	0,914729	0,108861	0,848609	0,151391
Age	−0,141942	0,263779	0,685527	0,559674	0,440326
Albumins	0,908303	−0,0949298	−0,167625	0,862124	0,137876
CRP_pre	−0,651832	0,514794	0,0364827	0,691229	0,308771
PCT_pre	−0,560482	0,371643	0,141625	0,472317	0,527683

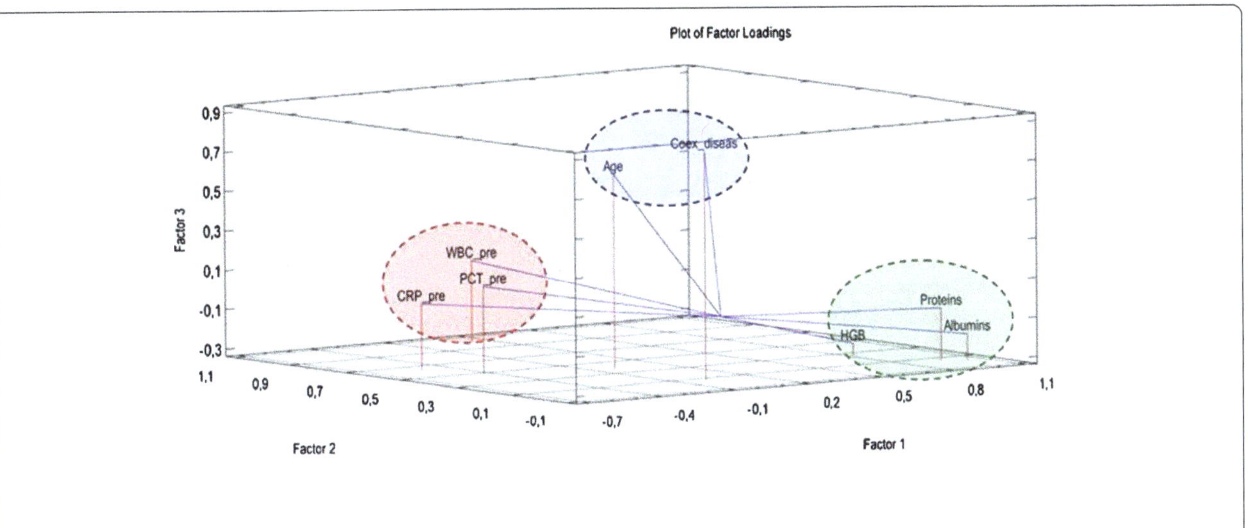

Figure 1 Plot of final factor loading after matrix rotation.

the analysis of "general risk" (i.e. F3). When plot (Figure 2) of "proteinic status" is analyzed, the value dividing recovery outcome from death is approximately −1,4 (F1). It should be understood as high probability of the patient's recovery if the score is higher than −1.4. In case of "inflammatory status" the caesura is located around +1.0 (F2). The prediction of survival is for patients with the score lower than +1.0. Respectively, "general risk" (F3) score lower than +0.4 is a prediction of recovery outcome (as presented in tab.5). The predictable result based on F1 is most of all in compliance with the observed result of the treatment (only 7 variances/44 results). The variances result from the application of 3 factors. It should be known that if 8 parameters are subject of analysis, the whole explanation of variability is possible with 8 factors. The same is visible in density traces (Figure 2) where full strict dichotomic separation of recovery from death outcome subpopulations is impossible. That kind of mutually penetrating subpopulations is often observed in biological sciences.

Discussion

Early recognition of septic complications, information about sepsis severity and thus, the ability to predict the prognosis can have a significant impact on the treatment strategy in AM. Access to such data can be of importance in establishing the urgency and type of surgical intervention, monitoring in postoperative period, necessity for repair, the kind of antibiotic-therapy and supportive treatment. In medicine, numerous prognostic scales have been created allowing to assess the prognosis in selected pathological states. However, in available literature we have not found a scale related to acute mediastinitis. Most probably it results from rare prevalence of this disease and difficulty in gathering appropriately rich material within one medical centre. The proposed prognostic method, based on the evaluation of 8 simple and easy to obtain parameters compiled in the form of 3 factors, allows dichotomic categorization of patients into 2 groups as regards the predicted prognosis: survival or death. When the calculated values of individual factors are combined, it is easy to distinguish within first few hours of hospitalization the patients whose prognosis is worse than that of the others. Obviously, the selection of proper parameters for the estimation of the predicted prognosis in the course of AM can be the subject of discussion.

In practice the first information about the patient's general condition is obtained during taking the history data. At this stage we can obtain the data regarding patient's age and coexisting diseases which in the proposed prognostic scale are important for calculating factor 3 values. In critically ill patients with sepsis, older age and coexisting diseases are associated with poor prognosis [18-20]. There are several prognostic scales considering the effectof coexisting diseases on the prognosis. The best known are: Charlson Comorbidity Index (CCI), Davies (Stokes) score and Index of Coexisting Diseases (ICED). They are widely applied in the patients dialyzed due to renal failure [21-24]. Charlson scale, which estimates similar parameters as our scale but it is based on different methodology, is used most frequently. It takes into account 19 coexisting diseases which are assigned with a score. CCI includes age as one of the evaluated elements and the age scores are counted according to the following scheme: 1 score for each decade over 40 years of age. The total score enables to predict the prognosis [25]. It was demonstrated in C-Y Wang's study that higher value of CCI (>2) in patients treated surgically due to stage I of lung cancer was associated with

Table 5 Factor scores

Case	Observed outcome	Factor1	Factor2	Factor3	Classification result
		Proteinic status	Inflammatory status	General risk	
		Recovery Prediction for > −1.4*	Recovery Prediction for <1.0*	Recovery Prediction for <0.4*	
1	Death	−8,61293	1,97822	2,03692	TN
2	Recovery	**−1,89787**	**1,01016**	**0,60735**	FN
3	Death	−5,67083	1,17312	3,18046	TN
4	Recovery	2,96689	0,0611059	−1,30167	TP
5	Death	−4,61678	**0,759947**	1,84367	TN
6	Death	−3,58174	3,35379	2,15131	TN
7	Recovery	1,24868	−0,0408765	0,219901	TP
8	Recovery	**−2,55507**	0,0101163	−0,12325	FN
9	Recovery	0,858724	0,588775	0,151806	TP
10	Recovery	**−1,95238**	0,0573994	0,216068	FN
11	Recovery	3,64292	−0,704072	−0,684944	TP
12	Recovery	2,6163	−1,34394	−2,25436	TP
13	Death	−4,19034	4,84986	0,915751	TN
14	Recovery	1,82354	0,0636333	−1,26561	TP
15	Recovery	3,03511	**1,12721**	−0,649727	TP
16	Recovery	3,37817	−1,38079	−2,2192	TP
17	Recovery	0,580244	−0,316079	−1,61708	TP
18	Death	−1,56375	**−2,27389**	**−0,389642**	TN
19	Death	−1,78795	**−0,0187813**	**−0,789484**	TN
20	Recovery	0,57392	**1,00331**	−0,714067	TP
21	Recovery	2,86891	−0,0531427	−1,05936	TP
22	Recovery	0,343636	0,293051	**0,970888**	TP
23	Recovery	1,14208	−0,965971	−1,6126	TP
24	Recovery	5,51418	−1,06023	−3,28449	TP
25	Death	−3,25473	1,29683	1,1493	TN
26	Death	−2,12645	2,29104	0,529981	TN
27	Recovery	2,29387	0,0084471	**1,6481**	TP
28	Death	**0,907509**	**−0,6706**	3,7267	FP
29	Recovery	1,29283	−1,69442	0,299441	TP
30	Recovery	3,45795	−1,35408	−2,1628	TP
31	Death	**2,96653**	**−1,47445**	**−0,86775**	FP
32	Recovery	0,0323576	−1,55881	**0,509574**	TP
33	Recovery	1,0745	0,26778	0,334441	TP
34	Death	−2,52481	2,36734	1,19426	TN
35	Recovery	1,32141	**1,05543**	**0,824733**	TP
36	Recovery	1,29592	−1,62119	−2,8627	TP
37	Death	−5,05654	**0,832591**	1,11692	TN
38	Recovery	2,11607	−0,960466	−0,634111	TP
39	Recovery	**−1,4526**	0,511999	1,41191	FN
40	Recovery	−0,871523	−1,93215	−0,779669	TP
41	Death	**3,87668**	**−2,0661**	**−0,280317**	FP
42	Recovery	−1,30349	−0,759654	**0,880723**	TP

Table 5 Factor scores *(Continued)*

43	Recovery	1,76721	−1,49925	−1,44593	TP
44	Recovery	0,0236466	−1,21219	**1,07856**	TP

This table shows the factor scores (prognostic) for each patient from our data file (observation). * – level of dichotomic division of subpopulation: recovery and death, see cross of the lines in density traces (Figure 2). **Bold**-lack of agreement between prediction and observation. Classification result: TP-true positive, TN-true negative, FP-false positive, FN-false negative.

higher mortality rate than in the group of patients with lower number of comorbidities; CCI < 2 [26]. The proposed by us prognostic scale is different because the data on the general state (F3) are only one of three estimated elements. If after substituting the data concerning age and coexisting diseases for the given formula for "F3" we obtain the value < +0.4, there increases the chance for the patient's survival. F3 is important for the whole scale but according to our calculations it has a lower diagnostic value compared to the remaining two factors (SNC = 73%, SPC = 71%). Anticipating the questions why there were not taken into account such obvious clinical risk factors as: etiology, delay in diagnosis or the type of pathogen, we want to explain that the introduction of these data, to our surprise, led in consequence to the weakening of the algorithm diagnostic value. It seems that additional parameters can act the opposite way in the whole pool. Presumably, the factor analysis eliminated less reliable variables leaving those which presented the highest predictive power in the proposed algorithm. For instance, the delay in diagnosis and the time of the introduction of the surgical treatment are not unequivocal parameters. It is worth emphasizing that majority of the patients were hospitalized earlier on other wards, where initially no proper diagnosis was established. Furthermore, they were then subjected to surgical procedures the effect of which could sometimes deteriorate their condition and sometimes improve it partially. Similar remarks concern the bacterial flora which changed in the course of the treatment and finally its distribution was the effect of coincidence, antibiotic therapy and/or infection. It was impossible to classify such internally unstable parameters by the method of factor analysis and attempts of their inclusion into the algorithm had a negative effect on the accuracy of the prediction.

Laboratory investigations are important elements of the proposed algorithm. The determination of other risk factors, found in already mentioned 2 factors: "proteinic status" and "inflammatory status" using 6 simple biochemical tests, supplements our prognostic method. F1 determines the initial state of the patient's protein metabolism on the basisof 3 parameters: total protein, albumin and HGB level. Malnutrition and hypoproteinemia are distinctly associated with increased death rate due to infection and neoplastic disease [27,28]. An objective estimation of malnutrition and protein metabolism is usually difficult, it is based on clinical observation, determination of BMI and biochemical investigations [29]. Among biochemical markers albumin level is most frequently used in malnutrition assessment. Hypoalbuminemia is associated with malnutrition and the decrease of protein level because liver reduces albumin production in favor of more important plasma proteins [16]. In 1988 Busby et al., first described the Nutritional Risk Index (NRI) to score the severity of postoperative complications [14,15]. It combines two nutritional indicators (albumin and weight loss), which are strictly correlated with higher morbidity and mortality risk in the population of elderly patients [30]. The need of determining ideal body weight, which is difficult in elderly or critically ill patients, is one of the limitations of this scale. Thus, it became necessary to find a formula enabling to calculate ideal body weight,

Table 6 Final statistics of factor scores

Parameter	Factor1	Factor2	Factor3
	Proteinic status	Inflammatory status	General risk
Count	44	44	44
Average	$9{,}55 \times 10^{-8}$	$5{,}11 \times 10^{-7}$	$1{,}36 \times 10^{-7}$
Median	0,72	−0,005	0,18
Standard deviation	2,98	1,50	1,52
Minimum	−8,61	−2,27	−3,28
Maximum	5,51	4,85	3,73
Range	14,13	7,12	7,01
Standardized skewness	−1,88	2,64	0,26
Standardized kurtosis	0,45	1,94	−0,01

Table 7 Final statistics of subgroups (factor scores)

	Factor1		Factor2		Factor3	
	Proteinic status		Inflammatory status		General risk	
	death	recovery	death	recovery	death	recovery
Count	14	30	14	30	14	30
Average	−2,52	1,17	0,89	−0,41	1,11	−0,52
Median	−2,89	1,27	1,00	−0,18	1,13	−0,64
Standard deviation	3,36	1,89	2,06	0,93	1,41	1,30
Minimum	−8,61	−2,56	−2,27	−1,93	−0,87	−3,28
Maximum	3,88	5,51	4,85	1,13	3,73	1,65
Range	12,49	8,07	7,12	3,06	4,59	4,93
Stnd. skewness	0,64	−0,19	0,16	0,18	0,41	−0,70
Stnd. kurtosis	0,20	−0,18	−0,28	−1,38	−0,43	−0,79

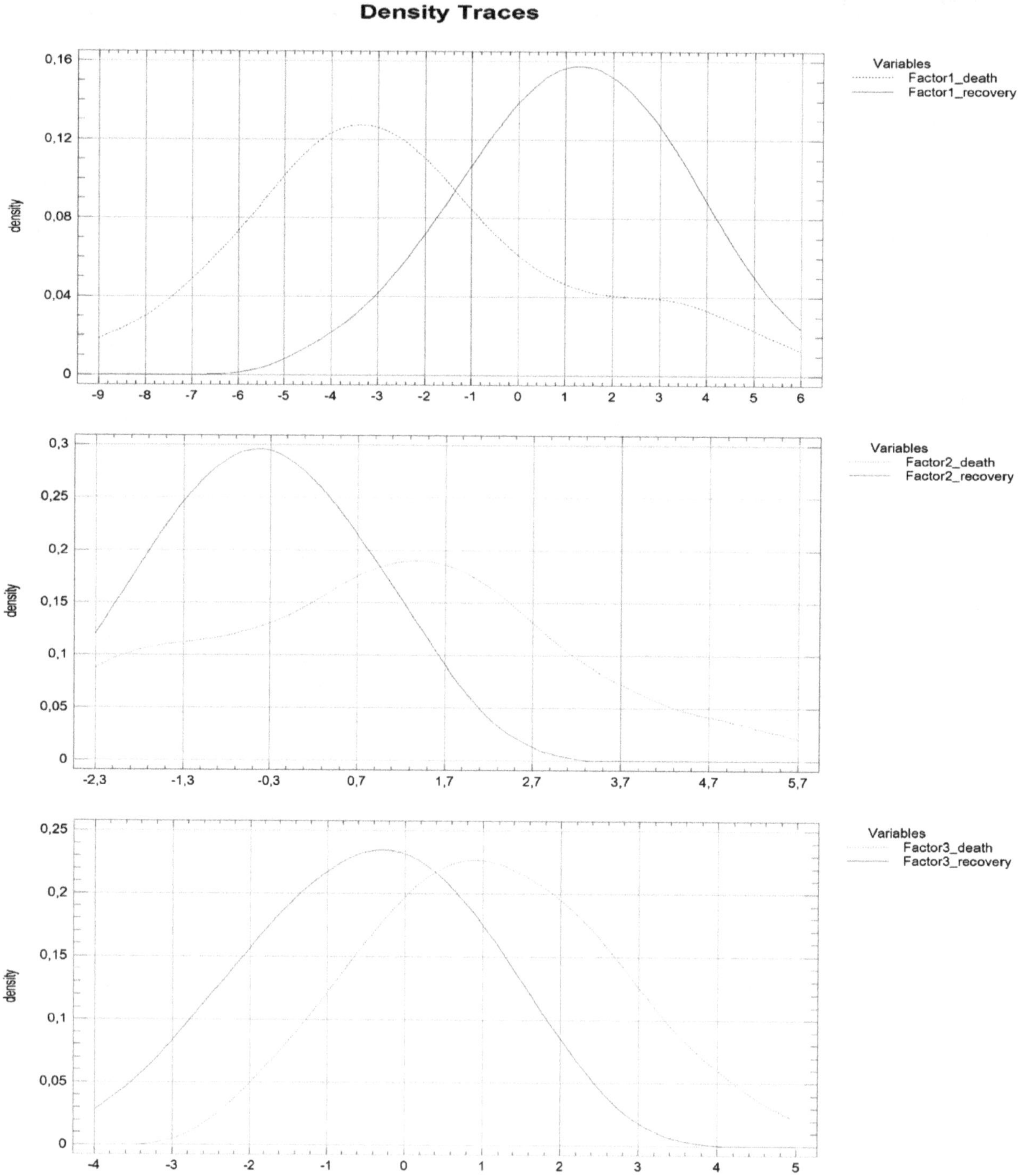

Figure 2 Comparison of Proteinic status (Factor 1), Inflammatory status (Factor 2), and General risk (factor 3) in subpopulation of recovery and lethal outcome of acute mediastinitis. The difference is statistically significant.

which led to creation of a new, more objective tool – the Geriatric Nutritional Risk Index (GNRI) [31]. Basing on the performed analysis we have demonstrated that there is also a need for inclusion of the hemoglobin level into the prognostic scale. It was included into the markers estimating "proteinic status". The presence of anemia is a known factor affecting poor prognosis, particularly in combination with other diseases [32,33]. The studies of

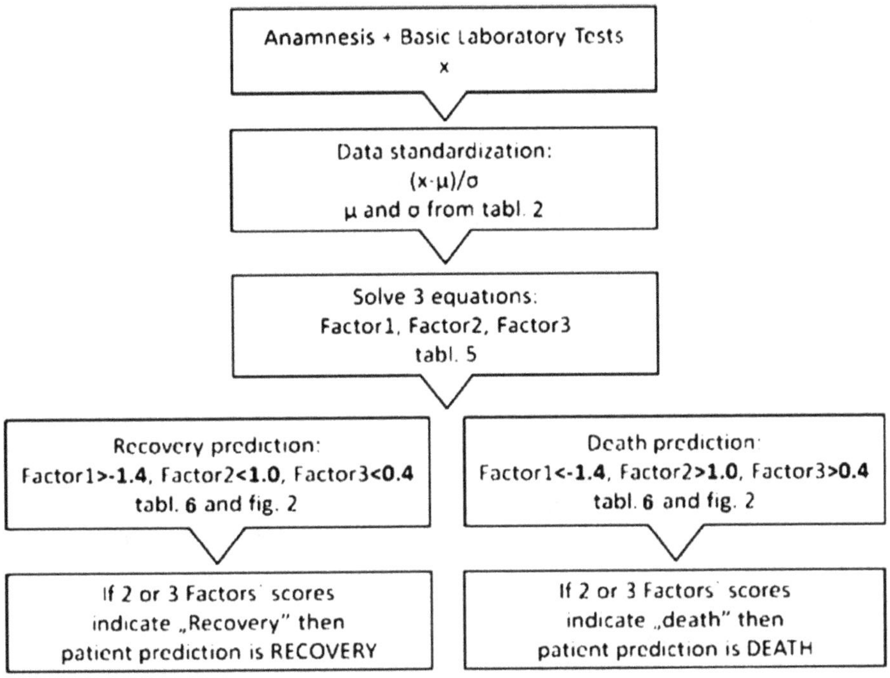

Figure 3 Schema of the application of the recovery prediction method.

Welch et al. demonstrated that general death risk increases with the decrease of HGB concentration and even benign forms of anemia can be associated with the increase of the death risk [34]. The advantage of the suggested prognostic method is the determination of protein metabolism in simpler way than in NRI or GNRI basing only on biochemical tests which is of importance in patients in critical condition. The obtained high diagnostic value for "proteinic status", corresponding with the final prognosis (SNC = 87%, SPC = 79%) should be . If the value of F1 calculated on the basis of the formula is lower than −1.4, it means a high death risk for the patient.

We are convinced that in the case of infectious diseases limitation to the assessment of protein metabolism, age and co-existing diseases is not sufficient for the prediction of the prognosis. It seems natural to extend the prognostic scale including biochemical markers of inflammation. White blood cell count (WBC) is the oldest widely used marker. It should be reminded that WBC value is one of the criteria of SIRS and sepsis diagnosis [35]. Fever in combination with elevated WBC count is a quick and cheap way of infection diagnosis but its low diagnostic value is its basic limitation [36]. This parameter in combination with other inflammatory markers still has a wide clinical application both in the diagnosis and monitoring of the results of the treatment. CRP remains one of the most important classic markers for inflammation. It is included into sensitive but little specific acute phase proteins, the level of which increases in inflammation and malignancy [37,38]. It has been confirmed that initial CRP values were directly associated with total mortality rate in neoplastic disease [39]. However, Matson et al. paid attention to the fact that "normal" plasma CRP level in critically ill patients is rarely the same as in healthy population [40]. The post-mortem studies demonstrated that in patients with cachexia related to malignant carcinoma, in the case of extensive tumor necrosis, significant deviations were observed in the behavior of acute phase proteins [41]. That is why in these cases the determination of CRP alone can appear to be insufficient in the monitoring of inflammation. PCT is a biochemical marker extremely useful in the diagnosis and differentiation of severe infections and septic complications [42-44]. The increase of PCT concentration induced by bacterial toxins (with preserved insensitivity to other pro-inflammatory stimuli) and close relation between serum PCT concentration and infection severity are the most important properties of this marker [45,46]. Taking into account the above mentioned properties we have included serum PCT concentration into F2 evaluation. We think that simultaneous determination of three biochemical markers will enable more precise and more objective assessment of "inflammatory status" eliminating errors resulting from heterogeneity of the investigated group and known deviations in the behavior of the selected markers in some critical morbid states.

Among the prognostic scales using inflammatory state markers we have not found any similar to ours. Our scale is unique due to the combination of biochemical data of inflammation with simultaneous assessment of the patient's general condition and protein metabolism. Ingenbleek and Carpentier Prognostic Inflammatory and Nutritional Index (PINI) deserves attention [16]. The scale is based on the evaluation of 4 parameters: 2 markers of malnutrition: albumin and prealbumin, and 2 markers of inflammatory state: CRP and α1acid glycoprotein (AAG). This scoring system may predict morbidity or mortality in hospitalized patients [24]. The normal PINI level in healthy population is <1. The value of PINI (>1) is associated with poor prognosis [16,47]. PINI has been found to be a reliable indicator of both nutritional status and prognosis in trauma, burns and infection [48,49] and lately in cancer [50]. PINI is slightly similar to the scale proposed by us, as it considers 2 of 3 analyzed groups of risk factors. In our investigations we did not determine AAG, which is not a marker commonly used in clinical practice in our country, and prealbumin due to its susceptibility to nutrition inhibition, which always occurs in the course of the treatment of AM patients. Other authors also confirmed that nutritional state can affect inflammatory response in patients with advanced carcinoma and the results of PINI prognostic scale [51,52]. Wunder et al. presented an interesting attempt of working out an independent indicator of early prediction of death in sepsis [53]. The authors, analyzing 33 patients with sepsis of different etiology, noticed that the deviations of the values of PCT and Acute Physiology and Chronic Health Evaluation (APACHE II) were correlated with poor prognosis. Novotny et al. carried out similar studies on a larger group of 160 patients with sepsis resulting from peritonitis or mediastinitis after an anastomotic leak and perforation of a hollow organ [54]. It should be noted that the clinical material presented in this study was to a great extent similar to our material. The authors, owing to combination of both indicators and calculations with the use of binary logistic regression analysis, were able to identify the groups of high and low death risk. In a multivariate analysis, both PCT and APACHE III score were identified as independent, early predictive indicators of sepsis lethality. While 71% of the high-risk patients died of sepsis, 77% of patients assigned to the low-risk group survived the septic complication (sensitivity 71%, specificity 77%) [54]. To compare, the diagnostic value for "inflammatory status" in the suggested method obtained higher sensitivity (87%) but lower specificity (50%). Poor prognosis should be suspected in patients whose value of F2 calculated from the formula is <1.0.

High death rate in the course of AM points to the need of further studies. Rare prevalence of the disease and high differentiation of the material within one medical centre are the limitations. Thus, introduction of multicentre register of the patients should be taken into consideration. A detailed analysis of the investigated cases in a large representative group of patients can have an influence on the determination of risk factors and on the improvement of the prognosis in patients treated surgically due to AM.

Conclusion

We do hope that the proposed prognostic method has a chance to be introduced into the clinical practice which can contribute to the modification of the treatment of patients with AM. It is based on mathematical assessment of own material and devoid of subjective interpretation. Its most important advantages are: inclusion into the assessment of 2 simple clinical data and 6 biochemical tests which can be obtained within first 2–3 hours after the patient's admission to hospital (duration of laboratory investigations), low costs and simple interpretation of the results. We think that the construction of the method, based on the evaluation of 3 groups of risk factors determining inflammatory, proteinic and general status, will be less sensitive to difficult to foresee deviations of the values of biochemical markers associated with the impact of factors such as: malnutrition, bacteriological etiology, comorbidities, surgical complications and others. To simplify the calculations, the scale can be prepared in a form of automatic electronic "calculator" which provides a ready result after entering appropriate data. The result proving poor prognosis should induce to more aggressive surgical treatment and to modification of antibiotic-therapy and supportive treatment.

Consent

Written informed consent was obtained from the patient for publication of this report and any accompanying images.

Abbreviations

AM: acute mediastinitis; APACHE: Acute Physiology and Chronic Health Evaluation; NRI: Nutritional Risk Index; PINI: Prognostic Inflammatory and Nutritional Index; CRP: C-reactive protein; PCT: Procalcitonin; HGB: Hemoglobin; WBC: White blood cell; pre: Preoperative; Coex_disease: coexisting diseases; SNC: Sensitivity; SPC: Specificity; P: Positive; N: Negative; T: True; F: False; TP: True positive; TN: True negative; FP: False positive; FN: False negative; F1: Factor1; F2: Factor2; F3: Factor3; CCI: Charlson Comorbidity Index; ICED: Index of Coexisting Diseases; BMI: Body mass index; GNRI: Geriatric Nutritional Risk Index; SIRS: Systemic Inflammatory Response Syndrome; PINI: Prognostic Inflammatory and Nutritional Index; AAG: α1acid glycoprotein.

Competing interests

The authors declare that they have no competing interests.

Acknowledgement
The authors wish to thank professor Marian Brocki and professor Jacek Rysz for making the hospitalized patients' data available, for their professional advice in preparing this article and for providing necessary support.

Author details
[1]Department of Thoracic Surgery, General and Oncological Surgery, Medical University of Lodz, 113 Żeromskiego St., 90-547, Łódź, Poland. [2]Department of Maxillofacial Surgery, Medical University of Lodz, 113 Żeromskiego St., 90-547, Łódź, Poland.

Authors' contribution
JS and KM are equally engaged into the study: Study design, data collection, statistical analysis, data interpretation, manuscript preparation, literature search, and funds collection. Both authors read and approved the final manuscript.

References

1. Marty-Ané CH, Berthet JP, Alric P, *et al*: **Management of descending necrotizing mediastinitis: an aggressive treatment for an aggressive disease.** *Ann Thorac Surg* 1999, **68**:212–217.
2. Muir AD, White J, McGuigan JA, McManus KG, Grahamoraz AN: **Treatment and outcomes of oesophageal perforation in a tertiary referral centre.** *Eur J Cardiothorac Surg* 2003, **23**:799–804.
3. Reeder LB, DeFilippi VJ, Ferguson MK: **Current results of therapy for esophageal perforation.** *Am J Surg* 1995, **169**:615–617.
4. Freeman RK, Vallières E, Verrier ED, Karmy-Jones R, Wood DE: **Descending necrotizing mediastinitis: an analysis of the effects of serial surgical debridement on patient mortality.** *J Thorac Cardiovasc Surg* 2000, **119**:260–267.
5. Bufkin BL, Miller JI Jr, Mansour KA: **Esophageal perforation: emphasis on management.** *Ann Thorac Surg* 1996, **61**:1447–1452.
6. Dubost C, Kaswin D, Duranteau A, Jehanno C, Kaswin R: **Esophageal perforation during attempted endotracheal intubation.** *J Thorac Cardiovasc Surg* 1979, **78**:44–51.
7. Akman C, Kantarci F, Cetinkaya S: **Imaging in mediastinitis: a systematic review based on aetiology.** *Clin Radiol* 2004, **59**:573–585.
8. El Oakley RM, Wright JE: **Postoperative mediastinitis: classification and management.** *Ann Thorac Surg* 1996, **61**:1030–1036.
9. Schroeyers P, Wellens F, Degrieck I, De Geest R, Van Praet F, Vermeulen Y, Vanermen H: **Aggressive primary treatment for poststernotomy acute mediastinitis: our experience with omental- and muscle flaps surgery.** *Eur J Cardiothorac Surg* 2001, **20**:743–746.
10. Jones WG, Ginsberg RJ: **Esophageal perforation: a continuing challenge.** *Ann Thorac Surg* 1992, **53**:534–543.
11. Leung TK, Lee CM, Lin SY, Chen HC, Wang HJ, Shen LK, *et al*: **Balthazar computed tomography severity index is superior to Ranson criteria and APACHE II scoring system in predicting acute pancreatitis outcome.** *World J Gastroenterol* 2005, **11**:6049–6052.
12. Blamey SL, Imrie CW, O'Neill J, Gilmour WH, Carter DC: **Prognostic factors in acute pancreatitis.** *Gut* 1984, **25**:1340–1346.
13. Bradley EL III: A clinically based classification system for acute pancreatitis. Summary of the International Symposium on Acute Pancreatitis, Atlanta, Ga., September 11 through 13, 1992. Arch Surg. 1993,128:586–590.
14. Buzby GP, Knox LS, Crosby LO, *et al*: **Study protocol: a randomized clinical trialof total parenteral nutrition in malnourished surgical patients.** *Am J Clin Nutr* 1988, **47**:366–381.
15. Buzby GP, Williford WO, Peterson OL, *et al*: **A randomized clinical trial of total parenteral nutrition in malnourished surgical patients: the rationale and impact of previous clinical trials and pilot study on protocol design.** *Am J Clin Nutr* 1988, **47**:357–365.
16. Ingenbleek Y, Carpentier YA: **A prognostic inflammatory and nutritional index scoring critically ill patients.** *Int J Vitam Nutr Res* 1985, **55**:91–101.
17. Estrera AS, Lanay MJ, Grisham JM, *et al*: **Descending necrotizing mediastinitis.** *Surg Gynecol Obstet* 1983, **157**:545–552.
18. Martin GS, Mannino DM, Moss M: **The effect of age on the development and outcome of adult sepsis.** *Crit Care Med* 2006, **34**:15–21.
19. Yang Y, Yang KS, Hsann YM, Lim V, Ong BC: **The effect of comorbidity and age on hospital mortality and length of stay in patients with sepsis.** *J Crit Care* 2010, **25**:398–405.
20. Azoulay E, Adrie C, De Lassence A, *et al*: **Determinants of postintensive care unit mortality: a prospective multicenter study.** *Crit Care Med* 2003, **31**:428–432.
21. Fried L, Bernardini J, Piraino B: **Charlson Comorbidity Index as a predictor of outcomes in incident peritoneal dialysis patients.** *Am J Kidney Dis* 2001, **37**:337–342.
22. Beddhu S, Bruns FJ, Saul M, Seddon P, Zeidel ML: **A simple comorbidity scale predicts clinical outcomes and costs in dialysis patients.** *Am J Med* 2000, **108**:609–613.
23. Athienites NV, Miskulin DC, Fernandez G, Bunnapradist S, Simon G, Landa M, *et al*: **Comorbidity assessment in hemodialysis and peritoneal dialysis using the Index of Coexistent Disease.** *Semin Dial* 2000, **13**:320–326.
24. Davies SJ, Russell L, Bryan J, Phillips L, Russell GI: **Comorbidity, urea kinetics and appetite in continuous ambulatory peritoneal dialysis patients: their interrelationship and prediction of survival.** *Am J Kidney Dis* 1995, **26**:353–361.
25. Charlson ME, Pompei P, Ales KL, MacKenzie CR: **A new method of classifying prognostic comorbidity in longitudinal studies: development and validation.** *J Chronic Dis* 1987, **5**:373–383.
26. Wang C-Y, Lin Y-S, Tzao C, Lee H-C, Huang M-H, Hsu W-H, Hsu H-S: **Comparison of Charlson comorbidity index and Kaplan—Feinstein index in patients with stage I lung cancer after surgical resection.** *Eur J Cardiothorac Surg* 2007, **32**:877–881.
27. Marti J, Armadans L, Vaque J, Segura F, Schwartz S: **Protein-calorie malnutrition and lymphocytopenia as predictors of hospital infection in the elderly.** *Med Clin (Barc)* 2001, **116**:446–450.
28. Chen MK, Souba WW, Copeland EM: **Nutritional support of the surgical oncology patient.** *Hematol Oncol Clin North Am* 1991, **5**:125–145.
29. Reynolds TM, Stokes A, Russell L: **Assessment of a prognostic biochemical indicator of nutrition and inflammation for identification of pressure ulcer risk.** *J Clin Pathol* 2006, **59**(3):308–310.
30. Naber HJ, de Bree A, Schermer TRJ, *et al*: **Specificity of indexes of malnutrition when applied to apparently healthy people: the effect of age.** *Am J Clin Nutr* 1997, **65**:1721–1725.
31. Bouillanne O, Morineau G, Dupont C, Coulombel I, Vincent J-P, Nicolis I, Benazeth S, Cynober L, Aussel Ch: **Geriatric Nutritional Risk Index: a new index for evaluating at-risk elderly medical patients.** *Am J Clin Nutr* 2005, **82**:777–783.
32. Carson JL, Noveck H, Berlin JA, Gould SA: **Mortality and morbidity in patients with very low postoperative Hb levels who decline blood transfusion.** *Transfusion* 2002, **42**(7):812–818.
33. Garson JL, Duff A, Poses RM, Berlin JA, Spence RK, Trout R, Noveck H, Strom BL: **Effect of anaemia and cardiovascular disease on surgical mortality and morbidity.** *Lancet* 1996, **348**:1055–1060.
34. Welch HG, Mehan KR, Goodnough LT: **Prudent strategies for elective red blood cell transfusion.** *Ann Intern Med* 1992, **116**:393–402.
35. American College of Chest Physicians/Society of Critical Care Medicine Consensus Conference: **definitions for sepsis and organ failure and guidelines on the use of innovative therapies in sepsis-Members of the American College of Chest Physicians/Society of Critical Care Medicine Consensus Conference Committee.** *Crit Care Med* 1992, **20**:864–874.
36. Weitzman M: **Diagnostic utility of white blood cell and differential cell counts.** *Am J Dis Child* 1975, **129**:1183–1189.
37. Okamura JM, Miyagi JM, Terada K, Hokama Y: **Potential clinical applications of C-reactive protein.** *J Clin Lab Anal* 1990, **4**:231–235.
38. Clark BA, Mayhew JL: **An inexpensive method of determining body composition by underwater weighing.** *Br J Nutr* 1979, **42**:173–183.
39. Balkwill F, Mantovani A: **Inflammation and cancer: back to Virchow?** *Lancet* 2001, **357**:539–545.
40. Matson A, Soni N, Sheldon J: **C-reactive protein as a diagnostic test of sepsis in the critically ill.** *Anaesth Intensive Care* 1991, **19**:182–186.
41. Warren S: **The immediate causes of death in cancer.** *Am J Med Sciences* 1932, **184**:610–615.
42. Brunkhorst FM, Wegscheider K, Forycki ZF, Brunkhorst R: **Procalcitonin for early diagnosis and differentiation of SIRS, sepsis, severe sepsis, and septic shock.** *Intensive Care Med* 2000, **26**(Suppl 2):148–252.

43. Bertsch T, Richter A, Hofheinz H, Bohm C, Hartel M, Aufenanger J: **Procalcitonin.A new marker for acute phase reaction in acute pancreatitis.** *Langenbecks Arch Chir* 1997, **382:**367–372.
44. de Werra I, Jaccard C, Corradin SB, *et al*: **Cytokines, nitrite/nitrate, soluble tumour necrosis factor receptors, and procalcitonin concentrations: comparisons in patients with septic shock, cardiogenic shock, and bacterial pneumonia.** *Crit Care Med* 1997, **25:**607–613.
45. Dalton H: **Procalticonin: a predictor of lung injury attributable to sepsis.** *Crit Care Med* 1999, **25:**2304–2308.
46. Whang KT, Vath SD, Becker KL, *et al*: **Procalticonin and proinflamatory cytokine interactions in sepsis.** *Shock* 2000, **4:**73–78.
47. Perier C, Granouillet R, Chamson A, Gonthier R, Frey J: **Nutritional markers, acute phase reactants and tissue inhibitor of matrix metalloproteinase 1 in elderly patients with pressure sores.** *Gerontology* 2002, **48:**298–301.
48. Gottschlich MM, Baumer T, Jenkins M, Khoury J, Warden GD: **The prognostic value of nutritional and inflammatory indices in patients with burns.** *J Burn Care Rehabil* 1992, **13:**105–113.
49. Bonnefoy M, Ayzac L, Ingenbleek Y, Kostka T, Boisson RC, Bienvenu J: **Usefulness of the prognostic inflammatory and nutritional index (PINI) in hospitalized elderly patients.** *Int J Vitam Nutr Res* 1998, **68:**189–195.
50. Walsh D, Mahmoud F, Barna B: **Assessment of nutritional status and prognosis in advanced cancer: interleukin-6, C-reactive protein, and the prognostic and inflammatory nutritional index.** *Support Care Cancer* 2003, **11:**60–62.
51. Slaviero KA, Clarke SJ, Rivory LP: **Inflammatory response: an nrecognized sourceof variability in the pharmacokinetics and pharmacodynamics of cancer chemotherapy.** *Lancet Oncol* 2003, **4:**224–232.
52. Rivory LP, Slaviero K, Clarke SJ: **Hepatic cytochrome P450 3A drug metabolism isreduced in cancer patients with an acute-phase response.** *Br J Cancer* 2002, **87:**277–280.
53. Wunder C, Eichelbronner O, Roewer N: **Are IL-6, IL-10 and PCT plasma concentrations reliable for outcome prediction in severe sepsis? A comparison with APACHE III and SAPS II.** *Inflamm Res* 2004, **53:**158–163.
54. Novotny A, Emanuel K, Matevossian E, Kriner M, Ulm K, Bartels H, Holzmann B, Weighardt H, Siwert J-R: **Use of procalcitonin for early prediction of lethal outcome of postoperative sepsis.** *Am J Surg* 2007, **194:**35–39.

17

Splenic artery embolization: technically feasible but not necessarily advantageous

F. Van der Cruyssen[1*] and A. Manzelli[2]

Abstract

Background: The spleen is the second most commonly injured organ in cases of abdominal trauma. Management of splenic injury depends on the clinical status of the patient and can include nonoperative management (NOM), splenic artery embolization (SAE), surgery (operative splenic salvage or splenectomy), or a combination of these treatments. In nonoperatively managed cases, SAE is sometimes used to control haemorrhage. However, the indications for SAE have not been clearly defined and, in some cases, the potential complications of the procedure may outweigh its benefits.

Review of the literature: Through review of the literature we address the question of when SAE is indicated in combination with NOM of splenic injury, and whether SAE may delay needed surgical treatment in some cases. This systematic review highlighted the use of imperfect and inconsistent scoring systems in the diagnosis of splenic injury, the lack of consensus regarding indications for SAE, and the potential for severe morbidities associated with this procedure. Based on current literature and evidence we provide a new, non-verified, decision algorithm.

Conclusions: NOM+ SAE involves potential risks and operative management may be preferable to SAE for certain patients. To clarify current literature, we propose a new algorithm for blunt abdominal trauma that should be validated prospectively. New evidence-based protocols should be developed to guide diagnosis and management of patients with splenic trauma.

Keywords: Splenic artery, Embolization, Blunt splenic injury, Nonoperative management, Operative splenic salvage, Splenectomy, Trauma

Background

Abdominal injury occurs in approximately 20–30 % of all trauma patients. The spleen is the second most commonly injured organ in both blunt and penetrating abdominal trauma [1, 2].

Raza et al. reviewed 1285 cases of abdominal trauma over a ten-year period; 26 % of these suffered a splenic injury. Of the patients in the initial study group, 89.91 % were managed without surgery and 30 % of these had a splenic injury. The initial presentation of splenic injury can be variable and depends on the severity of the associated injuries, the amount of blood lost, and the mechanism of trauma. Routine diagnostic workup of suspected splenic injury includes chest radiographs, abdominal ultrasound, a focused assessment with sonography for trauma (FAST) scan, or CT imaging. Abdominal CT imaging with intravenous contrast is the preferred imaging method in hemodynamically stable patients; when the patient is in an unstable condition, a FAST scan that shows the presence of free within the abdomen can indicate that emergency surgery is necessary. Physicians and surgeons should remain alert for concomitant injuries to the liver (the organ most frequently injured by blunt abdominal trauma) and other intra-abdominal organs.

Splenic artery embolization (SAE) is increasingly being used in medical practice. This trend started in the 1970s when Maddison reported the first successful SAE in a patient with esophageal varices, hepatic cirrhosis, and recurrent gastrointestinal bleeding [3]. In 1975, Chuang and Reuter reported successful SAE after splenic injury in ten dogs [4]. In 1985, Sclafani et al. reported that embolization of 107 arterial

* Correspondence: frederic.vandercruyssen@student.kuleuven.be
[1]Third year master's student, Faculty of Medicine, Catholic University of Leuven (KU Leuven), Gasthuisberg, Belgium

injuries yielded an 82.2 % success rate [5]. There was a further evolution towards proximal SAE or more distal and selective embolization of the branches of the splenic artery.

Until the 1990s splenectomy remained the treatment of choice for splenic injury, but nonoperative management (NOM) became increasingly popular in the pediatric setting around 1992 when Haller et al. reported on the safety of NOM of solid organ injuries in children [6]. Sclafani reported in 1995 a study of 172 patients and the use angiography with subsequent use of proximal embolization of the splenic artery when extravasation was present [7]. In his study NOM was used in stable patients with no extravasation on angiography, splenectomy or splenorrhaphy was performed in unstable patients or in patients with associated injuries or disease. Overall splenic salvage rate was 88 % with a splenic salvage rate of 97 % in the patients managed non-operatively.

The first large multi-institutional study was published in 2000 by Peitzman et al. [8]. In this EAST study 1488 patients with blunt splenic injury were reviewed. The authors report operative management in 38,5 % of the patients and immediate operative management was proportional to the grade of injury. In patient groups with a larger hemoperitoneum, more laparotomies were performed. They further report a NOM failure rate of 10,8 % of which 60,9 % within the first 24 h of admittance. 54,8 % of the patients were successfully managed nonoperatively.

In 2005 Haan reported on 648 patients in a single institution study with splenic salvage rates of 90 % after SAE and 100 % after planned NOM [9]. Failure of NOM increased with higher injury grades but 80 % of grade IV and V injuries were successfully managed nonoperatively. Interestingly, a 40 % failure rate was reported when an arteriovenous fistula was present, even after embolization.

Currently, between 60 and 80 % of splenic injuries are managed without surgery and the reported success rates for NOM range between 85 and 94 %. NOM can be combined with SAE when certain conditions are met, and retrospective studies have reported higher success rates and higher splenic salvage rates when NOM is combined with SAE [10–12]. However, no consensus has been reached on the correct indications for combining NOM and SAE, especially in higher grade splenic injuries. In the current literature, the use of NOM in combination with SAE for treatment of blunt splenic injury is dependent on multiple factors, which are: the grade of the splenic injury, the injury severity score (ISS), patient age, the presence of contrast blush on CT, active extravasation on angiography, need for transfusion, the presence of significant hemoperitoneum, and the presence of splenic artery pseudoaneurysms. Most trauma protocols consider hemodynamic instability or a high-grade splenic lesion (IV–V) to be indications for emergency laparotomy. Operative splenic salvage (OSS) or splenectomy can then be attempted. However, based on the currently available literature the use of NOM, SAE, or OSS is controversial. Retrospective review of data, small study groups, and changes in protocols or in standard practice make it difficult to draw conclusions regarding the optimal management of splenic injuries.

Methods & results

We reviewed the literature and used critical interpretive synthesis methodology in the following discussion. A search of the following databases was conducted during October 2015: Medline database, Trip database, EMBASE, Web of Science, Cochrane Library, and Scopus. We also manually searched the reference lists of the retrieved articles. Our search terms included: splenic injury, embolization, operative, management.

We included original research articles that reported on splenic injury in combination with embolization therapy, operative, and nonoperative management. Papers were excluded if they focused specifically on adolescent, pediatric, or neonatal populations and if they included specific diagnostic groups. Guidelines, surveys, and meta-analyses were also excluded. The search was executed sequentially and is documented in Table 1. All articles were assessed for relevance by reading the abstract and, where needed, the entire paper using the above criteria.

Duplicates were excluded and the final selection of articles was based on their relevance and quality. Papers were excluded if no full text could be obtained. To select high-quality studies, we assessed all articles following the Critical Review Form for Quantitative Studies and guidelines from Law et al. [13]. An overview of the selected articles is presented in Table 2. Excluded articles are also presented in Table 2 for reference. Despite the large amount of articles retrieved, we were not able to carry out a meta-analysis because of the heterogeneity of study methods, data and quality of articles.

In order to further support the literature review we propose a new, non-verified, algorithm for blunt abdominal trauma, based on existing algorithms presented in the literature and modified according to our findings (Fig. 1).

Discussion

Hemodynamically unstable patients

Abdominal trauma with hemodynamic instability is an absolute indication for operative management in most

Table 1 Search results and number of articles retrieved after applying the selection criteria. After the initial search, all articles were entered in a reference database (Mendeley)

Database searched	Search terms used and limits applied	Number of results	Number met inclusion criteria
Medline	(("splenic injury") AND "embolization") AND "operative"	50	29
Medline	(((splenic trauma) AND operative management) AND artery embolization) AND non operative management	15	5
Trip database	(title:splenic injury)(title:embolization)(operative)	8	7
EMBASE: Search 1	'splenic injury'/exp OR 'splenic injury' AND ('embolization'/exp OR embolization) AND operative	90	46
EMBASE: Search 2	#1 AND ([adolescent]/lim OR [adult]/lim OR [young adult]/lim)	46	26
EMBASE: Search 3	#2 AND ('clinical article'/de OR 'clinical trial'/de OR 'comparative study'/de OR 'controlled study'/de OR 'major clinical study'/de OR 'medical record review'/de OR 'multicenter study'/de OR 'observational study'/de OR 'outcomes research'/de OR 'prospective study'/de OR 'retrospective study'/de) AND ('article'/it OR 'review'/it)	26	21
Web of Science	TOPIC: (splenic injury) AND TOPIC: (embolization) AND TOPIC: (operative) Timespan: All years. Indexes: SCI-EXPANDED, SSCI, A&HCI, CPCI-S, CPCI-SSH.	91	45
Cochrane Library	splenic injury embolization	7	6
Cochrane Library	splenic injury operative	1	0
Scopus	TITLE-ABS-KEY (splenic injury) AND TITLE-ABS-KEY (embolization) AND TITLE-ABS-KEY (operative)	79	34
Manual search from reference list of retrieved articles	Number in reference list - 1 - 7 - 8 - 9 - 14 - 15 - 16 - 18 - 24 - 30 - 38 - 41 - 42 - 51 Not selected - Hartnett KL, Winchell RJ, Clark DE (2003) Management of adult splenic injury: a 20-year perspective. Am Surg 69:608–611. - Upadhyaya P (2003) Conservative management of splenic trauma: history and current trends. Pediatr Surg Int 19:617–627. - Todd SR, Arthur M, Newgard C et al. (2004) Hospital factors associated with splenectomy for splenic injury: a national perspective. J Trauma 57:1065–1071. - Galvan DA, Peitzman AB (2006) Failure of nonoperative management of abdominal solid organ injuries. Curr Opin Crit Care 12:590–594. - Watson GA, Rosengart MR, Zenati MS et al. (2006) Nonoperative management of severe BSI: are we getting better? J Trauma 61:1113–1119. - Sclafani SJ, Shaftan GW, Scalea TM et al. (1995) Nonoperative salvage of computed tomography-diagnosed splenic injuries: utilization of angiography for triage and embolization for hemostasis. J Trauma 39:818–827.	22	14
TOTAL		435	233

protocols. However, in cases of splenic injury, SAE and NOM is increasingly being performed even in patients that are hemodynamically unstable. The use of NOM or SAE in hemodynamically unstable patients is highly controversial and should be further studied. Delays in diagnostic testing and inappropriate selection of hemodynamically unstable patients for this treatment protocol could increase morbidity and mortality rates, as some authors have suggested [14–16]. Importantly, there has been little research on managing patients with transient hemodynamic stability, although Hagiwara et al. did report successful SAE in 15 patients with transient responses to fluid administration [17].

Table 2 Summary table of articles that met inclusion criteria after initial selection. Articles marked in bold were excluded

	Reference	Study design	Sample size and sites	Comments/key findings	Included/ excluded
1	A.P. E, B. I, M. R, M.C. M. The impact of splenic artery embolization on the management of splenic trauma: an 8-year review. *Am J Surg.* 2009	Retrospective study	304 + 416 Single center	4 years NOM versus 4 years NOM + SAE	Included
2	**Akinkuolie AA, Lawal OO, Arowolo OA, Agbakwuru EA, Adesunkanmi ARK. Determinants of splenectomy in splenic injuries following blunt abdominal trauma. *SOUTH AFRICAN J Surg.* 2010**	**Retrospective study**	**55 Single center**	**Poor overall quality, 1998–2007, small study group**	**Excluded**
3	**Albrecht RM, Schermer CR, Morris A. Nonoperative management of blunt splenic injuries: factors influencing success in age >55 years. *Am Surg.* 2002**	**Retrospective study**	**37 Single center**	**Small study group**	**Excluded**
4	**Bala M, Edden Y, Mintz Y, et al. Blunt splenic trauma: Predictors for successful non-operative management. *Isr Med Assoc J.* 2007**	**Prospective study**	**64 Single center**	**Admission systolic bloodpressure, extra-abdominal injury are predictors for succesfull NOM, small study group**	**Excluded**
5	Barquist ES, Pizano LR, Feuer W, et al. Inter- and intrarater reliability in computed axial tomographic grading of splenic injury: Why so many grading scales? *J TRAUMA-INJURY Infect Crit CARE.* 2004	Retrospective study	200 Single center	200 CT images were reviewed for inter- and intrarater reliability	Included
6	**Benissa N, Boufettal R, Kadiri Y, et al. Non operative management of blunt splenic trauma in adults. *J Chir (Paris).* 2008**	**Retrospective study**	**62 Single center**	**Overall poor quality paper**	**Excluded**
7	**Bhangu A, Nepogodiev D, Lal N, Bowley DM. Meta-analysis of predictive factors and outcomes for failure of non-operative management of blunt splenic trauma. *Inj J CARE Inj.* 2012**	**Meta-analysis**		**Meta-analysis**	**Excluded**
8	**Brillantino A, Iacobellis F, Robustelli U, et al. Non operative management of blunt splenic trauma: a prospective evaluation of a standardized treatment protocol. *Eur J Trauma Emerg Surg.* September 2015**	**Prospective**	**87**	**No full text available, epub ahead of print**	**Excluded**
9	**Brugère C, Arvieux C, Dubuisson V, et al. Early embolisation in non-operative management of blunt splenic injuries: a retrospective multicentric study. *J Chir (Paris).* 2008**	**Retrospective multicentric study**	**22**	**Full text no longer available, Use of Moore clasification, low power**	**Excluded**
10	C. R, A. A, G.P. S, et al. Management of splenic trauma: a single institution's 8-year experience. *Am J Surg.* 2015	Retrospective registry review	926		Included
11	Chastang L, Bège T, Prudhomme M, et al. Is non-operative management of severe blunt splenic injury safer than embolization or surgery? Results from a French prospective multicenter study. *J Chir Viscerale.* 2015	Prospective multicentric study	91		Included
12	**Clancy AA, Tiruta C, Ashman D, Ball CG, Kirkpatrick AW. The song remains the same although the instruments are changing: complications following selective nonoperative management of blunt spleen trauma: A retrospective review of patients at a level I trauma centre from 1996 to 2007**	**Retrospective**	**538**	**Single center study from 1996–2007, lack of data and statistical analysis**	**Excluded**
13	Claridge JA, Carter JW, McCoy AM, Malangoni MA. In-house direct supervision by an attending is associated with differences in the care of patients with a blunt splenic injury. *Surgery.* 2011	Retrospective review	506		Included
14	Cohn SM, Arango JI, Myers JG, et al. Computed Tomography Grading Systems Poorly Predict the Need for Intervention after Spleen and Liver Injuries. *Am Surg.* 2009		300		Included
15	Cooney R, Ku J, Cherry R, et al. Limitations of splenic angioembolization in treating blunt splenic injury. *J Trauma - Inj Infect Crit Care.* 2005	Retrospective	194		Included

Table 2 Summary table of articles that met inclusion criteria after initial selection. Articles marked in bold were excluded *(Continued)*

16	D. D, G. A, B.A. E, et al. Blunt splenic injuries: High nonoperative management rate can be achieved with selective embolization. *J Trauma - Inj Infect Crit Care*. 2004	Retrospective study	233 + 168		Included
17	D.C. O, J.S.K. L, P.P. DR, et al. Variation in treatment of blunt splenic injury in Dutch academic trauma centers. *J Surg Res*. 2015	Retrospective study	253		Included
18	Dehli T, Bagenholm A, Trasti NC, et al. The treatment of spleen injuries: a retrospective study. *Scand J TRAUMA Resusc Emerg Med*. 2015	Retrospective study	109	More splenic salvage after introduction of SAE	Included
19	Ekeh AP, Khalaf S, Ilyas S, et al. Complications arising from splenic artery embolization: A review of an 11-year experience. *Am J Surg*. 2013	Retrospective study	1383		Included
20	**Ekeh AP, McCarthy MC, Woods RJ, et al. Complications arising from splenic embolization after blunt splenic trauma. *Am J Surg*. 2005**	**Retrospective study**	**284**	**More recent studies were used.**	**Excluded**
21	Fu C-Y, Wu S-C, Chen R-J, et al. Evaluation of need for operative intervention in blunt splenic injury: intraperitoneal contrast extravasation has an increased probability of requiring operative intervention. *World J Surg*. 2010	Retrospective study	69		Included
22	G. T, E. B, A. B, et al. Nonoperative management of blunt splenic injury in adults: there is (still) a long way to go. The results of the Bologna-Maggiore Hospital trauma center experience and development of a clinical algorithm. *Surg Today*. 2015	Retrospective study	293	Development of a BSI protocol	Included
23	Gaarder C, Dormagen JB, Eken T, et al. Nonoperative management of splenic injuries: improved results with angioembolization. *J Trauma*. 2006	Prospective study compared to historic control group	61 + 64	Results after protocol implementation	Included
24	Gonzalez M, Bucher P, Ris F, Andereggen E, Morel P. Splenic trauma: predictive factors for failure of non-operative management. *J Chir (Paris)*. 2008	Retrospective study	190	Predictive factors	Included
25	Haan JM, Biffl W, Knudson MM, et al. Splenic Embolization Revisited: A Multicenter Review. *J Trauma - Inj Infect Crit Care*. 2004	Retrospective multicentric study	140	Complications SAE	Included
26	**Hsieh T-M, Tsai TC, Liang J-L, Lin CC. Non-operative management attempted for selective high grade blunt hepatosplenic trauma is a feasible strategy. *WORLD J Emerg Surg*. 2014**	**Retrospective study**	**150**	**Hepatosplenic group**	**Excluded**
27	J. F, M. R, C. A, et al. Blunt splenic injury: are early adverse events related to trauma, nonoperative management, or surgery? *DIAGNOSTIC Interv Radiol*. 2015	Retrospective study	136	OM worse outcomes but related to ISS	Included
28	J. S, T.L. T, J.B. D, et al. Preserved splenic function after angioembolisation of high grade injury. *Injury*. 2012	Retrospective study	58		Included
29	**K.K. T, M.T. C, A. V, Tan KK, Chiu MT, Vijayan A. Management of isolated splenic injuries after blunt trauma: An institution's experience over 6 years. *Med J Malaysia*. 2010**		**42**	**Did not meet Critical Review Form requirements**	**Excluded**
30	Koca B, Topgul K, Yuruker SS, Cinar H, Kuru B. Non-operative treatment approach for blunt splenic injury: is grade the unique criterion? *Ulus TRAVMA VE ACIL CERRAHI DERGISI-TURKISH J TRAUMA Emerg Surg*. 2013	Retrospective study	31	Factors to consider NOM	Included
31	**Koo T-Y, Ra Y-M, Lee SE, et al. Extension of Nonoperative Management on Spleen Injury with Judicious Selection and Embolization; 10 Years of Experience. *J KOREAN Surg Soc*. 2011**	**Retrospective study**	**151**	**Lack of statistical analysis, did not meet Critical Review Form requirements**	**Excluded**
32	**Kourabi M, Reibel N, Perez M, Grosdidier G. A serious late complication of non-operative management of splenic trauma: rupture of splenic artery aneurysm. *J Chir (Paris)*. 2008**	**Three case reports**	**3**	**Case reports**	**Excluded**

Table 2 Summary table of articles that met inclusion criteria after initial selection. Articles marked in bold were excluded *(Continued)*

33	L.A. O, D. S, C.M. D, et al. Implications of the "contrast blush" finding on computed tomographic scan of the spleen in trauma. *J Trauma - Inj Infect Crit Care*. 2001	Retrospective study	324	Contrast blush alone should not mandate management	Included
34	**Le Moine M-C, Aguilar E, Vacher C, et al. Splenic injury: Management in the Languedoc-Roussillon region. Survey of public hospital surgeons. *J Chir Viscerale*. 2010**	**Survey**	**/**	**Surveys are not considered**	**Excluded**
35	**Liu PP, Lee WC, Cheng YF, et al. Use of splenic artery embolization as an adjunct to nonsurgical management of blunt splenic injury. *J Trauma*. 2004**	**Retrospective?**	**39**	**Did not meet Critical Review Form requirements**	**Excluded**
36	**Lutz N, Mahboubi S, Nance ML, Stafford PW. The significance of contrast blush on computed tomography in children with splenic injuries. *J Pediatr Surg*. 2004**	**Retrospective study**	**133**	**Paediatric population, blush does not mandate SAE**	**Excluded**
37	Marmery H, Shanmuganathan K, Alexander MT, Mirvis SE. Optimization of selection for nonoperative management of blunt splenic injury: Comparison of MDCT grading systems. *Am J Roentgenol*. 2007	Retrospective observational study	496	Comparison of grading systems	Included
38	Marmorale C, Guercioni G, Siquini W, et al. Non-operative management of blunt abdominal injuries. *Chir Ital*. 2007	Retrospective study	123	Nonspecific patient group, low statistical power	Excluded
39	**Matsushima K, Kulaylat AN, Won EJ, Stokes AL, Schaefer EW, Frankel HL. Variation in the management of adolescent patients with blunt abdominal solid organ injury between adult versus pediatric trauma centers: an analysis of a statewide trauma database. *J Surg Res*. 2013**	**Retrospective study**	**1532**	**Paediatric study group**	**Excluded**
40	**Mayglothling JA, Haan JM, Scalea TM, J.A. M, J.M. H, T.M. S. Blunt splenic injuries in the adolescent trauma population: The role of angiography and embolization. *J Emerg Med*. 2009**	**Retrospective study**	**97**	**Adolescent study group**	**Excluded**
41	**Mikocka-Walus A, Beevor HC, Gabbe B, Gruen RL, Winnett J, Cameron P. Management of spleen injuries: the current profile. *ANZ J Surg*. 2010**	**Retrospective study**	**318**	**Unrepresentative patient population**	**Excluded**
42	Miller PR, Chang MC, Hoth JJ, et al. Prospective Trial of Angiography and Embolization for All Grade III to V Blunt Splenic Injuries: Nonoperative Management Success Rate Is Significantly Improved. *J Am Coll Surg*. 2014	Prospective study	168	Prospective use of angiography and SAE	Included
43	Olthof DCC, Sierink JCC, van Delden OMM, Luitse JSKSK, Goslings JCC. Time to intervention in patients with splenic injury in a Dutch level 1 trauma centre. *Inj J CARE Inj*. 2014	Retrospective study	96	Time to intervention	Included
44	Olthof DC, Joosse P, Bossuyt PMM, et al. Observation Versus Embolization in Patients with Blunt Splenic Injury After Trauma: A Propensity Score Analysis. *World J Surg*. December 2015	Propensity score analysis	206	Use of propensity score to contemperous patient groups	Included
45	Olthof DC, van der Vlies CHCH, van der Vlies CHCH, et al. Consensus strategies for the nonoperative management of patients with blunt splenic injury: A Delphi study. *J Trauma Acute Care Surg*. 2013	Delphi study between 30 experts	N/A		Included
46	P. R, T. G, B. S, et al. Management of blunt injuries to the spleen. *Br J Surg*. 2010	Retrospective study	206	Succes of NOM, age	Included
47	Parihar ML, Kumar A, Gamanagatti S, et al. Role of splenic artery embolization in management of traumatic splenic injuries: a prospective study. *Indian J Surg*. 2013	Prospective study	67	Prospective study of success rates with NOM	Included
48	**Ransom KJ, Kavic MS. Laparoscopic splenectomy for blunt trauma: a safe operation following embolization. *Surg Endosc OTHER Interv Tech*. 2009**	**Retrospective study**	**46**	**Laparoscopic splenectomy is safe, not considered for this review**	**Excluded**
49	**Requarth JA. Distal Splenic Artery Hemodynamic Changes During Transient Proximal Splenic Artery Occlusion in Blunt Splenic Injury Patients: A Mechanism of Delayed Splenic Hemorrhage. *J Trauma Inj Infect Crit Care*. 2010**	**Retrospective study**	**7**	**Distal versus proximal embolization, lack of statistical power**	**Excluded**
50	S.-C. W, R.-J. C, A.D. Y, et al. Complications associated with embolization in the treatment of blunt splenic injury. *World J Surg*. 2008	Retrospective study	152	Complications of SAE	Included

Table 2 Summary table of articles that met inclusion criteria after initial selection. Articles marked in bold were excluded *(Continued)*

51	Sabe AA, Claridge JA, Rosenblum DI, Lie K, Malangoni MA. The effects of splenic artery embolization on nonoperative management of blunt splenic injury: a 16-year experience. *J Trauma.* 2009	Retrospective study	815	Three groups, more success NOM when combined with SAE	Included
52	Shih H-C, Wang C-Y, Wen Y-S, et al. Spleen artery embolization aggravates endotoxin hyporesponse of peripheral blood mononuclear cells in patients with spleen injury. *J Trauma.* 2010	Observational study	16	Effect of SAE on splenic function	Included
53	**Shiping L, Jianyong L, Zhi Z, Yun Z. Management of Traumatic Splenic Rupture in Adults: A Single Center's Experience in Mainland China. *Hepatogastroenterology.* 2014**	**Retrospective study**	**125**	**No full text available**	**Excluded**
54	**Skattum J, Loekke RJV, Titze TL, et al. Preserved function after angioembolisation of splenic injury in children and adolescents: A case control study. *Inj J CARE Inj.* 2014**	**Case control**	**11**	**Pediatric and adolescent study group, case control**	**Excluded**
55	**Soo K-M, Lin T-Y, Chen C-W, et al. More Becomes Less: Management Strategy Has Definitely Changed over the Past Decade of Splenic Injury-A Nationwide Population-Based Study. *Biomed Res Int.* 2015**	**Retrospective study**	**578**	**Lack of statistical analysis, no added value to article**	**Excluded**
56	**Stassen NA, Bhullar I, Cheng JD, et al. Selective nonoperative management of blunt splenic injury: An Eastern Association for the Surgery of Trauma practice management guideline. *J Trauma Acute Care Surg.* 2012**	**Guideline**	**N/A**	**Guideline**	**Excluded**
57	Wahl WL, Ahrns KS, Chen S, et al. Blunt splenic injury: Operation versus angiographic embolization. *Surgery.* 2004	Retrospective study	164	Factors to consider for indication of SAE versus operative management	Included
58	Wei B, Hemmila MR, Arbabi S, et al. Angioembolization reduces operative intervention for blunt splenic injury. *J Trauma - Inj Infect Crit Care.* 2008	Retrospective study	317	less complications and better outcomes with SAE	Included
59	Wu S-C, Fu C-Y, Muo C-H, Chang Y-J. Splenectomy in trauma patients is associated with an increased risk of postoperative type II diabetes: a nationwide population-based study. *Am J Surg.* 2014	Retrospective study	3723	Increased risk for T2DM	Included
60	Zarzaur BL, Croce MA, Fabian TC. Variation in the Use of Urgent Splenectomy After Blunt Splenic Injury in Adults. *J TRAUMA-INJURY Infect Crit CARE.* 2011	Retrospective study	11.793	Mortality after splenectomy	Included
61	Zarzaur BL, Savage SA, Croce MA, Fabian TC. Trauma center angiography use in high-grade blunt splenic injuries: Timing is everything. *J Trauma Acute Care Surg.* 2014	Retrospective study	10.405	Use of angio and role in splenectomy	Included
62	Zarzaur BL, Kozar R, Myers JG, et al. The splenic injury outcomes trial. *J Trauma Acute Care Surg.* 2015	Prospective observational study	383	Risk of splenectomy after NOM + SAE, importance of blush on CT	Included

Most studies in the literature are retrospective case series that describe the immediate technical success of SAE without comparisons with surgical treatment or a purely conservative approach. Operative intervention by means of splenectomy is thought to increase morbidity and mortality rates, but this is biased by higher injury severity scores in patients that are surgically managed. A large study of 11,793 patients by Zarzaur et al. (2011) could not confirm a correlation between splenectomy and in-hospital mortality when the data were corrected for demographic, physiologic, and injury-related factors [18]. The risk of overwhelming post-splenectomy sepsis has been advocated as a concern and relative contraindication for splenectomy; however, this rare complication occurs in only approximately 0.9 % of splenectomy cases and is preventable by immunization [19]. A recent, large, population-based study classified 9719 patients with splenic injuries into two groups, splenectomy or non-splenectomy, and compared these against a control group of 30,413 patients with other abdominal injuries. This study warned of a two-fold increased risk of

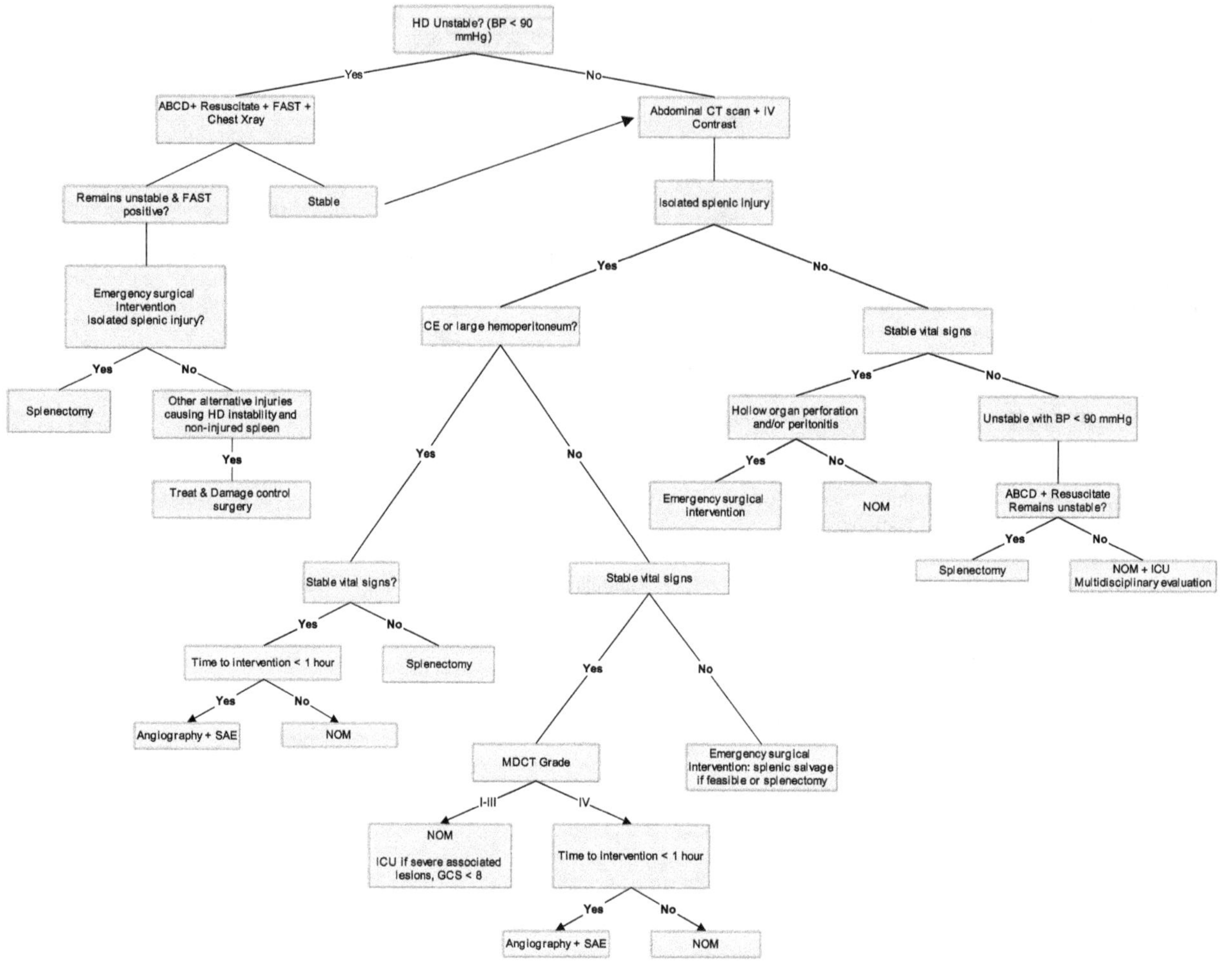

Fig. 1 Algorithm for management of splenic trauma modified from Ekeh and Tugnoli [8, 28]. Abbreviations: HD: hemodynamically; BP: blood pressure; FAST: Focused Assessment with Sonography for Trauma; ICU: Intensive Care Unit; SAE: splenic artery embolization; MDCT: Multidetector CT grading (Table 4); NOM: non operative management; CE: contrast extravasation; IV: intravenous

developing type II diabetes post-splenectomy [20]. In contrast, some authors have reported higher morbidity after SAE than after surgical intervention [21]. In addition, there is evidence of splenic functional alterations after SAE, although research suggests that no immunizations are necessary after NOM combined with SAE [22]. In a 2010 paper, Shih and colleagues demonstrated a cytokine hyporesponse after SAE [23] therefore, SAE should not be considered definitively safer than splenectomy.

Hemodynamically stable patients

SAE, as opposed to pure conservative management, is even more difficult to advocate in hemodynamically stable patients. In a 2015 study, Olthoff et al. looked at the management of 253 patients with splenic injury in Dutch trauma centers taking into account hemodynamic instability on admission, high-grade injury, and ISS [24]. Although the rate of NOM was comparable between the five trauma centers reviewed, the use of SAE for splenic injuries was highly variable between the centers, illustrating the lack of consensus that exists regarding the management of blunt splenic injury.

In hemodynamically stable patients, retrospective studies have shown that NOM has a reduced failure rate when combined with SAE [12, 25–30], but prospective studies and certain retrospective studies have failed to confirm these findings [11, 15]. Several studies have been published that show increased numbers of both minor and major complications, leading to an increase in time spent in the hospital, with the use of SAE [15, 31–33]. Moreover, there is no consensus on the follow-up management and imaging of patients with splenic injuries. Given the lack of evidence in the literature, Olthof et al. published a study in 2013 using the Delphi method to reach an expert opinion on the optimal management and follow-up protocol for blunt splenic injury [28]. In several questionnaires, trauma surgeons and interventional radiologists have tried to reach consensus on the indications for, and optimal follow-up management and imaging to use with, NOM combined with SAE. Almost all of the experts used the American Association for the Surgery of Trauma (AAST) scoring system to grade splenic injuries (Table 3). They all agreed on the use of NOM with or without SAE in small graded injuries (I–II) with no or only a small hemoperitoneum. In high-grade injuries (III–V) with a large hemoperitoneum and active contrast extravasation half of the experts would still attempt NOM + SAE, but most of them would not make a second attempt if the initial SAE failed. Most importantly, they all agreed that rapid intervention is needed for SAE to succeed. Current recommendations are that intervention should be performed within 60 min of admission in stable patients with active contrast extravasation and within 15 to 30 min when a large hemoperitoneum is present. No consensus was reached on management after failure of the initial NOM, or on the appropriate length of stay (LOS) in the hospital.

In search of better criteria for determining the need for intervention, Koca et al. correlated the results of NOM with the American Association for the Surgery of Trauma (AAST) splenic injury grade (see below) [34]. They found that hemodynamically stable patients can safely be treated with NOM, including patients with multi-organ injuries and higher grade splenic injuries. Most injuries are lower grade injuries (I–III), and not surprisingly transfusion is correlated with the injury grade. A 2008 article by Gonzalez et al. added the degree of hemoperitoneum and associated injuries as predictive factors for NOM failure [35]. In 2004, Wahl and colleagues retrospectively analyzed 164 patients with blunt splenic injuries; [36] after univariate analysis they found that lower blood pressure, higher ISS, lower pH, and more packed RBC transfusions are the best indicators of the need for operative intervention. Age, heart rate, splenic abbreviated injury scale score, and GCS did not significantly correlate with the need for operative management. Similarly, Tugnoli et al. (2014) presented the algorithm used in the Bologna-Maggiore Hospital; in 293 patients with splenic injuries admitted between 2009 and 2013 [37] they reported a NOM success rate of 95.8 %. All hemodynamically stable cases with active contrast extravasation or grade V injuries were embolized, preferably proximally within the splenic artery.

In a 2015 AAST prospective observational study, Zarzaur et al. investigated the risk of delayed splenectomy after NOM with or without SAE [38]. They found that the only risk factor for delayed splenectomy was the finding of active extravasation at presentation; thus calling for closer observation of patients with this finding irrespective of whether SAE was performed. Patients with grade I injury had no risk for delayed splenectomy. In cases with higher grade (II to V) injuries, the authors advocated close observation for 10–14 days. In the 2005 study of Haan et al. the presence of arteriovenous fistula on CT imaging was predictive for 40 % of failure rates in nonoperatively managed patients [9]. The presence of vascular lesions (arteriovenous fistulas, pseudoaneurysms) and impact on NOM success rates was further investigated by several authors. In a 2014 study, the Wake Forest University investigated failure rates after angiography with subsequent embolization, ignoring presence or absence of any vascular lesion, for all grade III to V splenic injuries in stable patients in a protocolized manner and comparing this to a historic control group [39]. From 168 patients 67 % were managed nonoperatively with an overall NOM failure rate of 5 %. In the patient group where protocol was violated the failure rate was 25 % compared to 3 % in the protocol group ($P = 0.03$). Comparing this to a historic control group, 52 % patients underwent NOM with a significant higher failure rate of 15 % ($P = 0.04$). For each injury grade they reported lower failure rates in the study

Table 3 Traditionally used American Association for the Surgery of Trauma (AAST) scoring system for splenic injuries

Grade	Hematoma	Laceration
I	Subcapsular < 10 % of surface area	Capsular tear < 1 cm deep into parenchyma
II	Subcapsular 10–50 % of surface area	Capsular tear 1–3 cm deep into parenchyma NO involvement of trabecular vessels
III	Subcapsular > 50 % of surface area OR Expanding, ruptured subcapsular or parenchymal hematoma OR Intraparenchymal hematoma > 5 cm or expanding	>3 cm deep into parenchyma or trabecular vessel involvement
IV		Segmental or hilar vessel involvement with major devascularization (>25 %) of spleen
V	Shattered spleen	Hilar vascular injury that devascularizes spleen

group compared to the control group and when protocol was followed. However, they did not reach statistical significance when comparing patients treated according to protocol or patients deviating from protocol in injury grades IV and V. The authors did not report on complications or on splenic function after embolization in their study group, no data is available whether proximal or distal embolization was used.

Another prospective study from Parihar et al. [40] found a shorter LOS in SAE patients (5.4 days compared with 6.6 days for NOM patients without SAE), as well as higher hemoglobin concentrations and systolic blood pressures. A recent study, which used propensity score analysis, found no statistically significant difference between observation and embolization in the subsequent splenectomy rate [41].

Scoring systems

Many scoring systems have been developed to grade splenic injuries, among which the AAST grading system for splenic injury (Table 3) is the most popular. Two separate studies have correlated CT findings with the AAST injury grade and subsequent need for intervention. In the study by Barquist et al. [42], four radiologists retrospectively reviewed 200 CT images of patients who had undergone splenectomy; the operative grading of the splenic injuries was used as a gold standard. The weighted kappa score for intrarater reproducibility was 0.15–0.77 and the interrater kappa score was 0–0.84 (mean 0.23). In the study by Cohn et al. [43], five radiologists reviewed CT scans of 300 patients with liver and splenic injuries using the AAST grading system. Twenty-one percent of the patients with splenic injuries visible on CT images required intervention. Cohn et al. reached the same conclusion as Barquist et al.; the sensitivity of the AAST injury grade for predicting the need for intervention is poor and interrater variability, even among experienced radiologists, is high. Both thus concluded that the AAST scoring system is unreliable because even experienced radiologists often underestimate the magnitude of the injury, and other factors should also be considered when evaluating indications for surgery or angiography. The authors also evaluated kappa scores for the reporting of contrast blush on CT imaging and found that they were similarly variable, although contrast blush on CT imaging is considered a major indication that intervention is needed.

In 2001, Protetch et al. reported that the incidence of contrast blush was related to the grade of injury, with 3.2 % of grade I/II injuries and up to 37.6 % of grade IV and V injuries showing a contrast blush in CT images [44]. Interventions were more frequent when a contrast blush was present, but multivariate regression analysis showed no correlation between finding a contrast blush and splenic intervention. This was confirmed by both Thompson et al. and Michailidou et al.; both also reported that the size of the contrast blush was correlated with the need for intervention [45, 46]. They both found that similar cut-off values (1 cm and 1.5 cm) indicated the need for intervention. Other factors that also correlated with the need for intervention in splenic injury were injury grade, hypotension on admission to the emergency department, and age. The findings of these studies support the need for better protocols and parameters to allow proper assessment of the need for intervention in cases of splenic trauma.

In 2007, Marmery et al. suggested a new grading system for splenic injury that takes into account active bleeding or splenic vascular injury (including splenic pseudoaneurysms and arteriovenous fistulas) [47]. Their new grading system was statistically significantly better than the AAST grading system in terms of its ability to predict the need for splenic arteriography ($P = 0.0036$) or the combination of arteriography and surgery ($P = 0.0006$). Table 4 presents the proposed new grading system.

Complications

There has been much research published, and work is still ongoing, to understand the complications after SAE compared with those after surgery and NOM. All of the treatment modalities for splenic injury are associated with high morbidity rates. Specific morbidities associated with SAE include pancreatitis, splenic infarction, post-embolization syndrome, and intestinal perforation.

Two retrospective studies examined the complications that occur after SAE [32, 33]. Ekeh et al. reviewed 1383 patients with blunt splenic injury over an 11-year period; 78.5 % were treated nonoperatively, and of this group 8.1 % underwent SAE. Major complications including splenic infarction, splenic abscess, contrast-induced

Table 4 Newly proposed Multi-Detector CT (MDCT) grading system, reproduced from Marmery et al. (2007)

Grade	
I	• Subcapsular hematoma < 1-cm thick • Laceration < 1 cm deep into parenchyma
II	• Subcapsular hematoma 1–3-cm thick • Parenchymal hematoma 1–3-cm diameter • Laceration 1–3 cm deep into parenchyma
III	• Splenic capsular disruption • Subcapsular hematoma > 3-cm thick • Parenchymal hematoma > 3-cm diameter • Laceration > 3 cm deep into parenchyma
IVa	• Active intraparenchymal and subcapsular splenic bleeding • Splenic vascular injury (pseudoaneurysm or arteriovenous fistula) • Shattered spleen
IVb	• Active intraperitoneal bleeding

renal insufficiency, and splenic cysts occurred in 14 % of the patients who underwent SAE. Wu et al. reported that 28.5 % of patients who underwent SAE experienced major complications. Distal embolization was associated with more major complications than proximal SAE. Minor complications (pleural effusion, coil migration, and fever) occurred in 34 % and 61.9 % of the patients in the SAE groups in the studies by Ekeh et al. and Wu et al., respectively.

In 2004, Haan et al. reported SAE complication rates in 140 patients and reported a splenic salvage rate of 87 % [31]. This rate indirectly correlated with injury severity scores. More than 80 % of the grade IV and V injuries in their study were successfully managed nonoperatively. No significant difference was noted in patients older than 55 years of age. The presence of a significant hemoperitoneum did not alter success rates; however, the presence of arteriovenous fistulas did. They concluded that complications after SAE are common, but do not seem to influence outcomes.

In 2008, Wei et al. published a retrospective study showing lower complication rates after SAE even with higher splenic Abbreviated Injury Scores in this group compared with the operatively managed group (6 % vs. 36 %, $P < 0.01$) [30]. They found that the introduction of SAE reduced operative interventions by 16 % between 2000 and 2006 in their Level 1 center. A French prospective multicenter study investigated complication rates in 91 patients [21]. Twenty percent underwent splenectomy with a postsurgical morbidity of 15 %. Fifteen patients (16 %) underwent embolization and 67 were initially managed nonoperatively. In the embolization group with severe injury (grade III–V), the morbidity was 73 %. The splenectomy group with severe injury had a total morbidity of 70 %. The NOM group had a morbidity of 58 %. Specific morbidities after NOM, surgery, and SAE were 10, 15, and 47 % ($P = 0.02$), respectively. The study concluded that embolization should not be used as a prophylactic measure, but should only be used in cases with active bleeding. We could not find well-designed studies comparing complication rates between the three treatment modalities.

Other factors to be considered

- Need for transfusion

In their 2015 study of 253 patients, Olthoff et al. found a very large variation but no significant difference in the need for transfusion between patients treated with SAE and those treated with NOM [24]. The mean number of transfused blood products was 5.5 units (±9.9) in the NOM group versus 9.1 units (±17.2) in embolized patients ($P = 0.75$). Rosati et al. reported on the need for transfusion in patients requiring immediate splenectomy (70 %), embolization (46.5 %), and NOM (25.9 %), but failed to adjust these data for injury severity and confounders [12]. They found that the need for transfusion was a major risk factor for mortality (adjusted OR = 2.63; CI 1.27 – 5.42, $P = 0.009$). Dent et al. compared transfusion rates between NOM, early embolization, and operative management [25]. They reported a 2.1-unit difference in the transfusion rate ($P < 0.01$) of the NOM group versus the operative management group, and found no statistically significant difference between transfusion rates in the early embolization and operative management groups without correcting for confounders. They also found no difference in transfusion rates when they compared patients who underwent early embolization versus late embolization.

- Impact of direct supervision

A retrospective review in 2011 investigated the impact of direct supervision (DS) or indirect supervision (IS) on the management of splenic injuries [48]. Using data from 506 cases the authors found significant differences in compliance with protocols (DS, 95 % vs. IS, 82 %, $P < 0.001$), operation rates (DS 16 %, vs. IS, 8 %, $P = 0.016$), ICU use (IS, 84.1 % vs. DS, 73.0 %, $P = 0.029$), hospital costs (IS, \$142.956 ± \$36.219 vs. DS, \$62.981 ± \$8.784, $P = 0.048$), and use of SAE without indication (IS, 8 vs. DS, 0). Interestingly, there were no reported differences in mortality or splenectomy rates.

- Time to intervention and volume of the centers.

In 2014, Olthof et al. retrospectively examined the time to intervention in patients undergoing SAE and patients undergoing surgery in a cohort of 96 adults [49]. In hemodynamically stable patients, the median time to intervention for patients in the SAE group was 117 min compared with 105 min for patients in the surgery group. The differences in time to intervention or reintervention, and the complication rates were not significantly different between the two patient groups. There was a higher transfusion rate for patients in the splenic surgery group; the median number of transfused units of packed RBCs was eight for hemodynamically unstable patients undergoing SAE versus 24 for patients undergoing splenic surgery ($P = 0.09$). A report published in 2015 reviewed 10,405 records in the National Trauma Data Bank to find a correlation between high and low angio centers and to investigate any relationship between angiography use and its timing or splenectomy after angiography [50]. They concluded that early angiography is associated with higher splenic salvage rates but found no statistically significant difference in splenectomy rates between the high and low angiography volume centers.

We could not find any articles comparing the relationship between time to intervention and success or complication rates between patients undergoing NOM, SAE, or splenic surgery.

- Costs & Length of stay

Different authors have investigated the costs of SAE versus surgical management. Wahl et al. reported no significant cost differences between these two treatment modalities (SAE, \$49.300 ± \$40.460 vs. OM, \$54.590 ± \$34.760) [36]. This was confirmed by Wei et al., who found the costs associated with SAE to be \$47,000 ± \$31,000 and the costs associated with OM to be \$40,000 ± \$34,000 [30]. Both authors assessed the LOS and differences in LOS in patients who received different treatments. Wahl et al. found an average LOS of 45 ± 26 days for patients who went directly to the operating theatre, compared with 14 ± 15 days for patients who underwent SAE ($P < 0.02$). Wei et al. found that the average LOS in the surgical group was 14 ± 10 days and in the SAE group was 12 ± 12 days ($P > 0.05$). Bruce et al. also came to the same conclusion in their 2011 study; [51] in that study the median total hospital charges were \$41,269 (± \$31,128) for the NOM + SAE group compared with \$46,356 (± \$11,334) for the OM group ($P = 0.545$). They did report higher procedure-related charges for OM patients compared with patients undergoing NOM + SAE (\$28,709 ± \$6941 vs. \$19,062 ± \$14,025; $P = 0.16$); however, this was offset by more charges for a greater number of radiological evaluations in the other group.

Summary

Based on the literature review we propose a new, non-verified, decision algorithm for splenic trauma. We hope this can further serve as a tree of order in the vast amount of publications concerning this topic. We stress that this algorithm is not verified and should be further verified in well designed, prospective studies, is it to be used in daily practice.

The term hemodynamically unstable is not clearly defined in most literature and it is often unclear if authors included or excluded transient responders. The nature of the patient's response to fluid therapy is important and should be considered in all splenic trauma protocols. Most authors agree that surgical intervention is indicated when the patient is hemodynamically unstable. In close relation with response to fluid resuscitation is time to intervention, which is an important factor to consider from the start. Higher splenic salvage rates are achieved when earlier intervention is possible and expert opinion states that intervention is recommended within one hour of admittance. In prospect, when the time to intervention will be several hours OM or NOM may be better options than SAE, depending on the clinical presentation. Clinicians and surgeons should always keep in mind that pre- and post-intervention delays make it increasingly difficult to operate because of the several surgical and nonsurgical issues that can develop (e.g., clotting of the intraperitoneal hemorrhage, infection, and development of comorbidities). Non responders should be triaged promptly with a minimal delay towards surgical intervention.

There is a distinction between major and minor complications and treatment-specific morbidities. While it is difficult to correlate complications with the embolization procedure, especially in small studies, it is interesting to look at treatment-specific complications and associated risk-benefit ratios; however, no well-designed studies compare NOM, NOM + SAE, and OM for the treatment of splenic trauma. Until such studies are available, we should look at the clinical value and possible risks of an intervention on a patient-specific level while considering all factors, and keeping in mind the relatively high complication rate after SAE. It is important to avoid the bias of expecting operative interventions to have higher complication rates than SAE, which seems like a less invasive procedure. Increased use of NOM with or without SAE should not erode clinical judgment and surgical skills.

Currently there is no evidence of reduced transfusion rates when SAE is used in conjunction with NOM compared with NOM alone. Transfusion rates are higher in patients who undergo an operative intervention and are a risk factor for mortality; however, no studies are available that compare similar patient groups and their corresponding transfusion rates.

Multiple studies have reported on the cost effectiveness of splenic injury management: operative intervention brings the costs of surgery and of higher transfusion rates; however, conversely NOM + SAE requires higher imaging costs and there is ultimately no significant difference between the costs of the two interventions.

We reviewed the different scoring systems and the use of imaging for diagnosing splenic injuries. As imaging modalities improve smaller bleeds are increasingly being visualized. It is known that these bleeds can be self-limiting; however, no studies have shown the clinical significance of these small bleeds and other radiological findings such as pseudoaneurysms and arteriovenous fistulas. Additional studies will be needed to assess whether embolization is superior to NOM in these cases. Studies have shown important interrater and intrarater differences in image evaluation in cases of splenic injury, and more specifically in the assessment of a contrast blush on CT imaging. Contrast blush is considered an important parameter for assessment of the need for intervention but recent studies have shown that the size of the contrast blush is what matters. Though whether a cut-off value of 1 cm or 1.5 cm is more suitable for determining the optimal treatment is not yet known. According to the literature, the presence of a hemoperitoneum does not alter the success rates of SAE.

The MDCT grading system proposed by Marmery et al. has shown a better correlation with the need for intervention than the conventionally used AAST grading system. Currently, there is no consensus on the use of one grading system that correlates well with the need for intervention, and most published studies have used the AAST grading system. Lack of standardized grading makes it difficult to compare older studies with recent and future studies. Interpreting CT images and grading the splenic injury is difficult and should be performed by experienced radiologists using the proposed grading system with a consistent technique. We propose the use of specific image analysis protocols to achieve a consistent approach and improve future studies. We propose the use of the MDCT grading system in our decision algorithm.

The treatment plan should be managed by experienced trauma surgeons or interventional radiologists using a multidisciplinary approach when possible. It should be clear who is responsible for assessing the indications for SAE, NOM, or OM. The literature has shown better results when protocols are in place; and ideally there should be consensus on who is responsible for initiating treatment.

Conclusions

The current literature is unclear on the correct indications for NOM ± SAE versus surgery for splenic trauma. To further clarify current evidence we propose, a non-verified, decision algorithm for blunt abdominal trauma. A prospective well designed study is needed to validate our decision algorithm. Consensus on the management of blunt splenic injury between radiologists, trauma surgeons and emergency medicine physicians could reduce conflicting data, improve current protocols, and avoid harm to patients. More prospective data and well-designed studies, taking into account other factors including long term results and morbidity, on the management of splenic trauma are needed.

Additional file

Additional file 1: Table 1. Search results and number of articles retrieved after applying the selection criteria.After the initial search, all articles were entered in a reference database (Mendeley). **Table 2.** Summary table of articles that met inclusion criteria after initial selection. Articles marked in grey were excluded. **Table 3.** Traditionally used American Association for the Surgery of Trauma (AAST) scoring system for splenic injuries. **Figure 1.** Algorithm for management of splenic trauma modified from Ekeh and Tugnoli.8, 32 Abbreviations: HD: hemodynamically; BP: blood pressure; FAST: Focused Assessment with Sonography for Trauma; ICU: Intensive Care Unit; SAE: splenic artery embolization; MDCT: Multidetector CT grading (Table 4); NOM: non operative management; CE: contrast extravasation; IV: intravenous.

Abbreviations

AAST: American Association for the Surgery of Trauma; BP: Blood pressure; CE: Contrast extravasation; DS: Direct supervision; FAST scan: Focused assessment with sonography for trauma; GCS: Glasgow coma scale; HD: Hemodynamically; ICU: Intensive care unit; IS: Indirect supervision; ISS: Injury severity score; IV: Intravenous; LOS: Length of stay; MDCT: Multidetector computer tomography; NOM: Nonoperative management; OM: Operative management; OR: Operating room; OSS: Operative splenic salvage; RBCs: Red blood cells; SAE: Splenic artery embolization

Acknowledgements

None.

Funding

None.

Authors' contributions

FvdC and AM were responsible for the study concept and design. FvdC carried out the literature search. Both authors critically reviewed the manuscript for important intellectual content. AM was the study supervisor. Both authors read and approved the final version of the manuscript.

Competing interests

The authors declare that they have no competing interests.

Author details

[1]Third year master's student, Faculty of Medicine, Catholic University of Leuven (KU Leuven), Gasthuisberg, Belgium. [2]Department of Upper Gastrointestinal Surgery, Royal Devon & Exeter Hospital, Exeter, UK.

References

1. Raza M, Abbas Y, Devi V, Prasad KV, Rizk KN, Nair PP. Nonoperative management of abdominal trauma – a 10 years review. World J Emerg Surg. 2013;8(1):14.
2. Søreide K. Epidemiology of major trauma. Br J Surg. 2009;96(7):697–8.
3. Maddison FE. Embolic therapy of hypersplenism. Invest Radiol. 1973;8(4):280–1.
4. Chuang VP, Reuter SR. Selective arterial embolization for the control of traumatic splenic bleeding. Invest Radiol. 1975;10(1):18–24.
5. Panetta T, Sclafani SJA, Goldstein AS, Phillips TF. Percutaneous transcatheter embolization for arterial trauma. J Vasc Surg. 1985;2(1):54–64.
6. Haller Jr JA, Papa P, Drugas G, Colombani P. Nonoperative management of solid organ injuries in children. Is it safe? Ann Surg. 1994;219(6):625–8. discussion 628–631.
7. Sclafani S, Shafan GW, Scalea TM, et al. Nonoperative salvage of computed tomography–diagnosed splenic injuries : utilization of angiography for triage and embolization for hemostasis. J Trauma Injury Infect Crit Care. 1995;39(5):818–27.

8. Peitzman AB, Heil B, Rivera L, et al. Blunt splenic injury in adults: multi-institutional study of the Eastern association for the surgery of trauma. J Trauma. 2000;49(2):177–87. discussion 187–189.
9. Haan JM, Bochicchio GV, Kramer N, Scalea TM. Nonoperative management of blunt splenic injury: a 5-year experience. J Trauma. 2005;58(3):492–8.
10. Fu C-Y, Wu S-C, Chen R-J, et al. Evaluation of need for operative intervention in blunt splenic injury: intraperitoneal contrast extravasation has an increased probability of requiring operative intervention. World J Surg. 2010;34(11):2745–51.
11. Ekeh AP, Izu B, Ryan M, McCarthy M. The impact of splenic artery embolization on the management of splenic trauma: an 8-year review. Am J Surg. 2009;197(3):337–41.
12. Rosati C, Ata A, Siskin GP, et al. Management of splenic trauma: a single institution's 8-year experience. Am J Surg. 2015;209(2):308–14.
13. Law M, Stewart D, Letts L, Pollock N, Bosch J, Westmorland M. Guidelines for critical review form : qualitative studies. McMaster Univ Occup Ther Evidence-Based Pract Res Gr. 2007;1–12.
14. Cooney R, Ku J, Cherry R, et al. Limitations of splenic angioembolization in treating blunt splenic injury. J Trauma. 2005;59(4):926–32.
15. Peitzman AB, Harbrecht BG, Rivera L, Heil B. Eastern Association for the Surgery of Trauma Multi institutional Trials Workgroup. Failure of observation of blunt splenic injury in adults: variability in practice and adverse consequences. J Am Coll Surg. 2005;201(2):179–87.
16. Peitzman AB, Ferrada P, Puyana JC. Nonoperative management of blunt trauma: have we gone too far? Surg Infect. 2009;10(5):427–33.
17. Hagiwara A, Fukushima H, Murata A, Matsuda H, Shimazaki S. Blunt splenic injury: usefulness of transcatheter arterial embolization in patients with a transient response to fluid resuscitation. Radiology. 2005;235(1):57–64.
18. Zarzaur BL, Croce MA, Fabian TC. Variation in the use of urgent splenectomy after blunt splenic injury in adults. J Trauma. 2011;71(5):1333–9.
19. Holdsworth R, Irving A, Cuschieri A. Postsplenectomy sepsis and its mortality rate: actual versus perceived risks. Br J Surg. 1991;78(9):1031–8.
20. Wu S-C, Fu C-Y, Muo C-H, Chang Y-J. Splenectomy in trauma patients is associated with an increased risk of postoperative type II diabetes: a nationwide population-based study. Am J Surg. 2014;208(5):811–6.
21. Chastang L, Bège T, Prudhomme M, et al. Is non-operative management of severe blunt splenic injury safer than embolization or surgery? Results from a French prospective multicenter study. J Visc Surg. 2015;152(2):85–91.
22. Skattum J, Titze TL, Dormagen JB, et al. Preserved splenic function after angioembolisation of high grade injury. Injury. 2012;43(1):62–6.
23. Shih H-C, Wang C-Y, Wen Y-S, et al. Spleen artery embolization aggravates endotoxin hyporesponse of peripheral blood mononuclear cells in patients with spleen injury. J Trauma. 2010;68(3):532–7.
24. Olthoff DC, Luitse JSK, de Rooij PP, et al. Variation in treatment of blunt splenic injury in Dutch academic trauma centers. J Surg Res. 2015;194(1):233–8.
25. Dent D, Alsabrook G, Erickson BA, et al. Blunt splenic injuries: high nonoperative management rate can be achieved with selective embolization. J Trauma. 2004;56(5):1063–7.
26. Dehli T, Bagenholm A, Trasti NC, et al. The treatment of spleen injuries: a retrospective study. Scand J Trauma Resusc Emerg Med. 2015;23(1):85.
27. Gaarder C, Dormagen JB, Eken T, et al. Nonoperative management of splenic injuries: improved results with angioembolization. J Trauma. 2006;61(1):192–8.
28. Olthof DC, van der Vlies CHCH, van der Vlies CHCH, et al. Consensus strategies for the nonoperative management of patients with blunt splenic injury: a Delphi study. J Trauma Acute Care Surg. 2013;74(6):1567–74.
29. Sabe AA, Claridge JA, Rosenblum DI, Lie K, Malangoni MA. The effects of splenic artery embolization on nonoperative management of blunt splenic injury: a 16-year experience. J Trauma. 2009;67(3):565.
30. Wei B, Hemmila MR, Arbabi S, et al. Angioembolization reduces operative intervention for blunt splenic injury. J Trauma. 2008;64(6):1472–7.
31. Haan JM, Biffl W, Knudson MM, et al. Splenic embolization revisited: a multicenter review. J Trauma. 2004;56(3):542–7.
32. Ekeh AP, Khalaf S, Ilyas S, et al. Complications arising from splenic artery embolization: a review of an 11-year experience. Am J Surg. 2013;205(3): 250–4.
33. Wu S-C, Chen R-J, Yang AD, et al. Complications associated with embolization in the treatment of blunt splenic injury. World J Surg. 2008; 32(3):476–82.
34. Koca B, Topgul K, Yuruker SS, Cinar H, Kuru B. Non-operative treatment approach for blunt splenic injury: is grade the unique criterion? J Trauma Emerg Surg. 2013;19(4):337–42.
35. Gonzalez M, Bucher P, Ris F, Andereggen E, Morel P. Splenic trauma: predictive factors for failure of non-operative management. J Chir (Paris). 2008;145(6):561–7.
36. Wahl WL, Ahrns KS, Chen S, et al. Blunt splenic injury: Operation versus angiographic embolization. Surgery. 2004;136(4):891–9.
37. Tugnoli G, Bianchi E, Biscardi A, et al. Nonoperative management of blunt splenic injury in adults: there is (still) a long way to go. The results of the Bologna-Maggiore Hospital trauma center experience and development of a clinical algorithm. Surg Today. 2015;45(10):1210–7.
38. Zarzaur BL, Kozar R, Myers JG, et al. The splenic injury outcomes trial. J Trauma Acute Care Surg. 2015;79(3):335–42.
39. Miller PR, Chang MC, Requarth JA, et al. Prospective Trial of Angiography and Embolization for All Grade III to V Blunt Splenic Injuries: nonoperative management success rate is significantly improved. J Am Coll Surg. 2014;218(4):644–8.
40. Parihar ML, Kumar A, Gamanagatti S, et al. Role of splenic artery embolization in management of traumatic splenic injuries: a prospective study. Indian J Surg. 2013;75(5):361–7.
41. Olthof DC, Joosse P, Bossuyt PMM, et al. Observation versus embolization in patients with blunt splenic injury after trauma: a propensity score analysis. World J Surg. 2016;40(5):1264–71.
42. Barquist ES, Pizano LR, Feuer W, et al. Inter- and intrarater reliability in computed axial tomographic grading of splenic injury: why so many grading scales? J Trauma. 2004;56(2):334–8.
43. Cohn SM, Arango JI, Myers JG, et al. Computed tomography grading systems poorly predict the need for intervention after spleen and liver injuries. Am Surg. 2009;75(2):133–9.
44. Omert LA, Salyer D, Dunham CM, Porter J, Silva A, Protetch J. Implications of the "contrast blush" finding on computed tomographic scan of the spleen in trauma. J Trauma. 2001;51(2):272–8.
45. Thompson BE, Munera F, Cohn SM, MacLean AA, Cameron J, Rivas L, et al. Novel computed tomography scan scoring system predicts the need for intervention after splenic injury. J Trauma. 2006;60(5):1083–6.
46. Michailidou M, Velmahos GC, van der Wilden G, Alam HB, de Moya M, Chang Y. "Blush" on trauma computed tomography: not as bad as we think! J Trauma Acute Care Surg. 2012;73(3):580–4.
47. Marmery H, Shanmuganathan K, Alexander MT, Mirvis SE. Optimization of selection for nonoperative management of blunt splenic injury: Comparison of MDCT grading systems. Am J Roentgenol. 2007;189(6):1421–7.
48. Claridge JA, Carter JW, McCoy AM, Malangoni MA. In-house direct supervision by an attending is associated with differences in the care of patients with a blunt splenic injury. Surgery. 2011;150(4):718–25.
49. Olthof DC, Sierink JC, van Delden OM, Luitse JSK, Goslings JC. Time to intervention in patients with splenic injury in a Dutch level 1 trauma centre. Injury. 2014;45(1):95–100.
50. Zarzaur BL, Savage SA, Croce MA, Fabian TC. Trauma center angiography use in high-grade blunt splenic injuries: timing is everything. J Trauma Acute Care Surg. 2014;77(5):666–71.
51. Bruce PJP, Helmer SD, Harrison PB, Sirico T, Haan JM. Nonsurgical management of blunt splenic injury: Is it cost effective? Am J Surg. 2011;202(6):810–6. doi:10.1016/j.amjsurg.2011.06.041.

18

Knowledge, awareness, and attitude towards infection prevention and management among surgeons: identifying the surgeon champion

Massimo Sartelli[1*], Yoram Kluger[2], Luca Ansaloni[3], Federico Coccolini[3], Gian Luca Baiocchi[4], Timothy C. Hardcastle[5], Ernest E. Moore[6], Addison K. May[7], Kamal M. F. Itani[8], Donald E. Fry[9,10], Marja A. Boermeester[11], Xavier Guirao[12], Lena Napolitano[13], Robert G. Sawyer[14], Kemal Rasa[15], Fikri M. Abu-Zidan[16], Abdulrashid K. Adesunkanmi[17], Boyko Atanasov[18], Goran Augustin[19], Miklosh Bala[20], Miguel A. Cainzos[21], Alain Chichom-Mefire[22], Francesco Cortese[23], Dimitris Damaskos[24], Samir Delibegovic[25], Zaza Demetrashvili[26], Belinda De Simone[27], Therese M. Duane[28], Wagih Ghnnam[29], George Gkiokas[30], Carlos A. Gomes[31], Andreas Hecker[32], Aleksandar Karamarkovic[33], Jakub Kenig[34], Vladimir Khokha[35], Victor Kong[36], Arda Isik[37], Ari Leppäniemi[38], Andrey Litvin[39], Eftychios Lostoridis[40], Gustavo M. Machain[41], Sanjay Marwah[42], Michael McFarlane[43], Cristian Mesina[44], Ionut Negoi[45], Iyiade Olaoye[46], Tadeja Pintar[47], Guntars Pupelis[48], Miran Rems[49], Ines Rubio-Perez[50], Boris Sakakushev[51], Helmut Segovia-Lohse[41], Boonying Siribumrungwong[52], Peep Talving[53], Jan Ulrych[54], András G. Vereczkei[55], Francesco M. Labricciosa[56] and Fausto Catena[57]

Abstract

Despite evidence supporting the effectiveness of best practices of infection prevention and management, many surgeons worldwide fail to implement them. Evidence-based practices tend to be underused in routine practice. Surgeons with knowledge in surgical infections should provide feedback to prescribers and integrate best practices among surgeons and implement changes within their team. Identifying a local opinion leader to serve as a champion within the surgical department may be important. The "surgeon champion" can integrate best clinical practices of infection prevention and management, drive behavior change in their colleagues, and interact with both infection control teams in promoting antimicrobial stewardship.

Keywords: Surgeon, Infection, Prevention, Antibiotic therapy

Background

In 2017, a global declaration for appropriate use of antimicrobials across the surgical pathway was shared by over 230 experts from 83 different countries [1]. Within this declaration, the authors highlighted the effects of antibiotic exposure, misuse, and overuse on antibiotic resistance and outlined the fundamental principles of appropriate antibiotic prophylaxis and therapy in surgery.

In that declaration, efforts to prevent healthcare-associated infections (HAIs) were not specifically highlighted [2]. HAIs including surgical site infection, ventilator-associated pneumonia, central line-associated bloodstream infection, and catheter-associated urinary tract infection are the most common nosocomial infections. Healthcare-associated infections continue to be of significant importance in surgical patients.

Surgical site infections (SSIs) are a major clinical problem in terms of morbidity, mortality, length of hospital

* Correspondence: massimosartelli@gmail.com
[1]Department of Surgery, Macerata Hospital, Via Santa Lucia, 62100 Macerata, Italy

stay, and overall direct and indirect costs globally [3, 4]. However, knowledge, attitudes, and awareness of infection prevention and control measures vary significantly among surgeons. Most significantly, a gap seems to exist between best evidence and clinical practice with regard to SSIs prevention.

The World Health Organization (WHO) [5], the Centers for Disease Control and Prevention (CDC) [6], and a combined effort by the American College of Surgeons/Surgical Infection Society [7, 8] have recently published guidelines for the prevention of SSIs. Despite clear evidence and guidelines to direct SSIs prevention strategies, compliance is unacceptably poor [9].

Preoperative antibiotic prophylaxis (PAP) is a cornerstone of SSIs prevention. The use of PAP contributes considerably to the total amount of antibiotics used in hospitals worldwide. PAP has been shown to be an effective measure for the prevention of SSIs, but its use should be limited to specific, well-accepted indications to avoid cost, toxicity, and antimicrobial resistance, and should never substitute for the good medical practice of infection prevention and control. Guidelines stress the importance of cessation of antibiotic prophylaxis immediately after surgery and refrain from the extension of prophylaxis outside the operating theater [5]. High rates of inappropriate use of prophylactic antibiotics in surgery continue to be reported in the literature [9]. In Appendix 1, seven strategies for correct antibiotic prophylaxis are illustrated.

Antibiotic therapy is an additional key component of daily surgical practice. Antibiotics are life-saving when treating bacterial infections but are often used inappropriately, specifically when not indicated. Antibiotic therapy plays an integral role in the management of surgical infections, especially in critically ill patients who require immediate empiric antibiotic therapy. Poor antibiotic coverage and inappropriate regimens are the variables most strongly associated with unfavorable outcomes [10, 11]. The timing, regimen, dose, route of administration, and duration of antibiotic therapy should be always optimized. In most patients with surgical infections, antibiotic therapy aims to treat any residual infection after adequate source control. In these patients, prolonging antibiotic treatment, which can lead to antibiotic resistance, does not prevent the persistence or recurrence of the infection. When source control is obtained, the duration of antibiotic therapy should be shortened as much as possible, unless there are special circumstances that require prolonging antimicrobial therapy, such as signs of an ongoing infection. Patients who have systemic signs of sepsis beyond 5 to 7 days of treatment warrant diagnostic investigation to determine an ongoing uncontrolled source of infection needing intervention [8]. In Appendix 2, ten strategies for correct antibiotic therapy are illustrated.

The surgeon as a champion in preventing and treating infections

Surgeons prescribing antibiotics have two opposing responsibilities. They have to (1) offer optimal therapy for the individual patient under their care and (2) restrain from overprescribing antibiotics to preserve their efficacy and minimize the rate of emergence of antimicrobial resistance, while also preventing collateral damage from antibiotics (such as *Clostridium difficile* infections) [12].

Because most surgeons have already established their attitudes and behaviors with regard to antibiotic usage, it is difficult to change their deeply established views and practice patterns. A range of factors such as diagnostic uncertainty, fear of clinical failure, time pressure, or organizational issues can influence prescribing decisions. However, due to cognitive dissonance (recognizing that an action is necessary but not implementing it), it is very challenging to change the prescribing behavior [1].

Surgeons should be aware of their role and responsibility for maintaining the effectiveness of current and future antibiotics. Although most of them are aware of the problem of antimicrobial resistance (AMR), many still underestimate this problem in their own hospital and in their patients. Inappropriate use of antibiotics, as well as poor prevention and control of infections such as hand hygiene, is contributing to the development of AMR. Surgeons are at the forefront in managing patients with infections and should take a proactive role in ensuring both effective antibiotic therapy and the avoidance of inappropriate and unnecessary antibiotic exposure [12].

Successful and cost-effective strategies to reduce AMR should involve a multi-faceted approach aimed at optimizing antibiotic use, strengthening surveillance and infection prevention and control, and improving clinician education regarding the appropriate use of antibiotics.

A growing body of evidence demonstrates that hospital-based programs dedicated to improving antibiotic use can both optimize the treatment of infections and reduce the adverse events associated with antibiotic use [1]. "Antibiotic stewardship programs" (ASPs) may significantly reduce the incidence of antimicrobial resistance and *Clostridium difficile* infections in hospitalized patients [1]. Every hospital worldwide should utilize the existing resources to create effective ASPs with a multi-disciplinary team. However, the best strategies to establish an ASPs are not well defined.

ASPs should be linked to infection control and prevention programs in order to improve antibiotic prescribing practices and to prevent infections.

Dedicated efforts, such as the establishment of locally adopted multi-disciplinary, evidence-based protocols and guidelines; unit specific antibiotic sensitivity data;

and compliance monitoring, are required to maximize the performance.

To investigate the effects of the antibiotic stewardship program on prevention and control of SSIs during clean surgery, Liu et al. [13] compared the effect before and after an antibiotic stewardship program intervention. From January 1, 2010, to December 31, 2016, 41,426 patients underwent clean surgeries in a grade III, class A hospital. The rate of prophylactic antibiotic use in the 41,426 clean surgeries was reduced from 82.9 to 28.0% after the interventions. The rate of antibiotic agents administered within 120 min of the first incision increased from 20.8 to 85.1%. The rate at which prophylactic antimicrobial agents were discontinued in the first 24 h after surgery increased from 22.1 to 60.4%. Appropriate antibiotic selection increased from 37.0 to 93.6%. Prophylactic antibiotic re-dosing increased from 3.8 to 64.8%. The SSI rate decreased from 0.7 to 0.5% ($p < 0.05$). The pathogen detection rate increased from 16.7 up to 41.8% after intervention. The intensity of antibiotic consumption reduced from 74.9 defined daily doses (DDDs) per 100 bed-days to 34.2 DDDs per 100 bed-days after the interventions.

Van Kasteren et al. [14] in a prospective multi-site study of elective procedures in 13 Dutch hospitals evaluated the quality of prophylaxis auditing before and after an intervention consisting of performance feedback and implementation of national clinical practice guidelines. Antimicrobial use decreased from 121 to 79 DDD/100 procedures, and costs reduced by 25% per procedure. After the intervention, the antibiotic choice was inappropriate in only 37.5% of the cases instead of in 93.5% expected cases prior to the intervention. Prolonged prophylaxis was observed in 31.4% instead of 46.8% expected cases and inappropriate timing in 39.4% instead of the expected 51.8%. Time series analysis showed that all improvements were statistically significant ($p < 0.01$). The overall SSI rates before and after intervention were 5.4% (95% CI 4.3–6.5) and 4.6% (95% CI 3.6–5.4), respectively.

Raising awareness is a crucial factor in changing behaviors. Efforts to improve educational programs are thus required, and this should preferably be complemented by active interventions such as prospective audits and feedback to clinicians to stimulate further changes. It would be advisable to introduce specific courses and training about antibiotics in the core curriculum of medical students, with emphasis on the rational prescription of antibiotics that emphasizes more the behavior of medical students towards antibiotics use rather than the advance of knowledge alone [15].

The best means of improving ASPs worldwide should involve collaboration among various specialties within a healthcare institution including prescribing clinicians. ASPs have many contributors, steps, and actions specifically related to the prevention and management of infection. The multidisciplinary approach reinforces the concept that all professionals bring with them their particular expertise and are responsible for their respective contributions. In this context, the direct involvement of surgeons can be highly effective.

Surgeons with adequate knowledge in surgical infection who are involved in an ASPs may provide feedback and integrate the best practices of infection prevention and treatment among surgeons.

Very few studies have focused on the relationship between ASPs and surgeons. In 2011, Dortch et al. [16] reported the results of a surgeon-led infection reduction and antibiotic stewardship program in two separate ICUs, one trauma and one surgical. Components of the program included unit-specific empiric and therapeutic antibiotic protocols for healthcare-acquired infections, prophylaxis guidelines, and numerous infection reduction strategies. They demonstrated a marked reduction in infectious complications, multidrug-resistant pathogens, and broad-spectrum antibiotic use.

In 2015, Çakmakçi [17] suggested that the engagement of surgeons in ASPs may be crucial to their success. However, Duane et al. [18] showed poor compliance of surgical services with ASP recommendations.

A retrospective study published in 2016 showed [19] that the implementation of an educational and surveillance-based ASP achieves a significant improvement in all antibiotic agent prescriptions and a reduction in antibiotics consumption. In a surgical unit performing mainly elective major abdominal surgery and emergency surgery, both a local protocol of surgical prophylaxis and a set of guidelines for management of intra-abdominal infections (IAIs) were introduced [20]. Moreover, a unit-specific control of antimicrobial agents used and surveillance of antimicrobial resistance were implemented. Comparing the pre-intervention and post-intervention periods, the mean total monthly antimicrobial use decreased significantly after the intervention. The model was based on the concept of the "surgeon champion." The "champion" was a surgeon who on a day-to-day basis worked within the surgical unit, promoting and maintaining a culture in which both infection prevention and management were given high priority. Such a champion model has been previously applied to surgical safety implementations in general, such as surgical checklists, and plays a key role in successful quality improvement at the hospital level [21].

Identifying a local opinion leader to serve as a champion may be important because the "surgeon champion" may integrate best clinical practices and drive their colleagues into changing behaviors while maintaining a tight collaboration with antimicrobial stewardship and infection control teams. The "champion" should possess a wide knowledge of surgical microbiology, as well as considerable expertise in the antibiotic management of surgical infections. Furthermore, the "champion" should increase the awareness of surgical infections in young staff surgeons and surgical residents.

We think that the concept of the "surgeon champion" can be a crucial way to improve the infection prevention and antibiotic prescribing practices across the surgical practice pathway.

Conclusions

Surgeons must be aware that appropriate antibiotic utilization is an integral part of any stewardship program and necessary to maximize clinical cure and minimize the emergence of antimicrobial resistance.

Antimicrobial restriction is not more effective than the persuasive strategy in achieving the goal of controlling antimicrobial use in the long term [22]. Moreover, in many settings, there may be inadequate personnel for a restrictive approach, and restriction strategies fail to consider the appropriateness of use of non-restricted antibiotics, which makes up the vast majority of antibiotics used in the hospital [23]. The impact on surgeon autonomy with antimicrobial restriction may also create barriers to collaboration with members of the ASP resulting in less communication about stewardship. Therefore, the emphasis needs to be on the incorporation of a surgeon champion in the ASPs.

Surgeons with good knowledge of surgical infections involved in ASPs may audit antibiotic prescriptions, provide feedback to the prescribers, and integrate the best practice of infection prevention and management among surgeons. We think that the concept of the "surgeon champion" is a crucial way to improve infection prevention and antibiotic prescribing practices across the surgical practice pathway.

Appendix 1

Strategies for a correct antibiotic prophylaxis [1]:

1. Antibiotics alone are unable to prevent surgical site infections. Strategies to prevent surgical site infections should always include attention to infection and prevention control strategies including correct and compliant hand hygiene practices
2. Antibiotic prophylaxis should be administered for operative procedures that have a high rate of postoperative surgical site infection, or when foreign materials are implanted.
3. Antibiotics given as prophylaxis should be effective against the aerobic and anaerobic pathogens most likely to contaminate the surgical site, i.e., Gram-positive skin commensals or normal flora colonizing the incised mucosae.
4. Antibiotic prophylaxis should be administered within 120 min prior to the incision. However, administration of the first dose of antibiotics beginning within 30–60 min before surgical incision is recommended for most antibiotics (e.g., cefazolin), to ensure adequate serum and tissue concentrations during the period of potential contamination. Obese patients require higher doses of antibiotic.
5. A single dose is generally sufficient. Additional antibiotic doses should be administered intraoperatively for procedures > 2–4 h (typically where duration exceeds two half-lives of the antibiotic) or with associated significant blood loss (> 1.5 L).
6. There is no evidence to support the use of postoperative antibiotic prophylaxis.
7. Each institution is encouraged to develop guidelines for the proper surgical prophylaxis.

Appendix 2

Strategies for a correct antibiotic therapy [1]:

1. The source of infection should always be identified and controlled as soon as possible.
2. Antibiotic empiric therapy should be initiated after a treatable surgical infection has been recognized, since microbiological data (culture and susceptibility results) may not be available for up to 48–72 h to guide the targeted therapy.
3. In critically ill patients, empiric broad-spectrum therapy to cover all likely pathogens should be initiated as soon as possible after a surgical infection has been recognized. Empiric antimicrobial therapy should be narrowed once the culture and susceptibility results are available and/or adequate clinical improvement is noted. In patients less severely ill, it may be pertinent to await culture results.
4. Empirical therapy should be chosen on the basis of local epidemiology, individual patient risk factors for multidrug-resistant bacteria, clinical severity, and infection source.
5. Specimens for microbiological evaluation from the site of infection are always recommended for patients with hospital-acquired or with community-acquired infections at risk for resistant pathogens (e.g., previous antimicrobial therapy, prior infection or colonization with multidrug-resistant pathogens) and in critically ill patients. Blood cultures should be performed before the administration of antibiotics in critically ill patients.
6. Antibiotics dose should be optimized to ensure that pharmacodynamic-pharmacokinetic targets are achieved

7. The appropriateness and need for antimicrobial treatment should be reassessed daily.
8. Once the source control is established, short courses of antibiotic therapy are as effective as longer courses regardless of the signs of inflammation according to the guidelines.
9. Failure of antibiotic therapy in patients having continued evidence of active infection may require a re-operation for a second source control intervention.
10. Biomarkers such as procalcitonin may be useful to guide the duration and/or cessation of antibiotic therapy in critically ill patients.

Abbreviations

AMR: Antimicrobial resistance; ASP: Antimicrobial stewardship program; HAIs: Healthcare-associated infections; PAP: Preoperative antibiotic prophylaxis; SSI: Surgical site infection

Authors' contributions

MS wrote the first draft of the manuscript. All the authors reviewed the manuscript and approved the final draft.

Competing interests

The authors declare that they have no competing interests.

Author details

[1]Department of Surgery, Macerata Hospital, Via Santa Lucia, 62100 Macerata, Italy. [2]Department of General Surgery, Division of Surgery, Rambam Health Care Campus, Haifa, Israel. [3]General Surgery Department, "M. Bufalini" Cesena Hospital, Cesena, Italy. [4]Department of Clinical and Experimental Sciences, University of Brescia, Brescia, Italy. [5]Department of Surgery, Trauma Service, Inkosi Albert Luthuli Central Hospital, Nelson R Mandela School of Clinical Medicine, Durban, South Africa. [6]Department of Surgery, Denver Health Medical Center, University of Colorado, Denver, CO, USA. [7]Division of Trauma and Surgical Critical Care, Vanderbilt University Medical Center, Nashville, TN, USA. [8]Department of Surgery, VA Boston Health Care System, Boston University, Harvard Medical School, Boston, MA, USA. [9]Department of Surgery, Northwestern University Feinberg School of Medicine, Chicago, IL, USA. [10]University of New Mexico School of Medicine, Albuquerque, NM, USA. [11]Department of Surgery, Academic Medical Center, Amsterdam, Netherlands. [12]Unit of Endocrine, Head, and Neck Surgery and Unit of Surgical Infections Support, Department of General Surgery, ParcTaulí, Hospital University, Sabadell, Spain. [13]Department of Surgery, University of Michigan, Ann Arbor, MI, USA. [14]Department of Surgery, Western Michigan University School of Medicine, Kalamazoo, MI, USA. [15]Department of Surgery, Anadolu Medical Center, Kocaali, Turkey. [16]Department of Surgery, College of Medicine and Health Sciences, UAE University, Al-Ain, United Arab Emirates. [17]Department of Surgery, College of Health Sciences, Obafemi Awolowo University, Ile-Ife, Nigeria. [18]Department of General Surgery, Medical University of Plovdiv, UMHAT Eurohospital, Plovdiv, Bulgaria. [19]Department of Surgery, University Hospital Centre Zagreb, Zagreb, Croatia. [20]Trauma and Acute Care Surgery Unit, Hadassah Hebrew University Medical Center, Jerusalem, Israel. [21]Department of Surgery, Hospital Clínico Universitario, Santiago de Compostela, Spain. [22]Department of Surgery and Obstetrics/ Gynaecology, Regional Hospital, Limbe, Cameroon. [23]Emergency Surgery Unit, San Filippo Neri Hospital, Rome, Italy. [24]Department of Surgery, Royal Infirmary of Edinburgh, Edinburgh, UK. [25]Department of Surgery, University Clinical Center of Tuzla, Tuzla, Bosnia and Herzegovina. [26]Department General Surgery, Kipshidze Central University Hospital, Tbilisi, Georgia. [27]Department of Digestive Surgery, Cannes Hospital, Cannes, France. [28]Department of Surgery, John Peter Smith Health Network, Fort Worth, TX, USA. [29]Department of General Surgery, Mansoura Faculty of Medicine, Mansoura University, Mansoura, Egypt. [30]Second Department of Surgery, Aretaieion University Hospital, National and Kapodistrian University of Athens, Athens, Greece. [31]Faculdade de Ciências Médicas e da Saúde de Juiz de Fora, Department of Surgery, Hospital Universitário Terezinha de Jesus, Juiz de Fora, Brazil. [32]Department of General and Thoracic Surgery, University Hospital Giessen, Giessen, Germany. [33]Clinic for Surgery, University Clinical Center "Zvezdara", Belgrade, Serbia. [34]Third Department of General Surgery, Jagiellonian University Medical College, Krakow, Poland. [35]Department of Emergency Surgery, City Hospital, Mozyr, Belarus. [36]Department of Surgery, Edendale Hospital, Pietermaritzburg, South Africa. [37]General Surgery Department, Magee Womens Hospital, UPMC, Pittsburgh, USA. [38]Abdominal Center, University Hospital Meilahti, Helsinki, Finland. [39]Surgical Disciplines, Immanuel Kant Baltic Federal University/Regional Clinical Hospital, Kaliningrad, Russian Federation. [40]1st Department of Surgery, Kavala General Hospital, Kavala, Greece. [41]Department of Surgery, II Cátedra de Clínica Quirúrgica, Universidad Nacional de Asunción, San Lorenzo, Paraguay. [42]Department of Surgery, Post-Graduate Institute of Medical Sciences, Rohtak, India. [43]Department of Surgery, Radiology, University Hospital of the West Indies, Kingston, Jamaica. [44]Second Surgical Clinic, Emergency Hospital of Craiova, Craiova, Romania. [45]Department of Surgery, Emergency Hospital of Bucharest, Bucharest, Romania. [46]Department of Surgery, University of Ilorin Teaching Hospital, Ilorin, Nigeria. [47]Department of Surgery, UMC Ljubljana, Ljubljana, Slovenia. [48]Department of General and Emergency Surgery, Riga East University Hospital "Gailezers", Riga, Latvia. [49]Department of General Surgery, Jesenice General Hospital, Jesenice, Slovenia. [50]Colorectal Surgery Unit, General Surgery Department, La Paz University Hospital, Madrid, Spain. [51]General Surgery Department, Medical University, University Hospital St George, Plovdiv, Bulgaria. [52]Faculty of Medicine, Department of Surgery, Thammasat University Hospital, Thammasat University, Amphoe Khlong Luang, Pathum Thani, Thailand. [53]Department of Surgery, North Estonia Medical Center, Tallinn, Estonia. [54]First Department of Surgery-Department of Abdominal, Thoracic Surgery and Traumatology, General University Hospital, Prague, Czech Republic. [55]Department of Surgery, Medical School University of Pécs, Pécs, Hungary. [56]Global Alliance for Infections in Surgery, Porto, Portugal. [57]Department of Emergency Surgery, Maggiore Hospital, Parma, Italy.

References

1. Global Alliance for Infections in Surgery Working Group. A Global Declaration on Appropriate Use of Antimicrobial Agents across the Surgical Pathway. Surg Infect (Larchmt). 2017;18:846-53.
2. Itani KMF, May AK. Surgical Infection Society: we endorse antimicrobial stewardship we stand by our international colleagues and societies in the fight for proper antimicrobial therapy. Surg Infect (Larchmt). 2017;18:843–5.
3. Zimlichman E, Henderson D, Tamir O, Franz C, Song P, Yamin CK, et al. Health care-associated infections: a meta-analysis of costs and financial impact on the US health care system. JAMA Intern Med. 2013;173:2039–46.
4. GlobalSurg Collaborative. Surgical site infection after gastrointestinal surgery in high-income, middle-income, and low-income countries: a prospective, international, multicentre cohort study. Lancet Infect Dis. 2018;18:516–25.
5. Allegranzi B, Zayed B, Bischoff P, Kubilay NZ, de Jonge S, de Vries F, et al. New WHO recommendations on intraoperative and postoperative measures for surgical site infection prevention: an evidence-based global perspective. Lancet Infect Dis. 2016;16:e288–303.
6. Berríos-Torres SI, Umscheid CA, Bratzler DW, Leas B, Stone EC, Kelz RR, et al. Centers for disease control and prevention guideline for the prevention of surgical site infection, 2017. JAMA Surg. 2017;152:784–91.
7. Ban KA, Minei JP, Laronga C, Harbrecht BG, Jensen EH, Fry DE, et al. American College of Surgeons and Surgical Infection Society: surgical site infection guidelines, 2016 update. J Am Coll Surg. 2017;224:59–74.
8. Ban KA, Laronga C, Harbrecht BG, Jensen EH, Fry DE, Itani KMF, et al. Executive summary of the American College of Surgeons/Surgical Infection Society Surgical Site Infection Guidelines-2016 update. Surg Infect. 2017;18:379–82.

9. Badia JM, Casey AL, Rubio-Pérez I, Crosby C, Arroyo-García N, Del Castillo JB. A survey to identify the breach between evidence and practice in the prevention of surgical infection: time to take action. Int J Surg. 2018;54(Pt A):290–7.
10. Sartelli M, Weber DG, Ruppé E, Bassetti M, Wright BJ, Ansaloni L, et al. Antimicrobials: a global alliance for optimizing their rational use in intra-abdominal infections (AGORA). World J Emerg Surg. 2016;11:33.
11. Rhodes A, Evans LE, Alhazzani W, Levy MM, Antonelli M, Ferrer R, et al. Surviving sepsis campaign: international guidelines for management of sepsis and septic shock: 2016. Intensive Care Med. 2017;43:304–77.
12. Sartelli M, Duane TM, Catena F, Tessier JM, Coccolini F, Kao LS, et al. Antimicrobial stewardship: a call to action for surgeons. Surg Infect. 2016;17:625–31.
13. Liu J, Li N, Hao J, Li Y, Liu A, Wu Y, Cai M. Impact of the antibiotic stewardship program on prevention and control of surgical site infection during peri-operative clean surgery. Surg Infect. 2018;19:326–33.
14. Van Kasteren ME, Mannien J, Kullberg BJ, de Boer AS, Nagelkerke NJ, Ridderhof M, et al. Quality improvement of surgical prophylaxis in Dutch hospitals: evaluation of a multi-site intervention by time series analysis. J Antimicrob Chemother. 2005;56:1094–102.
15. Huang Y, Gu J, Zhang M, Ren Z, Yang W, Chen Y, et al. Knowledge, attitude and practice of antibiotics: a questionnaire study among 2500 Chinese students. BMC Med Educ. 2013;13:163.
16. Dortch MJ, Fleming SB, Kauffmann RM, Dossett LA, Talbot TR, May AK. Infection reduction strategies including antibiotic stewardship protocols in surgical and trauma intensive care units are associated with reduced resistant gram-negative healthcare-associated infections. Surg Infect (Larchmt). 2011;12:15–25.
17. Çakmakçi M. Antibiotic stewardship programmes and the surgeon's role. J Hosp Infect. 2015;89:264–6.
18. Duane TM, Zuo JX, Wolfe LG, Bearman G, Edmond MB, Lee K, et al. Surgeons do not listen: evaluation of compliance with antimicrobial stewardship program recommendations. Am Surg. 2013;79:1269–72.
19. Sartelli M, Labricciosa FM, Scoccia L, Bellesi J, Mazzoccanti MR, Scaloni G, et al. Non-restrictive antimicrobial stewardship program in a general and emergency surgery unit. Surg Infect (Larchmt). 2016;17:485–90.
20. Sartelli M, Viale P, Catena F, Ansaloni L, Moore E, Malangoni M, et al. 2013 WSES guidelines for management of intra-abdominal infections. World J Emerg Surg. 2013;8:3.
21. Raval MV, Bentrem DJ, Eskandari MK, Ingraham AM, Hall BL, Randolph B, et al. The role of surgical champions in the American College of Surgeons National Surgical Quality Improvement Program--a national survey. J Surg Res. 2011;166:e15–25.
22. Davey P, Brown E, Charani E, Fenelon L, Gould IM, Holmes A, et al. Interventions to improve antibiotic prescribing practices for hospital inpatients. Cochrane Database Syst Rev. 2013;4:CD003543.
23. MacDougall C, Polk RE. Antimicrobial stewardship programs in health care systems. Clin Microbiol Rev. 2005;18:638–56.

19

Acute mesenteric ischemia: guidelines of the World Society of Emergency Surgery

Miklosh Bala[1*], Jeffry Kashuk[2], Ernest E. Moore[3], Yoram Kluger[4], Walter Biffl[5], Carlos Augusto Gomes[6], Offir Ben-Ishay[4], Chen Rubinstein[7], Zsolt J. Balogh[8], Ian Civil[9], Federico Coccolini[10], Ari Leppaniemi[11], Andrew Peitzman[12], Luca Ansaloni[10], Michael Sugrue[13], Massimo Sartelli[14], Salomone Di Saverio[15], Gustavo P. Fraga[16] and Fausto Catena[17]

Abstract

Acute mesenteric ischemia (AMI) is typically defined as a group of diseases characterized by an interruption of the blood supply to varying portions of the small intestine, leading to ischemia and secondary inflammatory changes. If untreated, this process will eventuate in life threatening intestinal necrosis. The incidence is low, estimated at 0.09–0.2% of all acute surgical admissions. Therefore, although the entity is an uncommon cause of abdominal pain, diligence is always required because if untreated, mortality has consistently been reported in the range of 50%. Early diagnosis and timely surgical intervention are the cornerstones of modern treatment and are essential to reduce the high mortality associated with this entity. The advent of endovascular approaches in parallel with modern imaging techniques may provide new options. Thus, we believe that a current position paper from World Society of Emergency Surgery (WSES) is warranted, in order to put forth the most recent and practical recommendations for diagnosis and treatment of AMI. This review will address the concepts of AMI with the aim of focusing on specific areas where early diagnosis and management hold the strongest potential for improving outcomes in this disease process.
Some of the key points include the prompt use of CT angiography to establish the diagnosis, evaluation of the potential for revascularization to re-establish blood flow to ischemic bowel, resection of necrotic intestine, and use of damage control techniques when appropriate to allow for re-assessment of bowel viability prior to definitive anastomosis and abdominal closure.

Keywords: Mesenteric ischemia, Mesenteric arterial occlusion, Mesenteric angiography, Mesenteric artery stenting, Small bowel ischemia, Guidelines, Recommendations

Background

Acute mesenteric ischemia (AMI) may be defined as a sudden interruption of the blood supply to a segment of the small intestine, leading to ischemia, cellular damage, intestinal necrosis, and eventually patient death if untreated [1]. AMI may be non-occlusive (NOMI) or occlusive, with the primary etiology further defined as mesenteric arterial embolism (50%), mesenteric arterial thrombosis (15–25%), or mesenteric venous thrombosis (5–15%) [2, 3]. The overall incidence is low (0.09 to 0.2% of all acute admissions to emergency departments), representing an uncommon cause of abdominal pain [4–6]. Prompt diagnostic and intervention are essential to reduce the high mortality rates (50 to 80%) [7–10].

There are currently no level 1 evidence to guide the evaluation and treatment of suspected AMI, and the published literature contains primarily institutional reviews, case series and personal recommendations with no clearly defined treatment guidelines.

Accordingly, this review aims to provide an update with recommendations based on the most currently accepted concepts in the management of AMI.

The current presentation evolved from the contributions of a group of experts in the field who submitted their evidence-based literature review of key points pertaining to diagnosis and management of AMI. Following preliminary preparation of these key points, a coordinated

* Correspondence: rbalam@hadassah.org.il
[1]Acute Care Surgery and Trauma Unit, General Surgery Department, Hadassah - Hebrew University Medical Center, Kiriat Hadassah, POB 12000, 91120 Jerusalem, Israel

presentation was organized during the WSES World Congress, May 2017 in Campinas, Brazil. The final version has taken into account the presentations at the congress as well as pertinent group discussions and comments on the various presentations.

The grading of recommendations was evaluated (Table 1).

Mesenteric vascular anatomy and physiology

The superior mesenteric artery (SMA) is the primary blood supply for the small bowel with some collateral flow from the celiac arterial system, via the superior and inferior pancreaticoduodenal arteries, as well as from the inferior mesenteric artery. Intestinal blood returns via the portal vein. The splanchnic circulation receives 15–35% of the cardiac output, depending on the feeding state, but oxygen extraction is relatively low, accounting for the oxygen delivery capacity of the portal vein to the liver. Thus, blood supply must be reduced by more than 50% before the small intestine becomes ischemic [11].

Furthermore, the intestines can autoregulate oxygen availability via enhanced oxygen extraction and perfusion due to vasodilation. Experimentally, it had been shown that mesenteric ischemia does not occur until the patient's mean arterial pressure is <45 mmHg [12]. Consequently, the small intestine is able to compensate for a 75% reduction in mesenteric blood flow for up to 12 h [13].

Pathophysiology and epidemiology

Acute mesenteric arterial embolism

Roughly, 50% of all cases of AMI are due to acute mesenteric embolism [2, 3]. Mesenteric emboli can originate from the left atrium, associated with cardiac dysrhythmias such as atrial fibrillation, left ventricle with global myocardial dysfunction associated with poor ejection fraction, or cardiac valves due to endocarditis. Occasionally emboli generated from an atherosclerotic aorta. Emboli typically lodge at points of normal anatomic narrowing, and the SMA is particularly vulnerable because of its relatively large diameter and low takeoff angle from the aorta. The majority of emboli lodge 3 to 10 cm distal to the origin of the SMA, thus classically sparing the proximal jejunum and colon. More than 20% of emboli to the SMA are associated with concurrent emboli to another arterial bed including the spleen, or kidney.

Table 1 Grading of recommendations

Grade of recommendation	Clarity of risk/benefit	Quality of supporting evidence	Implications
1A			
Strong recommendation, high-quality evidence	Benefits clearly outweigh risk and burdens, or vice versa	RCTs without important limitations or overwhelming evidence from observational studies	Strong recommendation, applies to most patients in most circumstances without reservation
1B			
Strong recommendation, moderate-quality evidence	Benefits clearly outweigh risk and burdens, or vice versa	RCTs with important limitations (inconsistent results, methodological flaws, indirect analyses, or imprecise conclusions) or exceptionally strong evidence from observational studies	Strong recommendation, applies to most patients in most circumstances without reservation
1C			
Strong recommendation, low-quality or very low-quality evidence	Benefits clearly outweigh risk and burdens, or vice versa	Observational studies or case series	Strong recommendation but subject to change when higher quality evidence becomes available
2A			
Weak recommendation, high-quality evidence	Benefits closely balanced with risks and burden	RCTs without important limitations or overwhelming evidence from observational studies	Weak recommendation, best action may differ depending on the patient, treatment circumstances, or social values
2B			
Weak recommendation, moderate-quality evidence	Benefits closely balanced with risks and burden	RCTs with important limitations (inconsistent results, methodological flaws, indirect or imprecise) or exceptionally strong evidence from observational studies	Weak recommendation, best action may differ depending on the patient, treatment circumstances, or social values
2C			
Weak recommendation, low-quality or very low-quality evidence	Uncertainty in the estimates of benefits, risks, and burden; benefits, risk, and burden may be closely balanced	Observational studies or case series	Very weak recommendation; alternative treatments may be equally reasonable and merit consideration

Thus, findings of changes in these organs on CTA suggest a proximal embolic source [14].

Acute mesenteric arterial thrombosis

Thrombosis of the SMA (approximately 25% of cases) is usually associated with pre-existing chronic atherosclerotic disease leading to stenosis. Many of these patients have a history consistent with chronic mesenteric ischemia (CMI), including postprandial pain, weight loss, or "food fear", and thus a systematic history is important when evaluating a patient suspected to have AMI. Thrombosis usually occurs at the origin of visceral arteries, moreover, an underlying plaque in the SMA usually progresses to a critical stenosis over years resulting in collateral beds. Accordingly, symptomatic SMA thrombosis most often accompanies celiac occlusion [15]. SMA thrombosis may also occur due to vasculitis, mesenteric dissection, or a mycotic aneurysm. Involvement of the ileocolic artery will result in necrosis of the proximal colon.

Pathophysiology of acute non-occlusive mesenteric ischemia

NOMI occurs in approximately 20% of cases and is usually a consequence of SMA vasoconstriction associated with low splanchnic blood flow [16]. The compromised SMA blood flow often involves the proximal colon as well due to involvement of the ileocolic artery. Patients with NOMI typically suffer from severe coexisting illness, commonly cardiac failure which may be precipitated by sepsis. Hypovolemia and the use of vasoconstrictive agents may precipitate NOMI.

Mesenteric venous thrombosis

Mesenteric venous thrombosis (MVT) accounts for less than 10% of cases of mesenteric infarction. Thrombosis is attributed to a combination of Virchow's triad, i.e., stagnated blood flow, hypercoagulability, and vascular inflammation, but approximately 20% are idiopathic. Hypercoagulabilty may be due to inherited disease such as Factor V Leiden, prothrombin mutation, protein S deficiency, protein C deficiency, antithrombin deficiency, and antiphospholipid syndrome. Additionally, recent work suggests that fibrinolysis shutdown (resistance to tissue plasminogen activator (tPA)) is a significant risk factor for hypercoagulability [17]. Thrombophilia may also be acquired due to malignancies, hematologic disorders, and oral contraceptives [18].

The additional components altering blood flow include portal hypertension, pancreatitis, inflammatory bowel disease, sepsis, and trauma. In these situations, the consequences of bowel edema and increased vascular resistance secondary to venous thrombosis result in reduced arterial blood flow, leading to bowel ischemia.

Severe abdominal pain out of proportion to physical examination findings should be assumed to be AMI until disproven. (Recommendation 1B)

The key to early diagnosis is a high level of clinical suspicion.

The clinical scenario of a patient complaining of excruciating abdominal pain with an unrevealing abdominal exam is classic for early AMI [19]. If the physical exam demonstrates signs of peritonitis, there is likely irreversible intestinal ischemia with bowel necrosis. In a study of AMI, 95% of patients presented with abdominal pain, 44% with nausea, 35% with vomiting, 35% with diarrhea, and 16% with blood per rectum [20]. Approximately one-third of patients present with the triad of abdominal pain, fever, and hemocult-positive stools. Other patients, particularly those with delayed diagnosis, may present in extremis with septic shock. Clinical signs of peritonitis may be subtle. Accordingly, one must have a high index of suspicion, because such findings almost always are predictive of intestinal infarction.

Clinical scenario differentiates AMI as mesenteric arterial emboli, mesenteric arterial thrombosis, NOMI or mesenteric venous thrombosis. (Recommendation 1B)

Phenotypes of AMI

A careful history is important because distinct clinical scenarios are associated with the pathophysiological form of AMI [21]. Patients with mesenteric arterial thrombosis often have a history of chronic postprandial abdominal pain, progressive weight loss, and previous revascularization procedures for mesenteric arterial occlusion. Patients with NOMI have pain that is generally more diffuse and episodic associated with poor cardiac performance. Patients with MVT present with a mixture of nausea, vomiting, diarrhea, and abdominal cramping. Gastrointestinal bleeding occurs in 10% [22].

Nearly 50% of patients presenting with embolic AMI have atrial fibrillation and approximately one-third of patients have a prior history of arterial embolus [20].

Risk factors for specific phenotypes of AMI presented in Table 2.

Conventional plain X-ray films have limited diagnostic value in evaluating AMI, although signs of intestinal perforation may be seen. (Recommendation 1B)

A radiograph is usually the initial test ordered in patients with acute abdominal pain but has a limited role in the diagnosis of mesenteric ischemia, especially in the early setting. A negative radiograph does not exclude mesenteric ischemia [23]. Plain radiography only becomes positive when bowel infarction

Table 2 Risk factors for specific phenotypes of AMI

	Pathogenesis of AMI			
	Acute mesenteric arterial embolism	Acute mesenteric arterial thrombosis	NOMI	Mesenteric venous thrombosis
Risk factors	Atrial fibrillation Recent MI cardiac thrombi Mitral valve disease Left ventricular aneurysm Endocarditis Previous embolic disease	Diffuse atherosclerotic disease Postprandial pain Weight loss	Cardiac failure Low flow states Multi-organ dysfunction Vasopressors	Portal hypertension History of VTE Oral contraceptives Estrogen use Thrombophilia pancreatitis

AMI acute mesenteric ischemia, *NOMI* non-occlusive mesenteric ischemia, *MI* myocardial infarction, *VTE* venous thromboembolism

has developed and intestinal perforation manifests as free intraperitoneal air.

There are no laboratory studies that are sufficiently accurate to identify the presence or absence of ischemic or necrotic bowel, although elevated l-lactate, and D-dimer may assist. (Recommendation 1B)

Although laboratory results are not definitive, they may help to corroborate clinical suspicion. More than 90% of patients will have an abnormally elevated leukocyte count. The second most commonly encountered abnormal finding is metabolic acidosis with elevated lactate level, which occurred in 88% [24].

Patients may present with lactic acidosis due to dehydration and decreased oral intake. Thus, differentiation of early ischemia versus irreversible bowel injury based upon the lactate level alone is not reliable unless accompanied by other clinical evidence. Elevated serum lactate levels >2 mmol/l was associated in irreversible intestinal ischemia (Hazard Ratio: 4.1 (95% CI: 1.4–11.5; $p < 0.01$) in established diagnosis of AMI [25].

It should be emphsized that the presence of lactic acidosis in combination of abdominal pain when the patient may not otherwise appear clinically ill should lead to consideration for early CTA.

Based on the current literature, no accurate biomarkers have been identified to date [26, 27]. D-dimer has been reported to be an independent risk factor of intestinal ischemia [27], reflecting ongoing clot formation and endogenous degradation via fibrinolysis. No patient presenting with a normal D-dimer had intestinal ischemia and D-dimer >0.9 mg/L had a specificity, sensitivity, and accuracy of 82, 60, and 79%, respectively [28]. Thus, D-dimer may well be useful in the early assessment. Elevated amylase has been reported in roughly a half of patients with AMI [29]. Other biomarkers reported to assist in the diagnosis of AMI include intestinal fatty acid binding protein (I-FABP), serum alpha-glutathione S-transferase (alpha–GST), and cobalt-albumin binding assay (CABA) [30, 31]. These biomarkers may offer improved diagnostic accuracy of acute mesenteric ischemia, however, further research is required to specify its accuracy and values.

Computed tomography angiography (CTA) should be performed as soon as possible for any patient with suspicion for AMI. (Recommendation 1A)

Delay in diagnosis is the dominant factor that accounts for continued mortality rates as high as 30–70% despite vast clinical experience and recognition of this entity [32, 33]. The multi-detector CTA has supplanted formal angiography as the diagnostic study of choice. Multidetector computed tomography (MDCT) scanners are essential for the early diagnosis of AMI, but often require specialized personnel to perform and interpret the findings. 3D reconstruction is frequently helpful (Fig. 1). Volume rendering as in this image is now a semiautomatic workflow component of many CT machines. These can aide remote communities with less experienced staff.

In the presence of advanced AMI, the CTA findings reflect irreversible ischemia (intestinal dilatation and thickness, reduction or absence of visceral enhancement, pneumatosis intestinalis, and portal venous gas) and free intraperitoneal air [34].

Comprehensive biphasic CTA includes the following important steps:

a) Pre-contrast scans to detect vascular calcification, hyper-attenuating intravascular thrombus and intramural hemorrhage.
b) Arterial and venous phases to demonstrate thrombus in the mesenteric arteries and veins, abnormal enhancement of the bowel wall, and the presence of embolism or infarction of other organs.
c) Multi-planar reconstructions (MPR) to assess the origin of the mesenteric arteries [35].

CTA should be performed despite the presence of renal failure, as the consequences of delayed diagnosis, missed diagnosis, or mismanagement are far more detrimental to the kidneys and the patient then exposure to the iodinated contrast agent. A recent study found that in 27 of 28 patients (96.4%) MDCT correctly diagnosed AMI (specificity of 97.9%) [16, 36]. A sensitivity of 93%, specificity of 100%, and positive

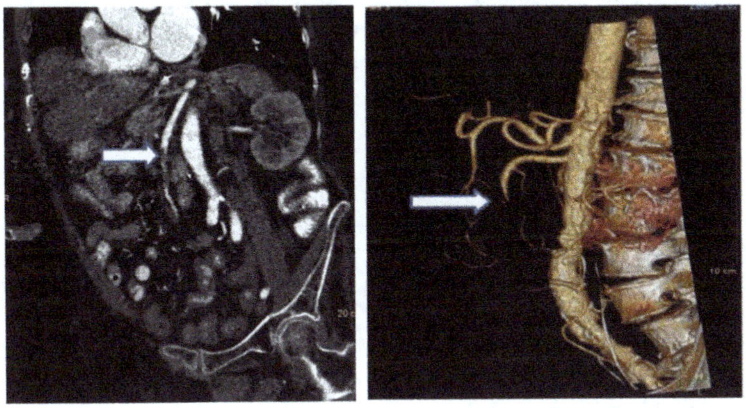

Fig. 1 Selected image from a CTA scan of a patient with acute mesenteric ischemia secondary to occluded SMA from an embolic source (arrow). 3D reconstruction is demonstrates mid occlusion of SMA (arrow)

and negative predictive values of 100 and 94%, respectively, were achieved [37, 38].

In NOMI CTA may demonstrate bowel ischemia and free fluid in the face of patent mesenteric vessels. In MVT, the most common positive radiological finding on venous phase CTA is thrombus in the superior mesenteric vein on venous phase CTA (Fig. 2). This has been described as the target sign [39].

Associated findings that suggest MVT include bowel wall thickening, pneumatosis, splenomegaly, and ascites [39]. Portal or mesenteric venous gas strongly suggests the presence of bowel infarction. Duplex ultrasonography has a limited role in this entity, but may be helpful if obtained early in chronic cases [22].

Non-occlusive mesenteric ischemia (NOMI) should be suspected in critically ill patients with abdominal pain or distension requiring vasopressor support and evidence of multi-organ dysfunction. (Recommendation 1B)

Unexplained abdominal distension or gastrointestinal bleeding may be the only signs of acute intestinal ischemia in NOMI and may be undetectable in sedated patients in the ICU in approximately 25% of cases [40, 41]. Patients surviving cardiopulmonary resuscitation who develop bacteremia and diarrhea (with or without abdominal pain) should be suspected of having NOMI. Right-sided abdominal pain associated with the passage of maroon or bright red blood in the stool is highly suggestive of NOMI in these patients.

Gastrointestinal perfusion is often impaired early in situations of critical illness, major surgery or trauma, all of which are characterized by increased demands on the circulation to maintain tissue oxygen delivery [42]. This relative mesenteric hypoperfusion is often aggravated by an underlying hypovolemic or a low-flow state. In cases of intraabdominal hypertension, all of the structures within the abdominal cavity are compressed, and this will lead to regional hypoperfusion to the organs in the splanchnic bed. Such an effect is most pronounced in the liver due to its size. Animal studies have shown that even with intraabdominal pressure of only 10 mmHg, portal venous blood flow is reduced considerably, and that at 20 mmHg, the portal venous flow and hepatic arterial flow are reduced by 35 and 55%, respectively [43].

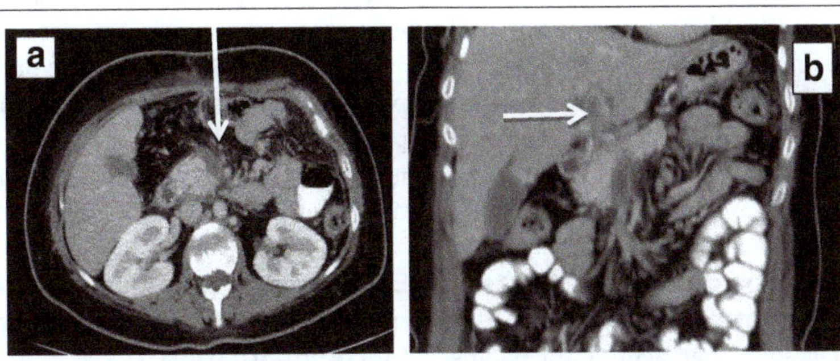

Fig. 2 30-year-old patient with acute superior mesenteric vein **a** and portal vein thrombosis **b** due to hypercoagulable state. No signs of bowel ischemia were noted, and the patient was treated successfully with long-term anticoagulation

Most of the symptoms listed in this section are often not clinically apparent in a critically ill ventilated patient on ICU. Accordingly, any negative changes in patient's physiology, including new onset of organ failure, increase in vasoactive support and nutrition intolerance should raise the suspicion of mesenteric ischemia.

When the diagnosis of AMI is made, fluid resuscitation should commence immediately to enhance visceral perfusion. Electrolyte abnormalities should be corrected, and nasogastric decompression initiated. (Recommendation 1B)

Fluid resuscitation with crystalloid and blood products is essential for the management of the patient with suspected AMI. Preoperatively resuscitation is important to prevent cardiovascular collapse on induction of anesthesia. To guide effective resuscitation, early hemodynamic monitoring should be implemented [44]. Assessment of electrolyte levels and acid–base status should be performed. This is especially true in patients with AMI, where severe metabolic acidosis and hyperkalemia may be present due to underlying bowel infarction and reperfusion [45]. Vasopressors should be used with caution, and only to avoid fluid overload and abdominal compartment syndrome. Dobutamine, low dose dopamine, and milrinone to improve cardiac function have been shown to have less impact on mesenteric blood flow [46, 47]. The fluid volume requirement in these patients may be high, due to extensive capillary leakage, but extensive crystalloid overload should be avoided to optimize bowel perfusion [48]. The endpoints of therapy should address physiologic levels of oxygen delivery with continued monitoring of lactate level as an indication of improvement. Although in the past, supra-physiologic levels were advocated, current evidence does not support this concept [49].

Broad-spectrum antibiotics should be administered immediately. Unless contraindicated, patients should be anticoagulated with intravenous unfractionacted heparin. (Recommendation 1B)

The high risk of infection among patients with AMI outweighs the risks of acquired antibiotic resistance, and therefore broad-spectrum antibiotics should be administered early in the course of treatment [50]. Intestinal ischemia leads to early loss of the mucosal barrier, which facilitates bacterial translocation and the risk of septic complications.

Prompt laparotomy should be done for patients with overt peritonitis. (Recommendation 1A)

When physical findings suggestive of an acute intraabdominal catastrophe are present, bowel infarction already occurred, and the chance of survival in this patient population with significant associated comorbidity is dramatically reduced. There is overwhelming evidence in literature that peritonitis secondary to bowel necrosis mandates surgery without delay.

The goal of surgical intervention for AMI includes:

1) Re-establishment blood supply to the ischemic bowel.
2) Resection of all non-viable regions.
3) Preservation of all viable bowel.

Intestinal viability is the most important factor influencing outcome in patients with AMI. Non-viable intestine, if unrecognized, results in multi-system organ dysfunction and ultimately death. Prompt laparotomy allows for direct assessment of bowel viability.

After initial resuscitation, midline laparotomy should be performed followed by assessment of all areas of the intestine with decisions for resection of all clearly necrotic areas. In cases of uncertainty, intraoperative Doppler may be helpful, as the presence of Doppler signals over distal branches of SMA facilitates bowel conservation, avoiding long-term disability. The SMA is easily palpated by placing fingers behind the root of the mesentery. The SMA is identified as a firm tubular structure, which may or may not have a palpable pulse. Otherwise, the SMA can also be reached by following the middle colic artery where it enters the SMA at the mesentery. Direct sharp dissection, exposing the artery from its surrounding mesenteric tissue, is required for proper exposure to perform revascularization. In cases of diagnostic uncertainties, arteriogram is the study of choice. It can be done intraoperatively especially in hybrid suites.

Different techniques of blood flow restoration are used depending on the pathophysiology of the AMI. Embolectomy and either primary or patch angioplasty is a well-established definitive treatment for SMA emboli. On the other hand, thrombosis of the SMA at the origin of aorta (a common pathology in diffuse aterosclerosis) will require a bypass procedure. However, it increases the magnitude of the procedure and may require prosthetics in the presence of contaminated field. One option is a retrograde bypass from the iliac artery to the distal SMA using the femoral vein or a synthetic graft (Fig. 3).

Neither NOMI nor MVT typically require vascular repair. Full dose anticoagulation should be initiated on all patients prior to the surgical procedure. Unfractioned heparin is effective and easy to manage, especially in patients with acute kidney failure.

Endovascular revascularization procedures may have a role with partial arterial occlusion. (Recommendation 1C)

Several case series using endovascular techniques in combination with pharmacologic therapy have been reported

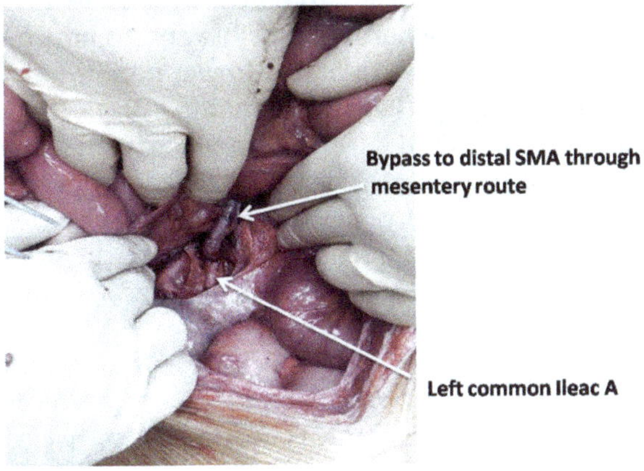

Fig. 3 Patient with acute thrombosis of SMA underwent left ileo–SMA bypass with a common femoral vein graft

recently. It should be emphasized, however, that any evidence of bowel ischemia or infarction precludes the use of thrombolytic therapy. At this time, these techniques have been attempted in very early, cases of AMI, and the role of such procedures remains to be determined [51, 52]. Other contraindications to thrombolytic therapy include recent surgery, trauma, cerebrovascular or gastrointestinal bleeding, and uncontrolled hypertension [53].

In recent retrospective series of 679 patients with AMI and vascular intervention (both open and endovascular) endovascular treatment performed in 24% (165 patients). The technique was successful in 87% of the patients, and in-hospital mortality was lower than among those who underwent open procedure (25 vs. 40%) [10]. Again, this report emphasized that only patients who did not require open emergent intervention are suitable for this technical approach to revascularization.

Endovascular embolectomy may be achieved by percutaneous mechanical aspiration or thrombolysis and permits percutaneous transluminal angioplasty, with or without stenting in case series of patients with CTA evidence of acute partial or complete occlusion of the SMA (either the main trunk or branch) and without no clinical or imaging evidence of advanced bowel ischemia. Complete technical success was achieved in 28% of cases; all of these had occlusion of the main SMA trunk [54–57].

There are no randomized controlled trials comparing laparotomy versus endovascular treatment as a first line strategy for the management AMI [10, 58, 59]. The most important argument in favor of the early laparotomy approach is the ability to assess bowel viability directly and thereby, minimizing delays in restoring mesenteric blood flow. In one retrospective series, the authors documented that 1/3 of patients managed with endovascular therapy avoided laparotomy [10]. In cases of endovascular approach, the use of laparoscopy to assess bowel function may be a reasonable addition [60].

Centers of excellence equipped with hybrid operating rooms may provide further data supporting the use of an endovascular strategy [61].

Damage control surgery (DCS) is an important adjunct for patients who require intestinal resection due to the necessity to reassess bowel viability and in patients with refractory sepsis. Planned re-laparotomy is an essential part of AMI management. (Recommendation 1B)

Damage control laparotomy strategy (abbreviated laparotomy) was accepted for trauma over 30 years ago and was found to be an important option in the patient with AMI. Damage control is the surgical modality of choice in the critically ill patient with AMI for physiological and technical reasons. The decision to implement the DCS mode should be made early based upon the response to resuscitation and ongoing physiology, as this has been associated with improved mortality [62]. Advanced age is not a contraindication to DCS as good outcomes have been observed in the elderly [63].

Planned second look techniques are required after restoration of SMA flow, with or without resection of ischemic bowel (and no anastomosis or stoma) following resuscitation in intensive care unit [64, 65]. Given frequent uncertainty with regard to bowel viability, the stapled off bowel ends should be left in discontinuity and re-inspected after a period of continued ICU resuscitation to restore physiological balance. Often, bowel which is borderline ischemic at the initial exploration will improve after restoration of blood supply and physiologic stabilization. Of note, however, multiple adjuncts have been suggested to assess intestinal viability, but none have proven to be uniformly reliable [66, 67].

Most often, re-exploration should be accomplished within 48 h and decisions regarding anastomosis, stoma, or additional resection can be made with plans for sequential abdominal closure.

In a review of 43 patients undergoing open mesenteric revascularization, the authors noted that 11 of the 23 patients undergoing a second-look operation required bowel resection [20]. The bowel in these patients is often very swollen and at high risk for anastomotic leak. Recent studies suggest that careful hand sewn techniques are preferable to the use of staples in this group [68, 69].

These patients often suffer from acidosis, hypothermia, and coagulation abnormalities, which require prompt and ongoing correction. Physiologic restoration is multifactorial and includes careful and limited crystalloid infusion to avoid abdominal compartment syndrome, frequent monitoring of lactate clearance and central venous oxygen saturation as an indication of satisfactory cardiac output, and the use of viscoelastic techniques (TEG, ROTEM) to assess coagulation status and guide ongoing blood product administration. Recent evidence suggests that peritoneal resuscitation techniques may aid in this process [70, 71].

Various techniques of open abdomen have been described. The author's preferred mechanism is a simple plastic drape over the bowel, covered with a sterile towel and the use of Ioban over the abdomen. After the initial laparotomy, abdominal closure via negative pressure wound therapy is most commonly used. The open abdomen may help reduce the risk of abdominal compartment syndrome in patients requiring prolonged resuscitation. Various abdominal closure techniques have been described, however, the guiding principle is constant traction on the fascia to facilitate closure [72–75].

Mesenteric venous thrombosis can often be successfully treated with a continuous infusion of unfractionated heparin. (Recommendation 1B)

MVT has a distinctive clinical finding on CTA scan, and when noted in a patient without findings of peritonitis, non-operative management should be considered. The first-line treatment for mesenteric venous thrombosis is anticoagulation. Systemic thrombolytic therapy is rarely indicated. When clinical signs demand operative intervention, one should resect only obvious necrotic bowel and employee damage control techniques liberally, since anticoagulation therapy may improve the clinical picture over the ensuing 24–48 h. Early use of heparin has been associated with improved survival [76].

Patients with peritonitis require emergency surgery. Intraoperative management is dictated by the surgical findings, which range from a segmental infarction of small bowel to necrosis of the entire bowel, with or without perforation. The aim of resection is to conserve as much bowel as possible. Second-look laparotomy, 24–48 h later, may avoid the resection of bowel that may be viable. A second-look procedure is mandatory in patients who have extensive bowel involvement.

Most published data on interventional radiological treatments for MVT are from small case series. Systemic intravenous tPA has been successfully reported [77]. Trans-jugular intrahepatic portosystemic shunt can be used for MVT with the rationale of decreasing portal pressure, which works as a vacuum of clot fragments and improves the effectiveness of thrombolysis in the case of acute thrombosis [78–80].

Supportive measures include nasogastric suction, fluid resuscitation, and bowel rest.

When NOMI is suspected, the focus is to correct the underlying cause wherever possible and to improve mesenteric perfusion. Infarcted bowel should be resected promptly. (Recommendation 1B)

Management of NOMI is based on treatment of the underlying precipitating cause. Fluid resuscitation, optimization of cardiac output, and elimination of vasopressors remain important primary measures. Additional treatment may include systemic anticoagulation and the use of catheter-directed infusion of vasodilatory and antispasmodic agents, most commonly papaverine hydrochloride [81]. The decision to intervene surgically is based on the presence of peritonitis, perforation, or overall worsening of the patient's condition [47].

If a patient presents with peritoneal signs, an exploratory laparotomy is required for resection of frankly necrotic bowel. Unfortunately, these patients are often in critical condition and the mortality remains very high (50–85%) [9]. Damage control mode is an important adjunct, given the critical state of these patients.

The finding of massive gut necrosis requires careful assessment of the patients underlying comorbidities and advanced directives in order to judge whether comfort carries the best treatment. (Recommendation 1C)

In cases of extensive infarction of most of the small bowel with or without a portion of the colon, the surgeon could face with a philosophical decision whether to do anything. Resection of the entire involved bowel will result in short bowel syndrome with its serious associated consequences. This may not be a preferable state, particularly in elderly infirm patients, who may not tolerate long-term parenteral nutrition. A preoperative discussion with the patient and the patient's family concerning these issues is warranted and often necessary peri-operatively as well so that an agreeable plan can be reached [82].

Conclusions

AMI is a true surgical emergency. First and foremost, important evidence is a high index of suspicion based on the combination of history of abrupt onset of abdominal pain, acidosis, and organ failure. This clinical scenario should prompt imaging (CTA) in order to establish the diagnosis. In parallel with rapid resuscitation and after careful assessment of the CTA, the patient should be explored to assess bowel viability, re-establish vascular flow, and resect non-viable bowel. Subsequently, the employment of damage control techniques and continued critical care resuscitation is essential. Planned re-assessment of the bowel with further resection or anastomosis and stoma as needed is integral. Close cooperation between acute care surgeons, radiologists, anesthetists, and the vascular surgeons is essential.

Appendix

Current recommendations:

Statement 1

Severe abdominal pain out of proportion to physical examination findings should be assumed to be AMI until disproven. (Recommendation 1B)

Statement 2

Clinical scenario differentiates AMI as mesenteric arterial emboli, mesenteric arterial thrombosis, NOMI, or mesenteric venous thrombosis. (Recommendation 1B)

Statement 3

Conventional plain X-ray films have limited diagnostic value in evaluating AMI, although signs of intestinal perforation may be seen. (Recommendation 1B)

Statement 4

There are no laboratory studies that are sufficiently accurate to identify the presence or absence of ischemic or necrotic bowel, although elevated l-lactate and D-dimer may assist. (Recommendation 1B)

Statement 5

Computed tomography angiography (CTA) should be performed as soon as possible for any patient with suspicion for AMI. (Recommendation 1A)

Statement 6

Non-occlusive mesenteric ischemia (NOMI) should be suspected in critically ill patients with abdominal pain or distension requiring vasopressor support and evidence of multi-organ dysfunction. (Recommendation 1B)

Statement 7

When the diagnosis of AMI is made, fluid resuscitation should commence immediately to enhance visceral perfusion. Electrolyte abnormalities should be corrected, and nasogastric decompression initiated. (Recommendation 1B)

Statement 8

Broad-spectrum antibiotics should be administered immediately. Unless contraindicated, patients should be anticoagulated with intravenous unfractionated heparin. (Recommendation 1B)

Statement 9

Prompt laparotomy should be done for patients with overt peritonitis. (Recommendation 1A)

Statement 10

Endovascular revascularization procedures may have a role with partial arterial occlusion. (Recommendation 1C)

Statement 11

Damage control surgery is an important adjunct for patients who require intestinal resection due to the necessity to reassess bowel viability and in patients with refractory sepsis. Planned re-laparotomy is an essential part of AMI management. (Recommendation 1B)

Statement 12

Mesenteric venous thrombosis can often be successfully treated with a continuous infusion of unfractionated heparin. (Recommendation 1B)

Statement 13

When NOMI is suspected, the treatment focus should be to correct the underlying cause and to restore mesenteric perfusion. Infarcted bowel should be resected promptly. (Recommendation 1B)

Statement 14

The finding of massive gut necrosis requires careful assessment of the patients underlying co-morbidities and advanced directives in order to judge whether comfort carries the best treatment. (Recommendation 1C)

Abbreviations

alpha–GST: Serum alpha-glutathione S-transferase; AMI: Acute mesenteric ischemia; CABA: Cobalt-albumin binding assay; CMI: Chronic mesenteric ischemia; CTA: Computed tomography angiography; DCS: Damage control surgery; I-FABP: Intestinal fatty acid binding protein; MDCT: Multi-detector computed tomography; MPR: Multi-planar reconstructions; NOMI: Non-occlusive mesenteric ischemia; NPWT: MVT: Mesenteric venous thrombosis; SMA: Superior mesenteric artery; tPA: Tissue plasminogen activator; WSES: World Society of Emergency Surgery

Acknowledgements

Not applicable.

Funding

Not applicable.

Authors' contributions

MB, EM, and JK are responsible for the manuscript conception and draft. YK, WB, CAG, OB, CR, ZB, IC, FC, AL, AP, LA, MS, MS, SDS, GF, and FC critically revised the manuscript. All authors gave the final approval.

Competing interests

The authors declare that they have no competing interests.

Author details
[1]Acute Care Surgery and Trauma Unit, General Surgery Department, Hadassah - Hebrew University Medical Center, Kiriat Hadassah, POB 12000, 91120 Jerusalem, Israel. [2]Assia Medical Group, Tel Aviv University Sackler School of Medicine, Tel Aviv, Israel. [3]Department of Surgery, Denver Health Medical Center, University of Colorado, Denver, USA. [4]Department of General Surgery, Rambam Health Care Campus, Haifa, Israel. [5]Department of Surgery, Queens Medical Center, Honolulu, Hi, USA. [6]Faculdade de Ciências Médicas e da Saúde de Juiz de Fora (SUPREMA), Federal University of Juiz de Fora (UFJF), Juiz de Fora, MG, Brazil. [7]Department of Vascular Surgery, Hadassah Hebrew University Medical Center, Jerusalem, Israel. [8]Department of Traumatology, John Hunter Hospital and University of Newcastle, Newcastle, NSW, Australia. [9]Department of Surgery, Auckland City Hospital, Auckland, New Zealand. [10]General Surgery I, Papa Giovanni XXIII Hospital, Bergamo, Italy. [11]Abdominal Center, University Hospital Meilahti, Helsinki, Finland. [12]Department of Surgery, UPMC, University of Pittsburgh School of Medicine, Pittsburgh, PA, USA. [13]Donegal Clinical Research Academy, Letterkenny University Hospital, Letterkenny, Ireland. [14]Department of Surgery, Macerata Hospital, Macerata, Italy. [15]Trauma Surgery Unit, Maggiore Hospital, Bologna, Italy. [16]Division of Trauma Surgery, Hospital de Clinica, School of Medical Sciences, University of Campinas, Campinas, Brazil. [17]Emergency Department, Maggiore University Hospital, Parma, Italy.

References

1. Patel A, Kaleya RN, Sammartano RJ. Pathophysiology of mesenteric ischemia. Surg Clin North Am. 1992;72:31–41.
2. Acosta S. Mesenteric ischemia. Curr Opin Crit Care. 2015;21:171–8.
3. Clair DG, Beach JM. Mesenteric Ischemia. N Engl J Med. 2016;374:959–68.
4. Acosta S, Bjorck M. Acute thrombo-embolic occlusion of the superior mesenteric artery: a prospective study in a well-defined population. Eur J Vasc Endovasc Surg. 2003;26:179–83.
5. Duran M, Pohl E, Grabitz K, Schelzig H, Sagban TA, Simon F. The importance of open emergency surgery in the treatment of acute mesenteric ischemia. World J Emerg Surg. 2015;26:10–45.
6. Stoney RJ, Cunningham CG. Acute mesenteric ischemia. Surgery. 1993;114: 489–90.
7. Chang RW, Chang JB, Longo WE. Update in management of mesenteric ischemia. World J Gastroenterol. 2006;12:3243–7.
8. Horton KM, Fishman EK. Multidetector CT angiography in the diagnosis of mesenteric ischemia. Radiol Clin N Am. 2007;45:275–88.
9. Schoots IG, Koffeman GI, Legemate DA, Levi M, van Gulik TM. Systematic review of survival after acute mesenteric ischaemia according to disease aetiology. Br J Surg. 2004;91:17–27.
10. Beaulieu RJ, Arnaoutakis KD, Abularrage CJ, Efron DT, Schneider E, Black JH. Comparison of open and endovascular treatment of acute mesenteric ischemia. J Vasc Surg. 2014;59:159–64.
11. Rosenblum JD, Boyle CM, Schwartz LB. The mesenteric circulation. Anatomy and physiology. Surg Clin North Am. 1997;77:289–306.
12. Haglund U, Bergqvist D. Intestinal ischemia—the basics. Langenbeck's Arch Surg. 1999;384:233–8.
13. van Petersen AS, Kolkman JJ, Meerwaldt R, Huisman AB, van der Palen J, Zeebregts CJ, Geelkerken RH. Mesenteric stenosis, collaterals, and compensatory blood flow. J Vasc Surg. 2014;60:111–9.
14. Acosta S, Ogren M, Sternby NH, Bergqvist D, Björck M. Clinical implications for the management of acute thromboembolic occlusion of the superior mesenteric artery: autopsy findings in 213 patients. Ann Surg. 2005;241:516–22.
15. Kärkkäinen JM, Acosta S. Acute mesenteric ischemia (part I) -incidence, etiologies, and how to improve early diagnosis. Best Pract Res Clin Gastroenterol. 2017;31:15–25.
16. Aschoff AJ, Stuber G, Becker BW, Hoffmann MH, Schmitz BL, Schelzig H, et al. Evaluation of acute mesenteric ischemia: accuracy of biphasic mesenteric multi-detector CT angiography. Abdom Imaging. 2009;34:345–57.
17. Moore HB, Moore EE, Lawson PJ, Gonzalez E, Fragoso M, Morton AP, Gamboni F, Chapman MP, Sauaia A, Banerjee A, Silliman CC. Fibrinolysis shutdown phenotype masks changes in rodent coagulation in tissue injury versus hemorrhagic shock. Surgery. 2015;158:386–92.
18. Cohn DM, Roshani S, Middeldorp S. Thrombophilia and venous thromboembolism: implications for testing. Semin Thromb Hemost. 2007;33:573–81.
19. Carver TW, Vora RS, Taneja A. Mesenteric ischemia. Crit Care Clin. 2016;32: 155–71.
20. Park WM, Gloviczki P, Cherry KJ Jr, Hallett JW Jr, Bower TC, Panneton JM, Schleck C, Ilstrup D, Harmsen WS, Noel AA. Contemporary management of acute mesenteric ischemia: Factors associated with survival. J Vasc Surg. 2002;35:445–52.
21. Acosta-Merida MA, Marchena-Gomez J, Hemmersbach-Miller M, Roque-Castellano C, Hernandez-Romero JM. Identification of risk factors for perioperative mortality in acute mesenteric ischemia. World J Surg. 2006;30: 1579–85.
22. Morasch MD, Ebaugh JL, Chiou AC, Matsumura JS, Pearce WH, Yao JS. Mesenteric venous thrombosis: a changing clinical entity. J Vasc Surg. 2001; 34:680–4.
23. Oliva IB, Davarpanah AH, Rybicki FJ, Desjardins B, Flamm SD, Francois CJ, Gerhard-Herman MD, Kalva SP, Ashraf Mansour M, Mohler ER 3rd, Schenker MP, Weiss C, Dill KE. ACR Appropriateness Criteria® imaging of mesenteric ischemia. Abdom Imaging. 2013;38:714–9.
24. Kougias P, Lau D, El Sayed HF, Zhou W, Huynh TT, Lin PH. Determinants ofmortality and treatment outcome following surgical interventions for acutemesenteric ischemia. J Vasc Surg. 2007;46:467–74.
25. Nuzzo A, Maggiori L, Ronot M, Becq A, Plessier A, Gault N, Joly F, Castier Y, Vilgrain V, Paugam C, Panis Y, Bouhnik Y, Cazals-Hatem D, Corcos O. Predictive factors of intestinal necrosis in acute mesenteric ischemia: prospective study from an intestinal stroke center. Am J Gastroenterol. 2017;112:597–605.
26. Evennett NJ, Petrov MS, Mittal A, Windsor JA. Systematic review and pooled estimates for the diagnostic accuracy of serological markers for intestinal ischemia. World J Surg. 2009;33:1374–83.
27. Powell A, Armstrong P. Plasma biomarkers for early diagnosis of acuteintestinal ischemia. Semin Vasc Surg. 2014;27:170–5.
28. Block T, Nilsson TK, Björck M, Acosta S. Diagnostic accuracy of plasma biomarkers for intestinal ischaemia. Scand J Clin Lab Invest. 2008;68: 242–8.
29. Wilson C, Imrie CW. Amylase and gut infarction. Br J Surg. 1986;73:219–21.
30. Matsumoto S, Sekine K, Funaoka H, Yamazaki M, Shimizu M, Hayashida K, Kitano M. Diagnostic performance of plasma biomarkers in patients with acute intestinal ischaemia. Br J Surg. 2014;101:232–8.
31. Treskes N, Persoon AM, van Zanten ARH. Diagnostic accuracy of novel serological biomarkers to detect acute mesenteric ischemia: a systematic review and meta-analysis. Intern Emerg Med. 2017. [Epub ahead of print].
32. Bradbury AW, Brittenden J, McBride K, Ruckley CV. Mesenteric ischaemia: a multidisciplinary approach. Br J Surg. 1995;82:1446–59.
33. Kassahun WT, Schulz T, Richter O, Hauss J. Unchanged high mortality rates from acute occlusive intestinal ischemia: six year review. Langenbeck's Arch Surg. 2008;393:163–71.
34. Kirkpatrick ID, Kroeker MA, Greenberg HM. Biphasic CT with mesenteric CTangiography in the evaluation of acute mesenteric ischemia: initial experience. Radiology. 2003;229:91–8.
35. Furukawa A, Kanasaki S, Kono N, Wakamiya M, Tanaka T, Takahashi M, Murata K. CT diagnosis of acute mesenteric ischemia from various causes. Am J Roentgenol. 2009;192:408–16.
36. Menke J. Diagnostic accuracy of multidetector CT in acute mesenteric ischemia: systematic review and meta-analysis. Radiology. 2010;256:93–101.
37. Hagspiel KD, Flors L, Hanley M, Norton PT. Computed tomography angiography and magnetic resonance angiography imaging of the mesenteric vasculature. Tech Vasc Interv Radiol. 2015;18:2–13.
38. Oliva IB, Davarpanah AH, Rybicki FJ, et al. ACR appropriateness criteria imaging of mesenteric ischemia. Abdom Imaging. 2013;38:714–9.
39. David RA, Erben Y, Kalra M. Clinical presentation, etiology, and diagnostic considerations. In: Oderich G, editor. Mesenteric Vascular Disease. New York: Springer; 2015. p. 199–209.
40. Daviaud F, Grimaldi D, Dechartres A, Charpentier J, Geri G, Marin N, Chiche JD, Cariou A, Mira JP, Pène F. Timing and causes of death in septic shock. Ann Intensive Care. 2015;5:16.
41. Guillaume A, Pili-Floury S, Chocron S, Delabrousse E, De Parseval B, Koch S, Samain E, Capellier G, Piton G. Acute mesenteric ischemia among post-cardiac surgery patients presenting with multiple organ failure. Shock. 2016. [Epub ahead of print].
42. Mastoraki A, Mastoraki S, Tziava E, Touloumi S, Krinos N, Danias N, Lazaris A, Arkadopoulos N. Mesenteric ischemia: pathogenesis and challenging

diagnostic and therapeutic modalities. World J Gastrointest Pathophysiol. 2016;7:125–30.

43. Mogilner JG, Bitterman H, Hayari L, et al. Effect of elevated intra-abdominal pressure and hyperoxia on portal vein blood flow, hepatocyte proliferation and apoptosis in a rat model. Eur J Pediatr Surg. 2008;18:380–6.
44. Wyers MC. Acute mesenteric ischemia: diagnostic approach and surgical treatment. Semin Vasc Surg. 2010;23:9–20.
45. Corcos O, Nuzzo A. Gastro-intestinalvascular emergencies. Best Pract Res Clin Gastroenterol. 2013;27:709–25.
46. Tendler DA, LaMont JT. Acute mesenteric ischemia. Uptodate. 2013. http://www.uptodate.com/contents/acute-mesentericischemia. Accessed 13 Aug 2016.
47. Sise MJ. Mesenteric ischemia: the whole spectrum. Scand J Surg. 2010;99: 106–10.
48. Oldenburg WA, Lau LL, Rodenberg TJ, Edmonds HJ, Burger CD. Acute mesentericischemia: a clinical review. Arch Intern Med. 2004;164:1054–62.
49. Helmerhorst HJ, Schultz MJ, van der Voort PH, de Jonge E, van Westerloo DJ. Bench-to-bedside review: the effects of hyperoxia during critical illness. Crit Care. 2015;19:284.
50. Silvestri L, van Saene HK, Zandstra DF, Marshall JC, Gregori D, Gullo A. Impactof selective decontamination of thedigestive tract on multiple organ dysfunctionsyndrome: systematic review of randomizedcontrolled trials. Crit Care Med. 2010;38:1370–6.
51. Schoots IG, Levi MM, Reekers JA, Lameris JS, van Gulik TM. Thrombolytic therapy for acute superior mesenteric artery occlusion. J Vasc Interv Radiol. 2005;16:317–29.
52. Landis MS, Rajan DK, Simons ME, Hayeems EB, Kachura JR, Sniderman KW. Percutaneous management of chronic mesenteric ischemia: outcomes after intervention. J Vasc Interv Radiol. 2005;16:1319–25.
53. Sarac TP. Techniques of endovascular revascularization for acute mesenteric ischemia. In: Oderich G, editor. Mesenteric Vascular Disease. New York: Springer; 2015. p. 241–52.
54. Kim BG, Ohm JY, Bae MN, Kim HN, Kim YJ, Chung MH, Park CS, Ihm SH, Kim HY. Successful percutaneous aspiration thrombectomy for acute mesenteric ischemia in a patient with atrial fibrillation despite optimal anticoagulation therapy. Can J Cardiol. 2013;29:1329.e5–7.
55. Schoenbaum SW, Pena C, Koenigsberg P, Katzen BT. Superior mesenteric artery embolism: treatment with intra arterial urokinase. JVIR. 1992;3:485–90.
56. Simó G, Echenagusia AJ, Camuñez F, Turégano F, Cabrera A, Urbano J. Superior mesenteric arterial embolism: local fibrinolytic treatment with urokinase. Radiology. 1997;204:775–9.
57. Jia Z, Jiang G, Tian F, Zhao J, Li S, Wang K, Wang Y, Jiang L, Wang W. Early endovascular treatment of superior mesenteric occlusion secondary to thromboemboli. Eur J Vasc Endovasc Surg. 2014;47:196–203.
58. Orr NT, Endean ED. Part two: against the motion. an endovascular first strategy is not the optimal approach for treating acute mesenteric ischemia. Eur J Vasc Endovasc Surg. 2015;50:276–9.
59. Arthurs ZM, Titus J, Bannazadeh M, Eagleton MJ, Srivastava S, Sarac TP, et al. A comparison of endovascular revascularization with traditional therapy for the treatment of acute mesenteric ischemia. J Vasc Surg. 2011;53:698–705.
60. Cocorullo G, Mirabella A, Falco N, Fontana T, Tutino R, Licari L, Salamone G, Scerrino G, Gulotta G. An investigation of bedside laparoscopy in the ICU for cases of non-occlusive mesenteric ischemia. World J Emerg Surg. 2017;12:4.
61. Björck M. Part one: for the motion. an endovascular first strategy is the optimal approach for treating acute mesenteric ischemia. Eur J Vasc Endovasc Surg. 2015;50:273–5.
62. Godat L, Kobayashi L, Costantini T, Coimbra R. Abdominal damage control surgery and reconstruction: world society of emergency surgery position paper. World J Emerg Surg. 2013;8:53.
63. Weber DG, Bendinelli C, Balogh ZJ. Damage control surgery for abdominal emergencies. Br J Surg. 2014;101:109–18.
64. Subramanian A, Balentine C, Palacio CH, Sansgiry S, Berger DH, Awad SS. Outcomes of damage-control celiotomy in elderly non trauma patients with intra-abdominal catastrophes. Am J Surg. 2010;200:783–8.
65. Weber DG, Bendinelli C, Balogh ZJ. Damage control surgery for abdominal emergencies. Br J Surg. 2014;101:e109–18.
66. Urbanavičius L, Pattyn P, de Putte DV, Venskutonis D. How to assess intestinal viability during surgery: a review of techniques. World J Gastrointest Surg. 2011;3:59–69.
67. Horgan PG, Gorey TF. Operative assessment of intestinal viability. Surg Clin North Am. 1992;72:143–55.
68. Worrell S, Mumtaz S, Tsuboi K, Lee TH, Mittal SK. Anastomotic complications associated with stapled versus hand-sewn anastomosis. J Surg Res. 2010; 161:9–12.
69. Brundage SI, Jurkovich GJ, Hoyt DB, Patel NY, Ross SE, Marburger R, Stoner M, Ivatury RR, Ku J, Rutherford EJ, Maier RV, WTA Multi-institutional Study Group, Western Trauma Association. Stapled versus sutured gastrointestinal anastomoses in the trauma patient: a multicenter trial. J Trauma. 2001;51: 1054–61.
70. Smith JW, Matheson PJ, Franklin GA, Harbrecht BG, Richardson JD, Garrison RN. Randomized controlled trial evaluating the efficacy of peritoneal resuscitation in the management of trauma patients undergoing damage control surgery. J Am Coll Surg. 2017;224:396–404.
71. Crafts TD, Hunsberger EB, Jensen AR, Rescorla FJ, Yoder MC, Markel TA. Direct peritoneal resuscitation improves survival and decreases inflammation after intestinal ischemia and reperfusion injury. J Surg Res. 2015;199:428–34.
72. Acosta S, Björck M, Petersson U. Vacuum-assisted wound closure and mesh-mediated fascial traction for open abdomen therapy—a systematic review. Anaesthesiol Intensive Ther. 2017.[Epub ahead of print].
73. Hofmann AT, Gruber-Blum S, Lechner M, Petter-Puchner A, Glaser K, Fortelny R. Delayed closure of open abdomen in septic patients treated with negative pressure wound therapy and dynamic fascial suture: the long-term follow-up study. Surg Endosc. 2017. [Epub ahead of print].
74. Willms A, Schaaf S, Schwab R, Richardsen I, Jänig C, Bieler D, Wagner B, Güsgen C. Intensive care and health outcomes of open abdominal treatment: long-term results of vacuum-assisted wound closure and mesh-mediated fascial traction (VAWCM). Langenbeck's Arch Surg. 2017;402:481–92.
75. Tolonen M, Mentula P, Sallinen V, Rasilainen S, Bäcklund M, Leppäniemi A. Open abdomen with vacuum-assisted wound closure and mesh-mediated fascial traction in tients with complicated diffuse secondary peritonitis: A single-center 8-year experience. J Trauma Acute Care Surg. 2017;82:1100–5.
76. Acosta S. Surgical management of peritonitis secondary to acute superior mesenteric artery occlusion. World J Gastroenterol. 2014;20:9936–41.
77. Hmoud B, Singal AK, Kamath PS. Mesenteric venous thrombosis. J Clin Exp Hepatol. 2014;4:257–63.
78. al Karawi MA, Quaiz M, Clark D, Hilali A, Mohamed AE, Jawdat M. Mesenteric vein thrombosis, non-invasive diagnosis and follow-up (US + MRI), and non-invasive therapy by streptokinase and anticoagulants. Hepato-Gastroenterology. 1990;37:507–9.
79. Semiz-Oysu A, Keussen I, Cwikiel W. Interventional radiological management of prehepatic obstruction of [corrected] the splanchnic venous system. Cardiovasc Intervent Radiol. 2007;30:688–95.
80. Sehgal M, Haskal ZJ. Use of transjugular intrahepatic portosystemic shunts during lytic therapy of extensive portal splenic and mesenteric venous thrombosis: long-term follow-up. J Vasc Interv Radiol. 2000;11:61–5.
81. Meilahn JE, Morris JB, Ceppa EP, Bulkley GB. Effect of prolonged selective intramesenteric arterial vasodilator therapy on intestinal viability after acute segmental mesenteric vascular occlusion. Ann Surg. 2001;234:107–15.
82. Lilley EJ, Cooper Z, Schwarze ML, Mosenthal AC. Palliative care in surgery: defining the research priorities. J Palliat Med. 2017;20:702–9.

20

2017 WSES guidelines for the management of iatrogenic colonoscopy perforation

Nicola de'Angelis[1*], Salomone Di Saverio[2], Osvaldo Chiara[3], Massimo Sartelli[4], Aleix Martínez-Pérez[5], Franca Patrizi[6], Dieter G. Weber[7], Luca Ansaloni[8], Walter Biffl[9], Offir Ben-Ishay[10], Miklosh Bala[11], Francesco Brunetti[1], Federica Gaiani[12], Solafah Abdalla[1], Aurelien Amiot[13], Hany Bahouth[10], Giorgio Bianchi[1], Daniel Casanova[14], Federico Coccolini[8], Raul Coimbra[15], Gian Luigi de'Angelis[12], Belinda De Simone[16], Gustavo P. Fraga[17], Pietro Genova[18], Rao Ivatury[19], Jeffry L. Kashuk[20], Andrew W. Kirkpatrick[21], Yann Le Baleur[13], Fernando Machado[22], Gustavo M. Machain[23], Ronald V. Maier[24], Alain Chichom-Mefire[25], Riccardo Memeo[26], Carlos Mesquita[27], Juan Carlos Salamea Molina[28], Massimiliano Mutignani[29], Ramiro Manzano-Núñez[30], Carlos Ordoñez[30], Andrew B. Peitzman[31], Bruno M. Pereira[17], Edoardo Picetti[32], Michele Pisano[8], Juan Carlos Puyana[33], Sandro Rizoli[34], Mohammed Siddiqui[1], Iradj Sobhani[13], Richard P. ten Broek[35], Luigi Zorcolo[36], Maria Clotilde Carra[37], Yoram Kluger[10] and Fausto Catena[38]

Abstract

Iatrogenic colonoscopy perforation (ICP) is a severe complication that can occur during both diagnostic and therapeutic procedures. Although 45–60% of ICPs are diagnosed by the endoscopist while performing the colonoscopy, many ICPs are not immediately recognized but are instead suspected on the basis of clinical signs and symptoms that occur after the endoscopic procedure. There are three main therapeutic options for ICPs: endoscopic repair, conservative therapy, and surgery. The therapeutic approach must vary based on the setting of the diagnosis (intra- or post-colonoscopy), the type of ICP, the characteristics and general status of the patient, the operator's level of experience, and surgical device availability.

Although ICPs have been the focus of numerous publications, no guidelines have been created to standardize the management of ICPs. The aim of this article is to present the World Society of Emergency Surgery (WSES) guidelines for the management of ICP, which are intended to be used as a tool to promote global standards of care in case of ICP. These guidelines are not meant to substitute providers' clinical judgment for individual patients, and they may need to be modified based on the medical team's level of experience and the availability of local resources.

Keywords: Iatrogenic colonoscopy perforation, Colonoscopy, Gastrointestinal endoscopy, Emergency surgery, Laparoscopy, Antibiotic therapy, Intra-abdominal infection, Open abdomen

Background

Iatrogenic colonic perforations (ICPs) are an infrequent but severe complication of colonoscopy. Globally, the incidence is estimated to be 0.016–0.8% for diagnostic colonoscopies and 0.02–8% for therapeutic colonoscopies [1–10], but considering the increasing numbers of screening, diagnostic, and therapeutic colonoscopies being performed every year, the frequency of ICP is not insignificant [11, 12].

Approximately 45–60% of ICPs are detected by the endoscopist while performing the colonoscopy, although a considerable number of ICPs are not recognized immediately, but rather are suspected on the basis of clinical signs and symptoms occurring after the endoscopic procedure. In this latter case, colonic perforations may lead to the development of secondary peritonitis, which is associated with significant morbidity and

* Correspondence: nic.deangelis@yahoo.it; nic.deangelia@yahoo.it
[1]Unit of Digestive, Hepato-Pancreato-Biliary Surgery and Liver Transplantation, Henri Mondor University Hospital, AP-HP, and University of Paris Est, UPEC, 51 Avenue du Maréchal de Lattre de Tassigny, 94010 Créteil, France

mortality [5, 13–18]. Depending on the delay in the management of the ICP and the pre-existing pathologies, ICP-related mortality is as high as 5–25% [5, 14–16, 18–22].

One of the most important issues in the management of ICPs is the time period between the diagnosis and the treatment. There are different treatment alternatives for ICP, including conservative, endoscopic, and surgical approaches. The therapeutic strategy varies based on the setting in which the ICP is diagnosed (i.e., intra- or post-colonoscopy), the specific characteristics of the perforation (e.g., size, location, and etiology), the patient's general status, and the skill level of the operator [8, 23, 24]. Although ICPs have been the subject of numerous publications, no randomized clinical trials have been conducted to evaluate the best treatment option and no guidelines have been defined to standardize its management. For this reason, the World Society of Emergency Surgery (WSES) convened a consensus conference to review the available literature, discuss the current controversies, and create guidelines for the management of ICP. The present article is the summary of the WSES consensus conference, including (1) the incidence of and risk factors for ICP, (2) the diagnosis of ICP, (3) the conservative and endoscopic treatments for ICP, (4) the surgical treatments for ICP, and (5) the follow-up after ICP treatment. Based upon the evidence emerging from the consensus conference, a decision-making algorithm was developed to guide clinicians and surgeons through the different medical, endoscopic, and surgical treatments for ICP.

Materials and methods: expert panel and consensus conference organization

On September 2016, the President of the WSES (Luca Ansaloni) appointed five WSES members (Nicola de'Angelis, Fausto Catena, Federico Coccolini, Salomone Di Saverio, Massimo Sartelli) to establish the project committee and determine the organization of an international multidisciplinary expert panel deputed to develop the WSES Guidelines for the management of ICP. The project committee agreed to develop practice guidelines by formal consensus, which consists of formalizing the degree of agreement among experts by identifying and selecting, through ratings and feedback, the points on which the experts agree and the points on which they disagree or are undecided. Additionally, it involves drafting a small number of concise and unambiguous recommendations that address the questions asked.

Briefly, the development of the WSES guidelines was structured upon two phases: the synthesis of the literature and the consensus conference. For phase I, the project committee identified 17 key questions regarding ICP risk, diagnosis, and treatments that would guide the literature search (Table 1). Then, an expert panel composed of surgeons, endoscopists, gastroenterologists, and anesthesiologists from five continents was invited to participate and answer the selected questions. The experts who agreed to participate ($n = 50$) were divided into 17 groups of at least 3 experts each who were asked to answer one of the selected key questions regarding ICP. For each group, a group leader was nominated; the group leader was

Table 1 Key questions used to develop the Consensus Conference on iatrogenic colonoscopy perforation (ICP)

Risk of ICP	
Q1	What are the general recommendations to minimize the risk of ICP during screening and therapeutic colonoscopies?
Q2	What is the maximum incidence of ICP considered acceptable for centers where diagnostic or therapeutic colonoscopies are performed?
Diagnosis of ICP	
Q3	What is the minimum information the endoscopist must report after diagnosing an ICP during a colonoscopy procedure?
Q4	What are the minimum biochemical and imaging investigations that should be requested in the case of suspected ICP?
Conservative and endoscopic treatments of ICP	
Q5	What are the indications for a conservative treatment or an immediate surgical intervention after an ICP diagnosis?
Q6	What is the minimum duration of the hospital observation period for patients who have undergone successful endoscopic closure or conservative management of ICP?
Q7	What investigations (clinical, biochemical, and imaging) should be performed during the observation period in patients who have undergone successful endoscopic closure or conservative management of ICP?
Q8	What is the recommended type and duration of antibiotic therapy in patients who have undergone successful endoscopic closure or conservative management of ICP?
Q9	What is the recommended type and duration of antithrombotic prophylaxis in patients who have undergone successful endoscopic closure or conservative management of ICP?
Q10	How long is the fasting time in patients who have undergone successful endoscopic closure or conservative treatments for ICP?
Surgical treatment of ICP	
Q11	Is explorative laparoscopy indicated in all patients with ICP?
Q12	What are the indications for conversion from laparoscopy to open surgery in patients with surgical ICP?
Q13	What are the key factors when choosing the best surgical approach for ICP?
Q14	What are the indications for performing a diverting or terminal stoma in patients with ICP?
Q15	What are the indications for drainages in patients with ICP?
Q16	What are the indications for the use of damage control surgery in patients with ICP?
Follow-up of ICP	
Q17	Is there any recommendation to perform a surveillance endoscopy after a successful ICP treatment? If so, what is the recommended timing for it?

responsible for coordinating the work of the experts in his/her group, providing a summary document that aligned the group's agreement upon answers to the specific question assigned, and meeting the assigned deadline. Experts were solicited to search the literature using a systematic approach within different databases (e.g., PubMed, EMBASE, and Scopus) and assess the level of evidence and the grade of the recommendation based on the recommendations of Guyatt et al. [25] (Table 2). For the literature search, the following keywords and MeSH terms were used: management of colonic/colon perforations, repair of iatrogenic large bowel perforations, abdominal imaging in colonic perforations, evolution of imaging, colonic perforation complications/outcomes, endoscopic treatment of colonic perforations, and peritonitis after colonoscopy.

Within each group, a scientific discussion ensued via email, and modifications were implemented when necessary based on feedback, consistent evidence from the literature, and, whenever pertinent, clinical experience (empirical evidence). The answers provided for each question constituted the provisional statements about the management of ICP that were submitted for review to all participants at the consensus conference (phase II). The Consensus Conference on ICP management was held in Campinas, Brazil, on May 20, 2017, during the 4th WSES World Congress. During the first part of the consensus conference, the group leaders presented the results of their group discussion with the answer to the key question assigned, the provisional statements along with the supporting literature, the level of evidence, and the grade of the recommendation. Each statement was then discussed and voted on by the audience. The percentage of agreement was recorded immediately; in cases of disagreement greater than 30%, the statement was modified after discussion. Furthermore, relevant comments about each statement were collected and used during the revision process. During the final portion of the consensus conference, a comprehensive algorithm for the management of ICP was developed based on the results of the literature review and the plenary discussion among the experts.

The revised statements, their level of evidence, and the recommendation grade are presented below. Please note that the WSES guidelines must be considered an adjunctive tool in the decision-making process regarding the management of ICP; they are not intended to substitute a provider's clinical judgment for an individual patient, and they may need to be modified based on the medical team's experience and the available local resources.

Table 2 Grading of recommendations (from Guyatt et al.)

Grade of recommendation	Description	Benefits vs. risks	Quality of supporting evidence	Implications
1A	Strong recommendation, high-quality evidence	Benefits clearly outweigh risks and burdens, or vice versa	RCTs without important limitations or overwhelming evidence from observational studies	Strong recommendation, applies to most patients in most circumstances without reservation
1B	Strong recommendation, moderate-quality evidence	Benefits clearly outweigh risk and burdens, or vice versa	RCTs with important limitations (inconsistent results, methodological flaws, indirect or imprecise) or exceptionally strong evidence from observational studies	Strong recommendation, applies to most patients in most circumstances without reservation
1C	Strong recommendation, low-quality or very low-quality evidence	Benefits clearly outweigh risk and burdens, or vice versa	Observational studies or case series	Strong recommendation based on limited evidence; recommendations may change when higher quality or more extensive evidence becomes available
2A	Weak recommendation, high-quality evidence	Benefits closely balanced with risks and burdens	RCTs without important limitations or overwhelming evidence from observational studies	Weak recommendation; best action may differ depending on circumstances, expertise of clinician, the patient in question, or other social issues
2B	Weak recommendation, moderate-quality evidence	Benefits closely balanced with risks and burdens	RCTs with important limitations (inconsistent results, methodological flaws, indirect or imprecise) or exceptionally strong evidence from observational studies	Weak recommendation; best action may differ depending on circumstances, expertise of clinician, the patient in question, or other social issues
2C	Weak recommendation, low-quality or very low quality evidence	Uncertainty in the estimates of benefits, risks, and burdens; benefits, risks, and burdens may be closely balanced	Observational studies or case series	Very weak recommendation; other alternatives may be equally reasonable

Results

Incidence of and risk factors for ICP

What are the general recommendations for minimizing the risk of ICP during screening and therapeutic colonoscopies?

There are a number of risk factors that have been related to ICP in the literature (Table 3). Older patients are more vulnerable to ICP, and the ages of 65, 75, and 80 years have been shown to be independent risk factors for ICPs [23, 26, 27]. Female gender [28, 29], low BMI [28, 30], low albumin level, the presence of comorbidities, diverticulosis, Crohn's disease, and admission to an ICU are also acknowledged to be risk factors in several studies [20, 23, 26, 28]. The endoscopist's level of experience may also be considered a risk indicator, as higher incidences of ICP have been reported for non-gastroenterologist endoscopists and low-volume endoscopy centers [31–33]. Finally, anesthesia during colonoscopy has been associated with an increased risk of ICP, in relation to the worsening of patient's comorbidities and the increasing technical complexity of these procedures [34, 35].

In a recent study of 56,882 colonoscopies, full-thickness large bowel perforation occurred in forty patients, corresponding to an incidence rate of 0.07% (0.05% in diagnostic/screening procedures and 0.17% in therapeutic colonoscopies) [18]. A greater risk of ICP was associated with low-volume practices, female gender (due to greater colonic length and a more mobile transverse colon), advanced age (reduced wall strength), history of diverticular disease, previous abdominal surgery (especially pelvic), and colonic obstruction (risk of over-insufflation).

Table 3 Principal risk factors for iatrogenic colonoscopy perforations (ICP)

Risk factors	References
Increasing age (> 65 years)	[18, 23, 26, 27, 36]
Female gender	[18, 28, 29, 36]
Low BMI	[28, 29]
Low albumin level	[20, 23, 26, 28]
Presence of comorbidities	[18, 36]
Crohn's disease and diverticulosis	[16, 18, 20, 23, 26, 28]
Admission in ICU	[20, 23, 26, 28]
Endoscopist's experience	[18, 29, 31–33]
Non-gastroenterologist endoscopists	[31, 33]
Low volume centers	[31, 33]
Previous abdominal surgery	[16, 36]
Colonic obstruction	[16, 18]
Bevacizumab therapy	[44, 46, 47]
Therapeutic vs. diagnostic procedure	[5, 10, 37–42, 44, 49]
Colonoscopy vs. sigmoidoscopy	[5, 29, 36]
General anesthesia	[34, 35]

In a Spanish study of 16,285 colonoscopies, ICPs were reported in 0.09% of cases [16]. Colonic obstruction, prior abdominal surgery, and sigmoid diverticular disease were indicated as potential risk factors.

A review from the Netherlands including 30,366 endoscopic procedures found that ICP occurred in 35 patients (0.12%) [5]. The authors described a 4-fold higher risk of ICP in colonoscopies compared with sigmoidoscopies and a 5-fold greater risk of ICP in therapeutic compared with diagnostic procedures.

A review of 10,486 colonoscopies performed in a single institution included 20 ICPs over a period of 10 years (corresponding to an incidence rate of 0.19%) [29]. During the same time interval, 46,501 flexible sigmoidoscopies were performed and only two ICPs occurred (0.004%). Female patients had significantly more ICPs compared with males and, although not statistically significant, the risk of ICP was numerically higher for endoscopists in training than experienced endoscopists [29].

In a review of studies published between 2001 and 2009 analyzing 969,913 colonoscopies [36], the incidence of ICP ranged from 0.032 to 0.14%. The risk factors for ICP included age over 75 years (4- to 6-fold increase), colonoscopy instead of sigmoidoscopy (2–4 times greater), female gender, diverticular disease, previous abdominal surgery, and multiple comorbidities, including diabetes mellitus, chronic pulmonary disease, congestive heart failure, myocardial infarction, cerebrovascular disease, peripheral vascular disease, renal insufficiency, liver disease, and dementia.

Therapeutic colonoscopies generally involved a higher risk for ICP, particularly the following procedures: polypectomy for large polyps, multiple polypectomies, pneumatic dilatation for Crohn's stricture [37], the use of argon plasma coagulation, and endoscopic mucosal resection (EMR) and endoscopic submucosal dissection (ESD) for colorectal neoplasia [38]. For endoscopic polypectomies, the related perforation risk has been related to the size of the polyp (larger than 10 mm in the right colon or 20 mm in the left colon) and a sessile morphology [38], and it is considered to be less than 1%, even when more challenging polypectomy techniques such as EMR are performed [39]. Complex procedures such as EMR and ESD are associated with a higher perforation incidence and should be considered to have a high risk of ICP. In 2014, a meta-analysis by Wang et al. comparing procedure-related complications in EMR and ESD for colorectal tumors (including 4 retrospective case-control studies) reported ESD-related perforations in 31/347 cases and EMR-related perforations in 33/566 cases [40]. The current literature demonstrates that the perforation risk for ESD is decreasing in higher volume centers to less than 5% [41, 42].

Perforation in colorectal stenting is the main early adverse event [43]. Use of a self-expandable metal stent

(SEMS) has been associated with an overall perforation rate of 7–8% [10, 44]. In cases of acute malignant colonic obstruction, retrospective studies have shown an SEMS-related perforation risk of 5–9% [45]. Stenting of either benign or neoplastic strictures has been associated with a 7.4% incidence of ICP in a recent meta-analysis [43]; the type of stent, benign etiology, bevacizumab therapy, and the need for re-dilation have been identified as risk factors for ICP [44, 46, 47].

Endoscopic balloon dilation may entail perforation rates up to 11%, even though the rate of iatrogenic perforation for Crohn's disease stricture treatment is less than 5% in the majority of retrospective studies [37, 45, 48]. Balloon dilation of rectal anastomotic strictures has been associated with a 1.1% rate of ICP [49].

The most common site of perforation is the sigmoid colon (53–65%), followed by the cecum, the ascending colon, the transverse colon, the descending colon, and the rectum [6, 13, 15, 29, 50] (Fig. 1). ICPs are generally intraperitoneal perforations; extra-peritoneal perforations may manifest as pneumoretroperitoneum, pneumomediastinum, or subcutaneous emphysema. Combined intra- and extra-peritoneal perforations have been reported anecdotally [51].

There is only one randomized study concerning the risk factors and preventive measures for ICP, whereas several reviews of large clinical series and meta-analyses to define the incidence and risk factors for ICP have been published [52, 53]. Recommendations for preventive measures derive from these studies and expert opinions [54].

Statement 1

1.1. *During diagnostic endoscopy training, a low threshold at which the senior endoscopist should assume manual control or abort the procedure should be established. Unusual difficulty in traversing the sigmoid colon, a difficult examination in a female or elderly patient, or the presence of diverticular disease or colonic obstruction should be considered alarming conditions (Recommendation Grade 1C).*

1.2. *During diagnostic or screening colonoscopies, endoscope progression should be gently performed and loop formation avoided. Alternative maneuvers (e.g., compression, decubitus changes) should be used in case of pain, but when difficulties in the progression are observed, it is recommended to abort the procedure (Recommendation Grade 1C).*

1.3. *Air should be insufflated judiciously to avoid barotrauma, especially if bowel obstruction is suspected. The use of CO_2 further minimizes bowel distension, abdominal discomfort, and the risk of perforation (Recommendation Grade 1B).*

1.4. *During en bloc endoscopic polypectomy, the maximum size of the tissue sample safely included in the SNARE should be 2 cm (especially if the lesion is proximal to the splenic flexure). Pre-polypectomy submucosal injection reduces the risk of electro-coagulative damage to the muscularis propria. Blended current mode limits the depth of tissue damage, and cold techniques are preferred for small polyps (≤5 mm) (Recommendation Grade 1C).*

1.5. *Endoscopic submucosal dissection (ESD) should be limited to selected cases because of the high rate of associated complications (Recommendation Grade 1C).*

1.6. *Stenting of a malignant disease should be discouraged in patients receiving bevacizumab. In the case of Crohn's disease, dilatation of a long stenotic area in the presence of active disease or a suspected fistula before or after stent placement is not advisable (Recommendation Grade 1C).*

1.7. *Whenever risky endoscopic procedures must be performed, the availability of and close collaboration with a hospital-based multidisciplinary team can improve patient outcomes (Recommendation Grade 1C).*

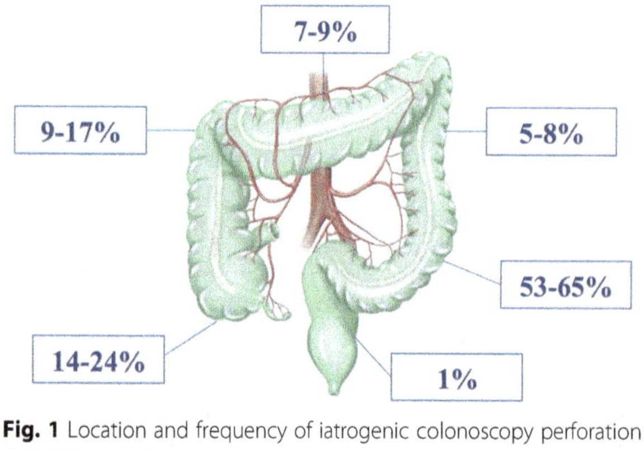

Fig. 1 Location and frequency of iatrogenic colonoscopy perforation

What is the maximum incidence of ICP considered acceptable for centers where diagnostic or therapeutic colonoscopies are performed?

Colonoscopy has been demonstrated to be the most cost-effective method for colorectal cancer screening. As the number of procedures performed worldwide is increasing, gastrointestinal professional societies have adopted strict safety standards for endoscopic practice, including the monitoring and auditing of complications to detect performance gaps and continuously improve the safety of colonoscopy [55]. The American Society for Gastrointestinal Endoscopy (ASGE)/American College of Gastroenterology (ACG) Task Force on Quality in Endoscopy recommends that post-colonoscopy perforation rates should be maintained at ≤ 1 per 500 colonoscopies (≤ 1/1000 in screening healthy subjects) [56]. For screening colonoscopies, the European Society of Gastrointestinal Endoscopy (ESGE) proposes that perforation should require surgery in ≤ 1/1000 [57]. In an audit of post-colonoscopy complications before starting national colorectal cancer screening, the British Society of Gastroenterology (BSG) reported post-colonoscopy perforation rates of 1/769 over a total of 9223 colonoscopies [58].

Statement 2

2.1. *The maximum acceptable incidence of ICP for diagnostic colonoscopies should not exceed 0.1% (Recommendation Grade 1A).*

2.2. *During therapeutic colonoscopy, the maximum acceptable incidence of ICP should be ≤ 1% for complex polypectomy (Recommendation 1A) and less than 7% for SEMS placement (Recommendation Grade 1C).*

Diagnosis of ICP

What is the minimum information the endoscopist must report after diagnosing an ICP during a colonoscopy procedure?

Perforation during diagnostic or screening endoscopic procedures may occur from one of these two main pathways: (a) direct mechanical damage to the colonic wall by the tip or the side of the endoscope as it is pushed forward or (b) a pneumatic distension due to barotrauma (Table 4). Direct mechanical trauma is the most frequent etiology of ICP, and perforations originating from mechanical trauma are commonly large and located in the sigmoid region. The injury is usually produced by direct trauma due to an inaccurate instrumental insertion, colonoscope movements toward the mucosal surface, retro-flexion maneuvers, or excessive torsion. Indirect injuries can also occur as the consequence of bowing or stretching the distal part of the colon. The presence of redundant colon diverticula or adhesions from previous surgeries can increase the risk of mechanical trauma during colonoscopy [16]. Barotrauma is instead produced by the excessive distension of the bowel due to over-insufflation, which produces linear lacerations at the colonic wall that may evolve into full-thickness defects. This type of perforation is more frequently located at the cecal region, where the thinner muscular layer and the larger lumen diameter make this region more vulnerable to pressure-related injuries [6, 16, 59, 60]. For interventional endoscopies, the mechanism of perforation can be the same as those occurring during diagnostic endoscopy, or they may be due to thermal/electrical injury of the colonic wall, manifesting as a wall ischemia. In this latter case, the perforation can occur with a delay of 24–72 h [18, 54]. Wall damage can be incomplete and the perforation concealed as it is confined by the surrounding tissues. During the following days or weeks, an abscess may develop that may delay the diagnosis.

Up to 60% of ICPs are detected by the endoscopist while performing the procedure [14, 16, 18, 60–62]. In a retrospective evaluation of a single institution, 68% of ICPs were identified on the day of endoscopy, 23% on day 1 or 2 after the endoscopy, and 9% were identified at least 2 weeks after the procedure [29]. The results of a survey of 30,336 colonoscopies showed a mean delay of 0.36 days for the diagnosis of ICP after diagnostic endoscopies and 1.5 days after therapeutic procedures [5].

Table 4 Main etiologies of iatrogenic colonoscopy perforation (ICP)

Type of injury
• Direct mechanical trauma
• Barotrauma
• Thermal/electrical injury
Endoscopic therapeutic procedures at risk for ICP
• Colorectal stenting
• Polypectomy
• Colonic dilation
• Argon plasma coagulation (APC)
• Endoscopic mucosal resection (EMR)
• Endoscopic submucosal dissection (ESD)

Statement 3

3.1. *If the ICP is detected during the procedure by the endoscopist, a detailed description should be provided including the following information:*

- *Colonoscopy indication (i.e., diagnostic or therapeutic)*
- *Associated colonic pathology (e.g., strictures, polyps, tumors)*
- *Administration of sedation, analgesia, or anesthesia for the colonoscopy*
- *Patient's general status and presence of comorbidities*
- *Gas type used for insufflation*
- *Quality of the colonic preparation*
- *Time of the ICP occurrence*
- *Most likely reason for ICP (e.g., thermal injury, mechanical injury)*
- *Injury localization and size*
- *Whether an endoscopic resolution was intended, attempted, or completed*
- *How the endoscopic repair was performed*
- *Presence of abdominal distention increasing the probability of abdominal compartment syndrome*

This recommendation was obtained by consensus after discussion with the panel experts (Recommendation Grade 2C).

Which are the minimum biochemical and imaging investigations that should be requested in the case of a suspected ICP?

A delay in the diagnosis of ICP is a critical issue for therapeutic outcomes; when the diagnosis is delayed more than 24 h, the chance increases that more invasive treatments (e.g., surgery) will be required [2, 63]. Physicians should therefore search for this potentially life-threatening complication and run clinical and biochemical tests if an ICP is suspected.

An ICP can be appreciated by direct visualization of the parietal defect or the view of intra-abdominal tissues through the colonic wall during the endoscopy [15]. Otherwise, the diagnosis of ICP is based on clinical, laboratory, and radiologic findings [64]. The clinical presentation of an ICP can vary widely, depending on the size of the perforation, the type of etiologic agent, the affected colonic location, the degree of intra-peritoneal contamination, and the patient's general status. In the majority of patients (91–92%), symptoms develop within the first 48 h following the completion of the endoscopy [14, 29]. The most common symptom is abdominal pain associated with distension, although painless cases of ICP or cases with severe cramp-like pain have been described [13, 16, 18]. In two large clinical series, the most consistent symptoms were abdominal pain (from 74 to 95%), guarding/rebound tenderness (82.5) with diffuse peritonitis, tachycardia (62.5%), leukocytosis (40%), fever (38%), rectal bleeding (15%), and isolated abdominal distension (6.6%) [16, 18]. Only a small number of patients with ICP (5%) remained asymptomatic [52, 59]. An unusual clinical sign (1/55 patients with ICPs) was a delayed subcutaneous emphysema and an ongoing necrotizing infection of the abdominal wall [16, 18]. It is a common belief that patients with diffuse peritonitis can be diagnosed and treated for perforation on a clinical basis, but peritonitis-like clinical scenarios can also occur in the absence of perforation. For instance, a transmural thermal injury after polypectomy with serosal irritation without any obvious perforation produces localized peritonitis that is amenable to non-operative management. Thus, biochemical and imaging studies are always indicated when an ICP is suspected.

Laboratory tests should be run for inflammatory markers that can reveal severe bacterial infections associated with the perforation [65], such as white blood cell count (WBC) and C-reactive protein (CRP) [66, 67]. In case of delayed presentation (> 12 h), the pro-calcitonin level (PCT) can be useful for ICP diagnosis.

Perforations of intra-peritoneal segments of the colon (e.g., the cecum, transverse colon, or sigmoid colon) more often lead to free intra-peritoneal fluid and air (large amounts in cases of barotrauma from insufflation), whereas perforations of the ascending and descending colon and rectum or wall injuries contained in the supplying mesentery result mainly in extra-peritoneal air. Mixed situations are possible if the perforation is in the middle between an intra- and extra-peritoneal portion [68]. Upright or decubitus abdominal radiographs can detect small amounts of free peritoneal air, but they are insensitive to the presence of fluid. Plain thoracic and abdominal radiographs have a positive predictive value (PPV) of 92% for ICPs [13]. Of note, the PPV has been shown to be higher for ICPs occurring during diagnostic procedures (PPV 100%) than for ICPs occurring during therapeutic procedures (PPV 45%) [2]. Alternatively, an ultrasound may be useful in cases in which the radiation burden should be limited, notably in children and pregnant women. However, this method should not be considered definitive in excluding a pneumoperitoneum [69].

If the clinical suspicion of ICP persists after a normal plain radiograph, a computed tomography (CT) scan with contrast enhancement should be requested, as this imaging tool can easily detect small amounts of both free intra-peritoneal air and fluids, in some cases with the foci of the gas congregating near the perforation site [68]. Air trapped in the mesenteric folds is found in perforation of the colon. A pneumoretroperitoneum is caused by extraperitoneal perforations such as perforations of the descending colon and rectum. Gas in the right anterior pararenal space indicates ascending colon perforation, whereas gas in the left pararenal space indicates descending or sigmoid colon perforations. Generally, rectal perforation causes bilateral pneumoretroperitoneum [70]. For extra-peritoneal perforations, the CT scan can show air tracking along the mesenteric and fascial planes, even in the mediastinum and abdominal, and chest and neck walls. Of note, the retro-peritoneal air dissecting the mediastinum and the retropharyngeal tissues can cause a change in the tone of the larynx, resulting in voice change [71].

Colonoscopy may also dissect within the wall of the colon with pneumatosis. Moreover, mucosal injury and intraluminal pressure may dissect air inside the mesenteric and portal venous system. For all these reasons, CT is much more effective in the diagnosis of extraluminal air compared to conventional radiography [15]. Double contrast CT (intravenous and rectal) is increasingly used in patients with clinical suspicion of ICP and without diffuse peritonitis. This diagnostic tool may be useful for detecting concealed or sealed perforations that are eligible for non-operative management [72]. Multi-detector CT (MDCT) is superior to single helical or conventional CT because it can provide rapid, high-volume coverage, and diagnostic images, even in patients who are unable to perform prolonged breath holds. One study showed that MDCT was 86% accurate in predicting the site of perforation [69].

The following recommendations were developed using a large clinical series and expert opinions, since randomized studies on this topic are lacking.

Statement 4

4.1. *After diagnostic or therapeutic colonoscopies, all patients who present with abdominal pain, and/or tenderness, and/or abdominal distension, and/or fever, and/or rectal bleeding should be investigated for ICP by laboratory tests and imaging exams (Recommendation Grade 1B).*

4.2. *The minimum biochemical markers that should be requested in the case of suspected ICP are white blood cell count and C-reactive protein (Recommendation Grade 1C).*

4.3. *ICP should be confirmed with the demonstration of free intra-peritoneal or extra-peritoneal air (Recommendation 1B). CT scan is more sensitive than standard abdominal radiographs to detect free air (Recommendation Grade 1C).*

4.4. *In the case of localized peritoneal signs, double contrast enhanced CT scan can be a useful adjunctive tool to confirm the feasibility of non-operative management of ICP (Recommendation Grade 1C).*

Conservative and endoscopic treatments for ICP

Which are the indications for conservative treatment or an immediate surgical intervention after an ICP diagnosis?

Once the diagnosis of perforation is confirmed by clinical and radiological examinations, the decision between surgical and non-operative treatments will depend on the type of injury, the quality of the bowel preparation, the underlying colonic pathology, and the clinical stability of the patient [6]. However, a surgical consultation should be obtained in all cases of perforation [73].

Whenever the risk of a large perforation is present and the patient presents with signs and symptoms of peritonitis, the emergency surgery approach is reasonable and safe [6]. Surgical management is also recommended in patients with concomitant colonic diseases requiring surgery, transplanted patients, and immunosuppressed patients [36, 74]. In selected patients with localized pain, free air without diffuse free fluids in radiographs, hemodynamic stability, and an absence of fever, non-operative management (conservative) may be appropriate [61, 68, 75–78] and is associated with low morbidity, low mortality, and short hospital stays. Conservative management is usually suitable for small, sealed-off perforations that occurred during a therapeutic colonoscopy in patients with an optimal bowel preparation [8, 23, 24].

Conservative treatment consists of serial clinical and imaging monitoring (every 3–6 h) with absolute bowel rest, intravenous fluids for hydration, intravenous administration of broad-spectrum antibiotics, and a close multidisciplinary team follow-up to promptly detect the development of sepsis and peritoneal signs [6, 78, 79]. Drainage of the peritoneal air through a Veress needle punction may be useful in relieving abdominal pain, improving respiratory function, and facilitating the closure of the perforation site [80]. The overall success rate of conservative treatments for colonic perforation varies from 33 to 90% [36].

An early success with non-surgical treatment does not rule out the potential need for surgery [52]. If the conservative treatment is successful, clinical improvement will gradually occur within 24 h, but a continuous and strict clinical and biochemical follow-up is recommended. In cases of clinical deterioration or progression to a septic condition or peritonitis, surgical treatment should not be delayed. The sole presence of subdiaphragmatic free air does not constitute an indication for urgent surgery. Of note, complication rates and lengths of hospital stay are significantly higher in patients who have undergone surgery after conservative management than in patients who were initially treated with surgery [81]. Indeed, when surgical treatment is delayed, the peritonitis and colonic wall inflammation could worsen, requiring a more invasive surgery that is associated with a poorer prognosis [13, 82]. Ideally, the decision to pursue surgery should be made as early as possible after the endoscopy [2].

Endoscopic treatment is possible when the perforation site is recognized intra-procedurally or within 4 h following the procedure and the bowel preparation is still adequate [45]. Urgent endoscopic therapy with clip placement and the use of CO_2 may limit the volume of extraluminal insufflation and subsequently the need for surgery [83–85]. Endoscopic clip closure of ICP was first reported in the literature in 1997 [86]. Today, it should be considered a valuable non-invasive method for ICP that is recognized during a colonoscopy. It has been shown to be effective in sealing and healing the perforation and avoiding surgery in most cases [2]. The decision to perform the endoscopic closure of colonic perforation depends on the size and the cause of the iatrogenic damage as well as the endoscopist's experience and the availability of appropriate endoscopic devices [45]. Clipping closure of ICP is recommended for small perforations (less than 1 cm) originating from either diagnostic or therapeutic colonoscopies [2, 24, 87], with a success rate of 59–100% [2, 4, 88, 89]. In larger or difficult perforations, a combination of endoclips and endoloops might be used. There are also few reports in the literature about closure with conventional clips for perforations larger than 1 cm [90–92]. A limitation of the endoscopic closure is the difficulty of evaluating the completeness of the colonic closure after the clip application. This might result in delayed complications such as intra-abdominal abscesses, which can occur due to the persistence of intestinal fluids in the peritoneal cavity or an intermittent leakage [2].

Over the last several years, new devices have been introduced to widen the spectrum of possibilities of performing an endoscopic closure of a gastrointestinal perforation. Through-the-scope (TTS) clips and over-the-scope clips (OTSC) are both effective for the early closure of defects smaller than 2 cm, with overall technical and clinical success rates of 93 and 89%, respectively [88, 93–95]. TTS clips are more suitable for closure of small therapeutic perforations (less than 1 cm), whereas OTSC may be used for larger defects. The OTSC is a nitinol clip shaped to mimic a trap that allows for the inclusion of more tissue and consequently closure of larger perforations than the conventional clips [96]. Recent studies focusing on the outcomes after OTSC placement revealed a rate of procedural success of 80–100% and clinical success rates of 57–100% [96–98].

The overstitch endoscopic suturing device (Apollo Endosurgery, Austin, TX, USA) was recently developed and might play a role in the future ICP closures [99]. Partially or totally covered stenting could potentially allow closing the perforation, but data supporting its clinical application are still lacking. A clear indication for surgery in the setting of endoscopic treatment of an ICP consists of a complicated procedure or a failed endoscopic closure with an ongoing leak that is causing fecal peritonitis [45].

Statement 5

5.1. *Non-operative (conservative) management of ICPs may be appropriate in selected patients, including patients who are hemodynamically stable, without sepsis, experiencing localized pain, and with no free fluid in radiographs (Recommendation Grade 1C).*

5.2. *Endoscopic treatment can be considered as an initial approach if it is feasible within 4 h following the procedure depending on the size and cause of the iatrogenic injury and the operator's level of experience (Recommendation Grade 2C).*

5.3. *Emergency surgery is recommended when the patient develops signs and symptoms of peritonitis, in cases of clinical deterioration, suspected large perforation, failure of conservative management, poor bowel preparation, or in the presence of an underlying colonic disease requiring surgery (Recommendation Grade 1A).*

What is the minimum duration of the hospital observation period for patients who have undergone successful endoscopic closure or conservative management of ICP?

After a successful endoscopic closure, it is advisable that a multidisciplinary team, including abdominal surgeons, endoscopists, gastroenterologists, and anesthesiologists, are involved in the patient's follow-up [52]. Fasting, broad-spectrum antibiotic therapy and intravenous hydration are the basis of treatment [3, 88, 100]. Close observation for signs of peritoneal irritation and monitoring of biochemical inflammatory parameters are crucial. When pain disappears and the inflammatory parameters and bowel function return to normal, oral intake can be resumed [100]. The duration of observation is subjective but obviously related to the patient's status and the response to the conservative (non-operative) or endoscopic treatment. The mean duration of hospital stay after non-surgical ICP management ranges from 9 to 13 days [88].

Statement 6

6.1. *After conservative or endoscopic treatment of ICP, monitoring and follow-up should be assured by a multidisciplinary team, including surgeons. There is no optimal duration of the observation period, but it depends on the patient's clinical status and response to treatment (Recommendation Grade 1C)*

Which investigations (clinical, biochemical, and imaging) should be performed during the observation period in patients who have undergone successful endoscopic closure or conservative management of ICP?

There are no studies in the literature focusing specifically on the clinical and biochemical follow-up of patients who have undergone endoscopic closure or conservative management of ICP.

The available evidence is mainly supported by retrospective series. During the observation period, the patient treated for ICP should be monitored clinically as well as through laboratory values and imaging. Clinically, peritoneal signs such as tenderness, rebound tenderness, and muscle guarding, as well as signs of infection, such as fever, nausea, vomiting, abdominal distension, and diarrhea, should be recorded [36, 69]. Frequent assessment of the physical status and vital signs should be completed by laboratory tests for WBC, CRP, Hb, blood urea nitrogen, PCT, and electrolytes [66]. As an imaging technique, the CT scan remains the most accurate tool to be performed in case of clinical deterioration, especially when the need for surgery is in question and before discharge for non-operative treatments.

Statement 7

7.1. *During the observation period, the patient treated for ICP should be monitored clinically, by laboratory tests (including WBC, PCT, CRP) and imaging (CT scan) (Recommendation Grade 2C).*

What is the recommended type and duration of antibiotic therapy in patients who have undergone successful endoscopic closure or conservative management of ICP?

In patients who have undergone endoscopic repair of ICP, infection control is usually attained with a short-term course of antibiotic therapy (3–5 days). Antibiotics should be stopped if there are no signs of systemic inflammation and/or peritonitis after the short-term treatment. Considering the composition of the intestinal microbiota in the large bowel, patients with ICP require antimicrobial coverage for Gram-negative bacteria as well as for anaerobes. The potential infecting organisms in colorectal procedures are derived from the bowel lumen, where *Bacteroides fragilis* and other obligate anaerobes as well as *Enterobacteriaceae* such as *Escherichia coli* are the most common bacteria [101]. If there is any sign of an ongoing infectious process, antibiotics should be continued. An abdominal CT is recommended after 5–7 days to exclude residual signs of peritonitis or abscess formation and to exclude the possible need for a surgical intervention.

The duration of antimicrobial therapy in patients with complicated intra-abdominal infections has been debated. Antibiotic therapy should be shortened in those patients demonstrating a positive response to treatment. A prospective trial published recently by Sawyer et al. demonstrated that, in patients with complicated intra-abdominal infections undergoing an adequate source-control procedure, the outcomes after approximately 4 days of fixed-duration antibiotic therapy were similar to those after a longer course of antibiotics that extended until after the resolution of physiological abnormalities [102].

Statement 8

8.1. *In patients who have undergone conservative management of ICP, even if there is no sign of diffuse peritonitis, antibiotic therapy covering Gram-negative bacteria and anaerobes is recommended (Recommendation Grade 1C).*

8.2. *In patients with perforation repaired by endoscopic closure, a short-term course of antibiotic therapy (3–5 days) covering Gram-negative bacteria and anaerobes is recommended. Antibiotics should be stopped if there are no signs of systemic inflammation and/or peritonitis after the short-term treatment. Abdominal CT is suggested to help rule out peritonitis or early abscess formation (Recommendation Grade 1C).*

8.3. *In patients who have undergone a surgical procedure with an adequate source-control procedure, postoperative therapy should be shortened as much as possible after the resolution of physiological abnormalities (Recommendation Grade 1C).*

Which is the recommended type and duration of antithrombotic prophylaxis in patients who have undergone successful endoscopic closure or conservative management of ICP?

Sepsis is associated with activation of blood coagulation (hypercoagulability) contributing to venous thromboembolism (VTE) [103–105]. Patients with abdominal sepsis may be at increased risk of VTE due to their premorbid conditions, surgical intervention, admitting diagnosis of sepsis, and events and exposures such as central venous catheterization, invasive tests and procedures, and drugs that potentiate immobility. A prospective cohort study using the National Surgical Quality Improvement Program database of the American College of Surgeons (ACS-NSQIP) was designed to evaluate the impact of preoperative sepsis on the risk of postoperative arterial and venous thrombosis. The study included 2,305,380 adults who underwent a range of surgical procedures [106]. The systemic inflammatory response syndrome was defined by the presence of two or more of the following: temperature > 38 or < 36 °C; heart rate > 90 beats/min; respiratory rate > 20 breaths/min or a $PaCO_2$ < 32 mmHg (< 4.3 kPa); white blood cell count > 12,000 cells/mm^3, < 4000 cells/mm^3, or > 10% immature band forms; or anion gap acidosis (> 12 mEq/L). Among all surgical procedures, patients with preoperative systemic inflammatory response syndrome or any sepsis had three times the odds of having an arterial or venous postoperative thrombosis. The risk of thrombosis increased with the severity of the inflammatory response and was higher in both emergent and elective surgical procedures. Thus, patients with ICP should be considered at risk, and thromboprophylaxis should be recommended.

Statement 9

9.1. *In patients with ICP undergoing a surgical procedure, thromboprophylaxis is generally recommended during hospitalization and thereafter according to the underlying disease and comorbidities (Recommendation Grade 1B).*

How long is it recommended that patients fast following successful endoscopic closure or conservative treatments for ICP?

There are no prospective clinical trials assessing the necessary duration of fasting following non-operative management or endoscopic repair of ICP. In the setting of conservative treatment, the general recommendations called for "bowel rest," but the duration is unclear. Retrospective studies reported fasting durations of between 2 and 6 days. In one of the largest series, 24 patients with ICP were managed with conservative treatment, which failed in 3 patients; 31 patients were initially clipped, of which 22 procedures were successful. Poor outcomes were related to patient age, ASA status, and failure of conservative treatment. The only significant predictor of failure of the conservative treatment was the perforation size. Fasting duration did not appear to impact the outcomes [81].

Park et al. [69] reported a single-center series on ICP including 15 patients managed with either conservative treatment ($n = 4$) or endoscopic repair ($n = 11$) and compared these patients with 35 patients managed surgically. The duration of fasting was significantly shorter in the non-surgery group than in the surgery group (3.8 vs. 5.6 days). The mean fasting time was also 1 day shorter for patients treated by endoscopic repair versus surgery in the study by Kim et al. [4]. Moreover, the fasting duration was not related to ICP treatment failure.

It has been suggested that a clear liquid diet can begin immediately after the endoscopic repair of ICP; the evidence is not strong, but there are no data to indicate that this practice is not feasible or unsafe [36]. Following open or laparoscopic repair of ICP, there is no restriction on oral intake, as supported by numerous studies that provided enteral nutrition in the early period after colorectal surgery [107].

Statement 10

10.1 *A liquid diet may begin within 1 to 2 days after the initiation of conservative management of ICP, according to the patient's clinical status (Recommendation Grade 1C)*

10.2 *A liquid diet may begin immediately after endoscopic repair of ICP, according to the patient's clinical status (Recommendation Grade 1C)*

Surgical treatment of ICP

Is explorative laparoscopy indicated in all patients with ICP?

Surgery is indicated as the first treatment in patients with ongoing sepsis, signs of diffuse peritonitis, large perforations, and failure of conservative management and in the presence of certain concomitant pathologies, such as unresected polyps with high suspicion of being a carcinoma [6, 60, 78].

The peri-operative morbidity and mortality related to surgery for ICP are considerable, with rates of 21–44% and 7–25%, respectively [5, 13–18]. Particularly frail patients, such as older patients and patients with low preoperative blood pressure, can have higher risks of mortality associated with colorectal perforation [108]. Thus, appropriate patient selection and surgical procedures are crucial in limiting the morbidity and mortality related to surgery for ICP.

In general, intraoperative findings determine the best technique to apply according to the different scenarios. Surgical procedures for the management of ICP include colorraphy, wedge resection, colostomy by exteriorization of the perforation, and colonic resection with or without primary anastomosis or stoma. The decision regarding the type of surgical procedure depends on (a) the size, location, and etiology of the ICP; (b) the viability of the surrounding colon and mesocolon; (c) the degree of and time from the development of peritonitis; (d) the patient's general status and the presence of comorbidities; (e) the quality of the colonic preparation; and (f) the presence of residual lesions not resected during the colonoscopy procedure [2, 8, 24, 60, 82, 109, 110].

The decision of which procedure to perform, therefore, depends on many variables, and it must be made after a careful inspection of the whole colon and peritoneal cavity. Explorative laparoscopy should be considered a minimally invasive technique useful for performing both diagnostic and potentially therapeutic procedures. A timely application of explorative laparoscopy may prevent ongoing inflammation and injury that would necessitate more invasive measures, such as open laparotomy and/or colonic diversion [82]. The use of laparoscopy allows for visualizing the parietal defect and its size and specific location, as well as for identifying the potential cause of the perforation (e.g., perforation caused by the shaft of the endoscope, cautery, presence of mesenteric hematomas, emphysema, or effusions), which, as previously stated, are the main factors influencing the choice of treatment option. Early diagnosis is mandatory, and when timely management is ensured, laparoscopy can be the best option, offering reduced morbidity and length of stay and faster postoperative recovery. If no underlying lesion requiring surgical resection is seen during the endoscopy, the size of the tear is small, and the colon is healthy and well perfused, then a laparoscopic primary repair can be safely performed [52, 111].

Moreover, laparoscopic exploration allows the presence of potential signs of peritonitis to be evaluated and eventually allows aspiration, culture, and irrigation of the peritoneal cavity to be performed. Indeed, peritoneal washout and drainage have gained acceptance in the treatment of more advanced cases of colonic infection, such as Hinchey grade 2–3 diverticulitis [112]. Accordingly, the treatment of less advanced inflammatory processes, such as ICP, seems reasonable and indicated.

To summarize, explorative laparoscopy is indicated:

- For both diagnostic and therapeutic purposes [5, 9, 13, 17, 52, 100, 109, 113–119], and depending on the surgeon's skills, the potential exists for definitive surgical procedures, including suturing the defect, wedge resection, and segmental resection with or without anastomosis and/or stomia
- In questionable situations to rule out the need for further treatments, including laparotomy [82, 118, 120]
- In the case of failure of endoscopic treatment or an inability to perform endoscopic clip application after visualization of the ICP intra-procedurally

- In the case of development of peritonitis after a defined period of observation following perforation

Explorative laparoscopy has a significantly lower morbidity and mortality compared with explorative laparotomy in the emergency setting [121]: specifically, the reported postoperative complication rate is 18.2% for laparoscopy vs. 53.5% for laparotomy. The postoperative mortality rate is 1.11% for laparoscopy vs. 4.22% for laparotomy; and the need for further procedures is significantly lower for laparoscopy (1.11%) than for laparotomy (8.45%).

Explorative laparoscopy may not be indicated when there is:

- A potential risk for anesthesia-related complications, particularly in elderly or frail patients [122, 123], or any contraindications to surgery in general (e.g., hemodynamic instability, coagulopathy, or associated co-morbidities) [9, 122, 123]
- Recent laparotomy or previous abdominal surgery (more than 4 laparotomies) with extensive adhesions and a high risk of iatrogenic injury (relative contraindication)
- The presence of massive bowel dilatation (relative contraindication)
- Aorto-iliac aneurysmal disease (relative contraindication)

The potential diagnostic/therapeutic value of explorative laparoscopy should also be compared with the role of a CT scan in the evaluation of ICP. There is no study in the literature focusing on whether explorative laparoscopy should be performed instead of CT scans in patients with highly suspected ICP. However, when comparing these two modalities for penetrating abdominal trauma, CT scans have a sensitivity/specificity rate of 95%/95%, whereas explorative laparoscopy can achieve a 67–100% sensitivity and 50–100% specificity [121]. Thus, a CT scan should be performed in all cases before contemplating explorative laparoscopy, with the only obvious impediment being hemodynamic instability.

Statement 11

11.1 *Explorative laparoscopy is safe and can be considered as the preferred first-line surgical approach for the management of ICP (Recommendation Grade 1C).*

11.2 *Explorative laparoscopy should be performed according to the surgeon's experience and skills, as well as the availability of adequate technology and surgical devices (Recommendation Grade 1C).*

Which are the indications for conversion from laparoscopy to open surgery in patients with surgical ICP?

Thanks to the improvements in minimally invasive surgery, the laparoscopic approach has been increasingly used in recent years, and it should currently be considered a safe and feasible technique for the management of ICP [9, 24, 82, 113, 124–126]. Current literature comparing outcomes of laparoscopy versus laparotomy for the treatment of ICP is scarce and consists mainly of small retrospective studies. The first relevant study was published in 2008 [110] and compared the perioperative outcomes between laparoscopic and open procedures for ICP by including only primary colonic closures without diversion. The authors found fewer complications and a shorter length of hospital stay for the patients in the laparoscopic group [110]. Other studies by Rothold et al. [125] and Schloricke et al. [127] also observed fewer postoperative complications and significantly shorter hospital stays when utilizing the laparoscopic approach. Similar studies with similar results were published by Coimbra et al. [124] and Kim et al. [128], although in these studies, delayed surgeries (> 24 h) and ostomy formation rates were more frequently observed in the open groups, with higher primary repair rates in the laparoscopic groups.

Due to its favorable short-term outcomes, laparoscopy should be considered the preferred approach for both exploration and repair of ICPs that are not manageable with medical treatments. However, the surgeon's experience and skills are the key factors limiting the applicability and feasibility of laparoscopic ICP management. Conversion from laparoscopy to laparotomy should be considered whenever necessary. The most frequent reasons for conversion are the inability of the surgeon to complete the procedure laparoscopically, the large size of the ICP defect, the extensive peritoneal contamination, the highly inflammatory or neoplastic conditions of the colon, and the patient's hemodynamic instability.

Statement 12

12.1 *Conversion from laparoscopy to laparotomy should be considered whenever necessary with regard to the ability of the operator to proceed laparoscopically, the tissue viability, and the patient's status (Recommendation Grade 1C).*

What are the key factors upon which to choose the best surgical approach for ICP?

The choice of the surgical approach and technique mainly depends on the underlying pathology (e.g., colon cancer, diverticulitis) and the size of the ICP. Primary surgical repair can be used if the colonic tissue appears healthy and well vascularized and if suturing the perforation edges could be performed without tension [24, 113]. Wedge resection is feasible if it does not imply an excessive narrowing of the colonic lumen (e.g., cecum) [108]. Whenever the perforation is too large, the edges appear devitalized, or an avulsion of the adjacent mesocolon is seen, colonic resection might constitute the best option. Generally, patients who undergo surgery within 24 h are more appropriate candidates for less invasive techniques, such as primary suturing of the defect or linear wedge resection. In cases of delayed surgery (> 24 h from the colonoscopy), extensive peritoneal contamination, important comorbidities, or a deterioration of the general status of the patient (i.e., sepsis), a staged repair or colostomy by exteriorization of the perforation (e.g., double-barreled colostomy) must be considered [36, 52].

Currently, there are no prospective or retrospective studies in the English literature comparing the different types of repair (primary suture or wedge resection vs. segmental resection). Therefore, the choice of the surgical technique appears to be mainly empirical, and it is left to the surgeon's discretion according to the intraoperative findings. Independent of the surgical approach, the main goal of the therapy is the rapid diagnosis, repair, and prevention of abdominal sepsis. If an ICP is to be repaired laparoscopically, the operating surgeon and the surgical team should be comfortable with the laparoscopic techniques, such as mobilization of the colon and intracorporeal suturing. A clinical algorithm mainly based on the size of the perforation and the necrotic area was proposed in 1999 to assist in choosing which type of repair to perform [8]. The maximal size for sutured repair was set at 1 cm. Between 1 and 2.5 cm, a transverse tangential stapled resection was recommended, whereas above 2.5 cm, a segmental resection was indicated [8, 129]. The condition of the bowel to be repaired and the level of contamination and inflammation are the most important factors in determining whether the laparoscopic approach is safe [109]. Both sutured and stapled repair techniques seem to be safe and feasible to repair defects of up to 4 cm [82].

In case of perforated colon cancer, surgery must follow the oncologic principles of cancer resection.

Statement 13

13.1.*The best surgical technique for the management of ICP should be decided after a careful inspection of the abdominal cavity and considering the underlying colonic pathology (Recommendation Grade 2C).*

13.2*Primary repair can be used if the colonic tissues appear healthy and well vascularized, and an approximation of perforation edges could be done without tension (Recommendation Grade 2C).*

13.3.*Wedge resection would be feasible if it does not imply an excessive narrowing of the colonic lumen (e.g., perforation of the cecum or sigmoid colon) (Recommendation Grade 2C).*

13.4.*Colonic resection may be indicated if the perforation is too large, the edges appear devitalized, or an avulsion of the adjacent mesocolon is seen (Recommendation Grade 2C).*

13.5*Staged repair or colostomy may be necessary in cases of delayed surgery (> 24 h from the colonoscopy), extensive peritoneal contamination, important comorbidities or a deterioration of the patient's general status (i.e., hemodynamically unstable or sepsis) (Recommendation Grade 2C).*

What are the indications for performing a diverting or terminal stoma in patients with ICP?

The formation of a stoma is often included in the overall surgical strategy for the management of ICP. However, no randomized controlled trials or other high-level evidence trials exist to guide this operative decision in this specific indication. Case series of ICP report variable rates of stoma formation (up to 59.7%) [59, 114, 116, 126, 130]. As such, the formation of a stoma forms an adjunct to the overall treatment strategy for these patients.

The precise clinical or operative reasons for stoma formation are incompletely reported in the case series on ICP. Furthermore, these reports are generally limited by their largely retrospective study designs and low event numbers, complicating subgroup analyses. Notwithstanding these limitations, some authors have established increased stoma formation rates in patients with delayed diagnoses, significant peritonitis, and patients with left-sided perforations [114, 126]. Apart from these observations, the limited publications in this area infer that surgical judgment remains essential in the decision-making surrounding the formation of a stoma. Finally, no data exist to specifically address the type of stoma formation in ICP.

Statement 14

14.1*Stoma formation is an accepted and practiced adjunct in the surgical management of ICP (Recommendation Grade 1C).*

14.2*Surgical judgment is crucial in the decision regarding stoma need: patient, disease, and situational/environmental factors need to be considered in the individual clinical circumstance (Recommendation Grade 1C).*

What are the indications for drainage in patients with ICP?

The placement of an intra-abdominal drainage after surgical management of an ICP can be justified by either the presence of peritoneal contamination or the early diagnosis of a potential bleeding or leakage of the repair used for the perforation (i.e., colorraphy, wedge resection, colonic resection) [131–133]. There are no studies available in the literature focusing on the indications of abdominal drainage after successful surgical treatment of ICP. The decision is left to the discretion of the surgeon according to the ICP setting, the intraoperative findings, the type of surgical procedure performed, the adequateness of infection source control, and the patient's general status [5, 14, 108].

Statement 15

15.1 *In the case of early surgery (< 24 h from colonoscopy) in a patient with good bowel preparation, minimal peritoneal contamination, and adequate infection source control, intra-abdominal drainage placement should be avoided (Recommendation Grade 2C).*

15.2 *In the case of delayed surgery (> 24 h from colonoscopy) in a patient with poor bowel preparation or extensive peritoneal contamination, drainage placement may be recommended (Recommendation Grade 2C).*

What are the indications for the use of damage control surgery in patients with ICP?

At present, no study concerning ICP and damage control surgery (DCS) is available in the literature. However, once colonic perforation has occurred, the course of sepsis will develop independent of the underlying disease. Thus, to evaluate the use of DCS in cases of ICP, we could analyze the experience in similar settings, such as in perforated diverticulitis (PD), equating ICP to PD [134, 135].

Damage control is a surgical technique originally used in trauma surgery consisting of three stages: (1) an abbreviated initial laparotomy with the aim of controlling hemorrhage and contamination with temporary abdominal closure (TAC); (2) resuscitation until normal physiology is improved; and (3) return to the operating room after 24–72 h for definitive injury repair and abdominal wall closure [136–138].

Untreated or misdiagnosed ICP can progress to peritonitis and sepsis, resulting in serious morbidity and a very poor prognosis. Notably, morbidity rates as high as 43% and mortality rates as high as 25% have been reported [17, 20, 36, 50, 60, 139]. Nearly one quarter of patients will receive a delayed diagnosis, with a 45% incidence of fecal peritonitis [140]. The resultant inflammatory process associated with peritonitis clearly limits the operative options, precluding a single-stage procedure and resulting in fecal diversion in 38% of patients with fecal peritonitis. Several studies reported that age > 67 years, ASA score, blunt injuries, poor bowel preparation, and steroids are risk factors for increased postoperative morbidity (Table 5) [20, 123, 141, 142].

Over the last decade, DCS has become a valuable technique in unstable patients with fecal peritonitis [36, 136, 143]. The potential progression of ICP in fecal peritonitis is as probable as it is in perforated diverticulitis. In accordance with the WSES guidelines for the management of acute left-sided colonic diverticulitis, DCS may be suggested for clinically unstable patients (severe sepsis/septic shock) [135]. Critically ill patients with severe sepsis, hemodynamically unstable patients with hypotension, and patients with myocardial depression combined with coagulopathy are not candidates for endoscopic treatment or immediate complex operative interventions. In such patients, DCS allows rapid source control, enhances physiologic optimization, improves primary anastomosis rates, and decreases the need for stoma formation [144]. Therefore, in patients with abdominal sepsis, the application of DCS is individualized but not routinely used, as suggested by current clinical guidelines [145], stressing the importance of a careful assessment by the surgeons. Clearly, an individual approach tailored to each patient's clinical status might be the most appropriate. In cases of ICP, DCS should be performed in combination with the resection of the perforated colonic segment to bridge the patient to the definitive injury and colonic continuity repair. DCS can represent a very resource-heavy procedure for institutions, however, because of the requirements for access to facilities (operating rooms and intensive care units) and committed staff.

Statement 16

16.1 *DCS following ICP may be indicated in hemodynamically unstable patients, patients receiving a delayed diagnosed of ICP, and patients*

Table 5 Risk factors to evaluate when considering damage control strategy for iatrogenic colonoscopy perforations (ICP)

Risk factors	Description	References
Age	> 67	[140]
Delayed diagnosis	> 24 h	[140, 142]
Hemodynamic instability	Need for vasopressors before or during surgery	[123, 143]
"Blunt" ICP	Perforation caused by excessive dilatation or during diagnostic procedures	[142]
Medication use	Chronic steroid therapy	[13, 140]
Severe sepsis	Peritonitis with organ failure	[135, 141]
High surgical risk	ASA III and IV	[142]

presenting with significant comorbidities (Recommendation Grade 2C).

16.2 *DCS can be a valid option in cases of staged procedures, particularly when oncologic resections are required (Recommendation Grade 2C).*

Follow-up of ICP

Is there any recommendation to perform a surveillance endoscopy after successful ICP treatment? If any, what is the recommended timing for it?

At present, there are no studies in the literature focusing on the indications and timing for surveillance endoscopy after successful ICP treatment. However, based on the available evidence and clinical experience, a surveillance colonoscopy may be performed based on the initial indication (e.g., benign or malignant pathology) and type (e.g., screening or interventional) of the primary colonoscopy (during which the ICP occurred) and considering the risk-benefit ratio of performing an endoscopic exam [146, 147].

Colonoscopy is specifically contraindicated in cases of known or suspected perforation [148]. Consequently, any endoscopy after ICP treatment should be performed once the colonic wall has completely healed. Assuming that the healing time after ICP treatment is comparable to that after surgical sutures or anastomosis, a surveillance endoscopy may be indicated after approximately 3 months from the successful ICP treatment, depending on the size of the perforation and the type of repair [149].

In general, prior to any surveillance colonoscopy, it is necessary to carefully re-evaluate the presence of specific conditions favoring perforation, including increasing age, female gender, low BMI, intensive care unit stay, inpatient setting, diverticular disease [150], Crohn's disease [30], obstruction as an indication for the primary colonoscopy, and invasive interventional colonoscopy [26]. Indeed, colonoscopy is contraindicated whenever the risks for the patient's health or life are judged to outweigh the most favorable benefits of the procedure [148].

Statement 17

17.1 *In cases of perforation occurring during a diagnostic colonoscopy for screening or surveillance of colorectal cancer, a repeat endoscopy is indicated within 3 to 6 months postoperatively if the screening or clearing colonoscopy was incomplete due to malignant obstruction or inadequate preparation (Recommendation Grade 1C).*

17.2 *In cases of perforation occurring during a colonoscopy for gastrointestinal bleeding, a surveillance endoscopy is indicated for diagnostic and therapeutic purposes; in cases of acute lower gastrointestinal bleeding, it is necessary to ascertain the resolution of the perforation (Recommendation Grade 1C).*

17.3 *In cases of perforation occurring during an operative colonoscopy (e.g., polypectomy, endoscopic mucosal resection, or endoscopic submucosal dissection), a surveillance colonoscopy should be performed according to the current guidelines to determine whether the resection during the primary endoscopy was complete. The surveillance endoscopy can be performed within 3 to 6 months from the operative colonoscopy during which the ICP occurred in cases of incomplete resection (Recommendation Grade 1C).*

Conclusions

Iatrogenic perforation is a potentially severe complication of colonoscopy that requires a prompt and specific treatment to avoid further morbidity and mortality. In general, a multidisciplinary management, involving gastroenterologists, endoscopists, surgeons, and anesthesiologists, is recommended. The treatment strategy must be chosen based on the clinical setting and the patient's characteristics, but it should also be adapted to the medical team's experience and local resources. The comprehensive algorithm presented in Fig. 2 summarizes the management strategies in cases of ICP.

The risk of ICP should be carefully evaluated before a procedure; whenever a risky endoscopy must be performed, the availability of a hospital-based multidisciplinary team can improve patient outcomes. Continuous monitoring and auditing of endoscopic standards and related complications is recommended in each endoscopic center to detect possible performance gaps and improve the safety of colonoscopy. Close collaboration between endoscopists and surgeons is advisable; whenever an ICP occurs, the endoscopist is expected to provide a detailed description of the perforation, procedure, and patient to determine the best treatment option.

Endoscopic repair should be attempted whenever the perforation is detected during the procedure, though outcomes depend on the size and cause of the iatrogenic injury, as well as on the operator's level of experience.

When the ICP is not immediately detected, it should be suspected and investigated in all patients who present with abdominal pain, tenderness, abdominal distension, fever, and/or rectal bleeding after a diagnostic or therapeutic colonoscopy. CT scan is the most accurate imaging tool to diagnose ICP. Non-operative (conservative) management may be appropriate in selected patients who remain hemodynamically stable in the absence of signs of sepsis. Conservative management consists of complete bowel rest, short-course broad-

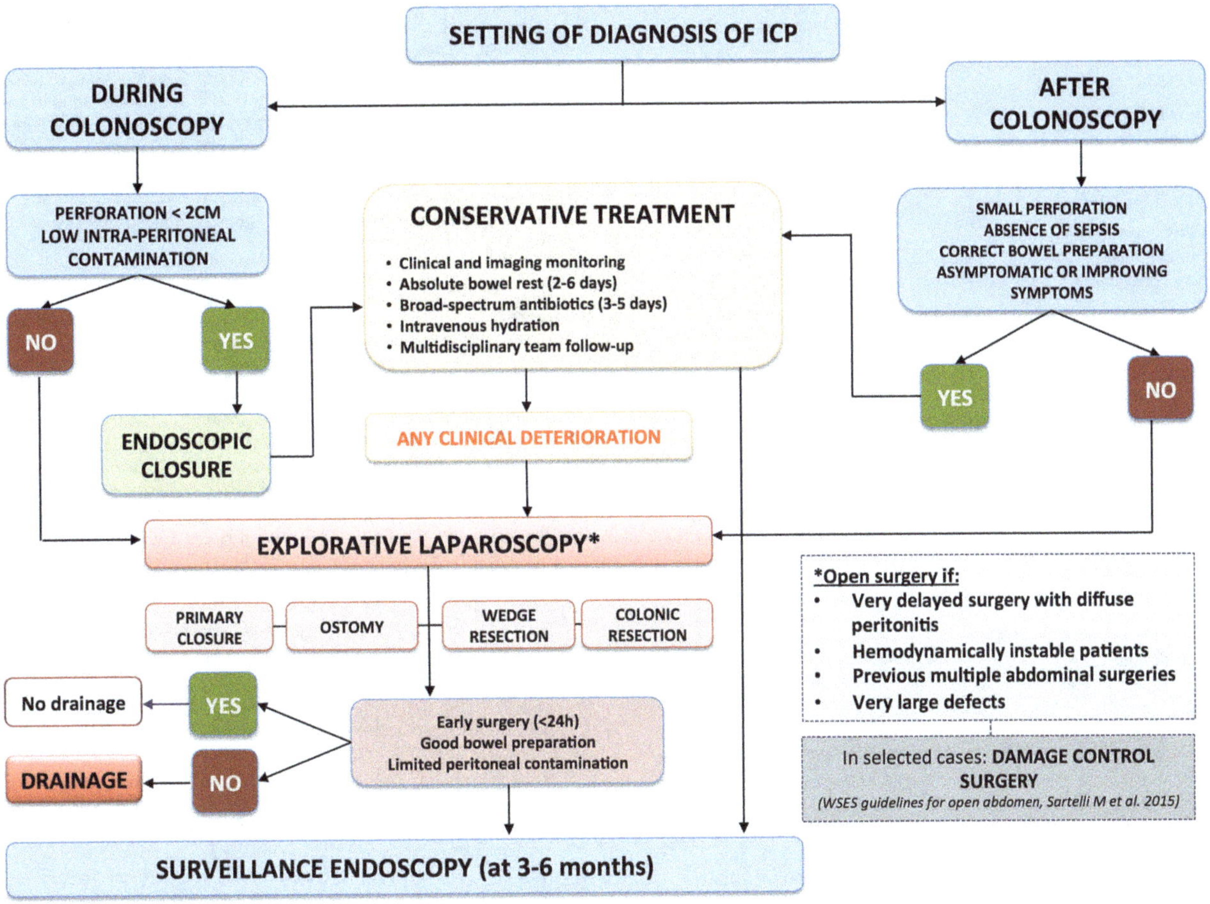

Fig. 2 Comprehensive algorithm for the management of iatrogenic colonoscopy perforation

spectrum antibiotics and intravenous hydration together with close clinical observation.

It must be stressed that early improvement with conservative treatment does not rule out the potential need for surgery. Close monitoring of the patient will allow detection of clinical deterioration, which may signal the need for emergency surgery. Where surgical intervention is required, timely decisions for proceeding with the operation are important. Ideally, these surgeries should occur early and within 24 h of the perforation, as further delays are related to a worse prognosis.

Colonic closure, wedge resection, ostomy, and colonic resection are the main surgical options for ICP management. No RCTs have assessed the superiority of one method over the others. Thus, the therapeutic decision remains essentially empirical, based on the perforation characteristics (e.g., size, time of evolution, and degree of peritoneal contamination), the patient's general status (e.g., comorbidities), and the availability of adequate technology and surgical devices. Explorative laparoscopy is safe and should be considered the first line approach to assess the perforation-related damages. In patients with good bowel preparation, minimal peritoneal contamination, and adequate infection source control, the perforation repair can possibly be performed by laparoscopy and without drainage placement. Alternatively, staged repair or, in extreme cases, damage control surgery may be required.

The present WSES guidelines contribute to clarifying the complex decision-making process for the management of ICP. Despite the large number of publications, evidence is often derived from observational and moderate to low quality studies. However, it is scarcely feasible to design RCTs for an infrequent complication often requiring emergency treatment. Prospective registries would be highly advantageous to defining the validity of the present recommendations and proposed guidelines.

Abbreviations

ASA: American Society of Anesthesiologist score; BMI: Body mass index; CRP: C-reactive protein; CT: Computed tomography; DCS: Damage control surgery; EMR: Endoscopic mucosal resection; ESD: Endoscopic submucosal dissection; ICP: Iatrogenic colonoscopy perforation; MDCT: Multidetector computed tomography; OTSC: Over-the-scope clips; PCT: Pro-calcitonin; PD: Perforated diverticulitis; PPV: Positive predictive value; RCT: Randomized controlled trial; TAC: Temporary abdominal closure; TTS: Through-the-scope clips; VTE: Venous thromboembolism; WBC: White blood cell

Acknowledgements
Not applicable.

Funding
No authors received funding or resources in relation to this article. The authors received a WSES institutional waiver for this publication.

Authors' contributions
NdeA wrote the first draft of the manuscript. All the authors reviewed the manuscript and approved the final draft.

Competing interests
The authors declare that they have no competing interests.

Author details
[1]Unit of Digestive, Hepato-Pancreato-Biliary Surgery and Liver Transplantation, Henri Mondor University Hospital, AP-HP, and University of Paris Est, UPEC, 51 Avenue du Maréchal de Lattre de Tassigny, 94010 Créteil, France. [2]Department of Surgery, Maggiore Hospital, Bologna, Italy. [3]General Surgery and Trauma Team, Niguarda Hospital, Milan, Italy. [4]Department of Surgery, Macerata Hospital, Macerata, Italy. [5]Department of General and Digestive Surgery, University Hospital Dr Peset, Valencia, Spain. [6]Unit of Gastroenterology and Endoscopy, Maggiore Hospital, Bologna, Italy. [7]Department of Trauma Surgery, Royal Perth Hospital, Perth, Australia. [8]General Surgery I, Papa Giovanni XXIII Hospital, Bergamo, Italy. [9]Acute Care Surgery at The Queen's Medical Center, John A. Burns School of Medicine, University of Hawaii, Honolulu, USA. [10]Department of General Surgery, Rambam Healthcare Campus, Haifa, Israel. [11]Trauma and Acute Care Surgery Unit, Hadassah Hebrew University Medical Center, Jerusalem, Israel. [12]Gastroenterology and Endoscopy Unit, University Hospital of Parma, Parma, Italy. [13]Department of Gastroenterology and Digestive Endoscopy, Henri Mondor Hospital, AP-HP, and University of Paris Est, UPEC, Creteil, France. [14]Unit of Digestive Surgery and Liver Transplantation, University Hospital Marqués de Valdecilla, University of Cantabria, Santander, Spain. [15]Department of Surgery, UC San Diego Health System, San Diego, CA, USA. [16]Unit of Digestive Surgery, Cannes Hospital, Cannes, France. [17]Division of Trauma Surgery, Department of Surgery, School of Medical Sciences, University of Campinas (Unicamp), Campinas, SP, Brazil. [18]Department of General and Oncological Surgery, University Hospital Paolo Giaccone, Palermo, Italy. [19]Virginia Commonwealth University, Richmond, VA, USA. [20]Assia Medical Group, Department of Surgery, Sackler School of Medicine, Tel Aviv University, Tel Aviv, Israel. [21]Department of Surgery, Critical Care Medicine and the Regional Trauma Service, Foothills Medical Center, Calgari, AB, Canada. [22]Department of Emergency Surgery, Hospital de Clínicas, School of Medicine, UDELAR, Montevideo, Uruguay. [23]II Cátedra de Clínica Quirúgica, Hospital de Clínicas, Facultad de Ciencias Medicas, Universidad National de Asuncion, Asuncion, Paraguay. [24]Department of Surgery, University of Washington, Seattle, WA, USA. [25]Department of Surgery and Obstetrics/Gynecologic, Regional Hospital, Limbe, Cameroon. [26]Unit of General Surgery and Liver Transplantation, Policlinico di Bari "M. Rubino", Bari, Italy. [27]Unit of General and Emergency Surgery, Trauma Center, Centro Hospitalar e Universitario de Coimbra, Coimbra, Portugal. [28]Department of Trauma and Emergency Center, Vicente Corral Moscoso Hospital, University of Azuay, Cuenca, Ecuador. [29]Digestive and Interventional Endoscopy Unit, Niguarda Ca'Granda Hospital, Milan, Italy. [30]Department of Surgery and Critical Care, Universidad del Valle, Fundacion Valle del Lili, Cali, Colombia. [31]Department of Surgery, UPMC, University of Pittsburg, School of Medicine, Pittsburg, USA. [32]Department of Anesthesiology and Intensive Care, University Hospital of Parma, Parma, Italy. [33]Critical Care Medicine, University of Pittsburg, School of Medicine, Pittsburg, USA. [34]Trauma and Acute Care Service, St Michael's Hospital, Toronto, ON, Canada. [35]Department of Surgery, Radboud University Medical Center, Nijmegen, The Netherlands. [36]Department of Surgery, Colorectal Surgery Unit, University of Cagliari, Cagliari, Italy. [37]University Paris Diderot, Rothschild Hospital, AP-HP, Paris, France. [38]Department of Emergency and Trauma Surgery of the University Hospital of Parma, Parma, Italy.

References

1. Carpio G, Albu E, Gumbs MA, Gerst PH. Management of colonic perforation after colonoscopy. Report of three cases. Dis Colon Rectum. 1989;32:624–6.
2. Cho SB, Lee WS, Joo YE, Kim HR, Park SW, Park CH, Kim HS, Choi SK, Rew JS. Therapeutic options for iatrogenic colon perforation: feasibility of endoscopic clip closure and predictors of the need for early surgery. Surg Endosc. 2012;26:473–9.
3. Gosen C, Poulose B, Trunzo J, Marks J. Endoscopic management of iatrogenic colon perforation during colonoscopy. Am Surg. 2009;75:184–6.
4. Kim JS, Kim BW, Kim JI, Kim JH, Kim SW, Ji JS, Lee BI, Choi H. Endoscopic clip closure versus surgery for the treatment of iatrogenic colon perforations developed during diagnostic colonoscopy: a review of 115,285 patients. Surg Endosc. 2013;27:501–4.
5. Luning TH, Keemers-Gels ME, Barendregt WB, Tan AC, Rosman C. Colonoscopic perforations: a review of 30,366 patients. Surg Endosc. 2007;21:994–7.
6. Panteris V, Haringsma J, Kuipers EJ. Colonoscopy perforation rate, mechanisms and outcome: from diagnostic to therapeutic colonoscopy. Endoscopy. 2009;41:941–51.
7. Shi X, Shan Y, Yu E, Fu C, Meng R, Zhang W, Wang H, Liu L, Hao L, Wang H, et al. Lower rate of colonoscopic perforation: 110,785 patients of colonoscopy performed by colorectal surgeons in a large teaching hospital in China. Surg Endosc. 2014;28:2309–16.
8. Wullstein C, Koppen M, Gross E. Laparoscopic treatment of colonic perforations related to colonoscopy. Surg Endosc. 1999;13:484–7.
9. Zhang YQ, Lu W, Yao LQ, Qin XY, Xu MD, Zhong YS, Li QL, Wu HF, Zhou PH. Laparoscopic direct suture of perforation after diagnostic colonoscopy. Int J Color Dis. 2013;28:1505–9.
10. Arezzo A, Balague C, Targarona E, Borghi F, Giraudo G, Ghezzo L, Arroyo A, Sola-Vera J, De Paolis P, Bossotti M, et al. Colonic stenting as a bridge to surgery versus emergency surgery for malignant colonic obstruction: results of a multicentre randomised controlled trial (ESCO trial). Surg Endosc. 2017; 31:3297–305.
11. European Colorectal Cancer Screening Guidelines Working G, von Karsa L, Patnick J, Segnan N, Atkin W, Halloran S, Lansdorp-Vogelaar I, Malila N, Minozzi S, Moss S, et al. European guidelines for quality assurance in colorectal cancer screening and diagnosis: overview and introduction to the full supplement publication. Endoscopy. 2013;45:51–9.
12. Force USPST, Bibbins-Domingo K, Grossman DC, Curry SJ, Davidson KW, Epling JW Jr, Garcia FA, Gillman MW, Harper DM, Kemper AR, et al. Screening for colorectal cancer: US preventive services task force recommendation statement. JAMA. 2016;315:2564–75.
13. Iqbal CW, Chun YS, Farley DR. Colonoscopic perforations: a retrospective review. J Gastrointest Surg. 2005;9:1229–35. discussion 1236.
14. Cobb WS, Heniford BT, Sigmon LB, Hasan R, Simms C, Kercher KW, Matthews BD. Colonoscopic perforations: incidence, management, and outcomes. Am Surg. 2004;70:750–7. discussion 757-758.
15. Iqbal CW, Cullinane DC, Schiller HJ, Sawyer MD, Zietlow SP, Farley DR. Surgical management and outcomes of 165 colonoscopic perforations from a single institution. Arch Surg. 2008;143:701–6. discussion 706-707.
16. Garcia Martinez MT, Ruano Poblador A, Galan Raposo L, Gay Fernandez AM, Casal Nunez JE. Perforation after colonoscopy: our 16-year experience. Rev Esp Enferm Dig. 2007;99:588–92.
17. Farley DR, Bannon MP, Zietlow SP, Pemberton JH, Ilstrup DM, Larson DR. Management of colonoscopic perforations. Mayo Clin Proc. 1997;72:729–33.

18. Samalavicius NE, Kazanavicius D, Lunevicius R, Poskus T, Valantinas J, Stanaitis J, Grigaliunas A, Gradauskas A, Venskutonis D, Samuolis R, et al. Incidence, risk, management, and outcomes of iatrogenic full-thickness large bowel injury associated with 56,882 colonoscopies in 14 Lithuanian hospitals. Surg Endosc. 2013;27:1628–35.
19. Teoh AY, Poon CM, Lee JF, Leong HT, Ng SS, Sung JJ, Lau JY. Outcomes and predictors of mortality and stoma formation in surgical management of colonoscopic perforations: a multicenter review. Arch Surg. 2009;144:9–13.
20. Gatto NM, Frucht H, Sundararajan V, Jacobson JS, Grann VR, Neugut AI. Risk of perforation after colonoscopy and sigmoidoscopy: a population-based study. J Natl Cancer Inst. 2003;95:230–6.
21. Levin TR, Zhao W, Conell C, Seeff LC, Manninen DL, Shapiro JA, Schulman J. Complications of colonoscopy in an integrated health care delivery system. Ann Intern Med. 2006;145:880–6.
22. Lohsiriwat V, Sujarittanakarn S, Akaraviputh T, Lertakyamanee N, Lohsiriwat D, Kachinthorn U. Colonoscopic perforation: a report from World Gastroenterology Organization endoscopy training center in Thailand. World J Gastroenterol. 2008;14:6722–5.
23. Lohsiriwat V, Sujarittanakarn S, Akaraviputh T, Lertakyamanee N, Lohsiriwat D, Kachinthorn U. What are the risk factors of colonoscopic perforation? BMC Gastroenterol. 2009;9:71.
24. Miranda L, Settembre A, Piccolboni D, Capasso P, Corcione F. Iatrogenic colonic perforation: repair using laparoscopic technique. Surg Laparosc Endosc Percutan Tech. 2011;21:170–4.
25. Guyatt G, Gutterman D, Baumann MH, Addrizzo-Harris D, Hylek EM, Phillips B, Raskob G, Lewis SZ, Schunemann H. Grading strength of recommendations and quality of evidence in clinical guidelines: report from an American College of Chest Physicians Task Force. Chest. 2006;129:174–81.
26. Arora G, Mannalithara A, Singh G, Gerson LB, Triadafilopoulos G. Risk of perforation from a colonoscopy in adults: a large population-based study. Gastrointest Endosc. 2009;69:654–64.
27. Day LW, Kwon A, Inadomi JM, Walter LC, Somsouk M. Adverse events in older patients undergoing colonoscopy: a systematic review and meta-analysis. Gastrointest Endosc. 2011;74:885–96.
28. Hamdani U, Naeem R, Haider F, Bansal P, Komar M, Diehl DL, Kirchner HL. Risk factors for colonoscopic perforation: a population-based study of 80118 cases. World J Gastroenterol. 2013;19:3596–601.
29. Anderson ML, Pasha TM, Leighton JA. Endoscopic perforation of the colon: lessons from a 10-year study. Am J Gastroenterol. 2000;95:3418–22.
30. Doran H, Marin IT, Iaciu M, Patrascu T. Iatrogenic perforations during colonoscopy. Chirurgia (Bucur). 2014;109:523–6.
31. Chukmaitov A, Bradley CJ, Dahman B, Siangphoe U, Warren JL, Klabunde CN. Association of polypectomy techniques, endoscopist volume, and facility type with colonoscopy complications. Gastrointest Endosc. 2013;77:436–46.
32. Bielawska B, Day AG, Lieberman DA, Hookey LC. Risk factors for early colonoscopic perforation include non-gastroenterologist endoscopists: a multivariable analysis. Clin Gastroenterol Hepatol. 2014;12:85–92.
33. Rabeneck L, Paszat LF, Hilsden RJ, Saskin R, Leddin D, Grunfeld E, Wai E, Goldwasser M, Sutradhar R, Stukel TA. Bleeding and perforation after outpatient colonoscopy and their risk factors in usual clinical practice. Gastroenterology. 2008;135:1899–906. 1906 e1891.
34. Goudra B, Nuzat A, Singh PM, Borle A, Carlin A, Gouda G. Association between type of sedation and the adverse events associated with gastrointestinal endoscopy: an analysis of 5 years' data from a tertiary center in the USA. Clin Endosc. 2017;50:161–9.
35. Wernli KJ, Brenner AT, Rutter CM, Inadomi JM. Risks associated with anesthesia services during colonoscopy. Gastroenterology. 2016;150:888–94. quiz e818.
36. Lohsiriwat V. Colonoscopic perforation: incidence, risk factors, management and outcome. World J Gastroenterol. 2010;16:425–30.
37. Hassan C, Zullo A, De Francesco V, Ierardi E, Giustini M, Pitidis A, Taggi F, Winn S, Morini S. Systematic review: endoscopic dilatation in Crohn's disease. Aliment Pharmacol Ther. 2007;26:1457–64.
38. Heldwein W, Dollhopf M, Rosch T, Meining A, Schmidtsdorff G, Hasford J, Hermanek P, Burlefinger R, Birkner B, Schmitt W, Munich Gastroenterology G. The Munich Polypectomy Study (MUPS): prospective analysis of complications and risk factors in 4000 colonic snare polypectomies. Endoscopy. 2005;37:1116–22.
39. Committee AT, Hwang JH, Konda V, Abu Dayyeh BK, Chauhan SS, Enestvedt BK, Fujii-Lau LL, Komanduri S, Maple JT, Murad FM, et al. Endoscopic mucosal resection. Gastrointest Endosc. 2015;82:215–26.
40. Wang J, Zhang XH, Ge J, Yang CM, Liu JY, Zhao SL. Endoscopic submucosal dissection vs endoscopic mucosal resection for colorectal tumors: a meta-analysis. World J Gastroenterol. 2014;20:8282–7.
41. Tanaka S, Terasaki M, Kanao H, Oka S, Chayama K. Current status and future perspectives of endoscopic submucosal dissection for colorectal tumors. Dig Endosc. 2012;24(Suppl 1):73–9.
42. Toyonaga T, Man-i M, East JE, Nishino E, Ono W, Hirooka T, Ueda C, Iwata Y, Sugiyama T, Dozaiku T, et al. 1,635 endoscopic submucosal dissection cases in the esophagus, stomach, and colorectum: complication rates and long-term outcomes. Surg Endosc. 2013;27:1000–8.
43. van Halsema EE, van Hooft JE, Small AJ, Baron TH, Garcia-Cano J, Cheon JH, Lee MS, Kwon SH, Mucci-Hennekinne S, Fockens P, et al. Perforation in colorectal stenting: a meta-analysis and a search for risk factors. Gastrointest Endosc. 2014;79:970–82. e977; quiz 983 e972, 983 e975.
44. Small AJ, Coelho-Prabhu N, Baron TH. Endoscopic placement of self-expandable metal stents for malignant colonic obstruction: long-term outcomes and complication factors. Gastrointest Endosc. 2010;71:560–72.
45. Paspatis GA, Dumonceau JM, Barthet M, Meisner S, Repici A, Saunders BP, Vezakis A, Gonzalez JM, Turino SY, Tsiamoulos ZP, et al. Diagnosis and management of iatrogenic endoscopic perforations: European Society of Gastrointestinal Endoscopy (ESGE) position statement. Endoscopy. 2014;46:693–711.
46. Cennamo V, Fuccio L, Mutri V, Minardi ME, Eusebi LH, Ceroni L, Laterza L, Ansaloni L, Pinna AD, Salfi N, et al. Does stent placement for advanced colon cancer increase the risk of perforation during bevacizumab-based therapy? Clin Gastroenterol Hepatol. 2009;7:1174–6.
47. Manes G, de Bellis M, Fuccio L, Repici A, Masci E, Ardizzone S, Mangiavillano B, Carlino A, Rossi GB, Occhipinti P, Cennamo V. Endoscopic palliation in patients with incurable malignant colorectal obstruction by means of self-expanding metal stent: analysis of results and predictors of outcomes in a large multicenter series. Arch Surg. 2011;146:1157–62.
48. de'Angelis N, Carra MC, Borrelli O, Bizzarri B, Vincenzi F, Fornaroli F, De Caro G, de'Angelis GL. Short- and long-term efficacy of endoscopic balloon dilation in Crohn's disease strictures. World J Gastroenterol. 2013;19:2660–7.
49. Ragg J, Garimella V, Cast J, Hunter IA, Hartley JE. Balloon dilatation of benign rectal anastomotic strictures—a review. Dig Surg. 2012;29:287–91.
50. Korman LY, Overholt BF, Box T, Winker CK. Perforation during colonoscopy in endoscopic ambulatory surgical centers. Gastrointest Endosc. 2003;58:554–7.
51. Dehal A, Tessier DJ. Intraperitoneal and extraperitoneal colonic perforation following diagnostic colonoscopy. JSLS. 2014;18:136–41.
52. Martinez-Perez A, de'Angelis N, Brunetti F, Le Baleur Y, Paya-Llorente C, Memeo R, Gaiani F, Manfredi M, Gavriilidis P, Nervi G, et al. Laparoscopic vs. open surgery for the treatment of iatrogenic colonoscopic perforations: a systematic review and meta-analysis. World J Emerg Surg. 2017;12:8.
53. Quintanilla E, Castro JL, Rabago LR, Chico I, Olivares A, Ortega A, Vicente C, Carbo J, Gea F. Is the use of prophylactic hemoclips in the endoscopic resection of large pedunculated polyps useful? A prospective and randomized study. J Interv Gastroenterol. 2012;2:99–104.
54. Manta R, Tremolaterra F, Arezzo A, Verra M, Galloro G, Dioscoridi L, Pugliese F, Zullo A, Mutignani M, Bassotti G. Complications during colonoscopy: prevention, diagnosis, and management. Tech Coloproctol. 2015;19:505–13.
55. Reumkens A, Rondagh EJ, Bakker CM, Winkens B, Masclee AA, Sanduleanu S. Post-colonoscopy complications: a systematic review, time trends, and meta-analysis of population-based studies. Am J Gastroenterol. 2016;111:1092–101.
56. Rex DK, Schoenfeld PS, Cohen J, Pike IM, Adler DG, Fennerty MB, Lieb JG 2nd, Park WG, Rizk MK, Sawhney MS, et al. Quality indicators for colonoscopy. Am J Gastroenterol. 2015;110:72–90.
57. Rembacken B, Hassan C, Riemann JF, Chilton A, Rutter M, Dumonceau JM, Omar M, Ponchon T. Quality in screening colonoscopy: position statement of the European Society of Gastrointestinal Endoscopy (ESGE). Endoscopy. 2012;44:957–68.
58. Bowles CJ, Leicester R, Romaya C, Swarbrick E, Williams CB, Epstein O. A prospective study of colonoscopy practice in the UK today: are we adequately prepared for national colorectal cancer screening tomorrow? Gut. 2004;53:277–83.
59. Gedebou TM, Wong RA, Rappaport WD, Jaffe P, Kahsai D, Hunter GC. Clinical presentation and management of iatrogenic colon perforations. Am J Surg. 1996;172:454–7. discussion 457-458.
60. Araghizadeh FY, Timmcke AE, Opelka FG, Hicks TC, Beck DE. Colonoscopic perforations. Dis Colon Rectum. 2001;44:713–6.

61. Hall C, Dorricott NJ, Donovan IA, Neoptolemos JP. Colon perforation during colonoscopy: surgical versus conservative management. Br J Surg. 1991;78:542–4.
62. Dixon P, Kowdley GC, Cunningham SC. The role of surgery in the treatment of endoscopic complications. Best Pract Res Clin Gastroenterol. 2016;30:841–51.
63. Kim HH, Kye BH, Kim HJ, Cho HM. Prompt management is most important for colonic perforation after colonoscopy. Ann Coloproctol. 2014;30:228–31.
64. Yang SK, Xiao L, Zhang H, Xu XX, Song PA, Liu FY, Sun L. Significance of serum procalcitonin as biomarker for detection of bacterial peritonitis: a systematic review and meta-analysis. BMC Infect Dis. 2014;14:452.
65. Pupelis G, Drozdova N, Mukans M, Malbrain ML. Serum procalcitonin is a sensitive marker for septic shock and mortality in secondary peritonitis. Anaesthesiol Intensive Ther. 2014;46:262–73.
66. Ortega-Deballon P, Radais F, Facy O, d'Athis P, Masson D, Charles PE, Cheynel N, Favre JP, Rat P. C-reactive protein is an early predictor of septic complications after elective colorectal surgery. World J Surg. 2010;34:808–14.
67. Hortmann M, Singler K, Geier F, Christ M. Recognition of infections in elderly emergency patients. Z Gerontol Geriatr. 2015;48:601–7.
68. Kim DH, Pickhardt PJ, Taylor AJ, Menias CO. Imaging evaluation of complications at optical colonoscopy. Curr Probl Diagn Radiol. 2008;37: 165–77.
69. Park JY, Choi PW, Jung SM, Kim NH. The outcomes of management for colonoscopic perforation: a 12-year experience at a single institute. Ann Coloproctol. 2016;32:175–83.
70. Furukawa A, Sakoda M, Yamasaki M, Kono N, Tanaka T, Nitta N, Kanasaki S, Imoto K, Takahashi M, Murata K, et al. Gastrointestinal tract perforation: CT diagnosis of presence, site, and cause. Abdom Imaging. 2005;30:524–34.
71. Kirkpatrick AW, Koo J, Zalev AH, Burnstein MJ, Warren RE. Endoscopic perforation of the rectum presenting initially as a change in voice. Can J Surg. 1999;42:305–6.
72. Shanmuganathan K, Mirvis SE, Chiu WC, Killeen KL, Scalea TM. Triple-contrast helical CT in penetrating torso trauma: a prospective study to determine peritoneal violation and the need for laparotomy. AJR Am J Roentgenol. 2001;177:1247–56.
73. Committee ASoP, Fisher DA, Maple JT, Ben-Menachem T, Cash BD, Decker GA, Early DS, Evans JA, Fanelli RD, Fukami N, et al. Complications of colonoscopy. Gastrointest Endosc. 2011;74:745–52.
74. de'Angelis N, Esposito F, Memeo R, Lizzi V, Martinez-Perez A, Landi F, Genova P, Catena F, Brunetti F, Azoulay D. Emergency abdominal surgery after solid organ transplantation: a systematic review. World J Emerg Surg. 2016;11:43.
75. Luigiano C, Consolo P, Scaffidi MG, Strangio G, Giacobbe G, Alibrandi A, Pallio S, Tortora A, Melita G, Familiari L. Endoscopic mucosal resection for large and giant sessile and flat colorectal polyps: a single-center experience with long-term follow-up. Endoscopy. 2009;41:829–35.
76. Fatima H, Rex DK. Minimizing endoscopic complications: colonoscopic polypectomy. Gastrointest Endosc Clin N Am. 2007;17:145–56. viii
77. Waye JD, Kahn O, Auerbach ME. Complications of colonoscopy and flexible sigmoidoscopy. Gastrointest Endosc Clin N Am. 1996;6:343–77.
78. Damore LJ 2nd, Rantis PC, Vernava AM 3rd, Longo WE. Colonoscopic perforations. Etiology, diagnosis, and management. Dis Colon Rectum. 1996; 39:1308–14.
79. Lo AY, Beaton HL. Selective management of colonoscopic perforations. J Am Coll Surg. 1994;179:333–7.
80. Broeders E, Al-Taher M, Peeters K, Bouvy N. Verres needle desufflation as an effective treatment option for colonic perforation after colonoscopy. Surg Laparosc Endosc Percutan Tech. 2015;25:e61–4.
81. An SB, Shin DW, Kim JY, Park SG, Lee BH, Kim JW. Decision-making in the management of colonoscopic perforation: a multicentre retrospective study. Surg Endosc. 2016;30:2914–21.
82. Hansen AJ, Tessier DJ, Anderson ML, Schlinkert RT. Laparoscopic repair of colonoscopic perforations: indications and guidelines. J Gastrointest Surg. 2007;11:655–9.
83. Riss S, Akan B, Mikola B, Rieder E, Karner-Hanusch J, Dirlea D, Mittlbock M, Weiser FA. CO_2 insufflation during colonoscopy decreases post-interventional pain in deeply sedated patients: a randomized controlled trial. Wien Klin Wochenschr. 2009;121:464–8.
84. Bassan MS, Holt B, Moss A, Williams SJ, Sonson R, Bourke MJ. Carbon dioxide insufflation reduces number of postprocedure admissions after endoscopic resection of large colonic lesions: a prospective cohort study. Gastrointest Endosc. 2013;77:90–5.
85. La Torre M, Velluti F, Giuliani G, Di Giulio E, Ziparo V, La Torre F. Promptness of diagnosis is the main prognostic factor after colonoscopic perforation. Color Dis. 2012;14:e23–6.
86. Yoshikane H, Hidano H, Sakakibara A, Ayakawa T, Mori S, Kawashima H, Goto H, Niwa Y. Endoscopic repair by clipping of iatrogenic colonic perforation. Gastrointest Endosc. 1997;46:464–6.
87. Jovanovic I, Zimmermann L, Fry LC, Monkemuller K. Feasibility of endoscopic closure of an iatrogenic colon perforation occurring during colonoscopy. Gastrointest Endosc. 2011;73:550–5.
88. Magdeburg R, Collet P, Post S, Kaehler G. Endoclipping of iatrogenic colonic perforation to avoid surgery. Surg Endosc. 2008;22:1500–4.
89. Taku K, Sano Y, Fu KI, Saito Y, Matsuda T, Uraoka T, Yoshino T, Yamaguchi Y, Fujita M, Hattori S, et al. Iatrogenic perforation associated with therapeutic colonoscopy: a multicenter study in Japan. J Gastroenterol Hepatol. 2007;22:1409–14.
90. Barbagallo F, Castello G, Latteri S, Grasso E, Gagliardo S, La Greca G, Di Blasi M. Successful endoscopic repair of an unusual colonic perforation following polypectomy using an endoclip device. World J Gastroenterol. 2007;13:2889–91.
91. Velchuru VR, Zawadzki M, Levin AL, Bouchard CM, Marecik S, Prasad LM, Park JJ. Endoclip closure of a large colonic perforation following colonoscopic leiomyoma excision. JSLS. 2013;17:152–5.
92. Trecca A, Gaj F, Gagliardi G. Our experience with endoscopic repair of large colonoscopic perforations and review of the literature. Tech Coloproctol. 2008;12:315–21. discussion 322.
93. Byeon JS. Colonic perforation: can we manage it endoscopically? Clin Endosc. 2013;46:495–9.
94. Ma MX, Bourke MJ. Complications of endoscopic polypectomy, endoscopic mucosal resection and endoscopic submucosal dissection in the colon. Best Pract Res Clin Gastroenterol. 2016;30:749–67.
95. Voermans RP, Le Moine O, von Renteln D, Ponchon T, Giovannini M, Bruno M, Weusten B, Seewald S, Costamagna G, Deprez P, et al. Efficacy of endoscopic closure of acute perforations of the gastrointestinal tract. Clin Gastroenterol Hepatol. 2012;10:603–8.
96. Wedi E, Gonzalez S, Menke D, Kruse E, Matthes K, Hochberger J. One hundred and one over-the-scope-clip applications for severe gastrointestinal bleeding, leaks and fistulas. World J Gastroenterol. 2016;22:1844–53.
97. Mangiavillano B, Caruso A, Manta R, Di Mitri R, Arezzo A, Pagano N, Galloro G, Mocciaro F, Mutignani M, Luigiano C, et al. Over-the-scope clips in the treatment of gastrointestinal tract iatrogenic perforation: a multicenter retrospective study and a classification of gastrointestinal tract perforations. World J Gastrointest Surg. 2016;8:315–20.
98. Weiland T, Fehlker M, Gottwald T, Schurr MO. Performance of the OTSC system in the endoscopic closure of iatrogenic gastrointestinal perforations: a systematic review. Surg Endosc. 2013;27:2258–74.
99. Stavropoulos SN, Modayil R, Friedel D. Current applications of endoscopic suturing. World J Gastrointest Endosc. 2015;7:777–89.
100. Raju GS, Saito Y, Matsuda T, Kaltenbach T, Soetikno R. Endoscopic management of colonoscopic perforations (with videos). Gastrointest Endosc. 2011;74:1380–8.
101. Sartelli M, Viale P, Catena F, Ansaloni L, Moore E, Malangoni M, Moore FA, Velmahos G, Coimbra R, Ivatury R, et al. 2013 WSES guidelines for management of intra-abdominal infections. World J Emerg Surg. 2013;8:3.
102. Sawyer RG, Claridge JA, Nathens AB, Rotstein OD, Duane TM, Evans HL, Cook CH, O'Neill PJ, Mazuski JE, Askari R, et al. Trial of short-course antimicrobial therapy for intraabdominal infection. N Engl J Med. 2015; 372:1996–2005.
103. Semeraro N, Ammollo CT, Semeraro F, Colucci M. Sepsis, thrombosis and organ dysfunction. Thromb Res. 2012;129:290–5.
104. Semeraro N, Ammollo CT, Semeraro F, Colucci M. Coagulopathy of acute sepsis. Semin Thromb Hemost. 2015;41:650–8.
105. Simmons J, Pittet JF. The coagulopathy of acute sepsis. Curr Opin Anaesthesiol. 2015;28:227–36.
106. Donze JD, Ridker PM, Finlayson SR, Bates DW. Impact of sepsis on risk of postoperative arterial and venous thromboses: large prospective cohort study. BMJ. 2014;349:g5334.
107. Osland E, Yunus RM, Khan S, Memon MA. Early versus traditional postoperative feeding in patients undergoing resectional gastrointestinal surgery: a meta-analysis. JPEN J Parenter Enteral Nutr. 2011;35:473–87.
108. Yamamoto T, Kita R, Masui H, Kinoshita H, Sakamoto Y, Okada K, Komori J, Miki A, Uryuhara K, Kobayashi H, et al. Prediction of mortality in patients

with colorectal perforation based on routinely available parameters: a retrospective study. World J Emerg Surg. 2015;10:24.
109. Makarawo TP, Damadi A, Mittal VK, Itawi E, Rana G. Colonoscopic perforation management by laparoendoscopy: an algorithm. JSLS. 2014;18:20–7.
110. Bleier JI, Moon V, Feingold D, Whelan RL, Arnell T, Sonoda T, Milsom JW, Lee SW. Initial repair of iatrogenic colon perforation using laparoscopic methods. Surg Endosc. 2008;22:646–9.
111. Di Saverio S, Patrizi F, Bassi M, Birindelli A, Nigro F, Cennamo V. Minimally invasive laparoscopic management of colonoscopic perforation avoiding laparotomy and colostomy: when and how to perform primary repair—a video vignette. Color Dis. 2016;18:817–8.
112. Cirocchi R, Di Saverio S, Weber DG, Tabola R, Abraha I, Randolph J, Arezzo A, Binda GA. Laparoscopic lavage versus surgical resection for acute diverticulitis with generalised peritonitis: a systematic review and meta-analysis. Tech Coloproctol. 2017;21:93–110.
113. Agresta F, Michelet I, Mainente P, Bedin N. Laparoscopic management of colonoscopic perforations. Surg Endosc. 2000;14:592–3.
114. Castellvi J, Pi F, Sueiras A, Vallet J, Bollo J, Tomas A, Verge J, Caballero F, Iglesias C, De Castro J. Colonoscopic perforation: useful parameters for early diagnosis and conservative treatment. Int J Color Dis. 2011;26:1183–90.
115. Gawlik V. Laparoscopic treatment of large intestinal injuries during colonoscopy. Rozhl Chir. 2011;90:182–3.
116. Oh JE, Shim SG. Colonoscopic perforation; a 10-year experience in single general hospital. Korean J Gastroenterol. 2009;54:371–6.
117. Shadis R, Zebley DM, Kim SY, Hofmann MT, Fassler SA. Laparoscopic repair of colonic anastomotic leak in an elderly patient. JSLS. 2011;15:555–7.
118. Shin DK, Shin SY, Park CY, Jin SM, Cho YH, Kim WH, Kwon CI, Ko KH, Hahm KB, Park PW, et al. Optimal methods for the management of iatrogenic colonoscopic perforation. Clin Endosc. 2016;49:282–8.
119. Vokurka J. Iatrogenic perforation during an endoscopic examination of the gastrointestinal tract. Bratisl Lek Listy. 2004;105:387–9.
120. Haas EM, Pedraza R, Ragupathi M, Mahmood A, Bartley Pickron T. Laparoscopic primary colorrhaphy for acute iatrogenic perforations during colonoscopy. Minim Invasive Surg. 2013;2013:823506.
121. O'Malley E, Boyle E, O'Callaghan A, Coffey JC, Walsh SR. Role of laparoscopy in penetrating abdominal trauma: a systematic review. World J Surg. 2013;37:113–22.
122. Ignjatovic M, Jovic J. Tension pneumothorax, pneumoretroperitoneum, and subcutaneous emphysema after colonoscopic polypectomy: a case report and review of the literature. Langenbeck's Arch Surg. 2009;394:185–9.
123. Mai CM, Wen CC, Wen SH, Hsu KF, Wu CC, Jao SW, Hsiao CW. Iatrogenic colonic perforation by colonoscopy: a fatal complication for patients with a high anesthetic risk. Int J Color Dis. 2010;25:449–54.
124. Coimbra C, Bouffioux L, Kohnen L, Deroover A, Dresse D, Denoel A, Honore P, Detry O. Laparoscopic repair of colonoscopic perforation: a new standard? Surg Endosc. 2011;25:1514–7.
125. Rotholtz NA, Laporte M, Lencinas S, Bun M, Canelas A, Mezzadri N. Laparoscopic approach to colonic perforation due to colonoscopy. World J Surg. 2010;34:1949–53.
126. Araujo SE, Seid VE, Caravatto PP, Dumarco R. Incidence and management of colonoscopic colon perforations: 10 years experience. Hepato-Gastroenterology. 2009;56:1633–6.
127. Schloricke E, Bader FG, Hoffmann M, Zimmermann M, Bruch HP, Hildebrand P. Open surgical versus laparoscopic treatment of iatrogenic colon perforation—results of a 13-year experience. Zentralbl Chir. 2013;138:257–61.
128. Kim J, Lee GJ, Baek JH, Lee WS. Comparison of the surgical outcomes of laparoscopic versus open surgery for colon perforation during colonoscopy. Ann Surg Treat Res. 2014;87:139–43.
129. Velez MA, Riff DS, Mule JM. Laparoscopic repair of a colonoscopic perforation. Surg Endosc. 1997;11:387–9.
130. Tan KK, Hong CC, Zhang J, Liu JZ, Sim R. Predictors of outcome following surgery in colonic perforation: an institution's experience over 6 years. J Gastrointest Surg. 2011;15:277–84.
131. Franklin ME Jr, Portillo G, Trevino JM, Gonzalez JJ, Glass JL. Long-term experience with the laparoscopic approach to perforated diverticulitis plus generalized peritonitis. World J Surg. 2008;32:1507–11.
132. Afshar S, Kurer MA. Laparoscopic peritoneal lavage for perforated sigmoid diverticulitis. Color Dis. 2012;14:135–42.
133. Angenete E, Thornell A, Burcharth J, Pommergaard HC, Skullman S, Bisgaard T, Jess P, Lackberg Z, Matthiessen P, Heath J, et al. Laparoscopic lavage is feasible and safe for the treatment of perforated diverticulitis with purulent peritonitis: the first results from the randomized controlled trial DILALA. Ann Surg. 2016;263:117–22.
134. Bruns BR, Ahmad SA, O'Meara L, Tesoriero R, Lauerman M, Klyushnenkova E, Kozar R, Scalea TM, Diaz JJ. Nontrauma open abdomens: a prospective observational study. J Trauma Acute Care Surg. 2016;80:631–6.
135. Sartelli M, Catena F, Ansaloni L, Coccolini F, Griffiths EA, Abu-Zidan FM, Di Saverio S, Ulrych J, Kluger Y, Ben-Ishay O, et al. WSES guidelines for the management of acute left sided colonic diverticulitis in the emergency setting. World J Emerg Surg. 2016;11:37.
136. Becher RD, Peitzman AB, Sperry JL, Gallaher JR, Neff LP, Sun Y, Miller PR, Chang MC. Damage control operations in non-trauma patients: defining criteria for the staged rapid source control laparotomy in emergency general surgery. World J Emerg Surg. 2016;11:10.
137. Bowley DM, Barker P, Boffard KD. Damage control surgery—concepts and practice. J R Army Med Corps. 2000;146:176–82.
138. Godat L, Kobayashi L, Costantini T, Coimbra R. Abdominal damage control surgery and reconstruction: world society of emergency surgery position paper. World J Emerg Surg. 2013;8:53.
139. Garbay JR, Suc B, Rotman N, Fourtanier G, Escat J. Multicentre study of surgical complications of colonoscopy. Br J Surg. 1996;83:42–4.
140. Iqbal CW, Askegard-Giesmann JR, Pham TH, Ishitani MB, Moir CR. Pediatric endoscopic injuries: incidence, management, and outcomes. J Pediatr Surg. 2008;43:911–5.
141. Blotiere PO, Weill A, Ricordeau P, Alla F, Allemand H. Perforations and haemorrhages after colonoscopy in 2010: a study based on comprehensive French health insurance data (SNIIRAM). Clin Res Hepatol Gastroenterol. 2014;38:112–7.
142. Hagel AF, Boxberger F, Dauth W, Kessler HP, Neurath MF, Raithel M. Colonoscopy-associated perforation: a 7-year survey of in-hospital frequency, treatment and outcome in a German university hospital. Color Dis. 2012;14:1121–5.
143. Kafka-Ritsch R, Birkfellner F, Perathoner A, Raab H, Nehoda H, Pratschke J, Zitt M. Damage control surgery with abdominal vacuum and delayed bowel reconstruction in patients with perforated diverticulitis Hinchey III/IV. J Gastrointest Surg. 2012;16:1915–22.
144. Ordonez CA, Sanchez AI, Pineda JA, Badiel M, Mesa R, Cardona U, Arias R, Rosso F, Granados M, Gutierrez-Martinez MI, et al. Deferred primary anastomosis versus diversion in patients with severe secondary peritonitis managed with staged laparotomies. World J Surg. 2010;34:169–76.
145. Kirkpatrick AW, Roberts DJ, De Waele J, Jaeschke R, Malbrain ML, De Keulenaer B, Duchesne J, Bjorck M, Leppaniemi A, Ejike JC, et al. Intra-abdominal hypertension and the abdominal compartment syndrome: updated consensus definitions and clinical practice guidelines from the world Society of the Abdominal Compartment Syndrome. Intensive Care Med. 2013;39:1190–206.
146. Lieberman DA, Rex DK, Winawer SJ, Giardiello FM, Johnson DA, Levin TR, United States Multi-Society Task Force on Colorectal C. Guidelines for colonoscopy surveillance after screening and polypectomy: a consensus update by the US Multi-Society Task Force on colorectal cancer. Gastroenterology. 2012;143:844–57.
147. Strate LL, Gralnek IM. ACG clinical guideline: management of patients with acute lower gastrointestinal bleeding. Am J Gastroenterol. 2016;111:755.
148. Committee ASoP, Early DS, Ben-Menachem T, Decker GA, Evans JA, Fanelli RD, Fisher DA, Fukami N, Hwang JH, Jain R, et al. Appropriate use of GI endoscopy. Gastrointest Endosc. 2012;75:1127–31.
149. Kahi CJ, Boland CR, Dominitz JA, Giardiello FM, Johnson DA, Kaltenbach T, Lieberman D, Levin TR, Robertson DJ, Rex DK. Colonoscopy surveillance after colorectal cancer resection: recommendations of the US Multi-Society Task Force on colorectal cancer. Am J Gastroenterol. 2016;111:337–46. quiz 347.
150. Levin B, Lieberman DA, McFarland B, Smith RA, Brooks D, Andrews KS, Dash C, Giardiello FM, Glick S, Levin TR, et al. Screening and surveillance for the early detection of colorectal cancer and adenomatous polyps, 2008: a joint guideline from the American Cancer Society, the US Multi-Society Task Force on Colorectal Cancer, and the American College of Radiology. CA Cancer J Clin. 2008;58:130–60.

21

Bologna guidelines for diagnosis and management of adhesive small bowel obstruction (ASBO): 2017 update of the evidence-based guidelines from the world society of emergency surgery ASBO working group

Richard P. G. ten Broek[1,39*†], Pepijn Krielen[1†], Salomone Di Saverio[2], Federico Coccolini[3], Walter L. Biffl[4], Luca Ansaloni[3], George C. Velmahos[5], Massimo Sartelli[6], Gustavo P. Fraga[7], Michael D. Kelly[8], Frederick A. Moore[9], Andrew B. Peitzman[10], Ari Leppaniemi[11], Ernest E. Moore[12], Johannes Jeekel[13], Yoram Kluger[14], Michael Sugrue[15], Zsolt J. Balogh[16], Cino Bendinelli[17], Ian Civil[18], Raul Coimbra[19], Mark De Moya[20], Paula Ferrada[21], Kenji Inaba[22], Rao Ivatury[21], Rifat Latifi[23], Jeffry L. Kashuk[24], Andrew W. Kirkpatrick[25], Ron Maier[26], Sandro Rizoli[27], Boris Sakakushev[28], Thomas Scalea[29], Kjetil Søreide[30,31], Dieter Weber[32], Imtiaz Wani[33], Fikri M. Abu-Zidan[34], Nicola De'Angelis[35], Frank Piscioneri[36], Joseph M. Galante[37], Fausto Catena[38] and Harry van Goor[1]

Abstract

Background: Adhesive small bowel obstruction (ASBO) is a common surgical emergency, causing high morbidity and even some mortality. The adhesions causing such bowel obstructions are typically the footprints of previous abdominal surgical procedures. The present paper presents a revised version of the Bologna guidelines to evidence-based diagnosis and treatment of ASBO. The working group has added paragraphs on prevention of ASBO and special patient groups.

Methods: The guideline was written under the auspices of the World Society of Emergency Surgery by the ASBO working group. A systematic literature search was performed prior to the update of the guidelines to identify relevant new papers on epidemiology, diagnosis, and treatment of ASBO. Literature was critically appraised according to an evidence-based guideline development method. Final recommendations were approved by the workgroup, taking into account the level of evidence of the conclusion.

(Continued on next page)

* Correspondence: Richard.tenbroek@radboudumc.nl; http://www.dutchadhesiongroup.org
†Richard P. G. ten Broek and Pepijn Krielen contributed equally to this work.
[1]Department of Surgery, Radboud University Medical Center, Nijmegen, The Netherlands
[39]Department of Surgery, Radboud University Nijmegen Medical Centre, P.O. Box 9101, 6500 HB Nijmegen, The Netherlands
Full list of author information is available at the end of the article

(Continued from previous page)
Recommendations: Adhesion formation might be reduced by minimally invasive surgical techniques and the use of adhesion barriers. Non-operative treatment is effective in most patients with ASBO. Contraindications for non-operative treatment include peritonitis, strangulation, and ischemia. When the adhesive etiology of obstruction is unsure, or when contraindications for non-operative management might be present, CT is the diagnostic technique of choice. The principles of non-operative treatment are *nil* per os, naso-gastric, or long-tube decompression, and intravenous supplementation with fluids and electrolytes. When operative treatment is required, a laparoscopic approach may be beneficial for selected cases of simple ASBO.
Younger patients have a higher lifetime risk for recurrent ASBO and might therefore benefit from application of adhesion barriers as both primary and secondary prevention.

Discussion: This guideline presents recommendations that can be used by surgeons who treat patients with ASBO. Scientific evidence for some aspects of ASBO management is scarce, in particular aspects relating to special patient groups. Results of a randomized trial of laparoscopic versus open surgery for ASBO are awaited.

Keywords: Small bowel obstruction, Adhesions, Surgery, Laparoscopy, Laparotomy

Background

Adhesive small bowel obstruction (ASBO) is one of the leading causes of surgical emergencies and in particular of surgical emergencies that require an emergent operations [1–4]. In the UK, small bowel obstruction was the indication for 51% of all emergency laparotomies [2]. Scott et al. reported on seven emergency surgical procedures that account for 80% of all general surgery emergency admissions, morbidity, deaths, and healthcare expenditures in the USA [3]. Adhesive small bowel obstruction was the most common diagnosis for both the top 2 (small bowel resection) and top 5 (adhesiolysis) procedures [3]. Post-operative adhesions are the leading cause of small bowel obstructions, accounting for 60% of cases [1].

ASBO causes considerable harm, resulting in 8 days of hospitalization on average and an in-hospital mortality rate of 3% per episode [5–8]. Between 20 and 30% of patients with adhesive small bowel obstruction require operative treatment [1, 9–11]. Length of hospitalization and morbidity depend on the need for surgical intervention. Average hospitalization after surgical treatment of ASBO is 16 days, compared to 5 days following non-operative treatment [12]. Associated costs in a Dutch study in 2016 were estimated at €16,305 for surgical and €2227 for non-operative treatment [12].

Although adhesive small bowel obstruction is a common condition, the prevention and treatment is often characterized by surgeons' personal preferences rather than standardized evidence-based protocols. There is a large amount of conflicting and low-quality evidence in publications regarding treatment of adhesive small bowel obstruction.

Therefore, the World Society of Emergency Surgery (WSES) working group on ASBO has developed evidence-based guidelines to support clinical decision making in diagnosis and management of ASBO [11, 13]. In the present revision of these guidelines, all recommendations were updated according to the latest evidence available from the medical literature. Further, we have introduced two new sections: prevention of ASBO and special patient groups.

Methods

The guideline was written under the auspices of the WSES by the ASBO working group. Systematic searches of the MEDLINE and Embase databases were carried out in October 2016 using the keywords relevant to each section. Terms relevant to each section of the guideline were mapped to MEDLINE Medical Subjects Headings (MeSH) terms, as well as searched for as text items. Articles describing randomized controlled trials and systematic reviews were searched for using the methodological filters of the Scottish Intercollegiate Guidelines Network (http://www.sign.ac.uk/methodological-principles.html). The bibliographies of included articles were subsequently hand-searched for other relevant references, and experts in the field were asked if they found any relevant reports missing.

Critical appraisal

Articles selected to support recommendations were assessed using the levels of evidence as published by the Centre for Evidence-Based Medicine of the University of Oxford (www.cebm.net; Table 1). Articles were classified according to the type of article and individually assessed for methodological quality using the GRADE method as proposed by the GRADE working group. That working group has developed a common, sensible, and transparent approach to grading the quality of evidence and strength of recommendations (http://www.gradeworkinggroup.org). The main literature on which the conclusion for each relevant topic is based is stated with the conclusion, accompanied by the level of evidence (Table 2) [14, 15].

Table 1 Classification of evidence per article

Level of evidence	Interventional research	Studies concerning diagnostic accuracy	Studies on complications or side effects, etiology, prognosis
A1	Systematic review/meta-analysis of at least 2 independently performed level A2 studies		
A2	Double-blind controlled randomized comparative clinical trial of good study quality with an adequate number of study participants	Diagnostic test compared to reference test; criteria and outcomes defined in advance; assessment of test results by independent observers; independent interpretation of test results; adequate number of consecutive patients enrolled; all patients subjected to both tests	Prospective cohort with sufficient amount of study participants and follow-up, adequately controlled for confounders; selection in follow-up has been successfully excluded
B	Comparative studies, but without all the features mentioned for level A2 (including patient-control studies, cohort studies)	Diagnostic test compared to reference test, but without all the features mentioned in A2	Prospective cohort study, but without all the features mentioned for level A2 or retrospective cohort study or case-control study
C	Noncomparative studies		
D	Expert opinion		

Conclusion and recommendations are graded according to the level of evidence from strong ("there is strong evidence for," level A) to weak ("we cannot be confident," level D). Recommendations were graded as strong recommendations (level I) or weak recommendation or suggestions (level II). Recommendations were considered strong recommendations if there is sufficient evidence (level A or B) demonstrating that the benefits of an intervention are of clinical importance and clearly outweigh the harm of the intervention. A concept guideline was sent to all involved for comment and approval after which internal consensus was reached between the members of the working group. Amendments were made based upon these comments, leading to the final version of this updated guideline.

Definitions

Peritoneal adhesions

The term "peritoneal adhesions" or simply "adhesions" is defined as fibrous tissue that connects surfaces or organs within the peritoneal cavity that are normally separated. Such adhesions are the results of a pathological healing response of the peritoneum upon injury, as opposed to the normal "ad integrum" repair [16]. Typical adhesions form after peritoneal injury from abdominal surgery. Other conditions that may cause peritoneal injury resulting in adhesion formation include radiotherapy, endometriosis, inflammation, and local response to tumors. Adhesions from a non-operative etiology are often part of a more complex pathology that can cause chronic pain and complications as the result of adhesions and other mechanisms [17]. Management of chronic abdominal complications by adhesiolysis is controversial [18, 19]. The scope of the present guideline is limited to diagnosis and management of acute bowel obstructions.

Table 2 Grading of the conclusions and recommendations according to the level of evidence and strength of recommendation

Level	Conclusion based on
A	Systematic review (A1) or at least 2 independent studies with evidence level A2 ("there is evidence that...")
B	One study with evidence level A2 or at least 2 independent studies with evidence level B ("it is likely that...")
C	One study with evidence level B or level C ("there are indications that...")
D	Expert opinion ("the working group recommends...")
Level	**Recommendation**
I	Strong recommendation
II	Weak recommendation (suggestion)

Adhesive small bowel obstruction

Small bowel obstruction is a surgical emergency in which the obstruction of the small intestine hinders passage of intestinal contents. Small bowel obstruction is characterized by abdominal pain, vomiting, distention, and constipation. Adhesions are the single most common cause for small bowel obstruction [1, 20]. Nonadhesive etiologies of bowel obstruction include incarcerated hernias, obstructive lesions (malignant and benign), and a number of infrequent causes for bowel obstruction such as bezoars, inflammatory bowel disease, and volvulus [21–25]. Definitive confirmation of the adhesive etiology of bowel obstruction is made during operative treatment. Methods to confirm the adhesive etiology of bowel obstruction non-invasively include a history of previous episodes of bowel obstruction by adhesions or exclusion of other causes of bowel obstruction by imaging (often CT scan).

Adhesiolysis

Adhesiolysis refers to releasing adhesions either by blunt or sharp dissection during surgery. It can be the primary indication for an operation, as in a reoperation for small bowel obstruction caused by adhesions. Adhesiolysis is also performed during reoperations for indications not related to adhesions in order to obtain sufficient access to the operative field. Complicated adhesiolysis refers to the event of inadvertent injury while performing adhesiolysis. Injuries during adhesiolysis are most frequently made to the bowel. These bowel injuries are classified as:

- Seromuscular injury: injury to the visceral peritoneum (serosa) and smooth muscle layer of the bowel. The lumen of the bowel or leakage of bowel contents is not visible.
- Enterotomy: a full thickness injury to the bowel. The mucous layer or lumen of the bowel is visible, or there may be leakage of intestinal contents.
- Delayed diagnosed perforation: bowel injuries made during surgery that initially go unrecognized. Typically, the abdomen is closed at the end of procedure with the bowel injury still in place, causing patients to deteriorate during the postoperative course.

Results

Epidemiology

The risk of SBO is highest following colorectal, oncologic gynecological, or pediatric surgery [1, 26–28]. One in ten patients develops at least one episode of SBO within 3 years after colectomy [7]. Reoperations for ASBO occur in between 4.2 and 12.6% of patients after pediatric surgery patients, and 3.2% of colorectal patients [1, 29]. Recurrence of ASBO is also frequent; 12% of non-operatively treated patients are readmitted within 1 year, rising to 20% after 5 years. The risk of recurrence is slightly lower after operative treatment: 8% after 1 year and 16% after 5 years [30].

Classification of adhesions

The most frequently used classification of adhesions in general surgery is the adhesion score according to Zühlke et al. (Table 3) [31]. The score is based on the tenacity and some morphologic aspects of the adhesions. The merits of this score are that it is easy to use and classifications are self-explanatory to most surgeons and gynecologists. The major drawback to the score is that it does not measure the extent of adhesions and that tenacity of adhesions can vary between different parts of the abdomen. The most used grading system in gynecological surgery is the American Fertility Society (AFS) score [32]. The score is designed for grading adhesions in the small pelvis. Adhesions are scored for extent and severity at four sites: right ovary, right tube, left ovary, and left tube. The scores for the right and left side are summed, and the final AFS score is the score for the side with the lowest summed score while discarding the score for the other side. Thus, a patient with an AFS score of 0 can still have adhesions. Further critiques for this score include a relatively low inter-observer reproducibility [33]. A modified AFS has therefore gained popularity in more recent studies [34].

A recently introduced score by the ASBO working group is the peritoneal adhesion index (PAI), which measures tenacity on a 1–3 scale at 10 predefined sites, to integrate tenacity and extent of adhesions in a single score (Fig. 1) [35]. This score is the only score that has been validated to be prognostic for convalescence after surgery for ASBO and the risk of injuries during adhesiolysis [36]. A limitation to all these adhesion scores is that they are only applicable to operative cases because they require operative assessment. Furthermore, none of them has yet been validated to correlate with the long-term risk for (recurrence of) adhesion-related complications.

A different type of classification in the field of ASBO is risk stratification that predicts the need for surgery. Zielinski reported on three radiological and clinical signs that correlate with the need for surgical exploration:

Table 3 Classification of adhesions according to Zühlke et al.

Grade 0	No adhesions or insignificant adhesions
Grade 1	Adhesions that are filmy and easy to separate by blunt dissection
Grade 2	Adhesions where blunt dissection is possible but some sharp dissection necessary, beginning vascularization
Grade 3	Lysis of adhesions possible by sharp dissection only, clear vascularization
Grade 4	Lysis of adhesions possible by sharp dissection only, organs strongly attached with severe adhesions, damage of organs hardly preventable

PERITONEAL ADHESION INDEX:

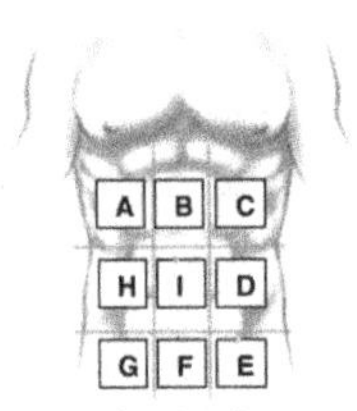

Regions:	Adhesion grade:	Adhesion grade score:
A Right upper	___	0 No adhesions
B Epigastrium	___	1 Filmy adhesions, blunt dissection
C Left upper	___	2 Strong adhesions, sharp dissection
D Left flank	___	3 Very strong vascularized adhesions, sharp dissection, damage hardly preventable
E Left lower	___	
F Pelvis	___	
G Right lower	___	
H Right flank	___	
I Central	___	
L Bowel to bowel	___	

PAI ☐

Fig. 1 Peritoneal adhesion index. Reproduced with permission from [35] mesenteric edema, absence of the small-bowel feces sign, and obstipation. The score was validated in 100 cases of ASBO and predicted the risk with a concordance index of 0.77 [37]. A more accurate model was reported by Baghdadi et al. This score comprises radiological findings, sepsis criteria, and comorbidity index. Although the score is somewhat complex to assess, it correlates with an area under the curve of 0.80 in a validation study of 351 cases [38].

Prevention

Surgical technique

The main principles of prevention of adhesion and related complications are minimizing surgical trauma and the use of adjuvants to reduce adhesion formation. Laparoscopy is often believed to reduce adhesion formation and the risk for ASBO. In a systematic review of cohort studies, the incidence of reoperation for ASBO was 1.4 (95% CI 1.0–1.8%) after laparoscopic and 3.8% (95% CI 3.1–4.4%) after open surgery. However, there were differences in both the type and indications for surgery [1]. In a recent meta-analysis of SBO after colorectal operations, the incidence of ASBO after laparoscopic surgery was somewhat lower than after open colorectal procedures (OR 0.62, 95% CI 0.54 to 0.72). However, no significant difference was found in the three randomized trials included in this review (OR 0.50, 95% CI 0.20 to 1.2) [39]. In summary, there is some evidence that the incidence of ASBO is lower after laparoscopy. However, the effect seems modest when correcting for type and indication of surgery. Thus, performing (colorectal) surgery by laparoscopy is not a complete solution to preventing adhesive SBO.

Many other aspects of surgical technique have been associated with adhesion formation, although there are little or no epidemiological data concerning their impact on the incidence of ASBO. Nevertheless, a number of important risk factors for aggravated adhesion formation are worth considering. One of the most important risk factors is the foreign body reaction, for example as seen with starch-powdered gloves, and meshes used for abdominal wall reconstruction [40, 41]. The choice of energy device might also impact adhesion formation. Peritoneal injury is lower in bipolar electrocautery and ultrasonic devices as compared to monopolar electrocautery [42, 43]. Animal data suggest that both systemic and intraperitoneal application of antibiotics, and metronidazole in particular, can reduce adhesion formation in septic conditions [44, 45].

Adhesion barriers

Adhesion barriers are adjuvants for peritoneal administration that can effectively reduce adhesion formation. Adhesion barriers are produced in several forms: solid membranes, gels, and liquids. The concept behind barriers is that they do not actively interfere with inflammation and wound healing. Rather, they act as a spacer which separates injured surfaces of the peritoneum, allowing these surfaces to heal without forming fibrinous attachments which eventually lead to adhesions. In order to accomplish this task, such barriers should ideally be inert to the human immune system and be slowly degradable.

There is moderate evidence that a hyaluronate carboxymethylcellulose adhesion barrier can reduce the incidence of reoperations for ASBO in colorectal surgery. In three trials involving 1132 patients undergoing colorectal surgery, hyaluronate carboxymethylcellulose reduced the incidence of reoperations for adhesive small bowel obstruction (RR 0.49, 95% CI 0.28–0.88) [46–48]. The use of such barriers seems cost-effective in open colorectal surgery [49]. An overview of common used adhesion barriers and their efficacy is found in Table 4.

Table 4 Overview of most common applied adhesion barriers and their impact on adhesion formation and incidence of ASBO

Barrier	Marketed as	Comments
Hyaluronate carboxymethylcellulose	Seprafilm®	Solid barrier most suitable for open surgery although laparoscopic placement has been described Studies in both general surgery and gynecological procedures Reduces adhesion formation, as well as the risk for reoperations for adhesive small bowel obstruction (relative risk 0.49, 95% CI 0.28–0.88)
Oxidized regenerated cellulose	Interceed®	Solid barrier most suitable for open surgery Only studied in gynecological procedures Reduces incidence of adhesion formation relative risk 0.51, 95% CI 0.31–0.86 No studies available on subsequent risk of ASBO This workgroup does not recommend the use of this barrier to prevent ASBO in general surgery
Icodextrin	Adept®	Liquid barrier, easy to apply in both open and laparoscopic surgery Good safety record in both general surgery and gynecological surgery Reduces recurrence of ASBO following surgery for ASBO in one trial (relative risk 0.20, 95% CI 0.04–0.88)
Polyethylene glycol	Sprayshield®/Spraygel®	Gel barrier, easy to apply in both open and laparoscopic surgery Reduces adhesion score in both general surgery and gynecological trials Relative few and small studies, impact on long-term adhesion-related complications not described

Adapted from [52]

Secondary prevention

Adhesion barriers might also be useful to prevent recurrence after surgical treatment of ASBO. One randomized trial with an adhesion barrier included patients undergoing surgery for ASBO [20]. In this trial, patients were randomized to a liquid 4% icodextrin adhesion barrier or standard operative treatment without an adhesion barrier. The ASBO recurrence rate was 2.19% (2/91) in the icodextrin groups versus 11.11% (10/90) in the control group after a mean follow-up period of 41.4 months ($p < 0.05$) [20]. In this trial, the barrier was applied in patients treated for ASBO by laparotomy. However, the icodextrin 4% adhesion barrier can also be administered in laparoscopic surgery. Other trials with icodextrin as an adhesion barrier indicated that it actually might not be the most potent barrier to prevent adhesion reformation, which is typically more challenging than prevention of de novo adhesions [50]. Favoring the use of icodextrin are its low costs and good safety record [51]. From the results of other trials, we suggest that a hyaluronate carboxymethylcellulose might be more efficacious, but this barrier is less practical in laparoscopic surgery [46–48, 52].

Approach to the patient with ASBO

An algorithm for the diagnostic and therapeutic approach to the patient with ASBO is presented in Fig. 2. The initial diagnosis of ASBO is of utmost importance. Failure to diagnose or having a delayed diagnosis represents 70% of malpractice claims in ASBO [53, 54].

The primary goals in the initial evaluation of patients in whom adhesive small bowel obstruction is suspected are:

- Differentiating between adhesive small bowel obstruction and other causes of bowel obstruction
- Assessing the need for urgent surgical exploration
- Identifying and preventing complications from bowel obstruction

History taking and physical examination

History taking in a patient suspected for ASBO includes assessment of potential causes of bowel obstruction (previous operations, radiotherapy) and nutritional status. Signs of dehydration should also be assessed. Traditionally, ASBO is clinically diagnosed in a patient with intermittent colicky abdominal pain, distention, and nausea (with or without vomiting), with or without absence of stools. Although diagnosis of small bowel obstruction is fairly certain in a patient in whom all of these symptoms are present, there are some specific pitfalls that can result in delayed or misdiagnosis of bowel obstruction upon initial presentation. In patients with incomplete obstruction, watery diarrhea may be present. The presence of watery diarrhea can cause an episode of ASBO to be mistaken for gastro-enteritis. Stools might also be present in patients with a relatively high obstruction who are admitted early after onset of symptoms. Moreover, not all of these symptoms may be present, especially in the elderly in whom pain is often less prominent [55, 56].

During physical examination, signs of peritonitis that might reveal strangulation or ischemia should be evaluated. Differential diagnostic considerations that can be assessed during physical examination include the presence of any abdominal wall or groin hernias. The evaluation of ASBO by history taking and physical examination has a low sensitivity for detecting bowel strangulation and ischemia. Sensitivity of physical examination for detection of strangulation is only 48%, even in experienced hands [57].

Laboratory tests

The minimum of laboratory tests include blood count, lactate, electrolytes, CRP, and BUN/creatinine. Laboratory values that might indicate peritonitis are a CRP > 75 and white blood cell count > 10.000/mm^3, although sensitivity and specificity of these tests are relatively low [6, 57, 58]. Electrolytes are often disturbed in patients with a bowel obstruction; in particular, low values of potassium are frequently found and need to be corrected. BUN/creatinine needs to be assessed as patients with ASBO are frequently dehydrated which could result in acute kidney injury.

Imaging studies

Plain X-rays

The value of plain X-rays complementary to physical examination is limited. In high-grade obstruction, a triad of multiple air-fluid levels, distention of small bowel loops, and absence of gas in the colon are pathognomonic for small bowel obstruction, but overall sensitivity and specificity of plain x-rays are low (sensitivity approximately 70%) [59, 60]. A large volume pneumoperitoneum secondary to bowel perforation in ASBO can also be detected on plain X-rays, preferably by an erect chest X-ray. Plain X-rays, however, do not detect the more early signs of peritonitis or strangulation [59–61]. Furthermore, a plain abdominal X-ray does not provide anatomical information that helps differentiate between the various causes of bowel obstruction.

Water-soluble contrast studies

Several systematic reviews and meta-analyses have established the usefulness of water-soluble contrast agents in the diagnostic work-up of ASBO [62–64]. If the contrast has not reached the colon on an abdominal X-ray taken 24 h following administration of the contrast, this is highly indicative of failure of non-operative management. Multiple studies have shown that the use of water-soluble contrast agents accurately predicts the need for surgery and reduces hospital stay [62, 63]. Some authors also suggest that water-soluble contrast studies reduce the need for

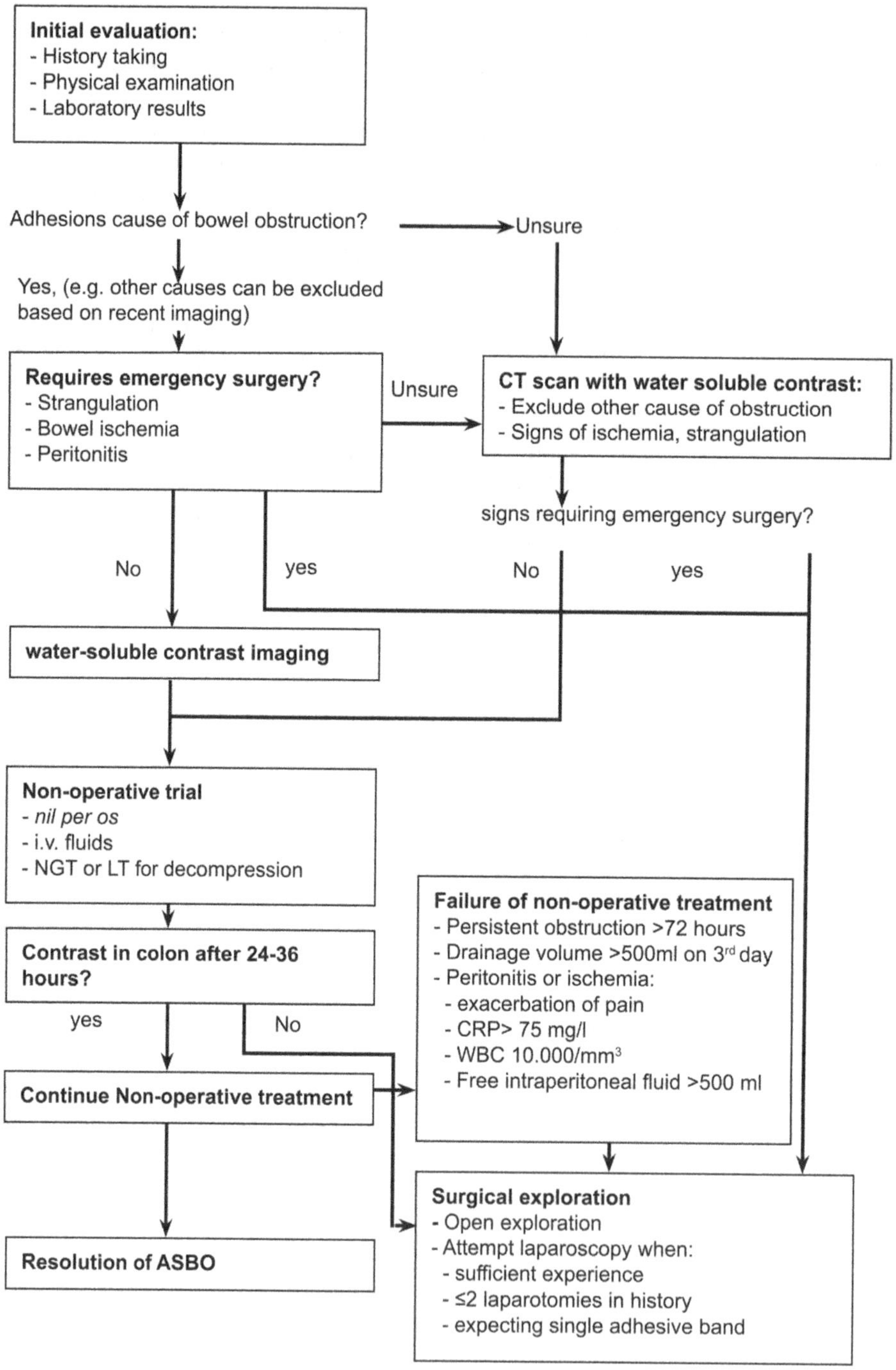

Fig. 2 Algorithm to diagnosis and treatment of ASBO

surgery, which is attributed to an active therapeutic role of the contrast [62, 63].

CT scans

Current helical CT scans not only have good test characteristics for diagnosing small bowel obstruction but also have approximately 90% accuracy in predicting strangulation and the need for urgent surgery [37, 60, 65–68]. Diagnostic value of CT scan can be enhanced with the use of water-soluble contract. As with water-soluble contrast studies, progress of the contrast can be evaluated by X-ray at 24 h after CT scan.

Although adhesions are not directly visible even on CT scan, a CT scan can differentiate accurately between different causes of bowel obstruction by excluding other causes. The workgroup therefore considers CT scan to be the preferred imaging technique if there is any doubt about the diagnosis of ASBO, and to assess the need for urgent surgery.

A CT scan should help to differentiate between a complete obstruction of the bowel and help facilitate the decision for a trial of non-operative management versus a decision to proceed to surgery. It may also help to define the location of the obstruction (e.g., high in the jejunum or deep in the pelvis). Signs of a closed loop, bowel ischemia, and free fluid are signs that suggest the need for surgery without delay. In addition, radiological and clinical scores can be used to predict the need for surgery as described above [37, 38].

Ultrasound and MRI

Although the working group considered CT scan to be the preferred technique for diagnosis of ASBO, ultrasound and MRI might be useful in specific situations. Ultrasound is operator dependent but in experienced hands can provide more information than plain X-rays, and is also available in most low income settings. Apart from distension of bowel loops, ultrasound enables detection of free fluid (that might indicate the need for urgent surgery) and assessment of the degree of shock in dehydrated patients [61, 69]. Ultrasound can also be of value in situations in which exposure to radiation is undesirable, such as in pregnant patients. In these cases, ultrasound might be complemented with MRI for more anatomical information if the diagnosis of bowel obstruction is confirmed [70].

Diagnosis: summary

Recommendations can be found in Table 5. In summary, CT scan with oral water-soluble contrast is the preferred technique of imaging in the initial evaluation. Progress

Table 5 Overview of conclusions and recommendation

Level A	Adhesive small bowel obstruction is a leading cause of morbidity, deaths, and healthcare expenditures in emergency surgery. *A2 Scott 2016; NELA project team 2016*
Level B	Adhesive small bowel obstruction causes high morbidity, with average hospital stay of 8 days and 3% in-hospital mortality per episode. Recurrence of adhesive small bowel obstruction is high. Risk for adhesive small bowel obstruction may be somewhat lower after laparoscopic compared to open colorectal surgery, but that results could not be confirmed in randomized trials. *A2 ten Broek 2013; Yamada 2016; B Krielen 2016; Foster 2006*
Level IB	Laparoscopic surgery reduces adhesion formation and might reduce subsequent incidence of ASBO. *B Lundorff 1992; ten Broek 2013; Yamada 2016*
Level IA	Hyaluronate carboxymethylcellulose reduces adhesion formation and the risk of subsequent reoperations of adhesive SBO. The use of this barrier seems cost-effective in open colorectal surgery. *A1 ten Broek 2014; A2 Fazio 2006; Park 2009; Kusunoki 205*
Level IIC	In the absence of signs that require emergent surgical exploration (i.e., peritonitis, strangulation, or bowel ischemia), non-operative management is the treatment strategy of choice. *C Fevang 2002; Fevang 2004; Ten Broek 2013; Jeppesen 2016*
Level IIB	A trial of non-operative management can be continued safely for 72 h. *B Keenan 2014; Sakakibara 2007*
Level IID	Initial evaluation should be complemented with assessment of nutritional status and laboratory tests evaluating at least blood count, lactate, electrolytes, and BUN/Creat *Expert opinion*
Level IIC	Plain X-rays have only limited value in the work-up of patients with small bowel obstruction and are not recommended. *B Maglinte 1996*
Level IB	Optimal diagnostic work-up should include CT scan in the assessment and water soluble oral contrast. In the absence of the need to perform immediate surgery, a follow-up abdominal X-ray should be made after 24 h. If the contrast has reach the colon, this is indicative for resolution of the bowel obstruction. *A2 Ceresoli 2016; Branco 2010; Abbas 2005; B Goussous 2013; Zielinski 2011; Zielinski 2010; Daneshmat 1999; Makita 1999; Zalcman 2000*
Level IIC	Long trilumen naso-intestinal tubes are more efficacious than naso-gastric tubes in non-operative management, but require endoscopic placement. *A2 Chen2012*
Level IIC	Laparoscopic adhesiolyis might reduce morbidity in selected cases of ASBO that require surgery. Results of a randomized trial are awaited. *B Sajid 2016; Farinella 2009; Sallinen 2014*
Level IIB	Adhesion barriers reduce the risk of recurrence for ASBO following operative treatment. *A2 Catena 2012*
Level IIC	Younger patients, and pediatric patients in particular, have higher lifetime risk of developing adhesion-related complications and might therefore benefit most from adhesion prevention. *A1 ten Broek 2013; A2 Strik 2016; B Fredriksson 2016*
Level C	More research is needed to the impact of comorbidities in elderly patients on optimal management of adhesive small bowel obstruction. Patients with diabetes might require more early operative intervention. *B Karamanos 2016*

of the contrast should be monitored after 24 h of non-operative treatment by X-ray. If the diagnosis of ASBO is certain (e.g., because other causes have been excluded with recent imaging), and there are no signs that immediate surgery might be warranted, only a water-soluble contrast study is considered sufficient. Ultrasound and MRI can be useful in specific situations, such as pregnancy or (in low income countries) when CT scan is unavailable.

Management

Initial decision making

Non-operative management should always be tried in patients with adhesive small bowel obstruction, unless there are signs of peritonitis, strangulation, or bowel ischemia [71]. Although the risk of recurrence is slightly lower after operative treatment, this is not a reason to opt for a primary surgical approach. Morbidity from emergency surgical exploration is high; there is a considerable risk for bowel injury, and surgical treatment may significantly reduce post-operative quality of life [1, 72–74].

Non-operative management

The cornerstone of non-operative management is *nil* per os and decompression using a naso-gastric tube or long intestinal tube. Non-operative management is effective in approximately 70–90% of patients with ASBO [1, 75, 76]. There has been some debate in the literature over the use of long intestinal tubes or naso-gastric tubes. In an older trial, no significant difference in failure rates was found between naso-gastric tubes and long intestinal tubes [77]. In a more recent trial, 186 patients were randomized between a newly designed trilumen long tube and a naso-gastric tube. Long tubes seemed more effective in this trial with a failure rate of 10.4% in this group compared with 53.3% in the naso-gastric tube group [78]. Results from this trial should be interpreted with care, because the failure rate of naso-gastric tube compression is much higher than would be expected from other literature. Moreover, a drawback of trilumen tubes is the need for endoscopic placement. Non-operative management should further include fluid resuscitation, correction of electrolyte disturbances, nutritional support, and prevention of aspiration.

Duration of the period in which non-operative management can be tried is subject to debate. Several retrospective series and databases have shown that delays in surgery increase morbidity and mortality [30, 71, 79, 80]. Evidence for the optimal duration of non-operative treatment is absent, but most authors and the panel consider a 72-h period as safe and appropriate [11, 58, 76, 79, 80]. Continuing non-operative treatment for more than 72 h in cases with persistent high output from a decompression tube, but no other signs of clinical deterioration, however, remains subject to debate. Common medical complications in patients with small bowel obstruction are dehydration with kidney injury, electrolyte disturbances, malnutrition, and aspiration.

Non-operative management: summary

The panel recommends a trial of non-operative management in all patients with ASBO, unless there are signs of peritonitis, strangulation, or bowel ischemia. Evidence for the optimal duration of non-operative is absent, but most authors and the panel consider a 72-h period as safe and appropriate. Further recommendations are found in Table 5.

Operative treatment

Historically, abdominal exploration through laparotomy has been the standard treatment for adhesive small bowel obstruction. In recent years, however, laparoscopic surgery for ASBO has been introduced. The potential benefits of laparoscopy include less extensive adhesion (re)formation, earlier return of bowel movements, reduced post-operative pain, and shorter length of stay [81–83]. In a recent systematic review and meta-analysis of 14 non-randomized studies, laparoscopic adhesiolysis reduced risk of morbidity, in-hospital mortality, and surgical infections [84]. However, there also seems strong selection bias in these series allocating mainly the less severe cases to laparoscopy. In a questionnaire among surgeons, 60% of the respondents reported to have performed laparoscopic adhesiolysis for ASBO in their practice, but half of them in less than 15% of cases [11].

Although laparoscopy might provide some benefits to some patients for ASBO, surgeons should carefully select candidates for laparoscopic treatment. Laparoscopy in an abdomen with very distended loops of bowel and multiple complex adhesions could increase the risk of severe complications such as enterotomies and delayed diagnosis of perforations [85, 86]. Indeed, some authors have reported bowel injury in 6.3 to 26.9% of patients treated with laparoscopic adhesiolysis for ASBO [87–89]. In a recent population-based study, bowel resections were significantly more frequent in laparoscopic surgery. Incidence of bowel resection was 53.5 versus 43.4% in laparoscopic versus open procedures [90]. Farinella et al. reported that predictors for a successful laparoscopic treatment of ASBO are the following: ≤ 2 laparotomies in history, appendectomy as the operation in history, no previous median laparotomy incision, and a single adhesive band [91]. Laparoscopic adhesiolysis also seems more difficult in patients who have previously been treated by radiotherapy [92].

More compelling evidence on the role of laparoscopy in surgery for ASBO is from an ongoing randomized trial and is still awaited [93]. In this trial, strict inclusion and exclusion criteria have been used to select candidates in whom simple single band adhesions are expected.

Operative management: summary

Laparoscopic surgery has been introduced in recent years and might decrease morbidity in subgroups of patients undergoing surgery for ASBO. The risk of bowel injuries seems higher in laparoscopic surgery for ASBO. Therefore, careful selection of patients for laparoscopic surgery is required. Further recommendations are found in Table 5.

Special patient groups

Young patients

The risk of adhesion-related complications is life-long. Although most small bowel obstructions will occur within the first 2 years after surgery, new cases continue to develop many years after the primary operation [1, 30, 72, 94, 95]. Also, the risk of requiring a future reoperation for unrelated causes is higher in younger patients [96]. Pediatric patients, who are at the extreme of young age, have a high risk for adhesion-related complications [1]. In a recent cohort of patients who underwent surgery at a pediatric age, the incidence of adhesive small bowel obstruction was 12.6% after a median follow-up of 14.7 years [29].

Young patients therefore might have the highest lifetime benefit from adhesion prevention [49]. No trials with adhesion barriers have been performed in pediatric surgery, but a recent cohort study in pediatric patients showed a significant reduction in ASBO with the use of a hyaluronate carboxymethylcellulose adhesion barrier [97]. After a follow-up of 24 months, 2.0% of pediatric patients operated with adhesion barrier versus 4.5% of patients operated on without adhesion barrier developed ASBO.

Elderly patients

In elderly patients, quality of life considerations are extremely important in decision making. Patients with a high frailty index have a prolonged recovery after a surgical procedure and may not be able to return to their previous functional state and quality of life [98, 99].

The principles of treatment for adhesive small bowel obstruction might interfere with comorbidities and medication in the elderly patients. There is a marked paucity of research on the consequences of stopping or withholding oral medications when a patient is put on *nil* per os for non-operative treatment of small bowel obstruction. A recent cohort showed that patients with diabetes might require earlier intervention although the level of evidence is rather low. Patients with diabetes were shown to suffer from a 7.5% incidence of acute kidney injury and 4.8% incidence of myocardial infarction if the operation was delayed more than 24 h [100]. The incidence of these complications was significantly higher when compared to diabetic patients that were operated within 24 h and non-diabetic patients with delayed operation.

Pregnancy

Small bowel obstruction in pregnancy is very rare but represents an important clinical challenge with significant risk of fetal loss. In a recent review, 46 cases of bowel obstruction during pregnancy were found in literature from case series and case reports [101]. Approximately half of cases were attributed to adhesions, most commonly from previous abdominal operations. Imaging studies performed to diagnose SBO in the case reports included ultrasound in ten cases (83%), abdominal X-ray in four patients (33%), MRI in four patients (33%), and a CT scan in three patients (25%). Strikingly, the failure rate of non-operative treatment in pregnant patients with ASBO was high. A total of 23 cases with ASBO were reported, in 17 of whom initial management was by a non-operative trial. Non-operative treatment failed in 16 cases (94%). Risk of fetal loss was 17% ($n = 8$) and risk of maternal death 2% ($n = 1$).

Conclusions

The conclusions and recommendations of this guideline have been summarized in Table 5. ASBO is a common surgical emergency, causing high morbidity and even some mortality. Surgeons should be aware that the adhesions causing such bowel obstructions are typically the footprints of previous abdominal surgical procedures or disease. Part of the adhesion formation can be prevented by application of minimal invasive surgical techniques and the use of adhesion barriers. Most cases of ASBO can be treated non-operatively. If operative treatment is required, a laparoscopic approach might be beneficial for simple cases. However, there is a considerable risk for conversion to an open laparotomy and care needs to be taken not to make bowel injury.

Authors' contributions

RtB, PK, and SdS performed the search for relevant literature, graded the level of evidence of available literature, contributed to the conception of the draft, contributed with important scientific knowledge, and gave the final approval of the manuscript. FCo, WB, LA, GV, MS, GF, MK, FM, AB, AL, EM, JJ, YK, MS, AB, CB, IC, RC, MdM, PF, KI, RI, RL, JK, AK, RM, SR, BS, TS, KS, DW, IW, FAZ, NdA, RP, JM, and FCa contributed to the manuscript draft, critically revised the manuscript, contributed with important scientific knowledge, and gave the final approval of the manuscript. HvG supervised the literature study, contributed to the conception of the draft, critically revised the manuscript, contributed with important scientific knowledge, and gave the final approval of the manuscript. All authors read and approved the final manuscript.

Competing interests

The authors declare that they have no competing interests.

Author details

[1]Department of Surgery, Radboud University Medical Center, Nijmegen, The Netherlands. [2]Addenbrooke's Hospital, Cambridge, UK. [3]General Emergency and Trauma Surgery, Bufalini hospital, Cesena, Italy. [4]Acute Care Surgery, The Queen's Medical Center, Honolulu, Hawaii, USA. [5]Department of Trauma, Emergency Surgery and Surgical Critical Care, Massachusetts General Hospital, Boston, MA, USA. [6]Department of Surgery, Macerata Hospital, Macerata, Italy. [7]Faculdade de Ciências Médicas (FCM), Unicamp Campinas, São Paulo, Brazil. [8]Albury Hospital, Albury, NSW, Australia. [9]University of Florida, Gainesville, USA. [10]Department of Surgery, Trauma and Surgical Services, University of Pittsburgh School of Medicine, Pittsburgh, USA. [11]Second Department of Surgery, Meilahti Hospital, Helsinki, Finland. [12]Trauma Surgery, Denver Health, Denver, CO, USA. [13]Erasmus MC, Rotterdam, The Netherlands. [14]Division of General Surgery Rambam Health Care Campus Haifa, Haifa, Israel. [15]General Surgery Department, Letterkenny Hospital, Letterkenny, Ireland. [16]Department of Traumatology, John Hunter Hospital and University of Newcastle, Newcastle, NSW, Australia. [17]John Hunter Hospital, New Lambton Heights, New Zealand. [18]Department of Vascular and Trauma Surgery, Auckland City Hospital, Auckland, New Zealand. [19]Department of Surgery, UC San Diego Health System, San Diego, USA. [20]Trauma, Acute Care Surgery Medical College of Wisconsin/Froedtert Trauma Center Milwaukee, Milwaukee, Wisconsin, USA. [21]Virginia Commonwealth University, Richmond, VA, USA. [22]Division of Trauma & Critical Care, LAC+USC Medical Center, University of Southern California, Los Angeles, CA, USA. [23]Department of General Surgery, Westchester Medical Center, Westchester, NY, USA. [24]Department of General Surgery, Assuta Medical Centers, Tel Aviv, Israel. [25]Department of Surgery, Foothills Medical Centre, Calgary, Canada. [26]Department of Surgery, Harborview Medical Centre, Seattle, USA. [27]Trauma & Acute Care Service, St Michael's Hospital, Toronto, ON, Canada. [28]Department of General Surgery, University of Medicine Plovdiv, Plovdiv, Bulgaria. [29]R Adams Crowley Shock Trauma Center, University of Maryland, Baltimore, USA. [30]Department of Gastrointestinal Surgery, Stavanger University Hospital, Stavanger, Norway. [31]Department of Clinical Medicine, University of Bergen, Bergen, Norway. [32]Department of General Surgery, Royal Perth Hospital, The University of Western Australia and The University of Newcastle, Perth, Australia. [33]Department of Surgery, Sheri-Kashmir Institute of Medical Sciences, Srinagar, India. [34]Department of Surgery, College of Medicine and Health Sciences, UAE University, Al-Ain, United Arab Emirates. [35]Unit of Digestive Surgery, HPB Surgery and Liver Transplant, Henri Mondor Hospital, Créteil, France. [36]Canberra Hospital, Canberra, Australia. [37]Trauma and Acute Care Surgery and Surgical Critical Care Trauma, Department of Surgery, University of California, Davis, USA. [38]Emergency and Trauma Surgery, Parma Maggiore hospital, Parma, Italy. [39]Department of Surgery, Radboud University Nijmegen Medical Centre, P.O. Box 9101, 6500 HB Nijmegen, The Netherlands.

References

1. Ten Broek RP, Issa Y, van Santbrink EJ, Bouvy ND, Kruitwagen RF, Jeekel J, et al. Burden of adhesions in abdominal and pelvic surgery: systematic review and met-analysis. BMJ. 2013;347:f5588.
2. NELA Project Team. The second patient report of the National Emergency Laparotomy Audit (NELA). London: The Royal College of Anaesthetists; 2016.
3. Scott JW, Olufajo OA, Brat GA, Rose JA, Zogg CK, Haider AH, et al. Use of national burden to define operative emergency general surgery. JAMA Surg. 2016;151(6):e160480.
4. Gale SC, Shafi S, Dombrovskiy VY, Arumugam D, Crystal JS. The public health burden of emergency general surgery in the United States: a 10-year analysis of the nationwide inpatient sample—2001 to 2010. J Trauma Acute Care Surg. 2014;77(2):202–8.
5. Kossi JA, Salminen PT, Laato MK. Surgical workload and cost of postoperative adhesion-related intestinal obstruction: importance of previous surgery. World J Surg. 2004;28(7):666–70.
6. Shih SC, Jeng KS, Lin SC, Kao CR, Chou SY, Wang HY, et al. Adhesive small bowel obstruction: how long can patients tolerate conservative treatment. World J Gastroenterol. 2003;9(3):603–5.
7. Parikh JA, Ko CY, Maggard MA, Zingmond DS. What is the rate of small bowel obstruction after colectomy? Am Surg. 2008 October;74(10):1001–5.
8. Shikata J, Ohtaki K, Amino K, Takeda Y. Nationwide investigations of intestinal obstruction in Japan. Jpn J Surg. 1990;20(6):660–4.
9. Pricolo VE, Curley F. CT scan findings do not predict outcome of nonoperative management in small bowel obstruction: retrospective analysis of 108 consecutive patients. Int J Surg. 2016;27:88–91.
10. Musiienko AM, Shakerian R, Gorelik A, Thomson BN, Skandarajah AR. Impact of introduction of an acute surgical unit on management and outcomes of small bowel obstruction. ANZ J Surg. 2016;86(10):831–5.
11. Di Saverio S, Coccolini F, Galati M, Smerieri N, Biffl WL, Ansaloni L, et al. Bologna guidelines for diagnosis and management of adhesive small bowel obstruction (ASBO): 2013 update of the evidence-based guidelines from the world society of emergency surgery ASBO working group. World J Emerg Surg. 2013;8(1):42.
12. Krielen P, van den Beukel BA, Stommel MW, Van GH, Strik C, Ten Broek RP. In-hospital costs of an admission for adhesive small bowel obstruction. World J Emerg Surg. 2016;11:49.
13. Catena F, Di SS, Kelly MD, Biffl WL, Ansaloni L, Mandala V, et al. Bologna guidelines for diagnosis and management of adhesive small bowel obstruction (ASBO): 2010 evidence-based guidelines of the World Society of Emergency Surgery. World J Emerg Surg. 2011;6:5.
14. Guyatt GH, Oxman AD, Kunz R, Vist GE, Falck-Ytter Y, Schunemann HJ. What is "quality of evidence" and why is it important to clinicians? BMJ. 2008; 336(7651):995–8.
15. Guyatt GH, Oxman AD, Kunz R, Falck-Ytter Y, Vist GE, Liberati A, et al. Going from evidence to recommendations. BMJ. 2008;336(7652):1049–51.
16. Duron JJ. Postoperative intraperitoneal adhesion pathophysiology. Color Dis. 2007;9(Suppl 2):14–24.
17. Kvaskoff M, Mu F, Terry KL, Harris HR, Poole EM, Farland L, et al. Endometriosis: a high-risk population for major chronic diseases? Hum Reprod Update. 2015;21(4):500–16.
18. Swank DJ, Swank-Bordewijk SC, Hop WC, van Erp WF, Janssen IM, Bonjer HJ, et al. Laparoscopic adhesiolysis in patients with chronic abdominal pain: a blinded randomised controlled multi-centre trial. Lancet. 2003;361(9365): 1247–51.
19. van den Beukel BA, de Ree R, van Leuven S, Bakkum EA, Strik C, Van Goor H, et al. Surgical treatment of adhesion-related chronic abdominal and pelvic pain after gynaecological and general surgery: a systematic review and meta-analysis. Hum Reprod Update. 2017;23(3):276–88.
20. Catena F, Ansaloni L, Di Saverio S, Pinna AD. P.O.P.A. study: prevention of postoperative abdominal adhesions by icodextrin 4% solution after laparotomy for adhesive small bowel obstruction. A prospective randomized controlled trial. J Gastrointest Surg. 2012;16(2):382–8.
21. Agresta F, Piazza A, Michelet I, Bedin N, Sartori CA. Small bowel obstruction. Laparoscopic approach. Surg Endosc. 2000;14(2):154–6.
22. Chowbey PK, Panse R, Sharma A, Khullar R, Soni V, Baijal M. Elective laparoscopy in diagnosis and treatment of recurrent small bowel obstruction. Surg Laparosc Endosc Percutan Tech. 2006;16(6):416–22.
23. Grassi R, Romano S, D'Amario F, Giorgio RA, Romano L, Pinto F, et al. The relevance of free fluid between intestinal loops detected by sonography in the clinical assessment of small bowel obstruction in adults. Eur J Radiol. 2004;50(1):5–14.
24. Nieuwenhuijzen M, Reijnen MM, Kuijpers JH, Van GH. Small bowel obstruction after total or subtotal colectomy: a 10-year retrospective review. Br J Surg. 1998;85(9):1242–5.
25. Zerey M, Sechrist CW, Kercher KW, Sing RF, Matthews BD, Heniford BT. The laparoscopic management of small-bowel obstruction. Am J Surg. 2007; 194(6):882–7.
26. Montz FJ. Small bowel obstruction following radical hysterectomy: risk factors, incidence, and operative findings. Gynecol Oncol. 1994;53(1):114–20.
27. Ellis H, Moran BJ, Thompson JN, Parker MC, Wilson MS, Menzies D, et al. Adhesion-related hospital readmissions after abdominal and pelvic surgery: a retrospective cohort study. Lancet. 1999;353(9163):1476–80.

28. Lower AM, Hawthorn RJ, Clark D, Boyd JH, Finlayson AR, Knight AD, et al. Adhesion-related readmissions following gynaecological laparoscopy or laparotomy in Scotland: an epidemiological study of 24 046 patients. Hum Reprod. 2004;19(8):1877–85.
29. Fredriksson F, Christofferson RH, Lilja HE. Adhesive small bowel obstruction after laparotomy during infancy. Br J Surg. 2016;103(3):284–9.
30. Foster NM, McGory ML, Zingmond DS, Ko CY. Small bowel obstruction: a population-based appraisal. J Am Coll Surg. 2006;203(2):170–6.
31. Zühlke HV, Lorenz EMP, Straub EM, Savvas V. Pathophysiology and classification of adhesions. Langenbecks Archiv fur Chirurgie. 1990:1009–16.
32. The American Fertility Society. The American Fertility Society classifications of adnexal adhesions, distal tubal occlusion, tubal occlusion secondary to tubal ligation, tubal pregnancies, mullerian anomalies and intrauterine adhesions. Fertil Steril. 1988;49(6):944–955.
33. The American Fertility Society. Improvement of interobserver reproducibility of adhesion scoring systems. Adhesion scoring group. Fertil Steril. 1994; 62(5):984–8.
34. Johns DB, Keyport GM, Hoehler F, diZerega GS. Reduction of postsurgical adhesions with Intergel adhesion prevention solution: a multicenter study of safety and efficacy after conservative gynecologic surgery. Fertil Steril. 2001;76(3):595–604.
35. Coccolini F, Ansaloni L, Manfredi R, Campanati L, Poiasina E, Bertoli P, et al. Peritoneal adhesion index (PAI): proposal of a score for the "ignored iceberg" of medicine and surgery. World J Emerg Surg. 2013;8(1):6.
36. Fugazzola P, Coccolini F, Nita GE, Montori G, Corman M, Adeskunkanmi AR, et al. Validation of peritoneal adhesion index as a standardized classification to universalize peritoneal adhesions definition. J Peritoneum (and other serosal surfaces). 2017;2:61–9.
37. Zielinski MD, Eiken PW, Heller SF, Lohse CM, Huebner M, Sarr MG, et al. Prospective, observational validation of a multivariate small-bowel obstruction model to predict the need for operative intervention. J Am Coll Surg. 2011;212(6):1068–76.
38. Baghdadi YMK, Morris DS, Choudhry AJ, Thiels CA, Khasawneh MA, Polites SF, et al. Validation of the anatomic severity score developed by the American Association for the Surgery of Trauma in small bowel obstruction. J Surg Res. 2016;204(2):428–34.
39. Yamada T, Okabayashi K, Hasegawa H, Tsuruta M, Yoo JH, Seishima R, et al. Meta-analysis of the risk of small bowel obstruction following open or laparoscopic colorectal surgery. Br J Surg. 2016;103(5):493–503.
40. Luijendijk RW, de L, Wauters CC, Hop WC, Duron JJ, Pailler JL, et al. Foreign material in postoperative adhesions. Ann Surg. 1996;223(3):242–8.
41. Schreinemacher MH, Emans PJ, Gijbels MJ, Greve JW, Beets GL, Bouvy ND. Degradation of mesh coatings and intraperitoneal adhesion formation in an experimental model. Br J Surg. 2009;96(3):305–13.
42. Ten Broek RP, Wilbers J, van Goor H. Electrocautery causes more ischemic peritoneal tissue damage than ultrasonic dissection. Surg Endosc. 2011; 25(6):1827–34.
43. Ten Broek RP, Kok-Krant N, Bakkum EA, Bleichrodt RP, van Goor H. Different surgical techniques to reduce post-operative adhesion formation: a systematic review and meta-analysis. Hum Reprod Update. 2013;19(1):12–25.
44. Kayaoglu HA, Ozkan N, Yenidogan E, Koseoglu RD. Effect of antibiotic lavage in adhesion prevention in bacterial peritonitis. Ulus Travma Acil Cerrahi Derg. 2013;19(3):189–94.
45. Wang XC, Gui CQ, Zheng QS. Combined therapy of allantoin, metronidazole, dexamethasone on the prevention of intra-abdominal adhesion in dogs and its quantitative analysis. World J Gastroenterol. 2003;9(3):568–71.
46. Fazio VW, Cohen Z, Fleshman JW, Van GH, Bauer JJ, Wolff BG, et al. Reduction in adhesive small-bowel obstruction by Seprafilm adhesion barrier after intestinal resection. Dis Colon Rectum. 2006;49(1):1–11.
47. Kusunoki M, Ikeuchi H, Yanagi H, Noda M, Tonouchi H, Mohri Y, et al. Bioresorbable hyaluronate-carboxymethylcellulose membrane (Seprafilm) in surgery for rectal carcinoma: a prospective randomized clinical trial. Surg Today. 2005;35(11):940–5.
48. Park CM, Lee WY, Cho YB, Yun HR, Lee WS, Yun SH, et al. Sodium hyaluronate-based bioresorbable membrane (Seprafilm) reduced early postoperative intestinal obstruction after lower abdominal surgery for colorectal cancer: the preliminary report. Int J Color Dis. 2009;24(3):305–10.
49. Ten Broek RP, Bakkum EA, Laarhoven CJ, van Goor H. Epidemiology and prevention of postsurgical adhesions revisited. Ann Surg. 2016;263(1):12–9.
50. Trew G, Pistofidis G, Pados G, Lower A, Mettler L, Wallwiener D, et al. Gynaecological endoscopic evaluation of 4% icodextrin solution: a European, multicentre, double-blind, randomized study of the efficacy and safety in the reduction of de novo adhesions after laparoscopic gynaecological surgery. Hum Reprod. 2011;26(8):2015–27.
51. Menzies D, Pascual MH, Walz MK, Duron JJ, Tonelli F, Crowe A, et al. Use of icodextrin 4% solution in the prevention of adhesion formation following general surgery: from the multicentre ARIEL registry. Ann R Coll Surg Engl. 2006;88(4):375–82.
52. Ten Broek RP, Stommel MW, Strik C, van Laarhoven CJ, Keus F, van Goor H. Benefits and harms of adhesion barriers for abdominal surgery: a systematic review and meta-analysis. Lancet. 2014;383(9911):48–59.
53. Ellis H, Crowe A. Medico-legal consequences of post-operative intra-abdominal adhesions. Int J Surg. 2009;7(3):187–91.
54. Choudhry AJ, Haddad NN, Rivera M, Morris DS, Zietlow SP, Schiller HJ, et al. Medical malpractice in the management of small bowel obstruction: a 33-year review of case law. Surgery. 2016;160(4):1017–27.
55. Laurell H, Hansson LE, Gunnarsson U. Acute abdominal pain among elderly patients. Gerontology. 2006;52(6):339–44.
56. Krause WR, Webb TP. Geriatric small bowel obstruction: an analysis of treatment and outcomes compared with a younger cohort. Am J Surg. 2015;209(2):347–51.
57. Sarr MG, Bulkley GB, Zuidema GD. Preoperative recognition of intestinal strangulation obstruction. Prospective evaluation of diagnostic capability. Am J Surg. 1983;145(1):176–82.
58. Loftus T, Moore F, VanZant E, Bala T, Brakenridge S, Croft C, et al. A protocol for the management of adhesive small bowel obstruction. J Trauma Acute Care Surg. 2015;78(1):13–9.
59. Maglinte DD, Reyes BL, Harmon BH, Kelvin FM, Turner WW Jr, Hage JE, et al. Reliability and role of plain film radiography and CT in the diagnosis of small-bowel obstruction. AJR Am J Roentgenol. 1996;167(6):1451–5.
60. Daneshmand S, Hedley CG, Stain SC. The utility and reliability of computed tomography scan in the diagnosis of small bowel obstruction. Am Surg. 1999;65(10):922–6.
61. Hefny AF, Corr P, Abu-Zidan FM. The role of ultrasound in the management of intestinal obstruction. J Emerg Trauma Shock. 2012;5(1):84–6.
62. Ceresoli M, Coccolini F, Catena F, Montori G, Di SS, Sartelli M, et al. Water-soluble contrast agent in adhesive small bowel obstruction: a systematic review and meta-analysis of diagnostic and therapeutic value. Am J Surg. 2016;211(6):1114–25.
63. Branco BC, Barmparas G, Schnuriger B, Inaba K, Chan LS, Demetriades D. Systematic review and meta-analysis of the diagnostic and therapeutic role of water-soluble contrast agent in adhesive small bowel obstruction. Br J Surg. 2010;97(4):470–8.
64. Abbas S, Bissett IP, Parry BR. Oral water soluble contrast for the management of adhesive small bowel obstruction. Cochrane Database Syst Rev. 2005;1:CD004651.
65. Goussous N, Eiken PW, Bannon MP, Zielinski MD. Enhancement of a small bowel obstruction model using the gastrografin(R) challenge test. J Gastrointest Surg. 2013;17(1):110–6.
66. Zielinski MD, Eiken PW, Bannon MP, Heller SF, Lohse CM, Huebner M, et al. Small bowel obstruction-who needs an operation? A multivariate prediction model. World J Surg. 2010;34(5):910–9.
67. Makita O, Ikushima I, Matsumoto N, Arikawa K, Yamashita Y, Takahashi M. CT differentiation between necrotic and nonnecrotic small bowel in closed loop and strangulating obstruction. Abdom Imaging. 1999;24(2): 120–4.
68. Zalcman M, Sy M, Donckier V, Closset J, Gansbeke DV. Helical CT signs in the diagnosis of intestinal ischemia in small-bowel obstruction. AJR Am J Roentgenol. 2000;175(6):1601–7.
69. Abu-Zidan FM. Optimizing the value of measuring inferior vena cava diameter in shocked patients. World J Crit Care Med. 2016;5(1):7–11.
70. Abu-Zidan FM, Abdel-Kader S, Abusharia MI, Mousa H. Role of magnetic resonance imaging in the management of intestinal obstruction during the first trimester of pregnancy. ANZ J Surg. 2016;
71. Fevang BT, Jensen D, Svanes K, Viste A. Early operation or conservative management of patients with small bowel obstruction? Eur J Surg. 2002; 168(8–9):475–81.
72. Fevang BT, Fevang J, Lie SA, Soreide O, Svanes K, Viste A. Long-term prognosis after operation for adhesive small bowel obstruction. Ann Surg. 2004;240(2):193–201.
73. Ten Broek RP, Strik C, Issa Y, Bleichrodt RP, van Goor H. Adhesiolysis-related morbidity in abdominal surgery. Ann Surg. 2013;258(1):98–106.

74. Jeppesen M, Tolstrup MB, Gogenur I. Chronic pain, quality of life, and functional impairment after surgery due to small bowel obstruction. World J Surg. 2016;40(9):2091–7.
75. Fazel MZ, Jamieson RW, Watson CJ. Long-term follow-up of the use of the Jones' intestinal tube in adhesive small bowel obstruction. Ann R Coll Surg Engl. 2009;91(1):50–4.
76. Schraufnagel D, Rajaee S, Millham FH. How many sunsets? Timing of surgery in adhesive small bowel obstruction: a study of the nationwide inpatient sample. J Trauma Acute Care Surg. 2013;74(1):181–7.
77. Fleshner PR, Siegman MG, Slater GI, Brolin RE, Chandler JC, Aufses AH Jr. A prospective, randomized trial of short versus long tubes in adhesive small-bowel obstruction. Am J Surg. 1995;170(4):366–70.
78. Chen XL, Ji F, Lin Q, Chen YP, Lin JJ, Ye F, et al. A prospective randomized trial of transnasal ileus tube vs nasogastric tube for adhesive small bowel obstruction. World J Gastroenterol. 2012;18(16):1968–74.
79. Keenan JE, Turley RS, McCoy CC, Migaly J, Shapiro ML, Scarborough JE. Trials of nonoperative management exceeding 3 days are associated with increased morbidity in patients undergoing surgery for uncomplicated adhesive small bowel obstruction. J Trauma Acute Care Surg. 2014;76(6): 1367–72.
80. Sakakibara T, Harada A, Yaguchi T, Koike M, Fujiwara M, Kodera Y, et al. The indicator for surgery in adhesive small bowel obstruction patient managed with long tube. Hepatogastroenterology. 2007;54(75):787–90.
81. Nordin A, Freedman J. Laparoscopic versus open surgical management of small bowel obstruction: an analysis of clinical outcomes. Surg Endosc. 2016;30(10):4454–63.
82. Szomstein S, Lo ME, Simpfendorfer C, Zundel N, Rosenthal RJ. Laparoscopic lysis of adhesions. World J Surg. 2006;30(4):535–40.
83. Hackenberg T, Mentula P, Leppaniemi A, Sallinen V. Laparoscopic versus open surgery for acute adhesive small-bowel obstruction: a propensity score-matched analysis. Scand J Surg. 2017;106(1):28–33.
84. Sajid MS, Khawaja AH, Sains P, Singh KK, Baig MK. A systematic review comparing laparoscopic vs open adhesiolysis in patients with adhesional small bowel obstruction. Am J Surg. 2016;212(1):138–50.
85. Strik C, Stommel MW, Ten Broek RP, Van GH. Adhesiolysis in patients undergoing a repeat median laparotomy. Dis Colon Rectum. 2015;58(8): 792–8.
86. Ten Broek RP, Strik C, Van GH. Preoperative nomogram to predict risk of bowel injury during adhesiolysis. Br J Surg. 2014;101(6):720–7.
87. Grafen FC, Neuhaus V, Schob O, Turina M. Management of acute small bowel obstruction from intestinal adhesions: indications for laparoscopic surgery in a community teaching hospital. Langenbeck's Arch Surg. 2010; 395(1):57–63.
88. Wullstein C, Gross E. Laparoscopic compared with conventional treatment of acute adhesive small bowel obstruction. Br J Surg. 2003;90(9):1147–51.
89. Johnson KN, Chapital AB, Harold KL, Merritt MV, Johnson DJ. Laparoscopic management of acute small bowel obstruction: evaluating the need for resection. J Trauma Acute Care Surg. 2012;72(1):25–30.
90. Behman R, Nathens AB, Byrne JP, Mason S, Look HN, Karanicolas PJ. Laparoscopic surgery for adhesive small bowel obstruction is associated with a higher risk of bowel injury: a population-based analysis of 8584 patients. Ann Surg. 2017;266(3):489–98.
91. Farinella E, Cirocchi R, La MF, Morelli U, Cattorini L, Delmonaco P, et al. Feasibility of laparoscopy for small bowel obstruction. World J Emerg Surg. 2009;4:3.
92. Nakamura T, Ishii Y, Tsutsui A, Kaneda M, Sato T, Watanabe M. Safety and indications of laparoscopic surgery for postoperative small-bowel obstruction: a single-center study of 121 patients. Surg Laparosc Endosc Percutan Tech. 2017;27(4):301–5.
93. Sallinen V, Wikstrom H, Victorzon M, Salminen P, Koivukangas V, Haukijarvi E, et al. Laparoscopic versus open adhesiolysis for small bowel obstruction—a multicenter, prospective, randomized, controlled trial. BMC Surg. 2014;14:77.
94. Duron JJ, Silva NJ, du Montcel ST, Berger A, Muscari F, Hennet H, et al. Adhesive postoperative small bowel obstruction: incidence and risk factors of recurrence after surgical treatment: a multicenter prospective study. Ann Surg. 2006;244(5):750–7.
95. Parker MC, Ellis H, Moran BJ, Thompson JN, Wilson MS, Menzies D, et al. Postoperative adhesions: ten-year follow-up of 12,584 patients undergoing lower abdominal surgery. Dis Colon Rectum. 2001;44(6):822–9.
96. Strik C, Stommel MW, Schipper LJ, Van GH, Ten Broek RP. Risk factors for future repeat abdominal surgery. Langenbeck's Arch Surg. 2016;401(6):829–37.
97. Inoue M, Uchida K, Otake K, Nagano Y, Ide S, Hashimoto K, et al. Efficacy of Seprafilm for preventing adhesive bowel obstruction and cost-benefit analysis in pediatric patients undergoing laparotomy. J Pediatr Surg. 2013; 48(7):1528–34.
98. Bruce J, Krukowski ZH. Quality of life and chronic pain four years after gastrointestinal surgery. Dis Colon Rectum. 2006;49(9):1362–70.
99. Bakker FC, Persoon A, Bredie SJ, van Haren-Willems J, Leferink VJ, Noyez L, et al. The CareWell in hospital program to improve the quality of care for frail elderly inpatients: results of a before-after study with focus on surgical patients. Am J Surg. 2014;208(5):735–46.
100. Karamanos E, Dulchavsky S, Beale E, Inaba K, Demetriades D. Diabetes mellitus in patients presenting with adhesive small bowel obstruction: delaying surgical intervention results in worse outcomes. World J Surg. 2016;40(4):863–9.
101. Webster PJ, Bailey MA, Wilson J, Burke DA. Small bowel obstruction in pregnancy is a complex surgical problem with a high risk of fetal loss. Ann R Coll Surg Engl. 2015;97(5):339–44.

22

The *Global Alliance for Infections in Surgery*: defining a model for antimicrobial stewardship

Massimo Sartelli[1*], Francesco M. Labricciosa[2], Pamela Barbadoro[2], Leonardo Pagani[3], Luca Ansaloni[4], Adrian J. Brink[5,6], Jean Carlet[7], Ashish Khanna[8], Alain Chichom-Mefire[9], Federico Coccolini[10], Salomone Di Saverio[11], Addison K. May[12], Pierluigi Viale[13], Richard R. Watkins[14,15], Luigia Scudeller[16], Lilian M. Abbo[17], Fikri M. Abu-Zidan[18], Abdulrashid K. Adesunkanmi[19], Sara Al-Dahir[20], Majdi N. Al-Hasan[21], Halil Alis[22], Carlos Alves[23], André R. Araujo da Silva[24], Goran Augustin[25], Miklosh Bala[26], Philip S. Barie[27], Marcelo A. Beltrán[28], Aneel Bhangu[29], Belefquih Bouchra[30], Stephen M. Brecher[31,32], Miguel A. Caínzos[33], Adrian Camacho-Ortiz[34], Marco Catani[35], Sujith J. Chandy[36], Asri Che Jusoh[37], Jill R. Cherry-Bukowiec[38], Osvaldo Chiara[39], Elif Colak[40], Oliver A. Cornely[41], Yunfeng Cui[42], Zaza Demetrashvili[43], Belinda De Simone[44], Jan J. De Waele[45], Sameer Dhingra[46,47], Francesco Di Marzo[48], Agron Dogjani[49], Gereltuya Dorj[50], Laurent Dortet[51], Therese M. Duane[52], Mutasim M. Elmangory[53], Mushira A. Enani[54], Paula Ferrada[55], J. Esteban Foianini[56], Mahir Gachabayov[57], Chinmay Gandhi[58], Wagih Mommtaz Ghnnam[59], Helen Giamarellou[60], Georgios Gkiokas[61], Harumi Gomi[62], Tatjana Goranovic[63], Ewen A. Griffiths[64], Rosio I. Guerra Gronerth[65], Julio C. Haidamus Monteiro[66], Timothy C. Hardcastle[67], Andreas Hecker[68], Adrien M. Hodonou[69], Orestis Ioannidis[70], Arda Isik[71], Katia A. Iskandar[72], Hossein S. Kafil[73], Souha S. Kanj[74], Lewis J. Kaplan[75], Garima Kapoor[76], Aleksandar R. Karamarkovic[77], Jakub Kenig[78], Ivan Kerschaever[79], Faryal Khamis[80], Vladimir Khokha[81], Ronald Kiguba[82], Hong B. Kim[83], Wen-Chien Ko[84], Kaoru Koike[85], Iryna Kozlovska[86], Anand Kumar[87], Leonel Lagunes[88], Rifat Latifi[89], Jae G. Lee[90], Young R. Lee[91], Ari Leppäniemi[92], Yousheng Li[93], Stephen Y. Liang[94], Warren Lowman[95], Gustavo M. Machain[96], Marc Maegele[97], Piotr Major[98], Sydney Malama[99], Ramiro Manzano-Nunez[100], Athanasios Marinis[101], Isidro Martinez Casas[102], Sanjay Marwah[103], Emilio Maseda[104], Michael E. McFarlane[105], Ziad Memish[106], Dominik Mertz[107], Cristian Mesina[108], Shyam K. Mishra[109], Ernest E. Moore[110], Akutu Munyika[111], Eleftherios Mylonakis[112], Lena Napolitano[113], Ionut Negoi[114], Milica D. Nestorovic[115], David P. Nicolau[116], Abdelkarim H. Omari[117], Carlos A. Ordonez[118], José-Artur Paiva[119], Narayan D. Pant[120], Jose G. Parreira[121], Michal Pędziwiatr[122], Bruno M. Pereira[123], Alfredo Ponce-de-Leon[124], Garyphallia Poulakou[125], Jacobus Preller[126], Céline Pulcini[127], Guntars Pupelis[128], Martha Quiodettis[129], Timothy M. Rawson[130], Tarcisio Reis[131], Miran Rems[132], Sandro Rizoli[133], Jason Roberts[134], Nuno Rocha Pereira[23], Jesús Rodríguez-Baño[135], Boris Sakakushev[136], James Sanders[137], Natalia Santos[138], Norio Sato[139], Robert G. Sawyer[140], Sandro Scarpelini[141], Loredana Scoccia[142], Nusrat Shafiq[143], Vishalkumar Shelat[144], Costi D. Sifri[145], Boonying Siribumrungwong[146], Kjetil Søreide[147,148], Rodolfo Soto[149], Hamilton P. de Souza[150], Peep Talving[151], Ngo Tat Trung[152], Jeffrey M. Tessier[153], Mario Tumbarello[154], Jan Ulrych[155], Selman Uranues[156], Harry Van Goor[157], Andras Vereczkei[158], Florian Wagenlehner[159], Yonghong Xiao[160], Kuo-Ching Yuan[161], Agnes Wechsler-Fördös[162], Jean-Ralph Zahar[163], Tanya L. Zakrison[164], Brian Zuckerbraun[165], Wietse P. Zuidema[166] and Fausto Catena[167]

* Correspondence: m.sartelli@virgilio.it
[1]Department of Surgery, Macerata Hospital, Macerata, Italy
Full list of author information is available at the end of the article

Abstract

Background: Antimicrobial Stewardship Programs (ASPs) have been promoted to optimize antimicrobial usage and patient outcomes, and to reduce the emergence of antimicrobial-resistant organisms. However, the best strategies for an ASP are not definitively established and are likely to vary based on local culture, policy, and routine clinical practice, and probably limited resources in middle-income countries. The aim of this study is to evaluate structures and resources of antimicrobial stewardship teams (ASTs) in surgical departments from different regions of the world.

Methods: A cross-sectional web-based survey was conducted in 2016 on 173 physicians who participated in the AGORA (Antimicrobials: A Global Alliance for Optimizing their Rational Use in Intra-Abdominal Infections) project and on 658 international experts in the fields of ASPs, infection control, and infections in surgery.

Results: The response rate was 19.4%. One hundred fifty-six (98.7%) participants stated their hospital had a multidisciplinary AST. The median number of physicians working inside the team was five [interquartile range 4–6]. An infectious disease specialist, a microbiologist and an infection control specialist were, respectively, present in 80.1, 76.3, and 67.9% of the ASTs. A surgeon was a component in 59.0% of cases and was significantly more likely to be present in university hospitals (89.5%, $p < 0.05$) compared to community teaching (83.3%) and community hospitals (66.7%). Protocols for pre-operative prophylaxis and for antimicrobial treatment of surgical infections were respectively implemented in 96.2 and 82.3% of the hospitals. The majority of the surgical departments implemented both persuasive and restrictive interventions (72.8%). The most common types of interventions in surgical departments were dissemination of educational materials (62.5%), expert approval (61.0%), audit and feedback (55.1%), educational outreach (53.7%), and compulsory order forms (51.5%).

Conclusion: The survey showed a heterogeneous organization of ASPs worldwide, demonstrating the necessity of a multidisciplinary and collaborative approach in the battle against antimicrobial resistance in surgical infections, and the importance of educational efforts towards this goal.

Keywords: Antibiotics, Infections, Surgery, Antimicrobial stewardship

Background

Antimicrobial Stewardship Programs (ASPs) have been promoted to optimize antimicrobial usage and patient outcomes and reduce the emergence of antimicrobial-resistant organisms. However, the best strategies for an ASP are not definitively established and are likely to vary based on local culture, policy and routine clinical practice, and probably limited resources in middle-income countries [1, 2]. Many hospitals remain without formal programs and those that do continue to struggle with gaining acceptance across service lines [3]. Moreover, identifying optimal efforts to impact system change has been challenging [4].

Restriction strategies may be effective at controlling use but raise issues of prescriber autonomy and require a large personnel commitment. Encouraging multidisciplinary collaboration within health systems to ensure that prophylactic, empirical, and targeted use of antimicrobial agents results in optimal patient outcomes is mandatory in the current era of antimicrobial resistance.

A panel of experts from the Surgical Infection Society (SIS) and World Society of Emergency Surgery (WSES) has recently published a review with the aim of defining the role of surgeons within the ASPs. The panel proposed that the best means of improving antimicrobial stewardship in surgical units worldwide should involve collaboration among various specialties within institutions including prescribing clinicians and pharmacists [5].

In 2016, a multidisciplinary task force from 79 different countries joined a global project to develop a consensus on the rational use of antimicrobials for patients with intra-abdominal infections (IAIs). The project has been termed AGORA (Antimicrobials: A Global Alliance for Optimizing their Rational Use in Intra-Abdominal Infections) [1].

Recently the *Global Alliance for Infections in Surgery* was founded and experts from 87 countries worldwide joined the highly diverse and skilled International Advisory Board. This alliance, promoted by the WSES, includes an interdisciplinary group of hospital administrators, epidemiologists, infection control specialists, infectious disease specialists, microbiologists, clinical pharmacologists and hospital pharmacists, surgeons, and intensivists. The mission of this alliance is to educate healthcare providers promoting the standards of care in managing infections in surgery worldwide [6]. Therefore, this study was conducted to evaluate the structure and resources of antimicrobial stewardship teams (ASTs) in surgical departments from different regions of the world.

Methods

We conducted a cross-sectional electronic survey evaluating the structure and resources of ASTs in surgical departments. The survey was designed by a multidisciplinary team of investigators including an epidemiologist, a surgeon, an infectious diseases physician, a pharmacologist, and a microbiologist. The questionnaire was piloted among five physicians for face and content validity.

The 24-item self-administered questionnaire collected information from multidisciplinary experts—mostly physicians—about characteristics and composition of the hospital team, implementation of local procedures, availability of antimicrobial use monitoring and surveillance systems, presence of an ASP, and related interventions (Additional file 1). An electronic invitation with a link to the survey was sent to 831 physicians: 173 physicians who participated in the AGORA project [1], and a large number (658) of international experts in the fields of antimicrobial stewardship, infection control, and infections in surgery identified after a thorough investigation using the PubMed database. The survey was Internet-based (using http://www.docs.google.com). Participation was voluntary but not anonymous; however, the confidentiality of respondents and their choices was ensured. No incentives were provided to the respondents. The study was open for 6 weeks between September 30 and November 11, 2016. Reminders were sent to all those who had not replied after 1 and 3 weeks. Due to the characteristics of the survey, a response rate ranging between 15 and 25% was expected.

Data were entered in an Excel database (Microsoft Corporation, Redmond, Washington, USA) and analyzed using Stata 11.0 software package (StataCorp, College Station, TX). Descriptive analyses included medians and interquartile ranges (IQR) for continuous variables or frequency (%) for categorical variables The two-sided chi-square or Fisher's exact test was used for categorical variables, as appropriate. All tests were two-sided, and p values of 0.05 or lower were considered statistically significant.

Results

Baseline data: coverage, response rate, working setting, and professional profile

A total of 161 (19.4%) of the 831 experts who were contacted by email completed the survey after two reminders. One incomplete survey was excluded from the study. In two cases the participants were from the same institution and only one survey was considered. One hundred fifty-eight responses were included in our analysis. Participants work settings and professional profiles are summarized in Table 1.

The response rate was similar to that of previous studies promoted by WSES [1, 7, 8].

As in the other WSES studies [1, 7, 8], participants were not homogeneously distributed across all geographic regions of the world due to the difficulty in recruiting participants in some areas of the world. However all geographic regions were represented in the survey.

Characteristics of the team

One hundred fifty-six (98.7%) participants stated their hospital had a multidisciplinary AST. Ninety participants (90/156, 57.7%) declared they were currently members of the team, with no difference in frequency between different WHO regions. The median number of physicians working inside the team was five [IQR 4–6]. Characteristics of the team are in Table 2.

One hundred thirty-five (135/158, 85.4%) participants had at least one surgeon with an interest or skills in surgical infections within the surgical department of their hospital; a surgeon was significantly more likely to be present in university hospitals (89.5%, two-sided chi-square test $p < 0.05$) compared to community teaching hospitals (83.3%) and community hospitals (66.7%).

Implementation of protocols and monitoring systems

Implementation of protocols and monitoring systems in 158 hospitals are reported in Table 3.

The vast majority of respondents (152/158, 96.2%) stated that their hospitals have a protocol for pre-operative prophylaxis. The protocol covered all surgical wards in 124 (78.5%) cases. A protocol for antimicrobial treatment of surgical infections was available in 130 (82.3%) hospitals; however, only 70 (44.3%) had it available in every surgical ward. One hundred twenty-eight (81.0%) hospitals had both a protocol for peri-operative prophylaxis and for antimicrobial treatment of surgical infections available, while four (4/158, 2.5%) hospitals lacked both.

Among 130 surgical wards implementing a protocol for antimicrobial treatment of surgical infections, 97 (74.6%) participants stated it included interventions to reduce the duration of therapy, 88 (67.7%) interventions to switch selected antimicrobials from intravenous-to-oral therapy, 78 (60.0%) interventions for alternative dosing strategies based on pharmacokinetics and pharmacodynamics, with significant difference between community hospitals (11.1%, two-sided Fischer's exact test $p < 0.05$) compared to university (57.0%) and community teaching (60.0%) hospitals. Thirty-five (26.9%) participants reported the use of biological markers - such as procalcitonin to decrease antimicrobial use in critically ill patients.

Implementations of ASPs and related interventions

One hundred fifty-five (155/158, 98.1%) participants declared their hospital had an ASP running.

Our survey showed that 30 (19.4%) hospitals have developed persuasive interventions, 17 (11.0%) restrictive interventions and 108 (69.7%) both of them.

Table 1 Participants' working settings and professional profiles

Characteristics	African region $n = 8$	Eastern- Mediterranean region $n = 13$	European region $n = 67$	Region of Americas $n = 47$	South-East Asia region $n = 8$	Western Pacific region $n = 15$	Total $n = 158$
Type of hospital, n (%)							
- University hospital	5 (62.5)	6 (46.1)	50 (74.6)	35 (74.5)	6 (75.0)	12 (80.0)	114 (72.1)
- Community teaching hospital	2 (25.0)	3 (23.1)	14 (20.9)	9 (19.1)	1 (12.5)	1 (6.7)	30 (19.0)
- Community hospital	0	2 (15.4)	3 (4.5)	1 (2.1)	1 (12.5)	2 (13.3)	9 (5.7)
- Other	1 (12.5)	2 (15.4)	0	2 (4.3)	0	0	5 (3.2)
Hospital setting, n (%)							
- Urban	5 (62.5)	10 (76.9)	65 (97.0)	44 (93.6)	6 (75.0)	14 (93.3)	144 (91.1)
- Suburban	3 (37.5)	3 (23.1)	2 (3.0)	1 (2.1)	2 (25.0)	0	11 (7.0)
- Rural	0	0	0	2 (4.3)	0	1 (6.7)	3 (1.9)
Hospital inpatient beds, n (%)							
- ≤100	0	2 (15.4)	3 (4.5)	1 (2.1)	0	0	6 (3.8)
- 101–500	3 (37.5)	5 (38.5)	15 (22.4)	10 (21.3)	2 (25.0)	3 (20.0)	38 (24.1)
- 501–1000	3 (37.5)	5 (38.5)	27 (40.3)	28 (59.6)	3 (37.5)	1 (6.7)	67 (42.4)
- ≥ 1000	2 (25.0)	1 (7.7)	22 (32.8)	8 (17.0)	3 (37.5)	11 (73.3)	47 (29.7)
Profession, n (%)							
Epidemiologist	1 (12.5)	0	2 (3.0)	1 (2.1)	0	0	4 (2.5)
Hospital administrator	0	0	0	0	0	0	0
Clinical pharmacologist	0	1 (7.7)	0	4 (8.5)	1(12.5)	1 (6.7)	7 (4.4)
Hospital pharmacist	0	0	1 (1.5)	1 (2.1)	1 (12.5)	1 (6.7)	4 (2.5)
Infection control specialist	0	0	1 (1.5)	1 (2.1)	0	0	2 (1.3)
Infectious diseases specialist	0	4 (30.8)	10 (14.9)	10 (21.3)	0	5 (33.3)	29 (18.4)
Intensivist	1 (12.5)	0	5 (7.5)	2 (4.3)	0	1 (6.7)	9 (5.7)
Microbiologist	3 (37.5)	3 (23.1)	1 (1.5)	1 (2.1)	3 (37.5)	0	11 (7.0)
Surgeon	3 (37.5)	5 (38.5)	44 (65.7)	24 (51.1)	3 (37.5)	6 (40.0)	85 (53.8)
Other	0	0	3 (4.5)	3 (6.4)	0	1 (6.7)	7 (4.4)

Twenty-three surgical departments (23/136, 16.9%) have developed persuasive interventions, 14 (10.3%) restrictive interventions and 99 (72.8%) both of them.

The most common types of interventions in surgical departments were dissemination of educational materials (62.5%), expert approval (61.0%), audit and feedback (55.1%), educational outreach (53.7%), and compulsory order forms (51.5%).

Types of ASPs and related interventions in surgical departments and in all hospital wards are described in detail in Table 4.

Six (6/41, 14.6%) surgical departments implementing a formulary restriction do not perform any monitoring system of used antimicrobials, and 4 (4/41, 9.8%) do not carry out any systematic reports about resistance data. Furthermore, 6 (7/70, 10.0%) surgical departments using a compulsory order form do not perform any monitoring system of used antimicrobials, and 11 (11/70, 15.7%) do not carry out any systematic reports about resistance data.

One hundred twenty-five (125/158, 79.1%) participants stated their hospital had carried out structural interventions to improve ASPs in the last 5 years. Sixty-nine (43.7%) changed from paper to computerized records, 74 (46.8%) implemented rapid laboratory testing, 32 (20.3%) introduced computerized decision support systems, 69 (43.7%) introduced organization of quality monitoring mechanisms and 29 (18.4%) implemented other structural interventions.

Characteristics of the implementation of protocols, monitoring systems, and ASPs interventions in surgical departments are detailed in Table 5.

Discussion

Antimicrobial stewardship programs (ASP) are a key strategy to curb the spread of antibiotic resistance [3, 9]. The best strategies for an ASP are not definitively established and are likely to vary based on local routine clinical practice [7], despite several guidelines on the topic [9, 10].

Table 2 Characteristics of the team in 156 hospitals

Characteristics	n (%)
Components	
- Epidemiologist	64 (41.0)
- Hospital administrator	73 (46.8)
- Clinical pharmacologist	8 (5.1)
- Hospital pharmacist	95 (60.9)
- Infection control specialist	106 (67.9)
- Infectious disease specialist	125 (80.1)
- Intensivist	76 (48.7)
- Microbiologist	119 (76.3)
- Surgeon	92 (59.0)
- Other	11 (7.1)
- Infectious disease specialist AND hospital pharmacologist/pharmacist	87 (55.8)
Frequency of meetings	
- More than once a week	15 (9.6)
- Once a week	26 (16.7)
- Twice a month	13 (8.3)
- Once a month	58 (37.2)
- Less than once a month	27 (17.3)
- Only as necessary	17 (10.9)

Successful ASPs should focus on collaboration between healthcare professionals in order to share knowledge and best practices. It is essential for an ASP to have at least one member who is an infectious diseases specialist. Pharmacists with advanced training or longstanding clinical experience in infectious diseases are also key actors for the design and implementation of the stewardship program interventions [11]. Infection control specialists and hospital epidemiologists should coordinate efforts on monitoring and preventing healthcare-associated infections and in analyzing and reporting "real-time" data to prevent infections, improve antimicrobial use, and minimize secondary spread of resistance. Microbiologists should actively guide the proper use of tests and the flow of laboratory results. Being involved in providing surveillance data on antimicrobial resistance, they should provide periodic reports on antimicrobial resistance data allowing the multidisciplinary team to determine the ongoing burden of antimicrobial resistance in the hospital. Moreover, timely and accurate reporting of microbiology susceptibility test results allows selection of more appropriate targeted therapy, and may help reduce broad-spectrum antimicrobial use.

Surgeons with adequate knowledge in surgical infections and surgical anatomy when involved in ASPs may audit antibiotic prescriptions, provide feedback to the prescribers and integrate best practices of antimicrobial use among surgeons, and act as champions among colleagues. Although many surgeons are aware of the problem of antimicrobial resistance, most underestimate it in their own hospital [1]. Very few studies have been published on the role of ASPs in general surgical departments. In 2015, Cakmakci [12] suggested that the engagement of surgeons in ASPs might be crucial to their success. In 2013, however, Duane et al. showed poor compliance of surgical services with ASP recommendations [13]. Surgeons need to take part in addressing the global issue of antimicrobial resistance. Failure to do so will be catastrophic to patients and programs [3].

Infections are the main factors contributing to mortality in intensive care units (ICU) [14].

Intensivists have a critical role in treating multidrug resistant organisms in ICUs in critically ill patients. They have a crucial role in prescribing antimicrobial agents for our most challenging patients and are at the forefront of a successful ASP [15].

Finally, without adequate support from hospital administration, the ASP will be inadequate or inconsistent since the programs do not generate revenue [16]. Engagement of hospital administration has been confirmed as a key factor for both developing and sustaining an ASP [17].

In most cases, our survey demonstrated that ASPs do not involve a true multi-disciplinary approach.

An infectious diseases specialist and a hospital pharmacist were part of the team in 125 (80.1%) and in 95 (60.9%) cases, respectively. Only 87 (55.8%) teams included both an infectious diseases specialist and a hospital pharmacist. An infection control specialist and a hospital epidemiologist were part of the team in 106 (67.9%) and in 64 (41.0%) cases, respectively. It is possible that in some hospitals,

Table 3 Implementation of protocols and monitoring systems in 158 hospitals

Implementation of protocols and monitoring systems	All hospital wards n (%)	Some hospital wards, including surgical wards n (%)		Some hospital wards, not including surgical wards n (%)	No hospital wards n (%)
		Every surgical wards	Some surgical wards		
- SAP protocol	NA	124 (78.5)	28 (17.7)	NA	6 (3.8)
- TIS protocol	NA	70 (44.3)	60 (38.0)	NA	28 (17.7)
- UAMS	84 (53.2)	45 (28.5)		9 (5.7)	20 (12.7)
- RDSR	104 (65.8)	26 (16.5)		7 (4.4)	21 (13.3)

SAP Surgical antimicrobial prophylaxis, *TIS* therapy for infections in surgery, *UAMS* used antimicrobial monitoring system, *RDSR* resistance data systematic report

Table 4 Difference in type of ASPs and related implemented types of interventions in surgical departments and non-surgical departments

Characteristics	Surgical departments, $n = 136$ n (%)	Other departments, $n = 19$ n (%)	P value	Total, $n = 155$ n (%)
Type of ASPs				
- Persuasive interventions	23 (16.9)	7 (36.8)	0.06[a]	30 (19.4)
- Restrictive interventions	14 (10.3)	3 (15.8)	0.44[a]	17 (11.0)
- Both	99 (72.8)	9 (47.4)	<0.05	108 (69.7)
Type of interventions				
- Dissemination of educational materials	85 (62.5)	8 (42.1)	0.15	93 (60.0)
- Reminders	56 (41.2)	8 (42.1)	1.00	64 (41.3)
- Audit and feedback	75 (55.1)	4 (21.1)	<0.05	79 (51.0)
- Educational outreach	73 (53.7)	10 (52.6)	1.00	83 (53.6)
- Other persuasive interventions	23 (16.9)	3 (15.8)	1.00[a]	26 (16.8)
- Compulsory order form	70 (51.5)	7 (36.8)	0.34	77 (49.7)
- Expert approval	83 (61.0)	5 (26.3)	<0.05	88 (56.8)
- Restriction by removal	41 (30.1)	2 (10.5)	0.13	43 (27.7)
- Review and make changes	36 (26.5)	1 (5.3)	<0.05[a]	37 (23.9)
- Other restrictive interventions	10 (7.4)	3 (15.8)	0.20[a]	13 (8.4)

All p values were calculated using two-sided chi-square test unless otherwise noted
ASP antimicrobial stewardship program
[a]Calculated using two-sided Fisher's exact test

AMS and infection prevention and control team are two separate entities, which collaborate. A microbiologist was part of the team in 119 (76.3%) cases. A surgeon was part of the team in 92 (59.0%) cases and an intensivist in 76 (48.6%) cases. A hospital administrator was part of the team only in 73 (46.8%) cases. Interestingly a surgeon was significantly more likely to be part of the team in university hospitals (89.5%, two-sided chi-square test $p < 0.05$) compared to community teaching (83.3%) and community non-teaching hospital (66.7%).

Strategies of ASPs should be tailored based on individual hospital characteristics and personnel and resources available. The Infectious Diseases Society of America/ Society for Healthcare Epidemiology of America (IDSA/ SHEA) guidelines identified two core proactive evidence-based strategies and several supplemental strategies for promoting antimicrobial stewardship [7, 8]: first, a restrictive strategy based on a proactive strategy of either formulary restriction or a requirement for pre-approval for specific drugs or both, and second, a persuasive strategy of performing prospective audit with intervention and feedback to the prescriber.

Our survey showed that 23 (16.9%) surgical departments have developed persuasive interventions, 14 (10.3%) restrictive interventions and 99 (72.8%) both of them. ASP policies should be based on both international/national antibiotic guidelines, and tailored to local microbiology and resistance patterns. Local clinical practice guidelines and algorithms can be an effective way to standardize prescribing practices based on the country's epidemiology. Standardizing a shared protocol of antimicrobial prophylaxis should represent the first step of any Antimicrobial Stewardship program.

One hundred fifty-two (96.2%) participants stated their hospitals have a protocol for surgical antibiotic prophylaxis. Among the 158 hospitals, a protocol for antibiotic prophylaxis is present in all surgical wards in 124 (78.5%) of hospitals while only in some surgical wards in 28 (17.7%) hospitals.

A protocol for antibiotic treatment was present in all surgical wards in 70 (44.3%) hospitals, while only in some surgical wards in 60 (38.0%) hospitals. Among 130 hospitals implementing a protocol for antimicrobial treatment of surgical infections, 97 (74.6%) participants stated that it included interventions to reduce the duration of therapy, 88 (67.7%) interventions to switch select antimicrobials from intravenous-to-oral therapy, 78 (60.0%) interventions for alternative dosing strategies based on pharmacokinetic and pharmacodynamic principles, with substantial difference between community hospitals (11.1%, two-sided Fischer's exact test $p < 0.05$), university (57.0%) and community teaching (60.0%) ones. Thirty-five (26.9%) participants admitted to the use of biological markers - such as procalcitonin - to decrease antimicrobial use in critically ill patients.

In any healthcare setting, a significant amount of time and energy should be spent on infection control. Surveillance studies can help clinicians to identify trends in

Table 5 Implementation of protocols, monitoring systems and ASPs interventions in surgical departments related to working setting and team components

Variables	PAP protocol implemented n. (%), p	TIS protocol implemented n. (%), p	Monitoring system of used antimicrobials n. (%), p	Resistance data systematic reports n. (%), p	ASP implemented n. (%), p	Structural intervention n. (%), p
Number of bed						
Less than 100, $n = 6$	5 (83.3) 1.00[a]	4 (66.7) 0.29[a]	4 (66.7) 0.30[a]	4 (66.7) 0.29[a]	3 (50.0) 0.58[a]	3 (50.0) 0.10[a]
101–500, $n = 38$	37 (97.4) 1.00[a]	32 (84.2) 0.57	29 (76.3) 0.80	30 (78.9) 1.00	32 (84.2) 0.75	22 (57.9) <0.05[a]
501–1000, $n = 67$	62 (92.5) 0.08[a]	53 (79.1) 0.49	53 (79.1) 0.62	56 (83.6) 0.87	56 (83.6) 0.75	58 (86.6) <0.05[a]
More than 1000, $n = 47$	47 (100.0) 0.18[a]	40 (85.1) 0.71	42 (89.4) 0.16	39 (83.0) 1.00	39 (83.0) 1.00	41 (87.2) 0.16
Hospital setting						
Urban, $n = 144$	140 (97.2) 0.09	118 (81.9) 1.00[a]	119 (82.6) 0.29[a]	122 (84.7) <0.05[a]	120 (83.3) 0.40[a]	97 (67.4) 0.17[a]
Suburban and rural, $n = 14$	12 (85.7) 0.09	12 (85.7) 1.00[a]	11 (78.6) 0.29[a]	9 (64.3) <0.05[a]	10 (71.4) 0.40[a]	9 (64.3) 0.17[a]
Type of hospital						
University hospital, $n = 114$	110 (96.5) 0.67[a]	92 (80.7) 0.55	94 (82.5) 0.84	98 (86.0) 0.08	92 (80.7) 0.84	95 (83.3) <0.05
Community teaching hospital, $n = 30$	29 (96.7) 1.00[a]	27 (90.0) 0.33	27 (90.0) 0.60	24 (80.0) 0.92	26 (86.7) 0.77[a]	22 (73.3) 0.54
Community hospital, $n = 9$	8 (88.9) 0.30[a]	8 (88.9) 1.00[a]	7 (77.8) 0.67[a]	5 (55.6) 0.05[a]	9 (100.0) 1.00[a]	3 (33.3) <0.05[a]
Other, $n = 5$	5 (100.0) 1.00[a]	3 (60.0) 0.21[a]	3 (60.0) <0.05[a]	4 (80.0) 0.21[a]	4 (80.0) 0.52[a]	4 (80.0) 1.00[a]
Components of the team						
Epidemiologist, $n = 64$	62 (96.9) 1.00[a]	53 (82.8) 1.00	52 (81.3) 1.00	59 (92.2) <0.05	52 (81.3) 1.00	53 (82.8) 0.46
Infection control specialist, $n = 106$	103 (97.2) 0.40[a]	90 (84.9) 0.31	91 (85.8) 0.08	89 (84.0) 0.57	89 (84.0) 1.00	82 (77.4) 0.79
Hospital administrator, $n = 73$	71 (97.3) 0.69[a]	65 (89.0) 0.06	61 (83.6) 0.71	61 (83.6) 0.86	63 (86.3) 0.29	59 (80.8) 0.49
Hospital pharmacologist, $n = 95$	94 (98.9) <0.05[a]	80 (84.2) 0.57	80 (84.2) 0.42	82 (86.3) 0.16	83 (87.4) 0.29	79 (83.2) 0.08
Hospital pharmacist, $n = 8$	7 (87.5) 0.27[a]	6 (75.0) 0.43[a]	7 (87.5) 0.55[a]	5 (62.5) 0.15[a]	7 (87.5) 0.36[a]	3 (37.5) <0.05[a]
Infectious diseases specialist, $n = 125$	120 (96.0) 1.00[a]	100 (80.0) v0.23	104 (83.2) 0.47	103 (82.4) 1.00	107 (85.6) 0.15[a]	95 (76.0) 0.50
Intensivist, $n = 76$	74 (97.4) 0.68[a]	65 (85.5) 0.41	66 (86.8) 0.16	63 (82.9) 1.00	66 (86.8) 0.80	60 (78.9) 1.00
Microbiologist, $n = 119$	119 (100.0) 0.64[a]	98 (82.4) 1.00	96 (80.7) 0.75	100 (84.0) 0.44	98 (82.4) 0.82	91 (76.5) 0.46
Surgeon, $n = 92$	88 (95.7) 1.00[a]	80 (87.0) 0.11	77 (83.7) 0.56	77 (83.7) 0.73	76 (82.6) 0.70	70 (76.1) 0.61
Other, $n = 11$	11 (100.0) 1.00[a]	9 (81.8) 1.00[a]	11 (100.0) 0.22[a]	10 (90.9) 0.69[a]	10 (90.9) 1.00[a]	8 (72.7) 0.70[a]

All *p* values were calculated using two-sided chi-square test unless otherwise noted
PAP pre-operative antimicrobial prophylaxis, *TIS* therapy for infections in surgery, *ASP* antimicrobial stewardship program
[a]Calculated using two-sided Fisher's exact test. *ASP* antimicrobial stewardship program

pathogens incidence and antimicrobial resistance, including identification of emerging pathogens at local level. The survey showed that 130 (83.3%) surgical departments had systematic reports about resistance data.

Hospital pharmacists inside the multidisciplinary team should negotiate with hospital administration to obtain adequate and necessary infrastructure to measure antimicrobial use. Regular feedback about antimicrobial consumption can be an important determinant for change for healthcare professionals and policy makers to expedite progress towards prudent use of antimicrobials. The survey showed that 129 (81.6%) surgical departments had an antimicrobial monitoring system.

Interestingly, 6 (6/41, 14.6%) surgical departments implementing a formulary restriction do not perform any monitoring system of used antimicrobials, and 4 (4/41, 9.8%) do not carry out any systematic reports about resistance data. Furthermore, 6 (7/70, 10.0%) surgical departments using a compulsory order form do not perform any monitoring system of used antimicrobials, and 11 (11/70, 15.7%) do not carry out any systematic reports about resistance data. In institutions that use restrictive interventions, monitoring overall trends in antimicrobial use and systematic reports about resistance data should be necessary to assess and respond to such shifts in use.

The ultimate goal of any stewardship program should be to stimulate a behavioral change in prescribing practices. In this context, education of prescribers is crucial to convince clinicians to use antibiotics judiciously. However, without concurrent interventions education alone is of little value. In this regard, various stewardship interventions have been implemented with the aim of improving adherence to guidelines. Where these interventions have been clinician focused, accumulating evidence suggests that educational interventions are mostly ineffective and result in insignificant changes to overall compliance [17]. It is possible that this might relate to cognitive dissonance, a process in which clinician-focused education fails to engage prescribers effectively, allowing them to ignore the evidence and to continue with their regular habits and practices. Alternative strategies of improving antibiotic management of surgical patients are needed and these may include guidance of clinicians in the institutional process of improvement, which has not as yet been addressed in guidelines [17]. The answer may lie within the principles and imperatives contained with the change of processes in hospitals.

It is highly important that faculty in academic medical centers and teaching hospitals focus on fundamental antibiotic stewardship principles in their preclinical and clinical curricula [18].

The survey found that dissemination of educational materials and educational outreach were developed respectively in 85 cases (62.5%) and 73 (53.7%) surgical departments.

This study has several limitations: with a response rate of just 19.4% we have to consider a response bias, and it is possible that non-participating physicians may have been less interested in ASPs than the participants and therefore it is possible that results are biased towards a better picture than it actually is. Furthermore, the study was conducted in a sample of physicians who participated in the AGORA project, and selecting international experts in the field again potentially resulting in an overrepresentation of hospitals with a considerably active ASP. No stratification or sampling according to medical specialty were pre-planned to ensure that all stakeholders were adequately represented, and finally our questionnaire was self-reported, has not been externally validated, and was evaluated in a single institution. The major strength of the study is its multinational (global) and multidisciplinary approach, to our best knowledge the first in this setting. Thus, our survey provides a benchmark to all interested stakeholders; it can be repeated over time to explore if better uniformity on a global platform of healthcare environments would develop in the future, and may be used to build consensus around the best practices in the field of prevention of surgical infections and rational use of antibiotics in a future project.

Conclusions

The results of the survey showed a heterogeneous organization of ASPs worldwide and demonstrated the need for a cohesive approach in order limit the emergence of antimicrobial resistance in surgical infections. Successful ASPs should focus on collaboration between all healthcare professionals in order to gain the wider-possible acceptance, share knowledge and spread best clinical practices. The main bias of the survey is the low response rate.

Abbreviation

ASP: Antimicrobial stewardship program

Acknowledgements

Not applicable.

Funding

None.

Authors' contributions

MS wrote the first draft of the manuscript. All the authors reviewed the manuscript and approved the final draft.

Competing interests

The authors declare that they have no competing interests.

Author details

[1]Department of Surgery, Macerata Hospital, Macerata, Italy. [2]Department of Biomedical Sciences and Public Health, Unit of Hygiene, Preventive Medicine and Public Health, Università Politecnica delle Marche, Ancona, Italy. [3]Infectious Diseases Unit, Bolzano Central Hospital, Bolzano, Italy. [4]General Surgery Department, Papa Giovanni XXIII Hospital, Bergamo, Italy. [5]Department of Clinical microbiology, Ampath National Laboratory Services, Milpark Hospital, Johannesburg, South Africa. [6]Division of Infectious Diseases and HIV Medicine, Department of Medicine, University of Cape Town, Cape town, South Africa. [7]World Alliance against Antibiotics Resistance, Rome, Italy. [8]Center for Critical Care, Anaesthesiology Institute and Department of Outcomes Research, Cleveland Clinic, Cleveland, OH, USA. [9]Department of Surgery and Obstetrics/Gynaecology, Regional Hospital, Limbe, Cameroon. [10]Department of Surgery, Infermi Hospital, Rimini, Italy. [11]Department of Surgery, Maggiore Hospital, Bologna, Italy. [12]Department of Surgery, Vanderbilt University Medical Center, Nashville, Tennessee, USA. [13]Infectious Diseases Unit, Department of Medical and Surgical Sciences, Sant'Orsola Hospital, University of Bologna, Bologna, Italy. [14]Division of Infectious Diseases, Cleveland Clinic Akron General, Akron, OH, USA. [15]Department of Medicine, Northeast Ohio Medical University, Rootstown, OH, USA. [16]Clinical Epidemiology Unit, IRCCS Policlinico San Matteo Foundation, Pavia, Italy. [17]Division of Infectious Diseases, Jackson Health System, University of Miami Miller School of Medicine, Miami, FL, USA. [18]Department of Surgery, College of Medicine and Health Sciences, UAE University, Al-Ain, United Arab Emirates. [19]Department of Surgery, College of Health Sciences, Obafemi Awolowo University, Ile-Ife, Nigeria. [20]Division of Clinical and Administrative Sciences, College of Pharmacy, Xavier University of Louisiana, New Orleans, LA, USA. [21]Department of Medicine, Division of Infectious Diseases, University of South Carolina School of Medicine, Columbia, SC, USA. [22]General Surgery Department, Bakirkoy Dr Sadi Konuk Training and Research Hospital, Instanbul, Turkey. [23]Unit of Prevention and Infection Control, Center of Hospital Epidemiology, São João Hospital Centre, Porto, Portugal. [24]Infection Control Committee, Prontobaby Hospital da Criança, Rio de Janeiro, Brazil. [25]Department of Surgery, University Hospital Center, Zagreb, Croatia. [26]Trauma and Acute Care Surgery Unit, Hadassah Hebrew University Medical Center, Jerusalem, Israel. [27]Department of Surgery, Weill Cornell Medicine, New York, NY, USA. [28]Department of General Surgery, Hospital San Juan de Dios de La Serena, La Serena, Chile. [29]Academic Department of Surgery, Queen Elizabeth Hospital, Birmingham, UK. [30]Department of Microbiology National Reference Laboratory Cheikh Khalifa Ibn Zaid Hospital, Mohammed 6th University of Health Sciences, Casablanca, Morocco. [31]Department of Pathology and Laboratory Medicine, VA Boston HealthCare System, Boston, MA, USA. [32]Department of Pathology and Laboratory Medicine, Boston University School of Medicine, Boston, MA, USA. [33]Department of Surgery, Hospital Clínico Universitario, Santiago de Compostela, Spain. [34]Hospital Epidemiology and Infectious Diseases, Hospital Universitario Dr Jose Eleuterio Gonzalez, Monterrey, Mexico. [35]Department of Emergency, Umberto I Hospital, Rome, Italy. [36]Department of Pharmacology, Pushpagiri Institute of Medical Sciences and Research Centre, Thiruvalla, Kerala, India. [37]Department of General Surgery, Kuala Krai Hospital, Kuala Krai, Kelantan, Malaysia. [38]Division of Acute Care Surgery, Department of Surgery, University of Michigan, Ann Arbor, MI, USA. [39]Niguarda Hospital, Milano, Italy. [40]Department of General Surgery, Health Sciences University, Samsun Training and Research Hospital, Samsun, Turkey. [41]Department of Internal Medicine and Infectious Diseases, University of Cologne, Cologne, Germany. [42]Department of Surgery, Tianjin Nankai Hospital, Nankai Clinical School of Medicine, Tianjin Medical University, Tianjin, China. [43]Department General Surgery, Kipshidze Central University Hospital, Tbilisi, Georgia. [44]Department of Digestive Surgery, Cannes Hospital, Cannes, France. [45]Department of Critical Care Medicine, Ghent University Hospital, Ghent, Belgium. [46]School of Pharmacy, Faculty of Medical Sciences, The University of the West Indies, St. Augustine, Trinidad and Tobago. [47]Eric Williams Medical Sciences Complex, Uriah Butler Highway, Champ Fleurs, Trinidad and Tobago. [48]Department of Surgery, Versilia Hospita, Lido di Camaiore, Italy. [49]Department of Surgery, University Hospital of Trauma, Tirana, Albania. [50]School of Pharmacy and Biomedicine, Mongolian National University of Medical Sciences, Ulaanbaatar, Mongolia. [51]Department of Microbiology, Bicêtre Hospital, Paris-Sud University, La Kremlin-Bicêtre, France. [52]Department of Surgery, John Peter Smith Health Network, Fort Worth, Texas, USA. [53]Sudan National Public Health Laboratory, Federal Ministry of Health, Khartoum, Sudan. [54]Department of Medicine, Infectious Disease Division, King Fahad Medical City, Riyadh, Saudi Arabia. [55]Department of Surgery, Virginia Commonwealth University, Richmond, VA, USA. [56]Department of Surgery, Clinica Foianini, Santa Cruz, Bolivia. [57]Department of Abdominal Surgery, Vladimir City Clinical Hospital of Emergency Medicine, Vladimir, Russia. [58]Department of Surgery, Bharati Vidyapeeth Deemed University Medical College and Hospital, Sangli, Maharashtra, India. [59]Department of General Surgery, Mansoura Faculty of Medicine, Mansoura University, Mansoura, Egypt. [60]Sixth Department of Internal Medicine, Hygeia General Hospital, Athens, Greece. [61]Second Department of Surgery, Aretaieion University Hospital, National and Kapodistrian University of Athens, Athens, Greece. [62]Center for Global Health, Mito Kyodo General Hospital, University of Tsukuba, Mito, Ibaraki, Japan. [63]University Department for Tumours, Sestre Milosrrdnice UHC, Zagreb, Croatia. [64]General and Upper GI Surgery, Queen Elizabeth Hospital, Birmingham, UK. [65]Peruvian Navy Medical Center, Lima, Peru. [66]Department of Gastrointestinal Surgery, Santa Casa Hospital, Campo Grande, Brazil. [67]Trauma and Trauma ICU, Inkosi Albert Luthuli Central Hospital and Department of Surgery, University of KwaZulu-Natal, Durban, South Africa. [68]Department of General and Thoracic Surgery, University Hospital Giessen, Giessen, Germany. [69]Department of Surgery, Faculty of Medicine, University of Parakou, BP 123 Parakou, Benin. [70]Fourth Surgical Department, General Hospital G. Papanikolaou, Medical School, Aristotle University of Thessaloniki, Thessaloniki, Greece. [71]Department of General Surgery, Erzincan University, Faculty of Medicine, Erzincan, Turkey. [72]Department of Pharmacy, Lebanese International University, Beirut, Lebanon. [73]Drug Applied Research Center, Tabriz University of Medical Sciences, Tabriz, Iran. [74]Division of Infectious Diseases, American University of Beirut, Beirut, Lebanon. [75]Department of Surgery Philadelphia VA Medical Center, Perelman School of Medicine, University of Pennsylvania, Philadelphia, PA, USA. [76]Department of Microbiology, Gandhi Medical College, Bhopal, India. [77]Clinic for Emergency Surgery, Medical Faculty University of Belgrade, Belgrade, Serbia. [78]Third Department of General Surgery, Jagiellonian University Medical College, Krakow, Poland. [79]Department of Abdominal Surgery, Regional Hospital of Tienen, Tienen, Belgium. [80]Department of Internal Medicine, Royal Hospital, Muscat, Oman. [81]Department of Emergency Surgery, City Hospital, Mozyr, Belarus. [82]Department of Pharmacology and Therapeutics, College of Health Sciences, Makerere University, Kampala, Uganda. [83]Department of Internal Medicine, Seoul National University Bundang Hospital, Seongnam, Republic of Korea. [84]Department of Internal Medicine, National Cheng Kung University Hospital, Tainan, Taiwan. [85]Department of Primary Care and Emergency Medicine, Kyoto University Graduate School of Medicine, Kyoto, Japan. [86]Department of Surgery n. 2, Higher educational institutions of Ukraine Bukovina State Medical University, Chernivtci City, Ukraine. [87]Section of Critical Care Medicine and Section of Infectious Diseases, Department of Medicine, Medical Microbiology and Pharmacology/Therapeutics, University of Manitoba, Winnipeg, MB, Canada. [88]Hospital Central Dr Ignacio Morones Prieto, San Luis Potosi, Mexico. [89]Department of Surgery, Division of Trauma, University of Arizona, Tucson, AZ, USA. [90]Department of Surgery, Yonsei University College of Medicine, Seoul, South Korea. [91]Texas Tech University, Health Sciences Center School of Pharmacy, Abilene, TX, USA. [92]Abdominal Center, University Hospital Meilahti, Helsinki, Finland. [93]Department of Surgery, Inling Hospital, Nanjing University School of Medicine, Nanjing, China. [94]Division of Infectious Diseases, Division of Emergency Medicine, Washington University School of Medicine, St. Louis, MO, USA. [95]Clinical Microbiology and Infectious Diseases, School of Pathology, Faculty of Health Sciences, University of the Witwatersrand, Johannesburg, South Africa. [96]Department of Surgery, Universidad Nacional de Asuncion, Asuncion, Paraguay. [97]Department for Traumatology and Orthopedic Surgery, Cologne

Merheim Medical Center (CMMC), University of Witten/Herdecke (UW/H), Cologne, Germany. [98]Second Department of General Surgery, Jagiellonian University Medical College, Krakow, Poland. [99]Health Research Program, Institute of Economic and Social Research, University of Zambia, Lusaka, Zambia. [100]Clinical Research Center, Fundacion Valle del Lili, Cali, Colombia. [101]First Department of Surgery, Tzaneion General Hospital, Piraeus, Greece. [102]Service of General Surgery, Hospital Complex of Jaén, Jaén, Spain. [103]Department of Surgery, Post-Graduate Institute of Medical Sciences, Rohtak, India. [104]Servicio de Anestesia y Reanimación, Hospital Universitario La Paz Madrid, Madrid, Spain. [105]Department of Surgery, Radiology, University Hospital of the West Indies, Kingston, Jamaica. [106]Infectious Diseases Division, Department of Medicine, Prince Mohamed Bin Abdulaziz Hospital, Ministry of Health, Riyadh, Saudi Arabia. [107]Departments of Medicine, Clinical Epidemiology and Biostatistics, and Pathology and Molecular Medicine, McMaster University, Hamilton, ON, Canada. [108]Second Surgical Clinic, Emergency Hospital of Craiova, Craiova, Romania. [109]Department of Microbiology, Tribhuvan University Teaching Hospital, Institute of Medicine, Kathmandu, Nepal. [110]Department of Surgery, University of Colorado, Denver Health Medical Center, Denver, CO, USA. [111]Department of Surgery, Onandjokwe Hospital, Ondangwa, Namibia. [112]Infectious Diseases Division, Warren Alpert Medical School of Brown University, Rhode Island Hospital, Providence, RI, USA. [113]Department of Surgery, University of Michigan, Ann Arbor, MI, USA. [114]Department of Surgery, Emergency Hospital of Bucharest, Bucharest, Romania. [115]Clinic for General Surgery, Clinical Centre, Nis, Serbia. [116]Center of Anti-Infective Research and Development, Hartford, CT, USA. [117]Department of Surgery, King Abdullah University Hospital, Irbid, Jordan. [118]Department of Surgery and Critical Care, Universidad del Valle, Fundación Valle del Lili, Cali, Colombia. [119]Intensive Care Medicine Department, Centro Hospitalar São João, University of Porto, Porto, Portugal. [120]Department of Microbiology, Grande International Hospital, Dhapasi, Kathmandu, Nepal. [121]Department of Surgery, Santa Casa de Sao Paulo School of Medical Sciences, São Paulo, Brazil. [122]Department of General and Emergency Surgery, University Hospital Kraków, Kraków, Poland. [123]Department of Surgery, University of Campinas, Campinas, Brazil. [124]Laboratory of Clinical Microbiology, Department of Infectious Diseases, Instituto Nacional de Ciencias Médicas y Nutrición Salvador Zubirán, Mexico City, Mexico. [125]Fourth Department of Internal Medicine and Infectious Diseases Unit, National and Kapodstrian University-Medical School, Attikon University General Hospital, Athens, Greece. [126]John Farman Intensive Care Unit, University Hospitals, NHS Foundation Trust, Cambridge, UK. [127]Infectious and Tropical Diseases Department, University Hospital of Nancy, and EA 4360 APEMAC, Lorraine University, Nancy, France. [128]Department of General and Emergency Surgery, Riga East University Hospital 'Gailezers', Riga, Latvia. [129]Department of Trauma, Hospital Santo Tomas, Panama, Panama. [130]National Institute for Health Research, Health Protection Research Unit in Healthcare Associated Infections and Antimicrobial Resistance, Imperial College London, Hammersmith Campus, London, UK. [131]Emergency Post-operative Department, Otavio de Freitas Hospital and Hosvaldo Cruz Hospital, Recife, Brazil. [132]Department of General Surgery, Jesenice General Hospital, Jesenice, Slovenia. [133]Trauma and Acute Care Service, St Michael's Hospital, University of Toronto, Toronto, Canada. [134]Burns, Trauma and Critical Care Research Centre, The University of Queensland, Brisbane, Queensland, Australia. [135]Unidad Clínica Intercentros de Enfermedades Infecciosas, Microbiología y Medicina Preventiva, Hospitales Universitarios Virgen Macarena y Virgen del Rocío-IBiS and Departamento de Medicina, Universidad de Sevilla, Seville, Spain. [136]General Surgery Department, Medical University, University Hospital St George, Plovdiv, Bulgaria. [137]JPS Health Network, Texas, TX, USA. [138]Hospital Center Tondela Viseu, Tondela, Portugal. [139]Department of Aeromedical Services for Emergency and Trauma Care, Ehime University Graduate School of Medicine, Ehime, Japan. [140]Department of Surgery, University of Virginia Health System, Charlottesville, VA, USA. [141]Department of Surgery, University of Sao Paulo, Ribeirao Preto, Brazil. [142]Unit of Hospital Pharmacy, Macerata Hospital, Macerata, Italy. [143]Department of Pharmacology, Postgraduate Institute of Medical Education and Research, Chandigarh, India. [144]Department of General Surgery, Tan Tock Seng Hospital, Tan Tock Seng, Singapore. [145]Office of Hospital Epidemiology/Infection Prevention and Control, University of Virginia Health System, Charlottesville, VA, USA. [146]Department of Surgery, Faculty of Medicine, Thammasat University Hospital, Thammasat University, Pathum Thani, Thailand. [147]Department of Gastrointestinal Surgery, Stavanger University Hospital, Stavanger, Norway. [148]Department of Clinical Medicine, University of Bergen, Bergen, Norway. [149]Department of Emergency Surgery and Critical Care, Centro Medico Imbanaco, Cali, Colombia. [150]Department of Surgery, School of Medicine, Pontifícia Universidade Católica do Rio Grande do Sul (PUCRS), Porto Alegre, Brazil. [151]Department of Surgery, North Estonia Medical Center, Tallinn, Estonia. [152]Department of Molecular Biology, Tran Hung Dao Hospital, No 1, Tran Hung Dao Street, Hai Ba Trung Dist, Hanoi, Vietnam. [153]Department of Infectious Diseases, John Peter Smith Health Network, Fort Worth, Texas, USA. [154]Institute of Infectious Diseases, Catholic University, Rome, Italy. [155]First Department of Surgery—Department of Abdominal, Thoracic Surgery and Traumatology, General University Hospital, Prague, Czech Republic. [156]Department of Surgery, Medical University of Graz, Graz, Austria. [157]Department of Surgery, Radboud University Nijmegen Medical Center, Nijmegen, The Netherlands. [158]Department of Surgery, Medical School University of Pécs, Pécs, Hungary. [159]Department of Urology, Pediatric Urology and Andrology, Medical Faculty of the Justus Liebig University Giessen, Giessen, Germany. [160]State Key Laboratory for Diagnosis and Treatment of Infectious Diseases, The First Affilliated Hospital, Zhejiang University, Zhejiang, China. [161]Trauma and Emergency Surgery Department, Chang Gung Memorial Hospital, Taoyuan City, Taiwan. [162]Department of Antibiotics and Infection Control, Rudolfstiftung Hospital, Vienna, Austria. [163]Infection Control Unit, Angers University, CHU d'Angers, Angers, France. [164]Division of Trauma and Surgical Critical Care, DeWitt Daughtry Family Department of Surgery, University of Miami, Miami, FL, USA. [165]Department of Surgery, University of Pittsburgh, Pittsburgh, PA, USA. [166]VU University Medical Center, Amsterdam, The Netherlands. [167]Department of General Surgery, Maggiore Hospital, Parma, Italy.

References

1. Sartelli M, Weber DG, Ruppé E, Bassetti M, Wright BJ, Ansaloni L, et al. Antimicrobials: a global alliance for optimizing their rational use in intra-abdominal infections (AGORA). World J Emerg Surg. 2016;11:33.
2. Davey P, Brown E, Charani E, Fenelon L, Gould IM, Holmes A, et al. Interventions to improve antibiotic prescribing practices for hospital inpatients. Cochrane Database Syst Rev. 2013;4:CD003543.
3. Howard P, Pulcini C, Levy Hara G, West RM, Gould IM, et al. An international cross-sectional survey of antimicrobial stewardship programmes in hospitals. J Antimicrob Chemother. 2015;70:1245–55.
4. Pollack LA, Plachouras D, Sinkowitz-Cochran R, Gruhler H, Monnet DL, Weber JT. Transatlantic taskforce on antimicrobial resistance (TATFAR) expert panel on stewardship structure and process indicators. A concise set of structure and process indicators to assess and compare antimicrobial stewardship programs among EU and US hospitals: results from a multinational expert panel. Infect Control Hosp Epidemiol. 2016;37:1201–11.
5. Sartelli M, Duane TM, Catena F, Tessier JM, Coccolini F, Kao LS, et al. Antimicrobial stewardship: a call to action for surgeons. Surg Infect. 2016;17:625–31.
6. Dellit TH, Owens RC, McGowan JE Jr, Gerding DN, Weinstein RA, Burke JP, et al. Infectious Diseases Society of America. Society for Healthcare Epidemiology of America Infectious Diseases Society of America and the Society for Healthcare Epidemiology of America guidelines for developing an institutional program to enhance antimicrobial stewardship. Clin Infect Dis. 2007;44:159–77.
7. Ben-Ishay O, Mitaritonno M, Catena F, Sartelli M, Ansaloni L, Kluger Y. Mass casualty incidents - time to engage. World J Emerg Surg. 2016;11:8.
8. Sartelli M, Catena F, Ansaloni L, Coccolini F, Corbella D, Moore EE, et al. Complicated intra-abdominal infections worldwide: the definitive data of the CIAOW study. World J Emerg Surg. 2014;9:37.
9. Barlam TF, Cosgrove SE, Abbo LM, MacDougall C, Schuetz AN, Septimus EJ, et al. Implementing an antibiotic stewardship program: guidelines by the Infectious Diseases Society of America and the Society for Healthcare Epidemiology of America. Clin Infect Dis. 2016;62:e51–77.
10. Molloy L, McGrath E, Thomas R, Kaye KS, Rybak MJ. Acceptance of pharmacist-driven antimicrobial stewardship recommendations with differing levels of physician involvement in a Children's hospital. Clin Pediatr (Phila). 2017;56(8):744–51.
11. Cakmakci M. Antibiotic stewardship programmes and the surgeon's role. J Hosp Infect. 2015;89:264–6.
12. Duane TM, Zuo JX, Wolfe LG, Bearman G, Edmond MB, Lee K, et al. Surgeons do not listen: evaluation of compliance with antimicrobial stewardship program recommendations. Am Surg. 2013;79:1269–72.

13. Angus DC, Linde-Zwirble WT, Lidicker J, Clermont G, Carcillo J, Pinsky MR. Epidemiology of severe sepsis in the United States: analysis of incidence, outcome, and associated costs of care. Crit Care Med. 2001;29:1303–10.
14. Luyt CE, Bréchot N, Trouillet JL, Chastre J. Antibiotic stewardship in the intensive care unit. Crit Care. 2014;18:480.
15. Battle SE, Bookstaver PB, Justo JA, Kohn J, Albrecht H, Al-Hasan MN. Association between inappropriate empirical antimicrobial therapy and hospital length of stay in gram-negative bloodstream infections: stratification by prognosis. J Antimicrob Chemother. 2017;72:299–304.
16. Goff DA, Karam GH, Haines ST. Impact of a national antimicrobial stewardship mentoring program: insights and lessons learned. Am J Health Syst Pharm. 2017;74:224–31.
17. Brink AJ, Messina AP, Feldman C, Richards GA, van den Bergh D, Netcare. Antimicrobial stewardship study alliance. From guidelines to practice: a pharmacist-driven prospective audit and feedback improvement model for peri-operative antibiotic prophylaxis in 34 south African hospitals. J Antimicrob Chemother. 2017;72:1227–34.
18. Pulcini C, Gyssens IC. How to educate prescribers in antimicrobial stewardship practices. Virulence. 2013;4:192–202.

23

Resuscitative endovascular balloon occlusion of the aorta deployed by acute care surgeons in patients with morbidly adherent placenta

Ramiro Manzano-Nunez[1,2*], Maria F. Escobar-Vidarte[6], Claudia P. Orlas[1,3], Juan P. Herrera-Escobar[2], Samuel M. Galvagno[4], Juan J. Melendez[5], Natalia Padilla[7], Justin C. McCarty[2], Albaro J. Nieto[6] and Carlos A. Ordoñez[3,5]

Abstract

Morbidly adherent placenta (MAP), which includes accreta, increta, and percreta, is a condition characterized by the invasion of the uterine wall by placental tissue. The condition is associated with higher odds of massive post-partum hemorrhage. Several interventions have been developed to improve hemorrhage-related outcomes in these patients; however, there is no evidence to prefer any intervention over another. Resuscitative endovascular balloon occlusion of the aorta (REBOA) is an endovascular intervention that may be useful and effective to reduce hemorrhage and transfusions in MAP patients. The objective of this narrative review is to summarize the evidence for REBOA in patients with MAP. We posit that acute care surgeons can perform REBOA for patients with MAP.

Keywords: Placenta accreta, Abnormal placentation, REBOA, Endovascular procedures

Background

Morbidly adherent placenta (MAP), which includes placenta accreta, increta, and percreta, is characterized by the abnormal invasion of the uterine wall by placental tissue [1]. MAP occurs in 1 per 333 to 533 deliveries and is a leading cause of post-partum hemorrhage (PPH) and maternal mortality worldwide [2, 3]. MAP may manifest at the moment of delivery when the invasive placenta does not readily detach from the uterus, precipitating potentially life-threatening PPH [1, 3].

The optimal management strategy for patients with MAP has been the subject of considerable debate [3–5]. Although several interventions have proven useful and effective for the management of abnormal placentation-associated PPH [1, 3, 6], early identification of patients at risk for catastrophic hemorrhage and aggressive multidisciplinary management is key for improving outcomes [4, 7]. Recent evidence suggests that resuscitative endovascular balloon occlusion of the aorta (REBOA) is a safe and effective intervention to improve hemorrhage-related outcomes in patients with MAP [8–11]. Acute care surgeons have increasing experience in performing REBOA in trauma patients and are optimally suited to, as part of a multidisciplinary team, perform REBOA in women with MAP undergoing either planned or emergent cesarean delivery.

Given the preventable nature of death from PPH, the active participation of acute care surgeons in providing the endovascular (REBOA) care to patients with MAP and at risk of massive hemorrhage could be a cornerstone of effective maternal mortality reduction worldwide, especially

* Correspondence: ramiro.manzano@correounivalle.edu.co; rmanzanonunez@bwh.harvard.edu
[1]Clinical Research Center, Fundacion Valle del Lili, Cali, Colombia
[2]Center for Surgery and Public Health - Brigham and Women's Hospital, Harvard Medical School & Harvard T.H. Chan School of Public Health, Boston, MA, USA

in low- to middle-income countries where 99% of all world PPH-related deaths occur [12].

The objective of this narrative review is to summarize the evidence for REBOA in patients with MAP. We posit that acute care surgeons can perform REBOA for women with MAP.

Morbidly adherent placenta

MAP is the global term encompassing the constellation of conditions resulting from varying levels of abnormal implantation of the placenta: placenta accreta, increta, and percreta. Placenta accreta occurs when the placenta becomes abnormally adherent to the uterine wall. Placenta increta is characterized by further invasion of the abnormal placental tissue into the myometrium. Placenta percreta results when the placenta penetrates the uterine serosa or surrounding tissues [1].

There are well-described risk factors for the development of MAP [1, 3]. The most common and relevant is previous cesarean delivery. Risk for MAP increases with each additional C-section as additional scar tissue develops [13]. The increasing incidence of MAP over the last 60 years has been attributed to increasing C-section rates. Recent estimates are that MAP occurs in 1 in every 300 to 500 pregnancies [2]. MAP thus accounts for a significant proportion of maternal morbidity and mortality cases as it carries a higher risk of catastrophic post-partum hemorrhage, especially in cases of placenta percreta with its deeper penetration [1–3, 14–16].

The primary peril with MAP occurs at the moment of delivery when the abnormally implanted placenta can result in major hemorrhage. Ninety percent of these patients will require transfusion of blood products, and at least 50% will receive a massive transfusion [3, 16, 17]. Despite prenatal surgical planning and perioperative resuscitation, maternal death may still occur in some cases [2, 3, 15].

The current recommendation for the surgical management of MAP at the moment of delivery is to perform a cesarean hysterectomy with the placenta left in situ [3, 5, 18]. Endovascular adjuvant strategies (i.e., prophylactic occlusion balloon catheters in both internal iliac arteries, uterine artery embolization) [19, 20] may be used to prevent and treat bleeding during cesarean hysterectomy. Although these interventions can prove life-saving, a considerable proportion of patients with MAP still end up requiring massive transfusion and post-op obstetrical critical care support. Furthermore, there is no evidence from randomized clinical trials to prefer any surgical intervention over another. Therefore, there is an urgent need for innovation and development of effective strategies to achieve expeditious hemorrhage arrest and prevent the occurrence of massive life-threatening bleeding.

Resuscitative endovascular balloon occlusion of the aorta in patients with MAP

REBOA is a minimally invasive procedure that introduces a balloon occlusion catheter via a percutaneous groin puncture or cutdown of the femoral artery into the aorta to obtain endovascular aortic occlusion [21, 22]. The physiologic rationale behind the use of REBOA is that it provides proximal control of bleeding and causes volume redistribution from the lower to the proximal vascular beds. These phenomena are hypothesized to ensure an adequate circulating volume and avoid the collapse of systemic circulation.

The use of REBOA in patients with MAP is not new: in 1995, a multidisciplinary team prophylactically deployed an aortic occlusion catheter in a patient with placenta percreta at 34 weeks' gestation undergoing a planned cesarean delivery. Neither massive transfusion nor admission to the intensive care unit was required, and the patient was discharged 1 week after C-section without any complications [23]. Since that initial case report, additional single cases [24, 25] and uncontrolled case series [10, 26, 27] of MAP patients undergoing C-section combined with temporary aortic balloon occlusion were published. In these reports, REBOA was used either as a rescue maneuver to stop the bleeding during an emergency peripartum hysterectomy [10, 24, 25] or as a prophylactic hemodynamic adjunct in elective cases [26, 27].

Data from retrospective comparative studies suggest that, compared to traditional planned cesarean delivery, planned C-section with the use of REBOA results in better maternal hemorrhage-related outcomes [8, 28–30]. Cui et al. [28] found that intraoperative blood loss was lower in women with placenta previa that underwent planned C-section plus REBOA, compared with patients that underwent C-section alone. These results were consistent with other studies [29, 30] which found that MAP patients benefited from REBOA in terms of average blood loss and transfusions. Moreover, a recent meta-analysis of observational data added additional validation to the finding that the prophylactic use of REBOA during elective C-section results in lower overall blood loss and fewer transfusions [9]. Thus, it seems reasonable to deploy REBOA in emergency and appropriate elective situations in patients with MAP [9].

Despite promising evidence of the potential effectiveness of REBOA in MAP [8, 9], this approach has not been routinely adopted likely due to the required involvement, time, and effort from multidisciplinary teams, including interventional radiologists or trained acute care surgeons, and because of the technical dexterity required.

REBOA deployed by acute care surgeons in pregnant women with MAP: is this feasible?

Within the field of trauma and emergency surgery, acute care surgeons have typically used REBOA in victims of traumatic truncal hemorrhage who present with hemodynamic instability [31–33]. Trauma surgeons are critical care providers and surgical rescuers [34]; hence, their role in REBOA applicable clinical scenarios has been limited only to those unstable patients who require urgent life-saving surgical interventions. There are, however, other clinical scenarios (i.e., elective care of abnormal placentation) where REBOA has proven feasible, safe, and effective [9], where acute care surgeons could play an active and integral role in the multidisciplinary care of pregnant women affected by MAP [9].

To date, three reports have shown that trauma and acute care surgeons can safely deploy a REBOA in pregnant women with MAP (Table 1) [9, 11, 35]. In these reports, pregnant women with MAP underwent a cesarean delivery with intraoperative REBOA deployment with the goal of either arresting ongoing bleeding [11] or preventing the onset of major hemorrhage [9, 35]. The REBOAs were deployed by acute care surgeons in hybrid suites or conventional operating rooms. No REBOA-related complications were reported, and all patients survived to discharge. Although these reports are case studies without a comparison group, they provide a glimpse into the potential benefits of REBOA in decreasing hemorrhage-related complications by having acute care surgeons be in charge of delivering the endovascular intervention. For example, our group [9] has previously described a case series of 12 pregnant women with a prenatal diagnosis of MAP scheduled for elective cesarean delivery with a multidisciplinary team in which a trauma surgeon was in charge of inserting, deploying, and removing the REBOA (Table 1). In this study, all patients survived, none required either massive transfusion or post-op obstetrical critical care, and no complications relating to REBOA use were noted. This compares with studies of MAP patients which found that they, on average, have blood loss of 3 to 5 l and a significant proportion require massive transfusion [3].

Traditionally, MAP patients have received endovascular care from interventional radiologists. Interventional radiologists are trained to deploy endovascular balloon occlusion catheters in the iliac arteries [19] or the aorta [8] and to perform selective arterial embolization when required. Although interventional radiologists' input in the multidisciplinary care of MAP patients has been remarkable, their participation and skill set demand the availability of modern interventional radiology suites. This infrastructure requirement is available in few well-equipped centers and is scarce in low- and middle-income countries, where PPH continues to be a leading cause of maternal death. In contrast, well-trained and qualified trauma and acute care surgeons can safely deploy a REBOA in a conventional operating room setting [9, 11]. Therefore, acute care surgeons with endovascular training and skills can be consulted either to rescue a pregnant patient who is dying in the operating room due to massive bleeding or to prophylactically deploy and inflate a REBOA in patients undergoing a planned C-section.

With the advent of smaller diameter catheters, REBOA may become more accessible for use in low-resource settings where neither interventional radiology suites nor blood supplies are available. In these scenarios, trauma surgeons with the ability to monitor all stages of REBOA technique may play a crucial role during the multidisciplinary surgical management of patients with MAP by providing the endovascular care which, in turn, could improve morbidity and mortality in these patients.

The REBOA procedure: how we do it

Previous research has established that the multidisciplinary team management of pregnant women with MAP is associated with a lower likelihood of prolonged maternal admission to the intensive care unit, less large-volume blood transfusion, decreased coagulopathy, fewer ureteral injuries, and less risk for early reoperation [7]. Therefore, in our institution, a multidisciplinary team composed of an obstetrician with training in critical care obstetrics, a urologist, an anesthesiologist, and a trauma and acute care surgeon manages the care of pregnant women with MAP.

With the goal of delivering appropriate care, a defined protocol for planned cesarean hysterectomy with simultaneous REBOA deployment has been established in our institution.

Pregnant women referred to our center with suspicion of MAP are initially evaluated by the obstetrician who makes a diagnosis based on findings from the ultrasonography and the MRI. If prenatal diagnosis of MAP is made, then the patient is scheduled for a planned cesarean delivery. At the time of C-section, the patients are taken to a conventional operating room equipped with a mobile C-arm and an ultrasound machine.

Regarding anesthesia, most centers would place an epidural catheter or use a combined spinal–epidural technique. Although neuraxial anesthesia would allow anesthesia for painless insertion of the REBOA, general anesthesia may be a better option for patients who are predicted to become hemodynamically unstable and require massive resuscitation [36].

After the induction of anesthesia and tracheal intubation, the assisting urologist inserts bilateral ureteral stents with cystoscopic guidance, and the acute care surgeon obtains endovascular access via the common femoral artery for REBOA deployment. Arterial access is obtained via the right groin under ultrasound guidance. The common femoral artery is punctured, and a guidewire is inserted and secured. A sheath (7 Fr) is then passed over the guidewire into the lumen. Finally, the guidewire is withdrawn leaving the introducer sheath in place through which 7 Fr catheter REBOA can be

Table 1 Studies reporting the deployment of REBOA in MAP patients by acute care surgeons

Author/year	Study type	*N*	Provider	Rem/Prop?	Shock?	Balloon/ sheath size	Access technique	Deployment method	Embo after REBOA	Blood loss	Transfusions of PRBCs	REBOA-related complications	Final outcome
Ordoñez 2018	CS	12	Trauma surgeon	Prop	No	Cook CODA/12 Fr	Per guided by US	Fluo	No	1500 ml (900–2750)*	2 U (0–3.5)*	None	All alive
Parra 2018	CR	1	Trauma surgeon	Rem	Yes	NR	NR	Fluo	Yes	Massive bleeding	Activation of the massive transfusion protocol	NR	Alive
Russo 2017	CR	1	Trauma surgeon	Prop	No	ER-REBOA/7 Fr	Per guided by US	External landmarks	No	3000 ml	None	None	Alive

NR not reported, *CS* case series, *CR* case report, *Prop* prophylactic, *Rem* remedial, *Per* percutaneous, *Fluo* fluoroscopy, *U* units
*Median (IQR)

introduced. The depth of REBOA advancement is determined by external landmarks, and C-arm fluoroscopy confirms correct positioning (aortic zone III). With REBOA in place and deflated, the obstetric team starts the cesarean hysterectomy.

The preferred abdominal entry technique is via midline vertical incision, and the hysterotomy is made away from the placenta. After fetal delivery and umbilical cord clamping, the placenta is left in place and the hysterotomy closed using a continuous suture, and a typical cesarean hysterectomy is performed. REBOA can be inflated either at the moment of umbilical cord clamping or when the obstetrician starts dissecting the most vascularized area [9]. We prefer, however, to inflate the REBOA immediately after umbilical cord clamping to provide a less bloody surgical field which in turn may accelerate the hysterectomy. With hysterectomy completed, the REBOA is deflated and removed along with the sheath with manual digital pressure applied to the groin puncture site for hemostasis.

There is currently no standard of care guideline regarding the appropriate care of pregnant women in the REBOA post-catheterization period. However, we recommend close monitoring for at least the first 24 h post-procedure. Examinations should be done every 15 min in the first 2 h post-REBOA and then every hour in the following 6 h. The surgeon in charge should examine the access site and assess extremity color, temperature, and pulses and must be aware of swelling and pain at the vascular access site, as well as of weak or absent distal pulses. Close monitoring during the first hours post-catheterization with the active participation of the bedside nurse is paramount for early identification and management of complications post-REBOA.

The role of acute care surgeons in MAP surgical protocols: beyond surgical rescue

Acute care surgeons can successfully be integrated into a multidisciplinary team responsible for the elective surgical care of otherwise healthy patients. Traditionally, acute care surgeons have been responsible for patients requiring emergency surgical care. However, with the growth of specific surgical fields, the scope of acute care surgeons has been reduced to simple surgical procedures. For example, Pottenger et al. [37] showed that among the ten procedures that trauma surgeons performed most frequently per year, seven could be performed at the bedside. It is clear that the field of acute care surgery requires expansion of horizons to survive the predominant model of excessive surgical specialization. In that sense, our proposal complements the five pillars of acute care surgery described by Pietzman and colleagues [34] as acute care surgeons can be consulted to rescue pregnant women with ongoing PPH or to provide elective endovascular care to patients at risk of catastrophic PPH.

Conclusion

REBOA is a feasible and safe surgical intervention that has proven effective in reducing the volume of blood loss and transfusions in pregnant women with morbidly adherent placenta undergoing cesarean delivery. This intervention can be safely delivered by acute care surgeons with endovascular training and experience in a conventional operating room. As PPH secondary to MAP continues to be a leading cause of maternal morbidity and mortality, we believe that our protocol could reduce the burden of mortality attributable to MAP worldwide.

Abbreviations

MAP: Morbidly adherent placenta; PPH: Post-partum hemorrhage; REBOA: Resuscitative endovascular balloon occlusion of the aorta

Acknowledgements

RMN, JPH, and CPO would like to express their gratitude to Dr. Carlos A. Ordoñez who not only have been a fantastic mentor but also taught them how to mentor other people. All the authors want to thank Dr. Fernando Rosso from the Clinical Research Center at La Fundacion Valle del Lili Hospital for his constant support.

Authors' contributions

Only authors who made substantive intellectual contributions were listed as authors. RMN, CPO, JPHE, SMG, JJM, AJN, NP, JCM, MFE, and CAO contributed equally to this work. CAO and RMN conceived the idea. CPO, JJM, and RMN performed the literature search. All authors wrote the report, made critical revisions to the manuscript, and approved the final version for submission.

Competing interests

The authors declare that they have no competing interests.

Author details

[1]Clinical Research Center, Fundacion Valle del Lili, Cali, Colombia. [2]Center for Surgery and Public Health - Brigham and Women's Hospital, Harvard Medical School & Harvard T.H. Chan School of Public Health, Boston, MA, USA. [3]Trauma and Acute Care Surgery Division, Department of Surgery, Fundacion Valle del Lili, Cali, Colombia. [4]R. Adams Cowley Shock Trauma Center, Baltimore, MD, USA. [5]Trauma Division and Trauma and Emergency Surgery Fellowship, Universidad del Valle, Cali, Colombia. [6]Critical Care Obstetrics, Department of Gynecology and Obstetrics, Fundacion Valle del Lili, Cali, Colombia. [7]School of Medicine, Universidad ICESI, Cali, Colombia.

References

1. Bauer ST, Bonanno C. Abnormal placentation. Semin Perinatol. 2009;33:88–96.
2. Wu S, Kocherginsky M, Hibbard JU. Abnormal placentation: twenty-year analysis. Am J Obstet Gynecol. 2005;192:1458–61.
3. Committee opinion no. 529: placenta accreta. Obstet Gynecol. 2012;120: 207–11.

4. Silver RM, Fox KA, Barton JR, Abuhamad AZ, Simhan H, Huls CK, et al. Center of excellence for placenta accreta. Am J Obstet Gynecol. 2015;212:561–8.
5. AG E, TF P, Soisson P, RM S. Optimal management strategies for placenta accreta. BJOG An Int J Obstet Gynaecol. 2009;116:648–54.
6. Dahlke JD, Mendez-Figueroa H, Maggio L, Hauspurg AK, Sperling JD, Chauhan SP, et al. Prevention and management of postpartum hemorrhage: a comparison of 4 national guidelines. Am J Obstet Gynecol. 2018;213:76 e1–76.e10.
7. Eller AG, Bennett MA, Sharshiner M, Masheter C, Soisson AP, Dodson M, et al. Maternal morbidity in cases of placenta accreta managed by a multidisciplinary care team compared with standard obstetric care. Obstet Gynecol. 2011;117:331–7.
8. Manzano-Nunez R, Escobar-Vidarte MF, Naranjo MP, Rodriguez F, Ferrada P, Casallas JD, et al. Expanding the field of acute care surgery: a systematic review of the use of resuscitative endovascular balloon occlusion of the aorta (REBOA) in cases of morbidly adherent placenta. Eur J Trauma Emerg Surg. 2018;44:519–26.
9. Ordoñez CA, Manzano-Nunez R, Parra MW, Rasmussen TE, Nieto AJ, Herrera-Escobar JP, et al. Prophylactic use of resuscitative endovascular balloon occlusion of the aorta in women with abnormal placentation: a systematic review, meta-analysis and case series. J Trauma Acute Care Surg. 2018;84:809–18.
10. Stensaeth KH, Sovik E, Haig INY, Skomedal E, Jorgensen A. Fluoroscopy-free resuscitative endovascular balloon occlusion of the aorta (REBOA) for controlling life threatening postpartum hemorrhage. PLoS One. 2017;12: e0174520.
11. Parra MW, Ordonez CA, Herrera-Escobar JP, Gonzalez-Garcia A, Guben J. Resuscitative endovascular balloon occlusion of the aorta for placenta percreta/previa. J Trauma Acute Care Surg. 2018;82:403–5.
12. Haeri S, Dildy GA. Maternal mortality from hemorrhage. Semin Perinatol. 2012;36:48–55.
13. Silver RM, Landon MB, Rouse DJ, Leveno KJ, Spong CY, Thom EA, et al. Maternal morbidity associated with multiple repeat cesarean deliveries. Obstet Gynecol. 2006;107:1226–32.
14. Eshkoli T, Weintraub AY, Sergienko R, Sheiner E. Placenta accreta: risk factors, perinatal outcomes, and consequences for subsequent births. Am J Obstet Gynecol. 2013;208:219.e1–7.
15. Hudon L, Belfort MA, Broome DR. Diagnosis and management of placenta percreta: a review. Obstet Gynecol Surv. 1999;54:509–17.
16. Brookfield KF, Goodnough LT, Lyell DJ, Butwick AJ. Perioperative and transfusion outcomes in women undergoing cesarean hysterectomy for abnormal placentation. Transfusion. 2014;54:1530–6.
17. Stotler B, Padmanabhan A, Devine P, Wright J, Spitalnik SL, Schwartz J. Transfusion requirements in obstetric patients with placenta accreta. Transfusion. 2011;51:2627–33.
18. Warshak CR, Ramos GA, Eskander R, Benirschke K, Saenz CC, Kelly TF, et al. Effect of predelivery diagnosis in 99 consecutive cases of placenta accreta. Obstet Gynecol. 2010;115:65–9.
19. Shrivastava V, Nageotte M, Major C, Haydon M, Wing D. Case-control comparison of cesarean hysterectomy with and without prophylactic placement of intravascular balloon catheters for placenta accreta. Am J Obstet Gynecol. 2007;197:1–5.
20. Gonsalves M, Belli A. The role of interventional radiology in obstetric hemorrhage. Cardiovasc Intervent Radiol. 2010;33:887–95.
21. Biffl WL, Fox CJ, Moore EE. The role of REBOA in the control of exsanguinating torso hemorrhage. J Trauma Acute Care Surg. 2015;78:1054–8.
22. Ordoñez CA, Manzano-Nunez R, del Valle AM, Rodriguez F, Burbano P, Naranjo MP, et al. Current use of resuscitative endovascular balloon occlusion of the aorta (REBOA) in trauma. Colomb J Anesthesiol. 2017;45:30–8.
23. Paull JD, Smith J, Williams L, Davison G, Devine T, Holt M. Balloon occlusion of the abdominal aorta during caesarean hysterectomy for placenta percreta. Anaesth Intensive Care. 1995;23:731–4.
24. Usman N, Noblet J, Low D, Thangaratinam S. Intra-aortic balloon occlusion without fluoroscopy for severe postpartum haemorrhage secondary to placenta percreta. Int J Obstet Anesth. 2014;23:91–3.
25. Bell-Thomas SM, Penketh RJ, Lord RH, Davies NJ, Collis R. Emergency use of a transfemoral aortic occlusion catheter to control massive haemorrhage at caesarean hysterectomy. BJOG An Int J Obstet Gynaecol. 2003;110:1120–2.
26. Duan X-H, Wang Y-L, Han X-W, Chen Z-M, Chu Q-J, Wang L, et al. Caesarean section combined with temporary aortic balloon occlusion followed by uterine artery embolisation for the management of placenta accreta. Clin Radiol. 2015;70:932–7.
27. Wei X, Zhang J, Chu Q, Du Y, Xing N, Xu X, et al. Prophylactic abdominal aorta balloon occlusion during caesarean section: a retrospective case series. Int J Obstet Anaesth. 2016;27:10–5.
28. Cui S, Zhi Y, Cheng G, Zhang K, Zhang L, Shen L. Retrospective analysis of placenta previa with abnormal placentation with and without prophylactic use of abdominal aorta balloon occlusion. Int J Gynecol Obstet. 2017;137: 265–70.
29. Wu Q, Liu Z, Zhao X, Liu C, Wang Y, Chu Q, et al. Outcome of pregnancies after balloon occlusion of the infrarenal abdominal aorta during caesarean in 230 patients with placenta praevia accreta. Cardiovasc Intervent Radiol. 2016;39:1573–9.
30. Xie L, Wang Y, Luo F-Y, Man Y-C, Zhao X-L. Prophylactic use of an infrarenal abdominal aorta balloon catheter in pregnancies complicated by placenta accreta. J Obstet Gynaecol (Lahore). 2017;37:557–61.
31. Morrison JJ, Galgon RE, Jansen JO, Cannon JW, Rasmussen TE, Eliason JL, et al. A systematic review of the use of resuscitative endovascular balloon occlusion of the aorta in the management of hemorrhagic shock. J Trauma Acute Care Surg. 2016;80:324–34.
32. Joseph JD, Thomas MS, Megan B, Dimitra S, Kenji I, Jeremy C, et al. The AAST prospective Aortic Occlusion for Resuscitation in Trauma and Acute Care Surgery (AORTA) registry: data on contemporary utilization and outcomes of aortic occlusion and resuscitative balloon occlusion of the aorta (REBOA). J Trauma Acute Care Surg. 2016;81:409–19.
33. Ordoñez CA, Parra MW, Manzano-Nunez R, Herrera-Escobar JP, Serna JJ, Rodriguez-Ossa P, et al. Intra-operative combination of resuscitative endovascular balloon occlusion of the aorta and a median sternotomy in hemodynamically unstable patients' with penetrating chest trauma: is this feasible? J Trauma Acute Care Surg. 2018;84:752–7.
34. Kutcher ME, Sperry JL, Rosengart MR, Mohan D, Hoffman MK, Neal MD, et al. Surgical rescue: the next pillar of acute care surgery. J Trauma Acute Care Surg. 2017;82:280–6.
35. Russo RM, Girda E, Kennedy V, Humphries MD. Two lives, one REBOA: hemorrhage control for urgent cesarean hysterectomy in a Jehovah's Witness with placenta percreta. J Trauma Acute Care Surg. 2017;83:551–3.
36. Lilker S, Meyer R, Downey K, Macarthur A. Anesthetic considerations for placenta accreta. Int J Obstet Anesth. 2011;20:288–92.
37. Pottenger BC, Galante JM, Wisner DH. The modern acute care surgeon: characterization of an evolving surgical niche. J Trauma Acute Care Surg. 2015;78:120–5.

24

Raising concerns about the Sepsis-3 definitions

Massimo Sartelli[1*], Yoram Kluger[2], Luca Ansaloni[3], Timothy C. Hardcastle[4,75], Jordi Rello[5], Richard R. Watkins[6,7], Matteo Bassetti[8], Eleni Giamarellou[9], Federico Coccolini[3], Fikri M. Abu-Zidan[10], Abdulrashid K. Adesunkanmi[11], Goran Augustin[12], Gian L. Baiocchi[13], Miklosh Bala[14], Oussema Baraket[15], Marcelo A. Beltran[16], Asri Che Jusoh[17], Zaza Demetrashvili[18], Belinda De Simone[19], Hamilton P. de Souza[20], Yunfeng Cui[21], R. Justin Davies[22], Sameer Dhingra[23], Jose J. Diaz[24], Salomone Di Saverio[22], Agron Dogjani[25], Mutasim M. Elmangory[26], Mushira A. Enani[27], Paula Ferrada[28], Gustavo P. Fraga[29], Sabrina Frattima[30], Wagih Ghnnam[31], Carlos A. Gomes[32], Souha S. Kanj[33], Aleksandar Karamarkovic[34], Jakub Kenig[35], Faryal Khamis[36], Vladimir Khokha[37], Kaoru Koike[38], Kenneth Y. Y. Kok[39], Arda Isik[40], Francesco M. Labricciosa[41], Rifat Latifi[42], Jae G. Lee[43], Andrey Litvin[44], Gustavo M. Machain[45], Ramiro Manzano-Nunez[46], Piotr Major[47], Sanjay Marwah[48], Michael McFarlane[49], Ziad A. Memish[50,76], Cristian Mesina[51], Ernest E. Moore[52], Frederick A. Moore[53], Noel Naidoo[54], Ionut Negoi[55], Richard Ofori-Asenso[56], Iyiade Olaoye[57], Carlos A. Ordoñez[58], Mouaqit Ouadii[59], Ciro Paolillo[60], Edoardo Picetti[61], Tadeja Pintar[62], Alfredo Ponce-de-Leon[63], Guntars Pupelis[64], Tarcisio Reis[65,77], Boris Sakakushev[66], Hossein Samadi Kafil[67], Norio Sato[68], Jay N. Shah[69], Boonying Siribumrungwong[70], Peep Talving[71], Cristian Tranà[1], Jan Ulrych[72,78], Kuo-Ching Yuan[73] and Fausto Catena[74]

Abstract

The Global Alliance for Infections in Surgery appreciates the great effort of the task force who derived and validated the Sepsis-3 definitions and considers the new definitions an important step forward in the evolution of our understanding of sepsis. Nevertheless, more than a year after their publication, we have a few concerns regarding the use of the Sepsis-3 definitions.

Keywords: Sepsis, Septic shock, Organ dysfunction, Infections

Background

The definition of sepsis has shifted over time.

Systemic inflammatory response syndrome (SIRS), sepsis, severe sepsis, and septic shock were initially defined in 1991 by a consensus panel convened by the American College of Chest Physicians (ACCP) and the Society of Critical Care Medicine (SCCM) [1]. The conference defined sepsis as a systemic inflammatory response syndrome (SIRS) due to infection. "Severe" sepsis was defined as sepsis associated with organ dysfunction, hypoperfusion, or hypotension, and "septic shock" was defined as sepsis with arterial hypotension despite adequate fluid resuscitation (Appendix 1).

The definitions were revisited in 2001 during the International Sepsis Definitions Conference, which included members from the ACCP, the SCCM, the American Thoracic Society (ATS), the European Society of Intensive Care Medicine (ESICM), and the Surgical Infection Society (SIS). [2] The consensus retained the definitions of sepsis as SIRS due to infection (presumed or confirmed) and severe sepsis as sepsis associated with acute organ dysfunction. However, the new criteria defining SIRS were greatly expanded from the 1991 original, and organ dysfunction variables indicative of severe sepsis were also defined. This new set of sepsis criteria also changed the diagnostic requirement from "more than 1" of the original 4 to "some" of the expanded list (Appendix 2).

* Correspondence: massimosartelli@gmail.com
[1]Department of Surgery, Macerata Hospital, Macerata, Italy

In February 2016, the Journal of the American Medical Association (JAMA) published a proposal for new definitions and criteria for sepsis, called Sepsis-3 [3], updating previous sepsis definitions [1, 2]. The new definitions were prepared by a task force appointed by the European Society of Intensive Care Medicine (ESICM) and the Society of Critical Care Medicine (SCCM) (Appendix 3). They were aimed at providing a standardized classification to facilitate clinical care, future research, and reporting.

In 2017, the Global Alliance for Infections in Surgery instituted an interdisciplinary task force of 76 experts from 50 different countries with different backgrounds to assess the clinical value of the Sepsis-3 definitions.

The Global Alliance for Infections in Surgery appreciates the great effort of the task force who derived and validated the Sepsis-3 definitions and considers the new definitions an important step forward in the evolution of our understanding of sepsis particularly in regard to what distinguishes sepsis from uncomplicated infection. Nevertheless, more than a year after their publication, we have a few concerns regarding the use of the Sepsis-3 definitions [3]. We hope our comments can encourage further discussion and debate on how to further optimize the definitions of the sepsis continuum.

Sepsis-3 definitions

The process for revising the Sepsis-3 definitions of sepsis and septic shock was a 2-year-long process that involved several components [3]. Critical efforts in this process included a discussion of the concept of sepsis, identification of criteria alerting clinicians for the patient's risk to develop sepsis, and the development of the criteria to identify septic shock.

The clinical criteria for sepsis were formulated by using a data-driven approach. Electronic health record data of 1.3 million encounters at 12 community and academic hospitals within the University of Pittsburgh Medical Center health system in southwestern Pennsylvania were studied, and among them, there were 148,907 patients with suspected infection. The power of the Sequential [sepsis-related] Organ Failure Assessment (SOFA) was equivalent to Logistic Organ Dysfunction Score (LODS) and higher than SIRS in predicting hospital mortality in the intensive care unit (ICU). The choice of the SOFA to measure organ dysfunction was due to its greater simplicity. The task force introduced the rapid bedside quick SOFA (qSOFA) tool for determined patients outside the ICU who likely develop sepsis from the retrospectively derived databases. Confirmatory analyses were performed by using data sets from the USA and Germany.

The clinical criteria for septic shock were formulated by using multiple methods: (a) a systematic literature review and meta-analysis of the criteria used in observational studies reporting sepsis epidemiology, (b) a Delphi process among the 19 members of the task force to achieve consensus on the new definitions, and (c) cohort studies to test variables identified by the Delphi process using the Surviving Sepsis Campaign registry, along with two other data sets from the USA.

Yet when they were published, these definitions, however, had not been prospectively validated in a generalizable population. Moreover, the patient data were all almost exclusively from adults in high-income countries and primarily contained information from patients in the USA and Germany, so the utility of these definitions in other geographic regions and particularly in settings with less resources is unknown.

In recent years, the SIRS criteria were criticized for being too non-specific. The current use of two or more SIRS criteria to identify sepsis was unanimously considered by the task force to be unhelpful.

However, the task force stated that, although SIRS was not helpful in identifying patients with organ dysfunction, non-specific SIRS criteria still might have utility in identifying patients having infection.

Sepsis is now defined as life-threatening organ dysfunction caused by a dysregulated host response to infection. The aim of this definition is to emphasize the primacy of the non-homeostatic host response to infection, the potential lethality, and the need for urgent recognition.

Organ dysfunction can be represented by an increase in the Sequential [sepsis-related] Organ Failure Assessment (SOFA) score of 2 points or more (Table 1) which is associated with an in-hospital mortality greater than 10%.

Septic shock is defined as a subset of sepsis and should be clinically identified by a vasopressor requirement to maintain a mean arterial pressure of 65 mmHg or greater and serum lactate level greater than 2 mmol/l (> 18 mg/dl) in the absence of hypovolemia. The term "severe sepsis" is now superfluous and has been removed from the current definitions.

The Sepsis-3 definitions suggest that patients with at least two of these three clinical variables may be prone for the poor outcome typical of sepsis: (1) low blood pressure (SBP ≤ 100 mmHg), (2) high respiratory rate (≥ 22 breaths per min), or (3) altered mentation (Glasgow coma scale < 15) (quick SOFA). It is supposed to be useful in out-of-hospital, emergency surgery (ED), or general hospital ward settings, and patients with positive qSOFA should be used to further investigate for organ dysfuntion. The qSOFA score should not be regarded as a diagnostic criterion for defining sepsis. Rather, it should be regarded as a warning for patients with suspected infection who are likely to have poor outcomes.

Table 1 SOFA score

PaO_2/FiO_2 (mmHg)	SOFA score
< 400	1
< 300	2
< 200 and mechanically ventilated	3
< 100 and mechanically ventilated	4
Glasgow coma scale	
13–14	1
10–12	2
6–9	3
< 6	4
Mean arterial pressure OR administration of vasopressors required	SOFA score
MAP < 70 mm/Hg	1
dop ≤ 5 or dob (any dose)	2
dop > 5 OR epi ≤ 0.1 OR nor ≤ 0.1	3
dop > 15 OR epi > 0.1 OR nor > 0.1	4
Bilirubin (mg/dl) [μmol/l]	
1.2–1.9 [> 20–32]	1
2.0–5.9 [33–101]	2
6.0–11.9 [102–204]	3
> 12.0 [> 204]	4
Platelets $\times 10^3/\mu l$	
< 150	1
< 100	2
< 50	3
< 20	4
Creatinine (mg/dl) [μmol/l] (or urine output)	
1.2–1.9 [110–170]	1
2.0–3.4 [171–299]	2
3.5–4.9 [300–440] (or < 500 ml/d)	3
> 5.0 [> 440] (or < 200 ml/d)	4

Raising concerns about the Sepsis-3 definitions

Sepsis is a multifaceted host response to an infecting pathogen that may be significantly amplified by endogenous factors. If left untreated, it may lead to the functional impairment of one or more vital organs or systems [4].There are many well-known risk factors for the infections that most commonly precipitate organ dysfunction, including acquired immunodeficiency syndrome, chronic obstructive pulmonary disease, many cancers, the use of immunosuppressive agents, and advanced age [5]. Although big steps forward have been made, the pathophysiological mechanisms for organ dysfunction are not entirely known, but it has become apparent that infection triggers a much more complex, variable, and prolonged host response, involving early activation of both pro- and anti-inflammatory responses.

Sepsis has variable clinical presentations depending on the initial site of infection, the causative organism, the pattern of acute organ dysfunction, and the underlying health status of the patient [5].

There is general consensus that early recognition and timely treatment largely determine outcome of sepsis.

Since the first classification in 1991 [1], the definition of sepsis, severe sepsis, and septic shock, though imprecise, have provided the clinicians a useful framework for clinical management, stressing the need for early recognition [6], and when these criteria are followed by the application of the Surviving Sepsis Campaign recommendations, they have an impressive history of success in reducing the mortality of sepsis in several areas of the world [7].

Several studies demonstrated that sepsis-related mortality reduced steadily over the years. A meta-analysis reported a reduction of sepsis 28-day mortality rates from 46.9% during the period 1991–1995 to 29% during 2006–2009 [8]. In the USA, mortality due to severe sepsis decreased by 51% from 1988 to 2012 [9]. In Australia and New Zealand, an overall decrease of 16.7% in hospital sepsis mortality was reported between 2000 and 2012 (from 35 to 18.4%) [10]. However, high mortality rates are still reported in low- and middle-income countries [11].

Despite decades of sepsis research, no specific therapies for sepsis have emerged. Without specific therapies, management is based on control of the infection and organ support.

Early antibiotics, source control, and fluid resuscitation support of vital organ function are the cornerstones for the treatment of patients with sepsis [12].

Timing and adequacy of source control are the most important issues in the management of patients with complicated intra-abdominal infections (cIAIs) because inadequate and late operation may have a negative effect on outcome. Source control was considered an essential element in the management of patients with complicated intra-abdominal infections (cIAIs) and should be considered and performed early after the diagnosis is established in most if not all patients [13]. Sotto et al. in 2002 found in a retrospective study that time between diagnosis and operation was associated with mortality [14]. In this study, the period between diagnosis and surgery was predictive of death within 30 days after diagnosis of peritonitis, emphasizing the importance of prompt surgical treatment. In the CIAOW (complicated intra-abdominal infections worldwide) observational study including 1898 consecutive patients older than 18 years undergoing surgery or interventional drainage to address IAI, a delayed initial intervention was found to be an independent variable predictive of mortality. In this study, the overall mortality rate was 10.5% (199/1898) [15].

To enable early interventions being effective, the diagnosis must be made as early as possible and treatment must be started early. The ability to identify septic patients who are at high risk for subsequent organ dysfunction and mortality, starting from pre-hospital care and ED, is crucial since timely recognition and appropriate, effective treatment substantially improves survival. This highlights the need for all healthcare workers to be vigilant about sepsis, so that the diagnosis can be made as early as possible [16].

One consequence of the new definitions is elimination of the concept of sepsis without organ dysfunction. Although the task force considered that the new definitions may better reflect the current understanding of sepsis pathophysiology, the literal interpretation of "sepsis" as a problem only when life-threatening organ dysfunction appears may be of limited utility in identifying patients who may benefit from early intervention.

The Sepsis-3 definitions requiring the presence of organ dysfunction to define sepsis may hinder the awareness of the importance of early recognition and treatment of infections before organ dysfunction appears, de-emphasizing intervention at earlier stages when it is most treatable.

Ideally, patients at risk for sepsis should be identified before organ dysfunction is established. Therefore, it may be questionable if it is helpful to have a definition that recognizes a patient once organ dysfunction has occurred and the patient already needs intensive care.

An observational study conducted at 132 medical institutions worldwide over a 4-month study period enrolled 4533 patients to validate a predictive score for patients with intra-abdominal infections [17]. Data from the WSES cIAIs Score Study (WISS) showed that mortality was significantly affected by the previous sepsis definition. Mortality with no sepsis was 1.2%, with sepsis only 4.4%, with severe sepsis 27.8%, and with septic shock was 67.8%. Severity of illness and the inherent mortality risk escalated from no sepsis, through sepsis, severe sepsis, and septic shock.

The previous stratification of the severity and consequent mortality due to infection that progressed from no sepsis to sepsis (infection meeting the criteria for systemic inflammatory response syndrome or SIRS), to severe sepsis (sepsis with organ failure, arterial hypertension, and/or hypoperfusion), to septic shock (arterial hypotension refractory to adequate volume resuscitation) is now reduced to simple infection, sepsis (infection and organ dysfunction), and septic shock (arterial hypotension defined as the use of vasopressors and hyperlactatemia). The previous concept of severe sepsis corresponds now to the definition of sepsis in the Sepsis-3 criteria, although this correlation is not absolute because sepsis, according to the new criteria, can include very different conditions, such as organ failure without hypotension nor hyperlactatemia [7].

The Sepsis-3 definitions exclude patients with isolated hypotension from the definition of sepsis because they would have a SOFA score of 1. Moreover, lactate is not part of the SOFA score, even though it is well documented to be a sensitive marker of severity of illness in patients with infection.

The Sepsis-3 definitions recommend using an increase in the SOFA score of 2 or more points to represent organ dysfunction. The SOFA score is intended to be used in the ICU and, to a lesser extent, the ED. Outside the ICU, SOFA was found only as good as the previous SIRS criteria (AUROC = 0.79 vs. AUROC = 0.76). Moreover, it is a valuable predictor of unfavorable outcome. The SOFA score was proposed in 1996 by the Working Group on Sepsis-Related Problems of the European Society of Intensive Care Medicine [18] to objectively describe the degree of organ dysfunction over time and to evaluate morbidity in patients in the ICU with sepsis. It was demonstrated to be a good indicator of prognosis in critically ill patients during the first few days of ICU admission [19]. The use of the SOFA score in research is commonly performed and constitutes a routine component of data collection for clinical trials in ICUs. However, the SOFA score is not universally accessible, especially for PaO_2, which would require an arterial blood gas measurement.

Recognizing these practical limitations, the task force described a simplified method termed the "quick SOFA" (qSOFA) score to facilitate easier identification of patients potentially at risk of dying outside of critical care settings [20]. This instrument, which had not been validated in clinical practice at the time of Sepsis-3 publication, comprises three clinical parameters that are easy to assess outside the ICU.

The prognostic accuracy for in-hospital mortality of qSOFA is an area of great debate. A recent multicenter prospective cohort study involving 879 patients with suspected infection treated in the ED reported that qSOFA may be better than previous criteria at predicting in-hospital mortality among patients with suspected infection [21]. Nevertheless, we calculated the positive predictive value (PPV) of qSOFA for in-hospital death in this study to be only 0.24. This indicates that only one-quarter of the patients who had a qSOFA equal or more than 2 died in the hospital.

A recent large retrospective cohort analysis of 184,875 patients in 182 Australian and New Zealand intensive care units (ICUs) found that SOFA score had superiority in prediction of in-hospital mortality and that SIRS criteria had a greater prognostic accuracy for in-hospital mortality than qSOFA score [22].

In an observational cohort study performed at one ED at an urban university teaching hospital in Norway [23], qSOFA failed to identify two thirds of the patients admitted to an ED with severe sepsis. Further, qSOFA failed to be a risk stratification tool as the sensitivity to predict 7-day and 30-day mortality was low. The sensitivity was poorer than the other warning scores already in use at the study site and the SIRS criteria.

In a study of 886 patients, Tusgul et al. showed that the qSOFA score, SIRS criteria, and sepsis definition have low identification sensitivity in selecting septic patients in the pre-hospital setting or upon arrival in the ED [24].

An important limitation of the new definitions is the poor sensitivity of the qSOFA scoring system. This leads to a high number of false negatives and, subsequently, to a delayed diagnosis in many patients, which likely excludes its use as a screening tool for early sepsis, the stage in which treatment is most effective.

In a recent analysis of three prospectively collected, observational cohorts of 7754 infected emergency department patients aged 18 years or older, Henning et al. [25] demonstrated that the mortality rate for patients with a qSOFA score greater than or equal to 2 was 14.2%, with a sensitivity of 52% and specificity of 86% to predict mortality. In comparison, the original SIRS-based Sepsis-2 definition had a mortality rate of 6.8%, a sensitivity of 83%, and a specificity of 50%. Both the Sepsis-2 and Sepsis-3 definitions stratified patients at risk for mortality, with differing performances. In terms of mortality prediction, the new definitions had improved specificity but had very low sensitivity.

Williams et al. prospectively studied 8871 consecutive patients who were admitted from the ED with presumed infection and compared the diagnostic accuracy of SIRS with qSOFA and Sepsis-2 with Sepsis-3 definitions for organ dysfunction [26]. SIRS was associated with increased risk of organ dysfunction and mortality in patients without organ dysfunction. SIRS and qSOFA showed similar discrimination for organ dysfunction. qSOFA was specific but poorly sensitive for organ dysfunction. Mortality for patients with organ dysfunction was similar for Sepsis-2 and Sepsis-3, although 29% of patients with Sepsis-3 organ dysfunction did not meet Sepsis-2 criteria. Increasing numbers of Sepsis-2 organ system dysfunctions were associated with greater mortality.

In another study in which 3346 patients with infection outside the ICU and 1058 patients with infection in the ICU were analyzed, qSOFA provided inadequate sensitivity for early risk assessment [27].

Peake et al. performed a post hoc analysis of 1591 adult patients presenting to the ED with early septic shock [28]. At baseline, 1139 patients had a qSOFA score of ≥ 2. In contrast, 1347 participants met the Sepsis-3 criteria for sepsis. Of these, 1010 participants had a qSOFA score of ≥ 2 and met the Sepsis-3 criteria for sepsis. A quarter of participants who met the new sepsis definitions did not fulfill the qSOFA screening criteria, potentially limiting its utility as a screening tool for sepsis in the ED.

Sepsis requires urgent recognition because delayed treatment increases mortality. To optimize the timing of therapy, a screening test should be as sensitive as possible. Thus, it is preferable to have a more sensitive test with lower false negative results in order to not miss cases of serious sepsis.

Although some patients with ongoing sepsis may not have elevated lactate levels at presentation or during their clinical course [29], lactate measurement is advised as an important component of the initial evaluation of patients with sepsis. Elevated lactate levels (even if > 4 mmol/l) are no longer part of organ dysfunction criteria to define organ failure.

In the new definition of septic shock, hyperlactatemia is a required component for septic shock, differently from Sepsis-1 and Sepsis-2 definitions in which just the presence of refractory hypotension to fluid loading was considered shock. Therefore, when lactate measurements are not available, the diagnosis of septic shock can be more challenging and patients with potential shock will be considered as having only sepsis.

Discussion

Sepsis was previously defined as a systemic inflammatory response syndrome (SIRS) in a patient with an infection but now reflects a significantly greater degree of illness, characterized by organ dysfunction, de-emphasizing intervention at earlier stages when it is most treatable.

Definition of organ failure based on SOFA ≥ 2 may be accurate and safe in the ICU, although reliance on the SOFA score can make it more challenging to diagnose a patient with sepsis outside the ICU environment.

The SOFA score is not globally accessible and not well known by emergency or ward healthcare professionals, and its applicability is complex outside the ICU, as it might demand the calculation of SOFA for subsequent days to verify if the patients fulfill the strict criteria and require laboratory tests [30].

The qSOFA is a tool for risk stratification, and it seems necessary to look for options to improve its low sensitivity. Until then, SIRS will still be helpful as a screening tool in ED to identify patients with infections that will most likely benefit from earlier and more aggressive interventions.

Clinicians should keep in mind the difference between a screening tool and a risk-stratification tool. A screening tool aims to identify patients with a particular disease from a larger pool of patients. Once these patients are identified, a risk-stratification tool can be applied to determine their likelihood of meeting a particular outcome.

We probably still need a good screening tool to identify patients at risk of developing organ dysfunction. However, this is not addressed in Sepsis-3.

The Sepsis-3 authors concluded that "These updated definitions and clinical criteria should clarify long-used descriptors and facilitate earlier recognition and more timely management of patients with sepsis or at risk of developing it." However, it seems to us that Sepsis3 definitions have the opposite outcome.

Sepsis 3 definitions exclude from the concept of sepsis those patients who are in transition from infection to sepsis and who have a SOFA score of 2 or more points.

Probably, a pre-sepsis scoring concept is missing [31] and should be mandatory.

Fever, tachypnea, tachycardia, and increased WBC count are consistent features of critical illnesses, including those induced by infection. Although the SIRS criteria have been criticized for their lack of specificity, since 1991, they have gained widespread acceptance among clinicians all over the world and are still used worldwide to recognize early sepsis in clinical practice.

Instead of replacing the SIRS score with the new qSOFA score to identify early patients with sepsis, why not use both of them together, taking advantage of the sensitivity of SIRS and the specificity of qSOFA?

The new definitions are based on a retrospective evaluation of large hospital databases from two countries (the USA and Germany).The majority of sources of infection were hospital patients in referral centers with respiratory and postoperative infections. The target reader is an intensive care unit (ICU) physician. Although these definitions are of help for research purposes, they may not be representative of the wider clinical community [32].

Major international differences exist in the prevalence of infections, types of infecting microorganisms, and mortality rates. EPIC II demonstrated significant differences in Eastern Europe as compared to Western Europe, in Australasia as compared to Asia, and in Latin America as compared to North America [33].

Early recognition of sepsis is a general principle of sepsis management and is very important in low- and middle-income countries where the priorities for improving the quality of care for critically ill patients are different. Documenting the burden of critical illness in low-resource settings is challenging [29]. In these settings, a triage system that quickly recognizes critically ill patients and transfers them immediately to an acute care unit is a vital component of the emergency services. The most important challenges in the management of sepsis in these areas are triage and pre-hospital diagnosis. It should be done by very sensitive and non-invasive methods outside the hospital setting.

As a consequence, any process of improving quality of sepsis care globally should focus on simple diagnostic criteria based on physical examination findings that can recognize patients needing critical care. In these settings, a feasible, low-cost method of rapidly identifying patients requiring critical care is crucial. Early warning system scores utilize physiological, easy-to-measure parameters, assessing physiological parameters such as systolic blood pressure, pulse rate, respiratory rate, temperature, oxygen saturations, and level of consciousness [34]. They are simple, non-invasive, and easy-to-repeat measurement bedside tools. Large multicenter trials will be needed to explore if these findings can be shared all over the world.

Conclusions

The pathogenesis of sepsis involves a complex interaction between the host immune system and the infecting microorganisms. Sepsis describes a broad-based syndrome covering many infectious agents, affecting various sites in patients of differing age, gender, and comorbidity. Its clinical manifestations are highly variable and may lead to severe organ dysfunction and death. Despite remarkable advances in the management of patients with sepsis, its recognition and timely, appropriate treatment remain of utmost importance.

The Sepsis-3 definitions underline the concept of a dysregulated immune response resulting in potentially modifiable life-threatening organ dysfunction. However, they may fail in identifying patients with serious infections before organ dysfunction ensues.

Downplaying infections that do not meet the current Sepsis-3 criteria may hinder their identification, resulting in an unnecessary increase in both morbidity and mortality due to their inexorable progression in the following hours.

Clear definitions for sepsis and septic shock should guide clinicians both to support early recognition of at-risk patients and to facilitate an understanding of the global epidemiology of sepsis.

Sepsis is a burden for global health. Its global nature calls for a global response, both in the geographic sense and across the whole range of sectors involved.

In this paper, we have raised our concerns regarding the Sepsis-3 definitions. We believe that in order for sepsis definitions to be universally accepted, they should facilitate clinical care on a global scale.

On Friday, May 26th, 2017, the World Health Assembly and the World Health Organization made sepsis a global health priority, by adopting a resolution to improve, prevent, diagnose, and manage sepsis [35].

The Global Alliance for Infections in Surgery suggests that future revisions have a more global perspective and include a wider range of representatives and expertise. We also hope our comments can serve as a basis for future discussions on how to further improve the definitions of the sepsis continuum.

Appendix 1

Sepsis-1 definitions

SIRS (systemic inflammatory response syndrome)

Presence of more than 1 of 4 findings:

- Body temperature > 38.0 or < 36.0 °C
- Heart rate > 90 beats/min
- Tachypnea > 20 breaths/min or hyperventilation with PaCO2 < 32 mmHg
- White blood cell (WBC) count > 12,000 cells/mm3 or < 4000 cells/mm3

Sepsis

SIRS in the presence of a confirmed or suspected infection.

Severe sepsis

Sepsis associated with organ dysfunction, hypoperfusion, or hypotension,

Septic shock

Sepsis with arterial hypotension despite adequate fluid resuscitation.

Appendix 2

Sepsis-2 definitions

Sepsis

Infection documented or suspected and some of the following parameters:

General parameters

- Fever (core temperature > 38.3 °C)
- Hypothermia (core temperature < 36 °C)
- Heart rate 90 bpm or > 2 SD above the normal value for age
- Tachypnea: > 30 bpm
- Altered mental status, significant edema or positive fluid balance (> 20 ml/kg over 24 h)
- Hyperglycemia (plasma glucose > 110 mg/dl or 7.7 mM/l) in the absence of diabetes

Inflammatory parameters

- Leukocytosis (white blood cell count > 12,000/µl)
- Leukopenia (white blood cell count < 4000/µl)
- Normal white blood cell count > 10% immature forms
- Plasma C reactive protein > 2 SD above the normal value
- Plasma procalcitonin > 2 SD above the normal value

Hemodynamic parameters

- Arterial hypotension (systolic blood pressure < 9 0 mmHg, mean arterial pressure < 70)
- Or a systolic blood pressure decrease > 40 mmHg in adults or < 2 SD below normal for age
- Mixed venous oxygen saturation > 70%
- Cardiac index > 3.5 l min^{-1} m^{-2}
- Organ dysfunction parameters
- Arterial hypoxemia ($PaO_2/FIO_2 < 300$)
- Acute oliguria (urine output > 0.5 ml/kg^{-1} h^{-1} or 45 mM/l for at least 2 h)
- Creatinine increase ≥ 0.5 mg/dl
- Coagulation abnormalities (international normalized ratio > 1.5 or activated partial thromboplastin time > 60 s)
- Ileus (absent bowel sounds)
- Thrombocytopenia (platelet count 4 mg/dl or 70 mmol/l)

Tissue perfusion parameters

- Hyperlactatemia (> 3 mmol/l)
- Decreased capillary refill or mottling

Appendix 3

Sepsis-3 definitions

Sepsis

Life-threatening organ dysfunction due to a dysregulated host response to infection.

Sepsis clinical criteria: organ dysfunction is defined as an increase of 2 points or more in the Sequential Organ Failure Assessment (SOFA) score.

Patients with suspected infection who are likely to have a prolonged ICU stay or to die in the hospital can be promptly identified at the bedside with qSOFA. Two or more of:

- Hypotension: SBP less than or equal to 100 mmHg
- Altered mental status (any GCS less than 15)
- Tachypnoea: RR greater than or equal to 22

Septic shock

Subset of sepsis in which underlying circulatory and cellular/metabolic abnormalities are profound enough to substantially increase mortality.

Septic shock clinical criteria: Sepsis and (despite adequate volume resuscitation) both of:

Persistent hypotension requiring vasopressors to maintain MAP greater than or equal to 65 mmHg, and lactate greater than or equal to 2 mmol/l.

Abbreviations

ED: Emergency department; IAI: Intra-abdominal infection; ICU: Intensive care unit; SIRS: Systemic inflammatory response syndrome; SOFA: Sequential [sepsis-related] Organ Failure Assessment

Acknowledgements

Not applicable.

Funding
None.

Authors' contributions
MS wrote the first draft of the manuscript. All the authors reviewed the manuscript and approved the final draft.

Competing interests
The authors declare that they have no competing interests.

Author details
[1]Department of Surgery, Macerata Hospital, Macerata, Italy. [2]Department of General Surgery, Division of Surgery, Rambam Health Care Campus, Haifa, Israel. [3]General Surgery Department, Bufalini Hospital, Cesena, Italy. [4]Trauma Service, Inkosi Albert Luthuli Central Hospital, Durban, South Africa. [5]Department of Clinical Research & Innovation in Pneumonia and Sepsis, Vall d'Hebron Institute of Research (VHIR), Barcelona, Spain. [6]Division of Infectious Diseases, Cleveland Clinic Akron General, Akron, OH, USA. [7]Department of Medicine, Northeast Ohio Medical University, Rootstown, OH, USA. [8]Infectious Diseases Division, Santa Maria Misericordia University Hospital, Udine, Italy. [9]6th Department of Internal Medicine, Hygeia General Hospital, Athens, Greece. [10]Department of Surgery, College of Medicine and Health Sciences, UAE University, Al-Ain, United Arab Emirates. [11]Department of Surgery, College of Health Sciences, Obafemi Awolowo University, Ile-Ife, Nigeria. [12]Department of Surgery, University Hospital Centre, Zagreb, Croatia. [13]Department of Clinical and Experimental Sciences, University of Brescia, Brescia, Italy. [14]Trauma and Acute Care Surgery Unit, Hadassah Hebrew University Medical Center, Jerusalem, Israel. [15]Department of Surgery, Bizerte Hospital, Bizerte, Tunisia. [16]Department of General Surgery, Hospital San Juan de Dios de La Serena, La Serena, Chile. [17]Department of General Surgery, Kuala Krai Hospital, Kelantan, Malaysia. [18]Department General Surgery, Kipshidze Central University Hospital, Tbilisi, Georgia. [19]Department of Digestive Surgery, Cannes Hospital, Cannes, France. [20]Department of Surgery, School of Medicine, Pontifícia Universidade Católica do Rio Grande do Sul (PUCRS), Porto Alegre, Brazil. [21]Department of Surgery, Tianjin Nankai Hospital, Nankai Clinical School of Medicine, Tianjin Medical University, Tianjin, China. [22]Colorectal Unit, Addenbrooke's Hospital, Cambridge University Hospitals NHS Foundation Trust, Cambridge, UK. [23]School of Pharmacy, Faculty of Medical Sciences, The University of the West Indies, St. Augustine, Eric Williams Medical Sciences Complex, Uriah Butler Highway, Champ Fleurs, Trinidad and Tobago. [24]Division of Acute Care Surgery, Program in Trauma, R Adams Cowley Shock Trauma Center, University of Maryland, Baltimore, MD, USA. [25]Department of Surgery, University Hospital of Trauma, Tirana, Albania. [26]Sudan National Public Health Laboratory, Federal Ministry of Health, Khartoum, Sudan. [27]Department of Medicine, Infectious Disease Division, King Fahad Medical City, Riyadh, Saudi Arabia. [28]Department of Surgery, Virginia Commonwealth University, Richmond, VA, USA. [29]Division of Trauma Surgery, Department of Surgery, School of Medical Sciences, University of Campinas (Unicamp), Campinas, SP, Brazil. [30]Istituto Clinico San Rocco di Franciacorta, Brescia, Italy. [31]Department of General Surgery, Mansoura Faculty of Medicine, Mansoura University, Mansoura, Egypt. [32]Department of Surgery, Hospital Universitário Terezinha de Jesus, Faculdade de Ciências Médicas e da Saúde de Juiz de Fora, Juiz de Fora, Brazil. [33]Division of Infectious Diseases, Department of Internal Medicine, American University of Beirut, Beirut, Lebanon. [34]Clinic for Emergency Surgery, Medical Faculty, University of Belgrade, Belgrade, Serbia. [35]Third Department of General Surgery, Jagiellonian University Medical College, Krakow, Poland. [36]Department of Internal Medicine, Royal Hospital, Muscat, Oman. [37]Department of Emergency Surgery, City Hospital, Mozyr, Belarus. [38]Department of Primary Care and Emergency Medicine, Graduate School of Medicine, Kyoto University, Kyoto, Japan. [39]Department of Surgery, The Brunei Cancer Centre, Jerudong Park, Jerudong, Brunei. [40]Department of General Surgery, Faculty of Medicine, Erzincan University, Erzincan, Turkey. [41]Global Alliance for Infections in Surgery, Porto, Portugal. [42]Department of Surgery, Division of Trauma, University of Arizona, Tucson, AZ, USA. [43]Department of Surgery, College of Medicine, Yonsei University, Seoul, South Korea. [44]Surgical Disciplines, Immanuel Kant Baltic Federal University/ Regional Clinical Hospital, Kaliningrad, Russian Federation. [45]Department of Surgery, Universidad Nacional de Asuncion, Asuncion, Paraguay. [46]Clinical Research Center, Fundacion Valle del Lili, Cali, Colombia. [47]2nd Department of General Surgery, Jagiellonian University Medical College, Krakow, Poland. [48]Department of Surgery, Post-Graduate Institute of Medical Sciences, Rohtak, India. [49]Department of Surgery, Radiology, University Hospital of the West Indies, Kingston, Jamaica. [50]Infectious Diseases Division, Department of Medicine, Prince Mohamed Bin Abdulaziz Hospital, Ministry of Health, Riyadh, Saudi Arabia. [51]Second Surgical Clinic, Emergency Hospital of Craiova, Craiova, Romania. [52]Department of Surgery, Denver Health Medical Center, University of Colorado, Denver, CO, USA. [53]Department of Surgery, Division of Acute Care Surgery, and Center for Sepsis and Critical Illness Research, College of Medicine, University of Florida, Gainesville, FL, USA. [54]Department of Surgery, University of KwaZulu-Natal, Durban, South Africa. [55]Department of Surgery, Emergency Hospital of Bucharest, Bucharest, Romania. [56]Research Unit, Health Policy Consult, Weija, Accra, Ghana. [57]Department of Surgery, University of Ilorin, Teaching Hospital, Ilorin, Nigeria. [58]Department of Surgery and Critical Care, Universidad del Valle, Fundación Valle del Lili, Cali, Colombia. [59]Department of Surgery, Hassan II University Hospital, Medical School of Fez, Sidi Mohamed Benabdellah University, Fez, Morocco. [60]Department of Emergency Medicine, Santa Maria Misericordia University Hospital, Udine, Italy. [61]Department of Anesthesia and Intensive Care, Azienda Ospedaliero-Universitaria Parma, Parma, Italy. [62]Department of Surgery, UMC Ljubljana, Ljubljana, Slovenia. [63]Laboratory of Clinical Microbiology, Department of Infectious Diseases, Instituto Nacional de Ciencias Médicas y Nutrición Salvador Zubirán, Mexico City, Mexico. [64]Department of General and Emergency Surgery, Riga East University Hospital "Gailezers", Riga, Latvia. [65]Emergency Post-Operative Department, Otavio De Freitas Hospital, Recife, Brazil. [66]General Surgery Department, Medical University, University Hospital St George, Plovdiv, Bulgaria. [67]Drug Applied Research Center, Tabriz University of Medical Sciences, Tabriz, Iran. [68]Department of Aeromedical Services for Emergency and Trauma Care, Graduate School of Medicine, Ehime University, Ehime, Japan. [69]Department of Surgery, Patan Hospital, Patan Academy of Health Sciences Lalitpur, Kathmandu, Nepal. [70]Department of Surgery, Faculty of Medicine, Thammasat University Hospital, Thammasat University, Rangsit, Pathum Thani, Thailand. [71]Department of Surgery, North Estonia Medical Center, Tallinn, Estonia. [72]First Department of Surgery, First Faculty of Medicine, Charles University in Prague, Prague, Czech Republic. [73]Department of Emergency and Critical Care Medicine, Taipei Medical University Hospital, Taipei, Taiwan. [74]Department of Emergency Surgery, Parma Maggiore Hospital, Parma, Italy. [75]Department of Surgery, Nelson R Mandela School of Clinical Medicine, Durban, South Africa. [76]College of Medicine, Alfaisal University, Riyadh, Saudi Arabia. [77]Osvaldo Cruz Hospital Recife, Recife, Brazil. [78]General University Hospital in Prague, Prague, Czech Republic.

References

1. Bone RC, Balk RA, Cerra FB, Dellinger RP, Fein AM, Knaus WA, et al. American College of Chest Physicians/Society of Critical Care Medicine consensus conference: definitions for sepsis and organ failure and guidelines for the use of innovative therapies in sepsis. Crit Care Med. 1992;20:864–74.
2. Levy MM, Fink MP, Marshall JC, Abraham E, Angus D, Cook D, et al. 2001 SCCM/ESICM/ ACCP/ATS/SIS international sepsis definitions conference. Crit Care Med. 2003;31:1250–6.
3. Singer M, Deutschman CS, Seymour CW, et al. The third international consensus definitions for sepsis and septic shock (Sepsis-3). JAMA. 2016;315: 801–10.
4. Sartelli M, Catena F, Di Saverio S, et al. Current concept of abdominal sepsis: WSES position paper. World J Emerg Surg. 2014;9:22.
5. Angus DC, van der Poll T. Severe sepsis and septic shock. N Engl J Med. 2013;369(9):840–51.
6. Simpson SQ. New sepsis criteria: a change we should not make. Chest. 2016;149:1117–8.
7. Carneiro AH, Póvoa P, Gomes JA. Dear Sepsis-3, we are sorry to say that we don't like you. Revista Brasileira de Terapia Intensiva. 2017;29(1):4–8.
8. Stevenson EK, Rubenstein AR, Radin GT, Wiener RS, Walkey AJ. Two decades of mortality trends among patients with severe sepsis: a comparative meta-analysis. Crit Care Med. 2014;42(3):625–31.

9. Zimmerman JE, Kramer AA, Knaus WA. Changes in hospital mortality for United States intensive care unit admissions from 1988 to 2012. Crit Care. 2013;17(2):R81.
10. Kaukonen KM, Bailey M, Suzuki S, Pilcher D, Bellomo R. Mortality related to severe sepsis and septic shock among critically ill patients in Australia and New Zealand, 2000–2012. JAMA. 2014;311(13):1308–16.
11. Schultz MJ, Dunser MW, Dondorp AM, Adhikari NK, Iyer S, Kwizera A, Global Intensive Care Working Group of the European Society of Intensive Care Medicine, et al. Current challenges in the management of sepsis in ICUs in resource-poor settings and suggestions for the future. Intensive Care Med. 2017;43(5):612–24.
12. Sartelli M, Catena F, Abu-Zidan FM, et al. Management of intra-abdominal infections: recommendations by the WSES 2016 consensus conference. World J Emerg Surg. 2017;12:22.
13. De Waele JJ. Early source control in sepsis. Langenbeck's Arch Surg. 2010; 395:489–94.
14. Sotto A, Lefrant JY, Fabbro-Peray P, Muller L, Tafuri J, Navarro F, et al. Evaluation of antimicrobial therapy management of 120 consecutive patients with secondary peritonitis. J Antimicrob Chemother. 2002;50:569–76.
15. Sartelli M, Catena F, Ansaloni L, et al. Complicated intra-abdominal infections worldwide: the definitive data of the CIAOW study. World J Emerg Surg. 2014;9:37.
16. Andaluz D, Ferrer R. SIRS, qSOFA, and organ failure for assessing sepsis at the emergency department. J Thorac Dis. 2017;9(6):1459–62. https://doi.org/10.21037/jtd.2017.05.36.
17. Sartelli M, Abu-Zidan FM, Catena F, Griffiths EA, Di Saverio S, Coimbra R, et al. Global validation of the WSES sepsis severity score for patients with complicated intra-abdominal infections: a prospective multicenter study (WISS study). World J Emerg Surg. 2015;10:61.
18. Vincent JL, Moreno R, Takala J, et al. The SOFA (sepsis-related organ failure assessment) score to describe organ dysfunction/failure. Intensive Care Med. 1996;22:707–10.
19. Ferreira FL, Bota DP, Bross A, et al. Serial evaluation of the SOFA score to predict outcome in critically ill patients. JAMA. 2001;286:1754–8.
20. Seymour CW, Liu VX, Iwashyna TJ, Brunkhorst FM, Rea TD, Scherag A, Rubenfeld G, Kahn JM, Shankar-Hari M, Singer M, et al. Assessment of clinical criteria for sepsis: for the third international consensus definitions for sepsis and septic shock (Sepsis-3). JAMA. 2016;315(8):762–74.
21. Freund Y, Lemachatti N, Krastinova E, Van Laer M, Claessens YE, Avondo A, Occelli C, Feral-Pierssens AL, Truchot J, Ortega M, et al. Prognostic accuracy of Sepsis-3 criteria for in-hospital mortality among patients with suspected infection presenting to the emergency department. JAMA. 2017;317(3):301–8.
22. Raith EP, Udy AA, Bailey M, et al. Prognostic accuracy of the SOFA score, SIRS criteria, and qSOFA score for in-hospital mortality among adults with suspected infection admitted to the intensive care unit. JAMA. 2017;317: 290–300.
23. Askim Å, Moser F, Gustad LT, Stene H, Gundersen M, Åsvold BO, Dale J, Bjørnsen LP, Damås JK, Solligård E. Poor performance of quick-SOFA (qSOFA) score in predicting severe sepsis and mortality—a prospective study of patients admitted with infection to the emergency department. Scand J Trauma Resusc Emerg Med. 2017;25(1):56.
24. Tusgul S, Carron PN, Yersin B, Calandra T, Dami F. Low sensitivity of qSOFA, SIRS criteria and sepsis definition to identify infected patients at risk of complication in the prehospital setting and at the emergency department triage. Scand J Trauma Resusc Emerg Med. 2017;25(1):108.
25. Henning DJ, Puskarich MA, Self WH, Howell MD, Donnino MW, Yealy DM, Jones AE, Shapiro NI. An emergency department validation of the SEP-3 sepsis and septic shock definitions and comparison with 1992 consensus definitions. Ann Emerg Med. 2017;70(4):544–552.e5.
26. Williams JM, Greenslade JH, McKenzie JV, Chu K, Brown AFT, Lipman J. Systemic inflammatory response syndrome, quick sequential organ function assessment, and organ dysfunction: insights from a prospective database of ED patients with infection. Chest. 2017;151(3):586 96.
27. Giamarellos-Bourboulis EJ, Tsaganos T, Tsangaris I, et al. Validation of the new Sepsis-3 definitions: proposal for improvement in early risk identification. Clin Microbiol Infect. 2017;23:104–9.
28. Peake SL, Delaney A, Bailey M, Bellomo R. ARISE investigators. Potential impact of the 2016 consensus definitions of sepsis and septic shock on future sepsis research. Ann Emerg Med. 2017 Oct;70(4):553–561.e1.
29. Sartelli M, Chichom-Mefire A, Labricciosa FM, Hardcastle T, Abu-Zidan FM, Adesunkanmi AK, et al. The management of intra-abdominal infections from a global perspective: 2017 WSES guidelines for management of intra-abdominal infections. World J Emerg Surg. 2017;12:29.
30. Machado FR, de Assunção MSC, Cavalcanti AB, Japiassú AM, de Azevedo LCP, Oliveira MC. Getting a consensus: advantages and disadvantages of Sepsis 3 in the context of middle-income settings. Revista Brasileira de Terapia Intensiva. 2016;28(4):361–5.
31. Bermejo-Martin JF, Martín-Fernandez M, Almansa R. Pre-sepsis: a necessary concept to complete the SEPSIS-3 picture? J Crit Care. 2017;44:148.
32. Rello J, Leblebicioglu H, members of ESGCIP. Sepsis and septic shock in low-income and middle-income countries: need for a different paradigm. Int J Infect Dis. 2016;48:120–2.
33. Vincent JL, Rello J, Marshall J, Silva E, Anzueto A, Martin CD, et al. International study of the prevalence and outcomes in infection in intensive care units. JAMA. 2009;302:2323–9.
34. Kruisselbrink R, Kwizera A, Crowther M, Fox-Robichaud A, O'Shea T, Nakibuuka J, Ssinabulya I, Nalyazi J, Bonner A, Devji T, Wong J, Cook D. Modified early warning score (MEWS) identifies critical illness among ward patients in a resource restricted setting in Kampala, Uganda: a prospective observational study. PLoS One. 2016;11(3):e0151408.
35. Reinhart K, Daniels R, Kissoon N, Machado FR, Schachter RD, Finfer S. Recognizing sepsis as a global health priority—a WHO resolution. N Engl J Med. 2017;377(5):414–7.

25

Predictors of Change in Functional Outcome at six months and twelve months after Severe Injury

Aidan Lyanzhiang Tan[1,2*], Yi Chiong[3], Nivedita Nadkarni[4], Jolene Yu Xuan Cheng[5], Ming Terk Chiu[5,6] and Ting Hway Wong[7,8]

Abstract

Background: There is increasing focus on long-term survival, function and quality-of-life for trauma patients. There are few studies tracking longitudinal changes in functional outcome over time. The goal of our study was to compare the Glasgow Outcome Scale-Extended (GOSE) at 6 months and 12 months in blunt trauma survivors with an Injury Severity Score (ISS) of more than 15.

Methods: Using the Singapore National Trauma Registry 2011–2013, patients with 6-month GOSE and 12-month GOSE scores were analysed. Patients were grouped into three categories—those with the same score at 6 months and 12 months, an improvement in score, and a worse score at 12 months. Ordinal regression was used to identify risk factors for improved score. Patients with missing scores at either 6 months or 12 months were excluded.

Results: We identified 478 patients: 174 had an improvement in score, 233 stayed the same, and 71 had worse scores at 12 months compared to 6 months. On univariate ordinal regression, the following variables were associated with same or better function at 12-months compared to 6-months: male gender, being employed pre-injury, thoracic Abbreviated Injury Scale (AIS) of 3 or more, anatomical polytrauma (AIS of 3 or more in 2 or more body regions), and road traffic injury mechanism. Older age, low fall, increasing Charlson comorbidity scores, new injury severity score, and head and neck AIS of 3 or more were associated with worse function at 12 months compared to 6 months. ISS and revised trauma score were not significant predictors on univariate or multivariable analysis.

On multivariable ordinal regression, motor vehicle mechanism (OR 2.78, 1.51–5.12, $p = 0.001$) was associated with improved function, while male gender (OR 1.36, 95% CI 1.02–1.82, $p = 0.039$) predicted improved function at 12 months.

Conclusions: Females experience worse functional outcomes at 12 months, potentially due to majority of female injuries being low falls in the elderly. In contrast, motor vehicle injury patients had better functional outcomes at 12 months. Additional interventional strategies for high-risk groups should be explored.

Keywords: Trauma, Quality of life, Functional outcomes, Severe injury, Singapore, Asia

* Correspondence: alt2163@columbia.edu
[1]Preventive Medicine, National University Hospital, Singapore, Singapore
[2]Health Services Research Unit, Singapore General Hospital, Singapore, Singapore
Full list of author information is available at the end of the article

Introduction

Trauma is a cause of chronic morbidity and disability [1]. Trauma survivors may suffer from activity limitations, reduced or inability to work in addition to other participation restrictions [1–4]. Socio-economic consequences are often present [3, 5, 6]. There are several scales that are available to measure quality of life in trauma survivors but few studies have tracked longitudinal changes in functional outcome over time. Glasgow Outcome Scale-Extended (GOSE) is a measure of overall disability, originally used to assess global outcome in traumatic brain injury survivors, and also used for overall outcomes for trauma survivors [7–12]. Recovery trajectories may differ based on patient characteristics and other factors [10, 12–23]. Outcomes have also been known to vary depending on healthcare system [22, 24–27]. Routine registry data can help provide a good reflection of trauma outcomes [8, 11, 23, 28–30].

In Singapore, trauma is the leading cause for hospitalisation, and one of the major causes of mortality [31]. Using the registry information from the Singapore National Trauma Registry, established in 2011, we aimed to evaluate factors associated with improvement in function, measured by change in GOSE score at 12 months post-trauma, for blunt trauma survivors with severe injuries. The secondary aim was to compare the characteristics of responders to non-responders, given that our registry GOSE scores are generally obtained during office hours.

Methods

Data source and data collection

A retrospective multi-centre cohort study was conducted using the Singapore National Trauma Registry data. It covered all patients admitted via the emergency department in all public-sector hospitals in Singapore from the year 2011 to 2013, regardless of nationality. Details of the registry data collection and processing have been described [32, 33].

GOSE scoring was conducted using the standardised structured interview via telephone call during office hours by registry officials unrelated to the study as part of the routine registry data collection process. This included indirect methods to interview patient caregivers, as direct interview with all patients was impracticable [13, 34]. The GOSE has been validated for administration via proxy or direct interview with the patient [35], with no difference when administered via telephone or otherwise [36, 37].

GOSE scoring was either performed face-to-face (if patients were still warded at the acute hospital at the time), or by phone. Consent for the GOSE scoring was obtained prior to proceeding with the scoring questions. The phone numbers were obtained from hospital records, which contain both home and cell phone numbers. In the event that the telephone call did not get through, another attempt was done at a separate time and day, for up to five separate occasions before a "missing" entry made.

Study design

Retrospective data from January 2011 to December 2013 was extracted. The association between change in GOSE scores and patient, injury, and clinical factors was examined.

Study population

We included adult patients (age 18 years and older) who sustained blunt injuries based on International Classification of Diseases, ninth revision, diagnostic codes 800–959.9, excluding 905–909.9. As the Singapore NTR only contains GOSE outcome data for patients with at least injury severity score (ISS) of 16, no data was available for those with ISS < 16 [38]. Patients with missing GOSE scores at either timepoint for the primary analysis were also excluded.

Outcome measures

The primary outcome measure was change in function at 12 months, compared to 6 months post-trauma. We measured and compared the GOSE score at 6 months and 12 months. These were categorised as similar (no change in scores), improved (increased), or worse (decreased) score at 12 months relative to the 6 month score.

Covariates

We extracted patient demographics and injury details (mechanism and severity) from the trauma registry.

Patient demographics were age, gender, and pre-injury employment status. Pre-injury employment status was a binary variable defined as "employed" or "unemployed". Patient comorbidity was measured using the Charlson comorbidity index (CCI) [39].

Injury mechanisms were coded in the registry as motor vehicle accident, fall, interpersonal violence, machinery, tools/objects, sports, unknown and others. We re-categorised injury mechanisms as 'low fall' (equivalent to falls from standing, chair or bed), [33, 40] 'high fall' (falls from heights greater than 0.5 m) [33, 40], 'road traffic' (motor vehicle accident, pedestrian, and motorcycle injuries), and 'others'.

We measured injury severity using the ISS, New Injury Severity Score (NISS) [26], Revised Trauma Score (RTS) [41]. The pattern of injury was described using an Abbreviated Injury Scale (AIS) score of 3 or greater at each AIS region [42].

Statistical testing

Patient characteristics at baseline were summarised by mean (standard deviation), median (inter-quartile range), or frequency (%) as appropriate. Univariate comparisons between change in GOSE scores and predictors of interest was conducted using two-sample t tests or

Mann-Whitney tests as appropriate, and chi-square tests, depending on variable type.

A multivariable ordinal regression model was fit to analyse patient group differences between those with similar/improved GOSE scores, and those with worse scores. Variables identified as having statistically significant associations ($p < 0.05$) in the univariate regression were included. Variables not statistically significant but deemed clinically meaningful were also included.

For the secondary analysis, we compared patient group differences between those without GOSE scores (non-responders to the registry calls), and those with GOSE scores (responders to registry calls). Univariate analysis using two-sample t tests or chi-square tests was conducted, depending on variable type.

STATA v.13 was used.

Ethical issues

Study and data collection protocols and processes were reviewed and approved by the respective hospital institutional review boards.

Results

Descriptive analysis

We identified 3013 potentially eligible patients from the registry and excluded 2072 as having no GOSE scores at all/non-responders to the telephone calls. Of the remaining 941 patients meeting the inclusion criteria, we further excluded 18 (1.9%) with missing 6-month GOSE scores and 445 (47.3%) with missing 12-month GOSE scores. Only 478 (50.8%) had complete GOSE scores at both 6-month and 12-month timepoints.

Of the 478 patients, compared to their 6-month score, one third had improved GOSE scores ($n = 174$, 36.4%), and 71 (14.9%) had worse GOSE scores at 12 months. The remainder ($n = 233$, 48.7%) had similar scores.

The mean age was 61.1 years, with males accounting for over two-thirds of the sample ($n = 331$, 69.2%). Majority were Singapore citizens or permanent residents ($n = 418$, 87.4%). Less than half were employed prior to their injury event ($n = 225$, 47.1%). The most common mechanism of injury was from low falls ($n = 214$, 44.8%). Majority had sustained head and neck injuries ($n = 363$, 75.9%). Summary statistics are presented in Table 1.

Table 1 Summary statistics

		Number (%)/median (IQR)/mean (SD)	
Demographics	Age	61.1	(19.9)
	Males	331	(69.2%)
Injury scores	Injury Severity Score (ISS)	22	(17, 26)
	New Injury Severity Score (NISS)	29	(22, 38)
	Revised Trauma Score (RTS)	7.84	(3.80, 7.84)
Charlson comorbidity score	0	339	(70.9%)
	1	93	(19.5%)
	2	31	(6.5%)
	> 2	15	(3.1%)
Citizenship	Singapore citizen/permanent resident	418	(87.4%)
Pre-injury employment status	Employed	225	(47.1%)
Mechanism of injury	Low fall	214	(44.8%)
	High fall	77	(16.1%)
	Pedestrian	13	(2.7%)
	Cyclist	13	(2.7%)
	Motorcycle	63	(13.2%)
	Motor vehicle	22	(4.6%)
Injury Region	Head and neck	363	(75.9%)
	Face	8	(1.7%)
	Chest	126	(26.4%)
	Abdomen and pelvic contents	48	(10.0%)
	Extremities and pelvic girdle	95	(19.9%)
	Polytrauma	135	(28.2%)

Table 2 Factors affecting functional-outcome change between 6 and 12 months

		Univariate				Multivariable			
	Variable	OR	95% CI		p	OR	95% CI		p
Demographics	Age	0.98	(0.97,	0.99)	0	0.99	(0.98,	1)	0.171
	Male	1.5	(1.03,	2.17)	0.032	1.36	(1.02,	1.82)	0.039
Injury score	New Injury Severity Score	0.99	(0.97,	1)	0.034	0.98	(0.96,	1)	0.136
Charlson comorbidity score	1	0.55	(0.36,	0.86)	0.008	0.65	(0.43,	1)	0.05
	2	0.37	(0.18,	0.74)	0.005	0.49	(0.21,	1.13)	0.094
	> 2	0.31	(0.12,	0.81)	0.017	0.38	(0.1,	1.42)	0.148
Pre-injury employment status	Employed	1.65	(1.17,	2.32)	0.005				
Injury mechanism	Pedestrian	0.99	(0.36,	2.71)	0.987				
	Motorcycle	1.45	(0.86,	2.42)	0.16				
	Motor vehicle	3.52	(1.48,	8.39)	0.004	2.78	(1.51,	5.12)	0.001
	Low fall	0.59	(0.42,	0.83)	0.003				
	High fall	1.09	(0.69,	1.72)	0.722				
Injury Region	Polytrauma (anatomical)	1.49	(1.02,	2.19)	0.041				
	Head and neck	0.64	(0.42,	0.97)	0.034				
	Chest	1.82	(1.23,	2.69)	0.003				

Univariate analysis

Functional outcomes at 12 months compared to 6 months were the same or better for male patients, or those who were employed prior to injury. Certain injuries and patterns were more likely to be associated with improved or similar functional outcomes: motor vehicle mechanism, those with injuries on the chest (AIS 3 or more), or patients with polytrauma (two or more body regions with AIS 3 or more). (Table 2, Fig. 1).

Older or higher comorbidity patients had worse functional outcomes. Severity scoring on NISS, head and neck injuries (AIS 3 or more), and injuries arising from low falls were predictors of worse function.

Injury scores ISS and RTS, other injury patterns or mechanisms were not significantly associated with functional outcomes.

Multivariable analysis

Male gender and injuries caused by motor vehicles were predictors of better outcome. All other variables (age, comorbidity, NISS), despite being significant on univariate analysis, were not significant on multivariable analysis (Table 2, Fig. 1).

Responder and non-responder comparison

Our response rate was 31.2% ($n = 941$), with 2072 non-responders to registry officials' telephone calls (Table 3). Non-responders tended to be foreign nationals and were younger than responders. Comorbidity scores tended to be lower for non-responders, although injury scores were similar. More non-responders suffered from polytrauma.

Discussion

Our study is the first study of factors associated with functional outcomes in patients with severe blunt trauma injuries in Singapore. Overall improvement rates from 6 to 12 months in our study (36%) were higher than similar studies using trauma registry data in Australia (26%) [13]. Comparison with other studies was difficult due to differences in instruments used to measure functional outcome.

Similar to international literature, we found that male gender was associated with improved functional outcomes. This approach was supported by the literature, where the female gender has been identified with worse outcomes [13, 14, 18, 25]. However, this is potentially confounded by age-related injury epidemiology. Majority of male trauma survivors were young and were involved in high-velocity injury but had good outcome. Whereas majority of female injury was associated with age-related falls, thus having worse outcome [33, 43, 44].

Although not statistically significant, patients with older age and higher comorbidity were more likely to experience deterioration in function by 12 months [12–15, 17–19, 25, 45]. This may be related to reduced physiological reserve and frail pre-injury status, thereby negatively affecting recovery. The decline in function in older patients and those with significant comorbidities could be due to natural progression of chronic disease, in addition to the impact of the injury.

Intuitively, more severe injuries would lead to worse outcomes. However, we found that trauma survivors with higher NISS, a measure of injury severity, improved better. This is likely to arise from age-related confounder

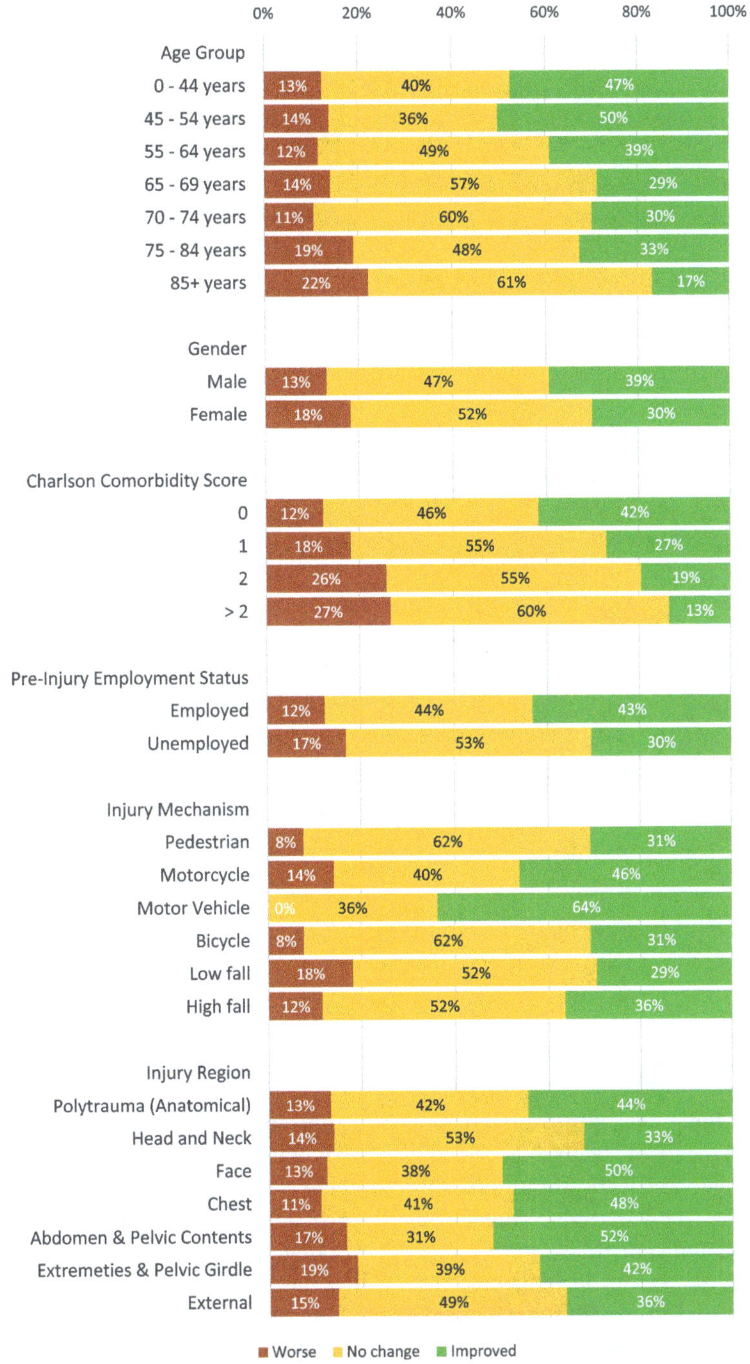

Fig. 1 Distribution of GOSE score change according to patient and clinical factors

as previously mentioned, and it is supported by previous literature, where long-term outcome (mortality) was not affected by NISS.

We found pre-injury employment status to be a significant predictor of improved functional outcomes. We used employment as a proxy for pre-incident functioning and socio-economic status, both of which have been previously found to be positive prognostic factors for functional improvement [6, 12, 14, 18, 20]. However, this is also potentially affected by age.

We found similar relationship patterns between anatomical injuries and functional outcomes [18]. Patients with head and neck injuries had worse outcomes, ostensibly due to concomitant spinal cord or central nervous system injury. This highlights the importance of preventive or protective strategies. Polytrauma patients were

Table 3 Responder and non-responder comparison

		Non-responder		Responder		
		Number (%)/median (IQR)/mean (SD)		Number (%)/median (IQR)/mean (SD)		*p* value
Total		2072		941		
Demographics	Age	54.1	(22.5)	59.2	(20.7)	< 0.001
	Males	1467	(71%)	671	(0.71%)	0.777
Injury scores	Injury Severity Score (ISS)	21	(17, 26)	21	(17, 26)	0.135
	New Injury Severity Score (NISS)	27	(21, 34)	27	(22, 34)	0.056
	Revised Trauma Score (RTS)	7.84	(2.63, 7.84)	7.84	(3.80, 7.84)	0.006
Charlson comorbidity score	0	1595	(77%)	692	(74%)	0.017
	1	331	(16%)	159	(17%)	
	2	104	(5%)	62	(7%)	
	> 2	42	(2%)	28	(3%)	
Citizenship	Singapore citizen/permanent resident	1536	(74%)	808	(86%)	< 0.001
Mechanism of injury	Low fall	799	(39%)	443	(47%)	< 0.001
	High fall	307	(15%)	119	(13%)	0.113
	Pedestrian	78	(4%)	31	(3%)	0.522
	Cyclist	0		31	(3%)	
	Motorcycle	424	(20%)	151	(16%)	0.004
	Motor vehicle	112	(5%)	46	(5%)	0.555
	Road traffic injury	0		228	(24%)	
Injury region	Head and neck	1512	(73%)	722	(77%)	0.029
	Face	38	(2%)	20	(2%)	0.59
	Chest	595	(29%)	231	(25%)	0.018
	Abdomen and pelvic contents	274	(13%)	90	(10%)	0.004
	Extremities and pelvic girdle	375	(18%)	152	(16%)	0.193
	External	3	(0.1%)	0		–
	Polytrauma	615	(30%)	234	(25%)	0.007

also found to experience functional improvement over time, possibly representing patients with high-velocity polytrauma requiring longer recovery time but with good rehabilitation potential. This may also explain our findings in relation to NISS and gender.

Our study also described the real-world functional outcome registry experience if majority of staff force made the calls during office hours. Our response rate at 12 months was lower than that of other countries (US 42%, UK 43%, Hong Kong 59%, and Australia 85.8%) [28, 30, 45, 46]. Younger patients and foreign nationals were more likely to be non-responders [28]. We postulate that younger patients were more likely to have recovered and returned to daily activity, hence not responding to the calls [16]. Foreign nationals may have departed the country, thereby also not responding. Conversely, patients with low falls were more likely to respond. This may be due to the fact that low falls occur more commonly in older patients who are more likely to be available during office hours or who have companions with them to answer calls. This is similar to what the Victoria State Trauma registry experienced, where the older or institutional patients tended to be captured during office hours interviews, while younger and working adults tended to be non-responders during office hours as they were working and therefore unavailable [34].

Our study was limited to trauma registry data, representing only hospitalised patients. However, as our focus was on severe injuries, we expect the majority if not all such cases to require inpatient care. Our study was able to cover all public-sector institutions nationwide, accounting for 80% of all hospital-based care in an urban multi-ethnic population. We also had issues of responder bias, where patients lacked GOSE scores at later timepoints. Nevertheless, we were able to demonstrate target groups for intervention in order to improve functional outcomes and recovery trajectories. Future studies should focus on longer-term follow-up as recovery processes may extend beyond 12 months, and on interventional strategies, such as our recent study showing that patients discharged to inpatient rehabilitation services were less likely to be readmitted [40].

Conclusion

Females experience worse functional outcomes at 12 months, potentially due to majority of female injuries being low falls in the elderly. In contrast, motor vehicle injury patients had better functional outcomes at 12 months. Additional interventional strategies for high-risk groups should be explored [40].

Abbreviations

AIS: Abbreviated Injury Scale; CCI: Charlson comorbidity index; GOSE: Glasgow outcome scaled-extended; ISS: Injury Severity Score; NISS: New Injury Severity Score; RTS: Revised Trauma Score

Acknowledgements

The authors would like to thank the National Trauma Committee, the National Trauma Registry working group, the National Trauma Unit, the trauma database coordinators, and colleagues at the National Registry of Diseases Office for maintaining the NTR. The collection and management of data for the National Trauma Registry is funded by the Ministry of Health, Singapore.

Funding

The authors received no specific individual funding for this work. The collection and management of data for the National Trauma Registry is funded by the Ministry of Health, Singapore.

Authors' contributions

THW conceived and designed the study. THW and NN performed the data analysis. ALT drafted the initial manuscript with all authors contributing substantially to the final manuscript. All authors read and approved the final manuscript. THW takes responsibility for the paper as a whole.

Competing interests

The authors declare that they have no competing interests.

Author details

[1]Preventive Medicine, National University Hospital, Singapore, Singapore. [2]Health Services Research Unit, Singapore General Hospital, Singapore, Singapore. [3]Department of Rehabilitation Medicine, Singapore General Hospital, Singapore, Singapore. [4]Centre for Quantitative Medicine, Duke-NUS Graduate Medical School, Singapore, Singapore. [5]National Trauma Unit, Tan Tock Seng Hospital, Singapore, Singapore. [6]Department of General Surgery, Tan Tock Seng Hospital, Singapore, Singapore. [7]General and Trauma Surgery, Singapore General Hospital, Singapore, Singapore. [8]Health Services and Systems Research, Duke-NUS Graduate Medical School, Singapore, Singapore.

References

1. Organization WH. Violence, injuries and disability: biennial report 2010–2011. 2012.
2. Soberg HL, Bautz-Holter E, Finset A, Roise O, Andelic N. Physical and mental health 10 years after multiple trauma: a prospective cohort study. J Trauma Acute Care Surg. 2015;78(3):628–33.
3. Soberg HL, Roise O, Bautz-Holter E, Finset A. Returning to work after severe multiple injuries: multidimensional functioning and the trajectory from injury to work at 5 years. J Trauma. 2011;71(2):425–34.
4. Evans JA, van Wessem KJ, McDougall D, Lee KA, Lyons T, Balogh ZJ. Epidemiology of traumatic deaths: comprehensive population-based assessment. World J Surg. 2010;34(1):158–63.
5. Hładki W, Lorkowski J, Trybus M, Brongel L, Kotela I, Golec E. Quality of life as a result of multiple injury in the aspect of limitations of handicaps--social roles. Przeglad lekarski. 2009;66(3):134–40.
6. Holbrook TL, Anderson JP, Sieber WJ, Browner D, Hoyt DB. Outcome after major trauma: 12-month and 18-month follow-up results from the trauma recovery project. J Trauma Acute Care Surg. 1999;46(5):765–73.
7. Neugebauer E, Bouillon B, Bullinger M, Wood-Dauphinee S. Quality of life after multiple trauma--summary and recommendations of the consensus conference. Restor Neurol Neurosci. 2002;20(3–4):161–7.
8. Gabbe BJ, Williamson OD, Cameron PA, Dowrick AS. Choosing outcome assessment instruments for trauma registries. Acad Emerg Med. 2005;12(8): 751–8.
9. Ardolino A, Sleat G, Willett K. Outcome measurements in major trauma--results of a consensus meeting. Injury. 2012;43(10):1662–6.
10. Gabbe BJ, Simpson PM, Sutherland AM, Wolfe R, Lyons RA, Cameron PA. Evaluating time points for measuring recovery after major trauma in adults. Ann Surg. 2013;257(1):166–72.
11. Williamson OD, Gabbe BJ, Sutherland AM, Wolfe R, Forbes AB, Cameron PA. Comparing the responsiveness of functional outcome assessment measures for trauma registries. J Trauma. 2011;71(1):63–8.
12. Gopinath B, Jagnoor J, Harris IA, Nicholas M, Casey P, Blyth F, et al. Prognostic indicators of social outcomes in persons who sustained an injury in a road traffic crash. Injury. 2015;46(5):909–17.
13. Gabbe BJ, Simpson PM, Harrison JE, Lyons RA, Ameratunga S, Ponsford J, et al. Return to work and functional outcomes after major trauma: who recovers, when, and how well? Ann Surg. 2016;263(4):623–32.
14. Polinder S, van Beeck EF, Essink-Bot ML, Toet H, Looman CW, Mulder S, et al. Functional outcome at 2.5, 5, 9, and 24 months after injury in the Netherlands. J Trauma. 2007;62(1):133–41.
15. Holtslag HR, van Beeck EF, Lindeman E, Leenen LP. Determinants of long-term functional consequences after major trauma. J Trauma. 2007;62(4):919–27.
16. Kaske S, Lefering R, Trentzsch H, Driessen A, Bouillon B, Maegele M, et al. Quality of life two years after severe trauma: a single centre evaluation. Injury. 2014;45:S100–S5.
17. Harcombe H, Langley J, Davie G, Derrett S. Functional status following injury: what recovery pathways do people follow? Injury. 2015;46(7):1275–80.
18. Gabbe BJ, Simpson PM, Cameron PA, Ponsford J, Lyons RA, et al. Long-term health status and trajectories of seriously injured patients: A population-based longitudinal study. PLoS Medicine. 2017;14(7):e1002322. https://doi.org/10.1371/journal.pmed.1002322.
19. Gabbe BJ, Harrison JE, Lyons RA, Edwards ER, Cameron PA. Comparison of measures of comorbidity for predicting disability 12-months post-injury. BMC Health Serv Res. 2013;13:30.
20. Gross T, Attenberger C, Huegli RW, Amsler F. Factors associated with reduced longer-term capacity to work in patients after polytrauma: a Swiss trauma center experience. J Am Coll Surg. 2010;211(1):81–91.
21. Hoffman K, Cole E, Playford ED, Grill E, Soberg HL, Brohi K. Health outcome after major trauma: what are we measuring? PLoS One. 2014;9(7):e103082.
22. Dinh MM, Curtis K, Mitchell RJ, Bein KJ, Balogh ZJ, Seppelt I, et al. Major trauma mortality in rural and metropolitan NSW, 2009-2014: a retrospective analysis of trauma registry data. Med J Aust. 2016;205(9):403–7.
23. Balogh ZJ, Martin AB. Prospective cohorts and risk adjusted outcomes for trauma. Injury. 2010;41(Suppl 1):S24–6.
24. Celso B, Tepas J, Langland-Orban B, Pracht E, Papa L, Lottenberg L, et al. A systematic review and meta-analysis comparing outcome of severely injured patients treated in trauma centers following the establishment of trauma systems. J Trauma. 2006;60(2):371–8 discussion 8.
25. Gabbe BJ, Simpson PM, Sutherland AM, Wolfe R, Fitzgerald MC, Judson R, et al. Improved functional outcomes for major trauma patients in a regionalized, inclusive trauma system. Ann Surg. 2012;255(6):1009–15.
26. Osler T, Baker SP, Long W. A modification of the injury severity score that both improves accuracy and simplifies scoring. J Trauma Acute Care Surg. 1997;43(6):922–6.
27. Wong TH, Lumsdaine W, Hardy BM, Lee K, Balogh ZJ. The impact of specialist trauma service on major trauma mortality. J Trauma Acute Care Surg. 2013;74(3):780–4.
28. Rios-Diaz AJ, Herrera-Escobar JP, Lilley EJ, Appelson JR, Gabbe B, Brasel K, et al. Routine inclusion of long-term functional and patient-reported outcomes into trauma registries: the FORTE project. J Trauma Acute Care Surg. 2017; 83(1):97–104.

29. Gabbe BJ, Cameron PA, Hannaford AP, Sutherland AM, McNeil JJ. Routine follow up of major trauma patients from trauma registries: what are the outcomes? J Trauma. 2006;61(6):1393–9.
30. Rainer TH, Yeung HH, Gabbe BJ, Yuen KY, Ho HF, Kam CW, et al. A comparison of functional outcome in patients sustaining major trauma: a multicentre, prospective, international study. PLoS One. 2014;9(8):e103396.
31. Singapore MoH. Singapore Health Facts 2017[updated 5 Dec 2017; cited 2018 23 July]. Available from: https://www.moh.gov.sg/resources-statistics.
32. Wong TH, Krishnaswamy G, Nadkarni NV, Nguyen HV, Lim GH, Bautista DCT, et al. Combining the new injury severity score with an anatomical polytrauma injury variable predicts mortality better than the new injury severity score and the injury severity score: a retrospective cohort study. Scand J Trauma Resusc Emerg Med. 2016;24(1):25.
33. Wong TH, Nguyen HV, Chiu MT, Chow KY, Ong MEH, et al. The Low Fall as a Surrogate Marker of Frailty Predicts Long-Term Mortality in Older Trauma Patients. PLoS ONE. 2015;10(9):e0137127. https://doi.org/10.1371/journal.pone.0137127.
34. Gabbe BJ, Sutherland AM, Hart MJ, Cameron PA. Population-based capture of long-term functional and quality of life outcomes after major trauma: the experiences of the Victorian state trauma registry. J Trauma. 2010;69(3):532–6 discussion 6.
35. Wilson JT, Pettigrew LE, Teasdale GM. Structured interviews for the Glasgow outcome scale and the extended Glasgow outcome scale: guidelines for their use. J Neurotrauma. 1998;15(8):573–85.
36. Pettigrew LE, Wilson JT, Teasdale GM. Reliability of ratings on the Glasgow outcome scales from in-person and telephone structured interviews. J Head Trauma Rehabil. 2003;18(3):252–8.
37. McMillan T, Wilson L, Ponsford J, Levin H, Teasdale G, Bond M. The Glasgow outcome scale — 40 years of application and refinement. Nat Rev Neurol. 2016;12:477.
38. Baker SP, O'Neill B. The injury severity score: An update. J Trauma Acute Care Surg. 1976;16(11):882–5.
39. Charlson ME, Pompei P, Ales KL, MacKenzie CR. A new method of classifying prognostic comorbidity in longitudinal studies: development and validation. J Chronic Dis. 1987;40(5):373–83.
40. Wong TH, Wong YJ, Lau ZY, Nadkarni N, Lim GH, Seow DCC, et al. Not all falls are equal: risk factors for unplanned readmission in older patients after moderate and severe injury—a National Cohort Study. J Am Med Dir Assoc. 2018. https://doi.org/10.1016/j.jamda.2018.08.006.
41. Champion HR, Sacco WJ, Copes WS, Gann DS, Gennarelli TA, Flanagan ME. A revision of the trauma score. J Trauma. 1989;29(5):623–9.
42. Gennarelli TA, Wodzin E. Abbreviated injury scale 2005: update 2008: Russ Reeder; 2008.
43. Haider AH, Crompton JG, Oyetunji T, Stevens KA, Efron DT, Kieninger AN, et al. Females have fewer complications and lower mortality following trauma than similarly injured males: a risk adjusted analysis of adults in the National Trauma Data Bank. Surgery. 2009;146(2):308–15.
44. James MK, Victor MC, Saghir SM, Gentile PA. Characterization of fall patients: does age matter? J Saf Res. 2018;64:83–92.
45. Rainer TH, Yeung JH, Cheung SK, Yuen YK, Poon WS, Ho HF, et al. Assessment of quality of life and functional outcome in patients sustaining moderate and major trauma: a multicentre, prospective cohort study. Injury. 2014;45(5):902–9.
46. Ahmed W, Alwe R, Wade D. One-year functional outcomes following major trauma: experience of a UK level 1 major trauma centre. Clin Rehabil. 2017; 31(12):1646–52.

Resuscitative Endovascular Balloon Occlusion of the Aorta in trauma

Emiliano Gamberini[1*], Federico Coccolini[2], Beatrice Tamagnini[3], Costanza Martino[1], Vittorio Albarello[1], Marco Benni[1], Marcello Bisulli[4], Nicola Fabbri[5], Tal Martin Hörer[6], Luca Ansaloni[2], Carlo Coniglio[7], Marco Barozzi[8] and Vanni Agnoletti[1]

Abstract

Aims: Resuscitative endovascular balloon occlusion of the aorta has been a hot topic in trauma resuscitation during these last years. The aims of this systematic review are to analyze when, how, and where this technique is performed and to evaluate preliminary results.

Methods: The literature search was performed on online databases in December 2016, without time limits. Studies citing endovascular balloon occlusion of the aorta in trauma were retrieved for evaluation.

Results: Sixty-one articles met the inclusion criteria and were selected for the systematic review. Overall, they included 1355 treated with aortic endovascular balloon occlusion, and 883 (65%) patients died after the procedure. In most of the included cases, a shock state seemed to be present before the procedure. Time of death and inflation site was not described in the majority of included studies. Procedure-related and shock-related complications are described. Introducer sheath size and comorbidity seems to play the role of risk factors.

Conclusions: Resuscitative endovascular balloon occlusion of the aorta is increasingly used in trauma victim resuscitation all over the world, to elevate blood pressure and limit fluid infusion, while other procedures aimed to stop the bleeding are performed. High mortality rate is probably due to the severity of the injuries. Time and place of balloon insertion, zone of balloon inflation, and inflation cutoff time are very heterogeneous.

Keywords: REBOA, Aortic balloon occlusion, Hemorrhagic shock, Severe trauma, Trauma system, Trauma center, Bleeding, Systematic review

Background

Hemorrhagic shock is a major cause of death [1, 2]. Although the main aims of resuscitation are to stop the hemorrhage and restore circulating blood volume, persistent hemorrhage can be rapidly fatal. In major trauma, uncontrolled bleeding is the first cause of potentially preventable death [3–5]. Resuscitative endovascular balloon occlusion of the aorta (REBOA) has been used in a variety of clinical settings (postpartum hemorrhage, upper gastrointestinal hemorrhage, pelvic hemorrhage during pelvic/sacral tumor surgery, traumatic abdomino-pelvic hemorrhage, ruptured aneurysm abdominal aorta [6–9]) to successfully elevate central blood pressure in the setting of shock, even if the evidence base is weak and devoid of clear indications. The effectiveness in this clinical target seems to have been confirmed by recent pooled analyses [10] that demonstrated an increase in mean systolic pressure following REBOA use; however, benefits in terms of overall reduction of trauma patient mortality are controversial [11, 12] (Table 1). Prospective data collection is underway in the form of an American Association for the Surgery of Trauma-sponsored observation study [13] and a European registry [14] which should permit the consistent recording of REBOA-specific data, including indications and outcome. The aortic level of balloon inflation is usually reported

* Correspondence: emiliano.gamberini@auslromagna.it
[1]Anesthesia and Intensive Care Department, AUSL Romagna Trauma Center "Maurizio Bufalini" Hospital, Viale Ghirotti 286, 47521 Cesena, Italy

Table 1 Report of included papers regarding REBOA in trauma, in chronological order, except for the last three to whom full text was recovered from other sources

Ref.	Year	Authors	Study type	No. of patients	Zone	Shock	Mortality
[26]	2016	Okada Y	Case report	1	I	Y	0/1 0%
[30]	2016	Uchino H	Case report	1	–	Y	1/1 100%
[28]	2016	Sadek S	Case report	1	III	Y	0/1 0%
[34]	2016	Matsumoto N	Case report	1	I	Y	0/1 0%
[29]	2016	DuBose JJ	Prospective observational study	46	8 × III 1 × II 33 × I 4 × converted to aortic open occlusion	Y	33/46 72%
[20]	2016	Costantini TW	Prospecting observational multicenter study	5	–	Y	3/5 60%
[5]	2016	Tsurukiri J	Retrospective study	13	4 × III 3 × II 6 × I	Y	3/13 23% Emergency room 6/13 46.1% 24 h 7/13 53.8% 60 g
[17]	2016	Inoue J	Retrospective cohort study	625	–	Y	386/625 61.8% intrahospital
[35]	2016	Hörer TM	Case series	3	1 × II 2 × I	Y	1/3 33.3%
[21]	2016	Hörer TM	Case series	7	–	Y	0/7 0%
[12]	2015	Moore LJ	Retrospective cohort study	24	5 × III 19 × I	Y	15/24 62.5%
[18]	2015	Saito N	Retrospective cohort study	24	I	Y	10/24 41.7% 24 h 17/24 70.8% 30 days
[11]	2015	Norii T	Observational prospective study	452	–	Y	343/452 75.9%
[19]	2015	Irahara T	Retrospective observational study	14	–	Y	9/14 64.3%
				1		N	0/1 0% TOT: 9/15 60%
[27]	2015	Ogura T	Case series	7 angioembolization + REBOA	–	Y	1/7 14.2% 28 days
				35 REBOA + other treatments			16/35 46%
[36]	2013	Brenner ML	Case series	6	3 × III 3 × I	Y	2/6 33.3%
[31]	2010	Martinelli T	Case series	13	III	Y	7/13 53.8%

Table 1 Report of included papers regarding REBOA in trauma, in chronological order, except for the last three to whom full text was recovered from other sources *(Continued)*

[37]	2009	Kataoka Y	Case series	3	–	Y	2/3 66.7%
[38]	2004	Long JA	Case report	1	–	Y	–
[39]	2003	Linsenmaier U	Case series	3	III	Y	2/3 66.7%
[40]	1995	Segol P	Case series	3	I	–	1/3 33.3%
[41]	1989	Gupta BK	Case series	21	I	Y	14/21 66.7%
[42]	1986	Low RB	Case series	15	–	Y	13/15 87%
[43]	1986	Wolf RK	Case report	1	III	Y	0/1 0%
[44]	1954	Hughes CW	Case series	2	I	Y	2/2 100%
[22]	2001	Matsuoka S	Case report	1	I	Y	0/1 0%
[32]	2016	Teeter WA	Retrospective review	33	I	Y	17/33 51% 24 h 19/33 58% 30 days

according to the three zone classifications: zone I thoracic aorta from left subclavian and celiac artery, zone II between celiac and renal artery, and zone III infra-renal placement [15, 16]. For bleeding in the abdominal cavity, the REBOA balloon is placed in zone I. For pelvic bleeding, generally from iliac artery branches, the balloon is placed in the distal aorta (zone III). Zone II is not currently in use. Prophylactic balloon placement in hemodynamically stable patients at risk of significant hemorrhage [10] has also been described. Positioning could lead to device-related morbidity (3.7%) and mortality (0.8%) due to arterial perforation or dissection, insertion site bleeding, and balloon-related thromboembolic events [10].

This aims to provide a systematic analysis of currently available literature regarding the use of REBOA in trauma victims.

Materials and methods

The methodological approach includes the development of selection criteria, definition of search strategies, and abstraction of relevant data. The PRISMA statement checklist for reporting a systematic review was followed.

Types of study included and criteria selection

All studies concerning REBOA use in trauma were retrieved and analyzed.

Review articles, systematic reviews, interventional trials, case series, and reports were considered eligible for inclusion in this systematic review. Conference abstracts, letters, experimental papers with animals, and commentaries were not considered.

Types of participants and intervention

Trauma victims who underwent REBOA during emergency department (ED) and operating room (OR) resuscitation phase were considered.

Types of outcome measures

The primary outcome was hospital mortality. All secondary parameters reported in the selected studies were evaluated.

Literature search and selection

Literature search was performed online on MEDLINE (through PubMed) and Cochrane Oral Health Group Specialized Register, with the addition of five articles identified from references of other works.

In order to facilitate the identification of relevant articles, the research equation was based on the following text words and criteria: "REBOA" or "resuscitative endovascular balloon occlusion of the aorta" or "ABO" or "aortic balloon" and "trauma" as *title/abstract.*

The literature search was performed in December 2016, with no time limit.

Out of the 144 initially identified articles, 61 met the inclusion criteria and were selected for the systematic review, 28 of which were actually analyzed for outcome measures and included in this review. The flow chart of study identification and the inclusion/exclusion process is shown in Fig. 1.

It was not possible to recover the full text of some articles; however, these have been included in the table (but not commented), when the data necessary for our analysis could be extrapolated from the abstracts.

Study characteristics/results

One thousand three hundred fifty-five patients treated with REBOA were included in this systematic review. Most of them were in a state of shock when REBOA was positioned; mortality was 65% (883 patients) and time of death was not always reported.

One hundred forty-nine patients were treated with REBOA in zone I, 5 in zone II, and 38 in zone III. In the majority of cases, REBOA zone was not described.

Criteria of inclusion/exclusion of patients

The studies were carried out mostly on an adult population (namely patients aged over 15 [5] or 16 [12, 17] or 18 years old, according to the explicit indications).

The studies are retrospective and used registries, so they refer to the time period in which the cases were selected (e.g., 2014 or from January 2007 to December 2013).

Inclusion criteria are heterogeneous. Patients included in the studies were analyzed for uncompressible trunk hemorrhage, intra-abdominal bleeding (e.g., liver or splenic injury), retroperitoneal hemorrhage (e.g., renal injury or pelvic fracture), and non-traumatic hemorrhage (e.g., obstetric or gastrointestinal that have been excluded from this review).

Patients' selection criteria vary depending on the studies, and they are usually indicated for example hemoperitoneum or pelvic ring fractures with potential imminent cardiac arrest or fluid resuscitation unresponsiveness state with a sustained SBP of less than 90 mmHg [18]. Some studies excluded patients who went into cardiac arrest during admission, were diagnosed with any terminal disease during the study period [5], or sustained what were defined as un-survivable injuries [17].

Lastly, some research excluded patients where REBOA was positioned to prevent shock (still hemodynamically stable); in the queue of their article, Irahara et al. [19]

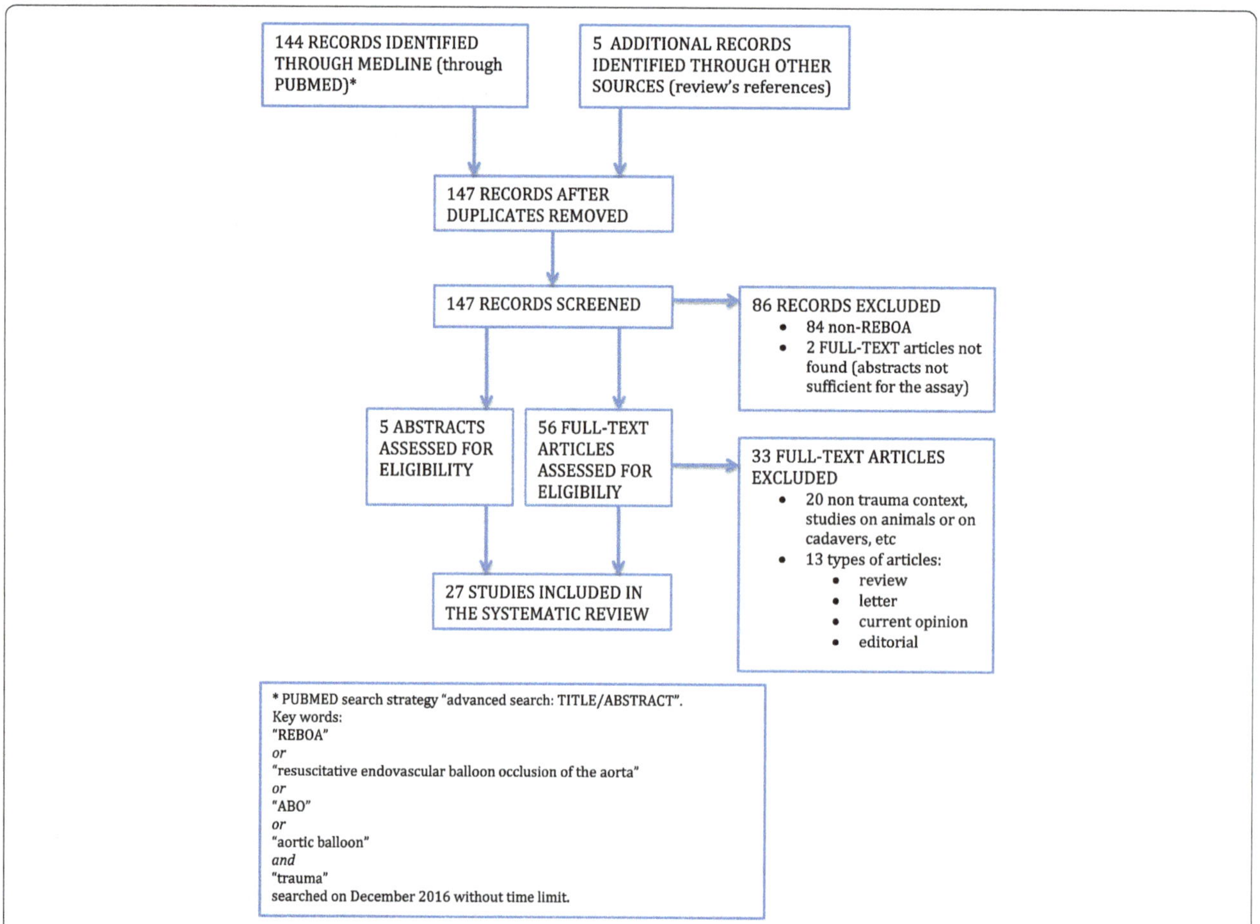

Fig. 1 Flow chart of the study search, selection, and inclusion/exclusion

described an interesting *case report* regarding the prophylactic use of REBOA in potentially evolutionary cases. While this practice is of great interest, other authors have confessed fears that they may become too invasive [18].

Many studies include patients undergoing treatment with REBOA for reasons other than trauma (e.g., bleeding of the gastrointestinal tract, post-partum bleeding); those only dealing with REBOA in non-traumatic cases were eliminated in the initial selection of this systematic review (Fig. 1), whereas articles including trauma patients were analyzed to extract data of interest.

Definition of shock

Some studies provided an explicit definition of shock (e.g., SBP < 90 mmHg or SI ≥ 1 [5]; SBP < 90 mmHg or HR > 120 bpm or base deficit < – 5 [20]; SBP < 80 mmHg and no response to fluid treatment [21]) while others did not; however, it was possible to deduce patient's vital parameters from the tables (mean patient SBP was often indicated in the tables, and for the purposes of this review, < 90 mmHg was defined as shock).

Vascular approach

Almost all REBOA was introduced from the femoral artery (which is considered as the ideal access point). Other access points are described in a limited number of cases described (e.g., left brachial artery or left common carotid artery [22]).

Access can be achieved using different techniques: percutaneous (with the Seldinger method), open exposure by surgical cutdown of the vessel, or exchange over a guidewire from an existing arterial line [16].

Imaging techniques can be used (e.g., eco guide for access and RX to confirm the balloon position), or it is also possible to work blindly, using only external landmarks; MacTaggart et al. describe the use of "morphometric roadmaps" to improve accurate device delivery for fluoroscopy-free REBOA, according to the patient physique [23].

REBOA insertion time in the simulation laboratory was under 5 min (Brenner et al.) [12–24]. Simulations were often videotaped in the *trauma center*, with a few performances under 3 min and some lasting up to 15 min when femoral access was difficult to obtain [12].

Operator and training

Operators who insert REBOA vary depending on the context; in a multidisciplinary team, the practice may be performed by an interventional radiologist, a vascular surgeon, a trauma surgeon, an intensive care unit expert, or an emergency department physician who is familiar with the endovascular approach.

The skill can be quickly acquired; for physicians with limited previous endovascular skills, attendance at procedural courses provides an opportunity to gain competence and it seems that the insertion of no. 3–5 REBOA under expert supervision [5], or a training period of some months, can be enough [11, 12].

There is no universal certification for REBOA positioning. For example, in order to become an emergency physician, the Japanese Association for Acute Medicine requires a minimum experience of no. 3 cases of REBOA insertion during residency training. It does not differ from the US "BEST" (Basic Endovascular Skills for Trauma) courses which include didactic lectures, virtual reality simulation, and cadaveric instruction, whereas "ESTARS" (Endovascular Skills for Trauma and Resuscitative Surgery) courses use simulations and live animal models to establish procedural competence [25].

There are also some courses in Europe, especially in London (Royal Medical Hospital and London's Air Ambulance) and in Örebro, Sweden ("EVTM" EndoVascular and hybrid Trauma and bleeding Management).

Type of device

In most of the studies, a 10 to 12 Fr introducer is used (Okada et al. considered the large size as a contributory cause of ischemic complications that led to lower limb amputation patients with a smaller build [26]).

Seven-French catheters are currently available (since 2014) and in use in Japan; Tsurukiri et al. have noted that this has enabled a reduction in complications coupled with 100% technical success [5].

Time and method of inflation

An ideal time of occlusion has not been established, although it is clear that it must be as short as it possible. There are several studies on animals (especially pigs and dogs) which identify 60–90 min as a cutoff time; however, it is difficult to adapt these data for human patients. Saito et al. define the golden time as 20 min of hemostasis as a goal for the future [18].

Some of the analyzed retrospective studies do not report occlusion time as it had not been recorded. However, it was found that occlusion time was shorter in survivors than in patients who died [19]. Mean occlusion time in the various articles ranged from 20 to 65 min.

During the CT scan, the balloon is partially deflated to let the contrast pass. It is interesting to note that when occlusion must necessarily exceed 20 min, Ogura et al. practiced a partial deflation for a few minutes and completed a rapid transfusion of blood products in order to take advantage of the ischemic preconditioning effect as a strategy to increase tissue tolerance. During this interval, if SBP was not maintained above 70 mmHg, the balloon was inflated again for a further 20 min. In this study, the total mean occlusion time is 80 min (although one patient did not tolerate deflation) and there were no complications related to the use of REBOA [27]. However, this approach does not seem to bring other advantages.

A significant correlation between total occlusion time, serum lactate concentration, and the shock index was noted [5].

The sheath can be left in place until it has been established with certainty that it is no longer required (although this could cause ischemic complications, especially patients with a smaller build [26]).

The development of new devices that do not require an oversized sheath or long guidewires is likely to reduce not only complications but also time to occlusion [5].

Insertion setting

REBOA is mostly positioned in emergency departments, in some cases in the operating room or, where available, in a hybrid room. There is also REBOA experience in prehospital settings (e.g., London's Air Ambulance, although limited to blind positioning in zone III only [28]).

Mortality (when, where, why)

As for mortality, several aspects must be considered: when, where (emergency department, operating room, intensive care unit), and why.

Some studies report mortality percentages with precise temporal references (e.g., mortality at 24 h, 30 days, 60 days, etc.), while others do not.

Saito et al. claim that mortality within 24 h is more relatable to REBOA because after this time, patients die from other causes [18].

Many studies compare the mortality of patients treated with REBOA versus resuscitative thoracotomy, matching patients with similar characteristics; most of them do not report favorable data for REBOA. However, Moore et al. [12] noted that the deaths of *REBOA patients* appear to be delayed and typically occur when the patient is already out of the emergency department and due to complications other than bleeding (especially multi-organ failure and brain injury). Post-REBOA deaths more commonly occurred in emergency or operatory room while a significantly larger portion of post-open aortic occlusion occurred in the intensive care unit [29].

Complications

In several series of patients, no complications have been related to the use of REBOA.

Eventually, complications may be related to the insertion, to the REBOA mechanism (pressure increases upstream from the occlusion), or to the failure of the technique itself.

Described complications are:

- 0.66% distal ischemia/thromboembolic events [18, 21, 26, 29] (with eventual need for amputation) [26]
- 0.07% intracranial massive hemorrhage [30]
- 0.22% pseudo-aneurysm in the access site [29]/arterial injury caused by puncture [18]
- 0.89% kidney failure [18]
- Spinal cord ischemia (no REBOA cases) [18]
- 0.15% balloon migration (e.g., in zone II) [29]
- 0.30% infections [29]
- 0.07% retroperitoneal hematoma following the blind insertion (the vessel was repaired a few days later without further complications); this is more common in obese patients in whom multiple attempts are performed; ultrasound-guided procedure, thanks to the widespread of portable devices, is useful as long as this does not cause an excessive elongation of the time [18, 21]
- 0.66% introducer insertion failure: especially in elderly patients (over 75 years, above all females) who had subsequently undergone resuscitative thoracotomy or REBOA in the angiography room and where the angiography revealed severe tortuosity or twisting of the femoral artery. [5]
- 0.07% rupture of the balloon (immediately replaced) [31]

The main risk factors are high body mass index, thrombocytopenia, emergency procedures, big size of the introducer, and use of anti-platelet drugs [5]. Complications seem to reduce significantly with 7-Fr catheter [32].

REBOA in combination with other techniques

REBOA is not considered as a permanent solution, rather it constitutes a bridge for patient stabilization until definitive hemostasis (angioembolization, surgery, or hybrid technique), eventually achieved during the diagnostic completion techniques (TC) and transfers.

However, in some circumstances, it was not enough by itself and it has been used in conjunction with other techniques to control bleeding, e.g., external fixator and pelvic packing. Sometimes, it was necessary to convert to an aortic open occlusion (e.g., 4 of 46 patients described by DuBose et al. [29]); other times, REBOA has been used in patients who have already undergone resuscitative thoracotomy; however, such cases have been excluded from the study (Saito et al. [18]) and from this review.

Table 1 shows the list of papers included, in chronological order, except for the last three to whom full text was recovered from other sources.

Conclusions

Resuscitative endovascular balloon occlusion of the aorta has been used increasingly during the last 10 years to elevate central arterial blood pressure in severely injured trauma victims with abdominal and/or pelvic bleeding, limiting infused fluid volume. Studies included in this review showed huge heterogeneity in patient selection, procedure performing time and environment, and balloon deflation cutoff time. However, there is homogeneity in using REBOA in severely injured patients using femoral artery access, with the aim to transiently stop or reduce distal aortic blood flow, while various procedures to finally control the bleeding are performed. Direct REBOA-related complications seem to have a minor role on mortality and are limited to local vascular injuries. High mortality rate is a feature of severely multiple injured patients, and REBOA role as a bridge to final bleeding control clearly emerges, even though not always effective. Pre-hospital REBOA role in trauma victim resuscitation, partial or intermittent balloon inflation, "prophylactic" REBOA insertion in selected cases, REBOA in combination with resuscitative thoracotomy for witnessed traumatic cardiac arrest, and resuscitative endovascular balloon occlusion of inferior vena cava to treat injuries in this site, should be interesting issues for the next future. Taking into account worldwide huge heterogeneity in trauma team composition and setting, considering also available literature concerning REBOA flow charts [33], an updated Trauma System should equip oneself of specific REBOA algorithm, included in severe trauma resuscitation protocol, accordingly with his own features. Different Trauma System benchmark will be the way to better understand and perform in severe hemorrhagic trauma resuscitation.

Abbreviations
ED: Emergency department; REBOA: Resuscitative endovascular balloon occlusion of the aorta

Acknowledgements
The authors would like to thank Dr. Magda Djellab for her help in revising the final version of the manuscript.

Funding
Nil.

Authors' contributions
EG and FC contributed to the concept of the study design, literature search, data analysis, data interpretation, and article drafting. BT contributed to the literature search, data collection, data analysis, and manuscript drafting. CM, VA, MBe, MBi, NF, LA, GG, and MB contributed to the literature search, data collection, data analysis, and manuscript revision. TMH and VA contributed to the concept of the study design, data analysis, data interpretation, and manuscript critical revision. All authors read and approve the final version of the manuscript.

Competing interests
The authors declare that they have no competing interests.

Author details
[1]Anesthesia and Intensive Care Department, AUSL Romagna Trauma Center "Maurizio Bufalini" Hospital, Viale Ghirotti 286, 47521 Cesena, Italy. [2]General and Emergency Surgery Department, ASST Trauma Center "Papa Giovanni XXIII" Hospital, Piazza OMS 1, 24127 Bergamo, Italy. [3]Emergency Medicine, University of Modena and Reggio Emilia, via Università 4, 41121 Modena, Italy. [4]Interventional Radiology Department, AUSL Romagna Trauma Center "Maurizio Bufalini" Hospital, Viale Ghirotti 286, 47521 Cesena, Italy. [5]General and Emergency Surgery Department, AUSL Romagna Trauma Center "Maurizio Bufalini" Hospital, Viale Ghirotti 286, 47521 Cesena, Italy. [6]Cardiothoracic and Vascular Surgery Department, Örebro University Hospital, Södra Grev Rosengatan, 701 85 Örebro, Sweden. [7]Anesthesia, Intensive Care and 118 Emergency System Department, AUSL Bologna Trauma Center "Maggiore" Hospital, Largo Nigrisoli 2, 40133 Bologna, Italy. [8]Emergency Medicine Department, AUSL Modena Trauma Center "Sant'Agostino" Hospital, Via Pietro Giardini 1355, 41126 Modena, Italy.

References
1. Davis JS, Satahoo SS, Butler FK, et al. An analysis of prehospital deaths: who can we save? J Trauma Acute Care Surg. 2014;77:213–8.
2. Morrison JJ, Ross JD, Houston R, et al. Use of resuscitative endovascular balloon occlusion of the aorta in a highly lethal model of noncompressible torso hemorrhage. Shock. 2014;41:130–7.
3. Bansal V, Fortlage D, Lee J, Costantini T, Potenza B, Coimbra R. Hemorrhage is more prevalent than brain injury in early trauma deaths: the golden six hours. Eur J Trauma Emerg Surg. 2009;35:26–30.
4. Tien HC, Spencer F, Tremblay LN, Rizoli SB, Brenneman FD. Preventable deaths from hemorrhage at a level I Canadian trauma center. J Trauma. 2007;62:142–6.
5. Tsurukiri, et al. Resuscitative endovascular balloon occlusion of the aorta for uncontrolled haemorrhagic shock as an adjunct to haemostatic procedures in the acute care setting. Scand J Trauma Resusc Emerg Med. 2016;24:13.
6. Morrison JJ, Rasmussen TE. Non compressible torso haemorrhage: are view with contemporary definitions and management strategies. Surg Clin North Am. 2012;92:843–85.
7. Laine L. Upper gastrointestinal bleeding. Clin Updat. 2007;14:1–4.
8. Carroli G, Cuesta C, Abalos E, Gulmezoglu AM. Epidemiology of post-partum haemorrhage: a systematic review. Best Pract Res Clin Obstet Gynaecol. 2008;22:999–1012.
9. Nordon IM, Hinchliffe RJ, Loftus IM, Thompson MM. Pathophysiology and epidemiology of abdominal aortic aneurysms. Nat Rev Cardiol. 2011;8:92–102.
10. Morrison JJ, Galgon RE, Jansen JO, Cannon JW, Rasmussen TE, Eliason JL. A systematic review of the use of resuscitative endovascular balloon occlusion of the aorta in the management of hemorrhagic shock. J Trauma Acute Care Surg. 2016;80:324–34.
11. Norii T, Crandall C, Terasaka Y. Survival of severe blunt trauma patients treated with resuscitative endovascular balloon occlusion of the aorta compared with propensity score-adjusted untreated patients. J Trauma Acute Care Surg. 2015;78:721–8.
12. Moore LJ, Brenner M, Kozar RA, Pasley J, Wade CE, Baraniuk MS, Scalea T, Holcomb JB. Implementation of resuscitative endovascular balloon occlusion of the aorta as an alternative to resuscitative thoracotomy for noncompressible truncal hemorrhage. J Trauma Acute Care Surg. 2015;79: 523–32.
13. American Association for the Surgery of Trauma. Multi-Institutional Studies Web Site. Available at: http://www.aast.org/Research/MultiInstitutional Studies.aspx. Accessed 1 July 2015.
14. ABOTrauma Registry Web Site. Available at: https://www.abotraumaregistry.com. Accessed 15 Aug 2015.
15. Guliani S, Amendola M, Strife B, Morano G, Elbich J, Albuquerque F, Komorowski D, Sydnor M, Malhotra A, Levy M. Central aortic wire confirmation for emergent endovascularprocedures: as fast as surgeon-performed ultrasound. J Trauma Acute Care Surg. 2015;79:549–54.
16. Stannard A, Eliason JL, Rasmussen TE. Resuscitative endovascular balloon occlusion of the aorta (REBOA) as an adjunct for hemorrhagic shock. J Trauma. 2011;71:1869–72.
17. Inoue J, Shiraishi A, Yoshiyuki A, Haruta K, Matsui H, Otomo Y. Resuscitative endovascular balloon occlusion of the aorta might be dangerous in patients with severe torso trauma: a propensity score analysis. J Trauma Acute Care Surg. 2016;80(4):559–66.

18. Saito N, Matsumoto H, Yagi T, Hara Y, Hayashida K, Motomura T, Mashiko K, Iida H, Yokota H, Wagatsuma Y. Evaluation of the safety and feasibility of resuscitative endovascular balloon occlusion of the aorta. J Trauma Acute Care Surg. 2015;78(5):897–903.
19. Irahara T, Sato N, Moroe Y, Fukuda R, Iwai Y, Unemoto K. Retrospective study of the effectiveness of intra-aortic balloon occlusion (IABO) for traumatic haemorrhagic shock. World J Emerg Surg. 2015;6(10(1)):1.
20. Costantini TW, Coimbra R, Holcomb JB, Podbielski JM, Catalano R, Blackburn A, Scalea TM, Stein DM, Williams L, Conflitti J, Keeney S, Suleiman G, Zhou T, Sperry J, Skiada D, Inaba K, Williams BH, Minei JP, Privette A, Mackersie RC, Robinson BR, Moore FO, AAST Pelvic Fracture Study Group. Current management of hemorrhage from severe pelvic fractures: results of an American Association for the Surgery of Trauma multi-institutional trial. J Trauma Acute Care Surg. 2016;80(5):717–23.
21. Hörer TM, Skoog P, Pirouzram A, Nilsson KF, Larzon T. A small case series of aortic balloon occlusion in trauma: lessons learned from its use in ruptured abdominal aortic aneurysms and a brief review. Eur J Trauma Emerg Surg. 2016;42(5):585–92.
22. Matsuoka S, Uchiyama K, Shima H, Ohishi S, Nojiri Y, Ogata H. Temporary percutaneous aortic balloon occlusion to enhance fluid resuscitation prior to definitive embolization of posttraumatic liver haemorrhage. Cardiovasc Intervent Radiol. 2001;24:274–6.
23. MacTaggart JN, Poulson WE, Akhter M, Seas A, Thorson K, Phillips NY, Desyatova AS, Kamenskiy AV. Morphometric roadmaps to improve accurate device delivery for fluoroscopy-free resuscitative endovascular balloon occlusion of the aorta. J Trauma Acute Care Surg. 2016;80(6):941–6.
24. Brenner M, Hoehn M, Pasley J, Dubose J, Stein D, Scalea T. Basic endovascular skills for trauma course: bridging the gap between endovascular techniques and the acute care surgeon. J Trauma Acute Care Surg. 2014;77(2):286–91.
25. Qasim Z, Brenner M, Menaker J, Scalea T. Resuscitative endovascular balloon occlusion of the aorta. Resuscitation. 2015;96:275–9.
26. Okada Y, Narumiya H, Ishi W, Ryoji I. Lower limb ischemia caused by resuscitative balloon occlusion of aorta. Surg Case Rep. 2016;2(1):130.
27. Ogura T, Lefor AT, Nakano M, Izawa Y, Morita H. Nonoperative management of hemodynamically unstable abdominal trauma patients with angioembolization and resuscitative endovascular balloon occlusion of the aorta. J Trauma Acute Care Surg. 2015;78(1):132–5.
28. Sadek S, Lockey DJ, Lendrum RA, Perkins Z, Price J, Davies GE. Resuscitative endovascular balloon occlusion of the aorta (REBOA) in the pre-hospital setting: an additional resuscitation option for uncontrolled catastrophic haemorrhage. Resuscitation. 2016;107:135–8.
29. DuBose JJ, Scalea TM, Brenner M, Skiada D, Inaba K, Cannon J, Moore L, Holcomb J, Turay D, Arbabi CN, Kirkpatrick A, Xiao J, Skarupa D, Poulin N, AAST AORTA Study Group. The AAST prospective aortic occlusion for resuscitation in trauma and acute care surgery (AORTA) registry: data on contemporary utilization and outcomes of aortic occlusion and resuscitative balloon occlusion of the aorta (REBOA). J Trauma Acute Care Surg. 2016; 81(3):409–19.
30. Uchino H, Tamura N, Echigoya R, Ikegami T, Fukuoka T. "REBOA"—is it really safe? A case with massive intracranial hemorrhage possibly due to endovascular balloon occlusion of the aorta (REBOA). Am J Case Rep. 2016;1(17):810–3.
31. Martinelli T, Thony F, Decléty P, Sengel C, Broux C, Tonetti J, Payen JF, Ferretti G. Intra-aortic balloon occlusion to salvage patients with life-threatening hemorrhagic shocks from pelvic fractures. J Trauma. 2010;68(4):942–8.
32. Teeter WA, Matsumoto J, Idoguchi K, Kon Y, Orita T, Funabiki T, Brenner ML, Matsumura Y. Smaller introducer sheaths for REBOA may be associated with fewer complications. J Trauma Acute Care Surg. 2016 Dec;81(6):1039–45.
33. Biffl WL, Fox CJ, Moore EE. The role of REBOA in the control of exsanguinating torso hemorrhage. J Trauma Acute Care Surg. 2015;78(5):1054–8.
34. Matsumoto N, Sogabe O, Yoshida O, Endo I, Yamamoto S, Inokawa H, Kubo M, Udaka T, Maeda H, Mizuta M. The usefulness of resuscitative endovascular balloon occlusion of the aorta in detecting the source of a hemorrhage due to abdominal blunt trauma. Am J Emerg Med. 2016;34(10):2057.
35. Hörer TM, Hebron D, Swaid F, Korin A, Galili O, Alfici R, Kessel B. Aorta balloon occlusion in trauma: three cases demonstrating multidisciplinary approach already on patient's arrival to the emergency room. Cardiovasc Intervent Radiol. 2016;39(2):284–9.
36. Brenner ML, Moore LJ, DuBose JJ, Tyson GH, McNutt MK, Albarado RP, Holcomb JB, Scalea TM, Rasmussen TE. A clinical series of resuscitative endovascular balloon occlusion of the aorta for hemorrhage control and resuscitation. J Trauma Acute Care Surg. 2013;75(3):506–11.
37. Kataoka Y, Minehara H, Shimada K, Nishimaki H, Soma K, Maekawa K. Sepsis caused by peripelvic soft tissue infections in critically injured patients with multiple injuries and unstable pelvic fracture. J Trauma. 2009;66(6):1548–54.
38. Long JA, Descotes JL, Terrier N, Faucheron JL, Pecher M, Francony G, Sengel C, Rambeaud JJ. Endovascular aortic balloon catheter occlusion for severe renal trauma. Prog Urol. 2004;14(3):394–7.
39. Linsenmaier U, Kanz KG, Rieger J, Krötz M, Mutschler W, Pfeifer KJ, Reiser M. CT-guided aortic balloon occlusion in traumatic abdominal and pelvic bleeding. Rofo. 2003;175(9):1259–63.
40. Segol P, Salame E, Auvray S, Marchand P, Tartière J. Major liver injury. Role of preoperative transcutaneous endoluminal aortic clamping. Presse Med. 1995;7(24(1)):29–30.
41. Gupta BK, Khaneja SC, Flores L, Eastlick L, Longomore W, Shaftan GW. The role of intra-aortic balloon occlusion in penetrating abdominal trauma. J Trauma. 1989;29(6):861–5.
42. Low RB, Longmore W, Rubinstein R, Flores L, Wolvek S. Preliminary report on the use of the Percluder occluding aortic balloon in human beings. Ann Emerg Med. 1986;15(12):1466–9.
43. Wolf RK, Berry RE. Transaxillary intra-aortic balloon tamponade in trauma. J Vasc Surg. 1986;4(1):95–7.
44. Hughes CW. Use of an intra-aortic balloon catheter tamponade for controlling intra-abdominal hemorrhage in man. Surgery. 1954;36:65–8.

27

Emergency abdominal surgery after solid organ transplantation

Nicola de'Angelis[1*], Francesco Esposito[1], Riccardo Memeo[2], Vincenzo Lizzi[1], Aleix Martìnez-Pérez[1], Filippo Landi[1], Pietro Genova[1], Fausto Catena[3], Francesco Brunetti[1] and Daniel Azoulay[1]

Abstract

Aims: Due to the increasing number of solid organs transplantations, emergency abdominal surgery in transplanted patients is becoming a relevant challenge for the general surgeon. The aim of this systematic review of the literature is to analyze morbidity and mortality of emergency abdominal surgery performed in transplanted patients for graft-unrelated surgical problems.

Methods: The literature search was performed on online databases with the time limit 1990–2015. Studies describing all types of emergency abdominal surgery in solid organ transplanted patients were retrieved for evaluation.

Results: Thirty-nine case series published between 1996 and 2015 met the inclusion criteria and were selected for the systematic review. Overall, they included 71671 transplanted patients, of which 1761 (2.5 %) underwent emergency abdominal surgery. The transplanted organs were the heart in 65.8 % of patients, the lung in 22.1 %, the kidney in 9. 5 %, and the liver in 2.6 %. The mean patients' age at the time of the emergency abdominal surgery was 49.4 ± 7. 4 years, and the median time from transplantation to emergency surgery was 2.4 years (range 0.1–20). Indications for emergency abdominal surgery were: gallbladder diseases (80.3 %), gastrointestinal perforations (9.2 %), complicated diverticulitis (6.2 %), small bowel obstructions (2 %), and appendicitis (2 %). The overall mortality was 5.5 % (range 0–17.5 %). The morbidity rate varied from 13.6 % for gallbladder diseases to 32.7 % for complicated diverticulitis. Most of the time, the immunosuppressive therapy was maintained unmodified postoperatively.

Conclusions: Emergency abdominal surgery in transplanted patients is not a rare event. Although associated with relevant mortality and morbidity, a prompt and appropriate surgery can lead to satisfactory results if performed taking into account the patient's immunosuppression therapy and hemodynamic stability.

Keywords: Emergency abdominal surgery, General surgery, Solid organ transplantation, Liver transplantation, Kidney transplantation, Heart transplantation, Lung transplantation, Systematic review

Abbreviations: CT, Computed tomography; EAS, Emergency abdominal surgery

Background

Organ transplantation is considered as the most effective treatment for end-stage disease of the heart, lung, pancreas, liver, and kidney, with approximately 28000 solid organs transplanted every year in Europe and USA, and overall 114690 organs transplanted in 2012 worldwide [1]. The high number of transplantations per year and the long-term graft survival had contributed to drastically increase the likelihood for an emergency surgeon to encounter a transplanted patient with a graft-unrelated surgical problem [2–5].

The management of graft-unrelated acute abdominal disease in transplanted patients generally adheres to the fundamental principles of any surgical treatment. Preoperative evaluation should consider that transplanted patients are chronically immunosuppressed, and although most of them achieve an excellent functional capacity and are able to live normal productive lives, they remain at increased risk for any surgical complication, particularly infectious. Moreover, the clinical presentation of many disease may be different from the general population,

* Correspondence: nic.deangelis@yahoo.it
[1]Department of Digestive, Hepatobiliary Surgery and Liver Transplantation, "Henri Mondor" University Hospital, Université Paris Est - UPEC, 51, Avenue du Maréchal de Lattre de Tassigny, 94010 Créteil, France

sometimes leading to misdiagnosis or underestimation of the disease severity [5]. Another important issue is the potential impact of any operative procedure on the functional capacity of the transplanted organ, which shows to have a reduced clinical reserve compared to the native organ. Even modest intra-operative insults, such as hypotension, may negatively affect the transplanted organ, and thus, when several options are available, the most cautious, conservative, minimally invasive, and standardized surgical approach should be preferred in these patients [5].

When considering the incidence of several common general surgical problems and the ever-larger cohort of transplanted patients living and functioning under chronic immunosuppression [6], it becomes apparent that all general surgeons, especially outside of transplant centers, should be familiar with the factors that influence the surgical outcomes in this particular subset of patients, along with the issues that are likely to affect the optimal surgery timing and the postoperative cares [6].

The aim of the present systematic review is to provide an exhaustive analysis of the current available literature about the outcomes of emergency abdominal surgery (EAS) performed in transplanted patients for graft-unrelated abdominal diseases. The evidence-based assessment of EAS morbidity and mortality in transplanted patients may help the surgeon and clinician in the decision making process face to the challenging management of acute abdominal disease in this particular subset of patients.

Materials and methods

The methodological approach included the development of selection criteria, definition of search strategies, assessment of study quality, and abstraction of relevant data. The PRISMA statements checklist for reporting a systematic review was followed [7].

Study inclusion criteria

The study selection criteria were defined before initiating data collection for proper identification of studies eligible for the analysis. All studies in which the primary objective was to describe EAS for graft-unrelated diseases in transplanted patients were retrieved and analyzed.

Types of study

Epidemiological studies, interventional trials, case–control studies, cross-sectional studies and case series including more than four patients [8] were considered eligible for inclusion in this systematic review. Case reports, review articles, systematic reviews, meta-analyses, conference abstracts, letters and commentaries were not considered.

Types of participants

Patients who had received a solid organ transplantation (heart, lung, liver, pancreas, or kidney) presenting with graft-unrelated surgical abdominal diseases were considered.

Types of intervention

All types of surgical abdominal emergencies (e.g. appendectomy, cholecystectomy, colectomy, bowel resection, gastric resection, surgical repair of incisional hernia, explorative laparotomy) were considered.

Types of outcome measures

The primary outcomes were the post-operative 90-day morbidity and mortality following EAS. All secondary parameters (e.g. hospital stay and immunosuppressive therapy) reported in the selected studies were also evaluated.

Literature search strategy

A literature search was performed on the following online databases: MEDLINE (through PubMed), EMBASE, Scopus, Cochrane Oral Health Group Specialized Register, and ProQuest Dissertations and Thesis Database. To increase the probability of identifying all relevant articles, a specific research equation was formulated for each database, using the following keywords and/or MeSH terms: emergency, emergency surgery, urgent surgery, appendicitis, diverticulitis, perforation, cholecystectomy, colectomy, appendectomy, cholecystitis, humans, adult, transplant, transplantation, solid organ transplantation, transplant patient, transplanted patient.

In addition, the reference lists from the eligible studies and relevant review articles (not included in the systematic review) were crosschecked to identify additional records. The literature search was performed on January 2016 and was restricted to articles published since 1990. Only studies written in English and meeting the selection criteria were reviewed.

Study selection and quality assessment

The titles and abstracts of the retrieved studies were independently and blindly screened for relevance by two reviewers (FE and VL). To enhance sensitivity, records were removed only if both reviewers excluded the record at the title screening level. All disagreements were resolved by discussion with a third and fourth reviewers (NdeA and RM). Subsequently, both reviewers performed a full-text analysis of the selected articles. Two reviewers independently assessed the risk of bias and study quality by using appropriate tools. Precisely, The NICE guidelines [9] was used for the quality assessment of case series, which was rated on a 8 points scale by answering eight questions concerning the following aspects:, study setting (i.e. uni or multicentric), study hypothesis/objective, case definition, outcome definition, data collection, patient recruitment, result description and analysis. Additionally, the Grading of Recommendations Assessment Development and Evaluation (GRADE) system [10] was used to enable consistent judgment of the "body of evidence" included in the systematic review. GRADE specifies four categories: high, moderate, low, and very low. In the context of a systematic review, the quality of evidence reflects the confidence that the estimates of the effect are correct and overpasses the individual study risk of bias by evaluating the following aspects: study design, imprecision, inconsistency, indirectness of study results, and publication bias.

Data extraction

Data extracted from the studies included in the systematic review were processed for qualitative and possibly quantitative analyses. Outcome measures (mean and median values, standard deviation, and ranges) were extracted for each variable. Average morbidity and mortality rates were calculated.

Results

Literature search and selection

Out of the 1428 articles initially identified, 39 articles [2, 4, 11–47] met the inclusion criteria and were selected for the systematic review. The flow chart of studies identification and inclusion/exclusion process is shown in Fig. 1.

Study characteristics

The selected studies were published between 1996 and 2015 and they were all case series [2, 4, 11–47]. They were carried out in ten different countries, particularly in Europe ($n = 11$) [13, 14, 18, 24, 28–30, 34, 35, 38, 40], North America ($n = 24$) [2, 4, 11, 12, 15–17, 19, 21–23, 25–27, 31, 33, 36, 37, 39, 41, 43–46], Asia and Pacific ($n = 4$) [20, 32, 42, 47]. The overall number of transplanted patients considered was 71671. Of these patients, 1761 (2.5 %) underwent EAS for graft-unrelated acute diseases. The mean age of the patients undergoing EAS was 49.4 ± 7.4 years, and the median time from transplantation to the required emergency operation was 2.4 years (range 0.1–20). The

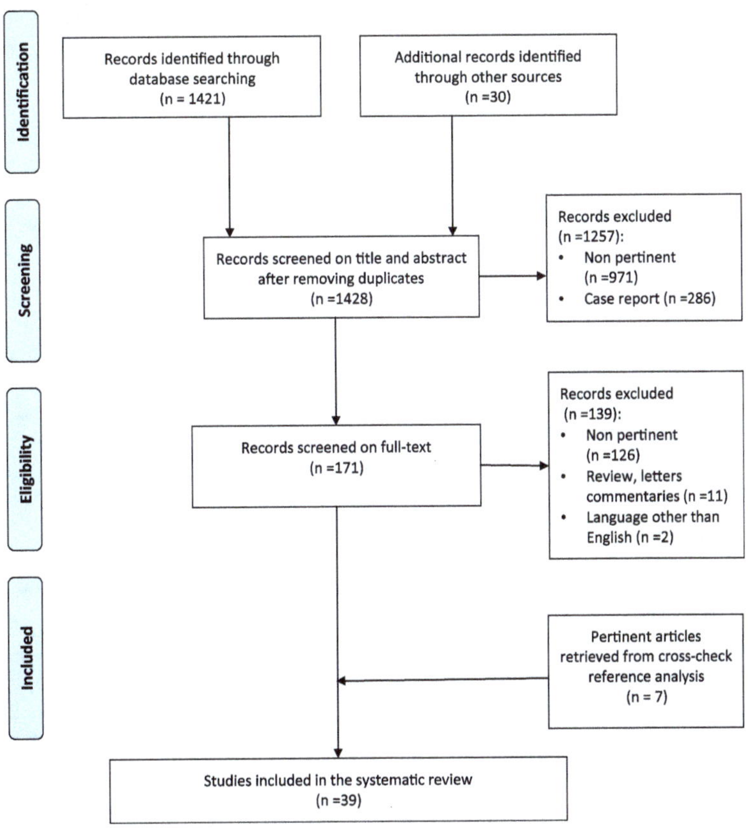

Fig. 1 Flow chart of the study search, selection, and inclusion. Example of search equation: emergency[Title/Abstract]) OR emergency surgery[Title/Abstract]) OR urgent surgery[Title/Abstract]) OR appendicitis[Title/Abstract]) OR diverticulitis[Title/Abstract]) OR perforation[Title/Abstract]) OR cholecystectomy[Title/Abstract]) OR colectomy[Title/Abstract]) OR appendectomy[Title/Abstract]) OR cholecystitis[Title/Abstract]) AND Humans[Mesh] AND English[lang] AND adult[MeSH]) AND (((((transplant[Title/Abstract]) OR transplantation[Title/Abstract]) OR solid organ transplantation[Title/Abstract]) OR transplant patient[Title/Abstract]) OR transplanted patient[Title/Abstract])

organ transplanted was the heart in 65.8 % of cases, the lung in 22.1 %, the kidney in 9.5 % and the liver in 2.6 %. EAS was necessary because of the following conditions: gallbladder diseases (80.3 %), gastrointestinal perforations (9.2 %), complicated diverticulitis (6.2 %), small bowel obstruction (2 %), appendicitis (2 %), and miscellaneous (0.3 %). The overall mortality rate was 5.5 %.

The studies concerning gallbladder diseases [4, 11–23] requiring EAS in transplanted patients are displayed in Table 1. Acute cholecystitis, with and without gallstones (including hydrops, empyema, gangrene and perforation), was the most common primary diagnosis, followed by gallstones without cholecystitis, and chronic cholecystitis. Laparoscopic cholecystectomy was performed in 72 % of EAS cases and laparotomy in 23.1 %. In 1.9 % of patients a surgical cholecystostomy was carried out. In 42 patients, the type of surgery performed was not precisely described. The morbidity rate was 13.6 %. The most frequent EAS-related complications included: respiratory failure, pneumonia, deep venous thrombosis, pulmonary embolism, postoperative haemorrhage, and surgical site infection. The overall mortality was 3.4 %. The median hospital stay was 9.3 days (range 1–38).

The studies concerning gastrointestinal perforations requiring EAS in transplanted patients [4, 13, 18, 21, 23–36] are shown in Table 2. The most frequent causes of perforation were: diverticulitis (this disorder and its complications are described below and in Table 3); peptic disease; ischemia; chronic inflammatory bowel disease; iatrogenic factors; post-transplantation lymphoproliferative disorders; enteritis and colitis caused by Clostridium difficile or Cytomegalovirus. In immunosuppressed transplanted patients, the signs and symptoms of perforation were often absent or non-specific. Therefore, the interval from clinical onset to surgery was very large, ranging from 2 to 8 days. The diagnosis of perforation was confirmed by an abdominal and pelvic

Table 1 Reports of gallbladder diseases requiring EAS after solid organ transplantation

Authors, Year	Transplanted organ (n)				EAS characteristics and outcomes				
	Heart	Lung	Heart-Lung	Kidney	Patients undergoing EAS (n)	EAS Rate (%)	Surgical procedures (n)	Morbidity [n(%)]	Mortality [n(%)]
Taghavi S et al., 2015 [11]		9186			258	2.81	OC (58), LC (190), n/a (10)	48 (18.6)	0 (0)
Kilic A et al., 2013 [12]	23854				1054	4.42	OC (233), LC (795), CS (26)	126 (12.0)	37 (3.5)
Lahon B et al., 2011 [13]		351			11	3.13	OC (11)	n/a	1 (9.1)
Paul S et al., 2009 [4]		208			13	6.25	OC (4), LC (9)	n/a	0 (0)
Sarkio S et al., 2007 [14]				1608	17	1.06	n/a (17)	n/a	1 (5.9)
Takeyama H et al., 2006 [15]	402				2	0.50	n/a (2)	n/a	0 (0)
Englesbe MJ et al., 2005 [16]	168				7	4.17	LC (7)	2 (28.6)	1 (14.3)
Richardson WS et al., 2003 [17]	518				19	3.67	OC (4), LC (15)	9 (47.4)	1 (5.3)
Hoekstra HJ et al., 2001 [18]		125			1	0.80	LC (1)	n/a	0 (0)
Gupta D et al., 2000 [19]	143	30	5		6	3.37	OC (6)	3 (50)	3 (50)
Lord RV et al., 1998 [20]	455	133	57		13	2.02	n/a (13)	4 (30.8)	1 (7.7)
Bhatia DS et al., 1997 [21]	349				5	1.43	OC (5)	n/a	2 (40)
Milas M et al., 1996 [22]	175				5	2,86	OC (5)	0 (0)	0 (0)
Sharma S et al., 1996 [23]	240				2	0.83	OC (1), CS (1)	0 (0)	1 (50)
Total	26304	10033	62	1608	1413	3.72	OC (327), LC (1017), CS (27), n/a (42)	192 (13.6)	48 (3.4)

EAS emergency abdominal surgery, *OC* open cholecystectomy, *LC* laparoscopic cholecystectomy, *CS* cholecystostomy, *n/a* not available

Table 2 Reports of gastrointestinal perforations requiring EAS after solid organ transplantation

	Transplanted organ (n)				EAS characteristics and outcomes				
Authors, Year	Liver	Heart	Lung	Kidney	Patients undergoing EAS (n)	EAS Rate (%)	Surgical procedures (n)	Morbidity [n (%)]	Mortality [n (%)]
Timrott K et al., 2014 [24]		342	1074		21[a]	1,48	BR (21)	n/a	n/a
Lee JT et al., 2014 [25]				2406	10	0.42	CR (10)	6 (60)	3 (30)
Cruz RJ Jr et al., 2012 [26]	5677				6	0.11	n/a (6)	n/a	2 (33.3)
Boutros M et al., 2012 [27]				814	2	0.25	CR (2)	n/a	0 (0)
Boutros M et al., 2012 [27]	430				3	0.70	CR (3)	n/a	1 (33.3)
Jorgensen KK et al., 2012 [28]	69				4	5.80	CR (4)	n/a	0 (0)
Lahon B et al., 2011 [13]			351		2	0.57	CR (2)	n/a	0 (0)
Paul S et al., 2009 [4]			208		8	3.85	n/a[c] (7), CR (1)	n/a	3 (37.5)
Catena F et al., 2008 [29]				1611	46	2.86	CR (21), BR (15), UC (10)	n/a	11 (23.9)
Ho GT et al., 2005 [30]	413				4	0.97	CR (4)	n/a	0 (0)
Keven K et al., 2004 [31]				702	2	0.28	CR (2)	1 (50)	1 (50)
Karakayali H et al., 2002 [32]				1038	6	0.58	UC (4), CR (2)	n/a	0 (0)
Hoekstra HJ et al., 2001 [18]			125		2	1.60	BR (1), CR (1)	n/a	0 (0)
Andreoni KA et al., 1999 [33]				1417	26	1.83	CR (26)	n/a	1 (3,8)
Mueller XM et al., 1999 [34]		93			2[b]	2.15	UC (1), CS (1)	0 (0)	0 (0)
Bhatia DS et al., 1997 [21]		349			7	2.01	CR (7)	3 (42.9)	0 (0)
Wekerle T et al., 1997 [35]			124		4	3.23	n/a[c] (2), CR (2)	n/a	4 (100)
Beaver TM et al., 1996 [36]			60		3	5.00	HP (3)	0 (0)	1 (33,3)
Sharma S et al., 1996 [23]		240			2	0.83	n/a[c] (2)	0 (0)	1 (50)
Total	6589	1024	1942	7988	160	0.91	BR (37), CR (87), HP (3), UC (15), CS (1), n/a (17)	n/a	28 (17.5)

EAS emergency abdominal surgery, *BR* bowel resection, *CR* colon resection, *UC* ulcer closure, *CS* colostomy, *HP* hartmann procedure, *n/a* not available
[a]3out of 21 were after heart transplantation; [b]1 Duodenal ulcer perforation and 1 iatrogenic colon perforation; [c]Peptic ulcer disease

computed tomography (CT) scan in most of the cases, whereas abdominal X-rays were sufficient in some cases.

The perforation was located at the level of colon in 58.4 % of patients, small bowel (including jejunum and ileum) in 33.8 %, stomach and duodenum in 7.8 %. All operations were performed by open approach. The surgical procedures carried out were: colon resection with primary anastomosis in 54.3 % of cases; small bowel resection with anastomosis in 23.2 %; stomach and duodenum ulcer closure in 9.4 %; Hartmann's procedure in 1.9 %; and colostomy in 0.6 %. In 10.6 % of cases, the type of surgery performed could not be traced back. Generally, the immunosuppressive therapy was maintained unmodified postoperatively. The median hospital stay was 22.2 days (range 9–87), with an overall mortality rate of 17.5 %.

Table 3 Reports of complicated diverticulitis after solid organ transplantation

	Transplanted organ (n)					EAS characteristics and outcomes				
Authors, Year	Liver	Heart	Lung	Heart-Lung	Kidney	Patients undergoing EAS (n)	EAS Rate (%)	Surgical procedures (n)	Morbidity [n (%)]	Mortality [n (%)]
Larson ES et al., 2014 [37]			314			7	2.23	HP (7)	n/a	1 (14.3)
Scotti A et al., 2014 [38]					717	9	1.26	HP (9)	5 (55.6)	0 (0)
Reshef A et al., 2012 [39]		5329[a]				9	0.17	CR (9)	5 (55.6)	2 (22.2)
Reshef A et al., 2012 [39]					5329[a]	12	0.23	CR (12)	6 (50)	0 (0)
Reshef A et al., 2012 [39]	5329[a]					4	0.08	CR (4)	3 (75)	1 (25)
Reshef A et al., 2012 [39]			5329[a]			12	0.23	CR (12)	9 (75)	4 (33.3)
Paul S et al., 2009 [4]			208			2	0.96	CR (2)	n/a	2 (100)
Dalla Valle R et al., 2005 [40]					875	8	0.91	HP (5), S (2), n/a (1)	6 (75)	1 (12.5)
Miller CB et al., 2006 [41]			229			3	1.31	HP (3)	n/a	0 (0)
Goldberg JH et al., 2006 [2]		530	435	47		11	1.09	HP (11)	n/a	1 (9.1)
Qasabian RA et al., 2004 [42]		639	248	66		9	0.94	HP (6), S (1), S + DLI (2)	0 (0)	1 (11.1)
Karakayali H et al., 2002 [32]					1038	2	0.19	CR (2)	n/a	0 (0)
Hoekstra HJ et al., 2001 [18]			125			5	4	HP (3), S (2)	n/a	0 (0)
Khan S et al., 2001 [43]		233	35			2	0.75	HP (2)	1 (50)	0 (0)
Lederman ED et al., 1998 [44]					1137	13	1.14	HP (13)	1 (7.7)	1 (7.7)
Sharma S et al., 1996 [23]		240				2	0.83	S (2)	n/a	1 (50)
Total	5329[a]	1642	1594	113	3767	110	0.88	HP (59), CR (41), S + DLI (2), S (7), n/a (1)	36 (32.7)	15 (13.6)

EAS emergency abdominal surgery, *HP* hartman procedure, *S* Sigmoidectomy, *S + DLI* sigmoidectomy + diverting loop ileostomy, *CR* colonic resection, *n/a* not available
[a]All transplant patients poled together

The studies specifically dealing with complicated diverticulitis [2, 4, 18, 23, 32, 37–44] occurring in transplanted patients and requiring EAS are displayed in Table 3. Among the most frequent clinical manifestations, there were fever, abdominal pain, signs of localized or diffuse peritonitis, anorexia, diarrhea and leukocytosis. Abdominal and pelvic CT scan was performed for all patients, showing complicated diverticulitis, including free perforations, phlegmons and abscesses. The surgical approach was laparotomy in all cases. It consisted in: Hartman's procedure in 53.6 % of patients; colon resection with primary anastomosis in 37.3 %; sigmoidectomy in 6.4 %; and sigmoidectomy with diverting loop ileostomy in 1.8 %. In 0.9 % of cases the type of surgery performed was not clearly reported. The immunosuppressive therapy was maintained unmodified postoperatively. The morbidity rate was 32.7 %, with the most frequent complications being severe respiratory diseases and wound infection. The overall mortality rate was 13.6 %, in most cases due to sepsis. No case of acute transplant rejection was reported.

The studies concerning small bowel obstructions occurring in transplanted patients and requiring EAS [4, 13, 21, 26, 32, 33, 41] are shown in Table 4. The most frequent causes of small bowel obstruction were post-transplantation lymphoproliferative disorders and mechanical obstruction due to intestinal adhesions. Abdominal pain, chronic diarrhea and lower gastrointestinal bleeding were the most common clinical signs and symptoms. Abdominal-pelvic CT scan was performed in most of the patients. In some cases, the

Table 4 Reports of small bowel obstructions requiring EAS after solid organ transplantation

Authors, Year	Transplanted organ (n)				EAS characteristics and outcomes				
	Liver	Heart	Lung	Kidney	Patients undergoing EAS (n)	EAS Rate (%)	Surgical procedures (n)	Morbidity [n (%)]	Mortality [n (%)]
Cruz RJ Jr et al., 2012 [26]	5677				7	0,12	BR (7)	n/a	2 (28.6)
Lahon B et al., 2011 [13]			351		3	0.85	BR (3)	n/a	0 (0)
Paul S et al., 2009 [4]			208		14	6.73	LA (14)	n/a	1 (7.1)
Miller CB et al., 2006 [41]			229		2	0.87	BR (1), LA (1)	n/a	1 (50)
Karakayali H et al., 2002 [32]				1038	1	0.10	BR (1)	n/a	0 (0)
Andreoni KA et al., 1999 [33]				1417	4	0.28	BR (4)	n/a	1 (25)
Bhatia DS et al., 1997 [21]		349			5	1.43	BR (5)	1 (20)	0
Total	5677	349	788	2455	36	0.39	BR (21), LA (15)	n/a	5 (13.9)

EAS emergency abdominal surgery, *BR* bowel resection, *LA* lysis of adhesions *n/a* not available

diagnosis was based on abdominal X-rays. Surgery consisted in exploratory laparotomy, with small bowel resection in 57.1 % of cases and lysis of adhesions in 42.9 %. The immunosuppressive therapy was maintained post-operatively or reduced in some patients. The overall mortality rate was 14.3 %, mostly because of sepsis or as a direct consequence of surgical complications.

The studies dealing with appendicitis in transplanted patients requiring EAS [18, 23, 24, 32, 41, 45, 46] are displayed in Table 5. Abdominal pain was present in 95.5 % of patients, with associated nausea, vomiting, fever, diarrhea, and leukocytosis. Physical examination demonstrated right lower quadrant tenderness in 90.1 % of the patients. Abdominal and pelvic CT scan was performed in all cases and showed signs of acute appendicitis, including a non-filling appendix, appendicolith, pericecal stranding, or free fluid. Furthermore, the 36.3 % of patients underwent ultrasound examination revealing appendicitis.

The time from abdominal pain onset to appendectomy varied from 14 h to 4 days. Pathologic examination demonstrated appendicitis in 81.8 % of cases. Appendicular perforation occurred in 22.7 % of patients, more frequently in those ones operated belatedly. Negative appendectomy was observed in four specimens (18.2 %). The levels of calcineurin inhibitors were titrated in the post-operative period and maintained at pre-operative values. Patients receiving steroids or mycophenolate resumed their pre-operative dosing immediately after surgery. All patients received a minimum of 24 h intravenous antibiotic treatment, with longer duration for patients with intraperitoneal contamination. The median duration of hospitalization was 6.3 days (range 1–20). No mortality was reported.

Other disorders necessitating EAS in transplanted patients included complicated incisional hernia, pancreatic abscess, and splenic infarction. These studies [23, 47] are shown in Table 6.

Table 5 Reports of appendicitis requiring EAS after solid organ transplantation

Authors, Year	Transplanted Organ (n)						EAS characteristics and outcomes			
	Liver	Heart	Lung	Kidney	Pancreas	Small Bowel	Patients undergoing EAS (n)	EAS Rate %	Morbidity [n (%)]	Mortality [n (%)]
Timrott K et al., 2014 [24]		342					2	0.58	n/a	n/a
Miller CB et al., 2006 [41]			229				2	0.87	n/a	0 (0)
Abt PL et al., 2005 [45]	n/a						7	n/a	2 (28.6)	0 (0)
Savar A et al., 2005 [46]	3287	1336	231	3053	6	10	17	0.21	4 (23.5)	0 (0)
Karakayali H et al., 2002 [32]				1038			5	0.48	n/a	0 (0)
Hoekstra HJ et al., 2001 [18]			125				2	1.6	n/a	0 (0)
Sharma S et al., 1996 [23]		240					1	0.42	n/a	0 (0)
Total	3287[a]	1918	585	4091	6	10	36	0.29[a]	n/a	0 (0)

[a]excluding Abt PL et al.'s study for lack of the number of recipients; *EAS* emergency abdominal surgery, *n/a* not available

Table 6 Reports of EAS for various indications after solid organ transplantation

Authors, Year	Transplanted organ (n)		EAS characteristics and outcomes					
	Liver	Heart	Indication for EAS	Patients undergoing EAS (n)	EAS Rate (%)	Surgical procedures (n)	Morbidity [n (%)]	Mortality [n (%)]
Ozgor D et al., 2014 [47]	173		IH	3	1.73	HRP (3)	1 (33.3)	0 (0)
Sharma S et al., 1996 [23]		240	PA	2	0.83	DD (2)	n/a	0 (0)
Sharma S et al., 1996 [23]		240	SI	1	0.42	SP (1)	n/a	0 (0)
Total	173	240		6	1.45	HRP (3), DD (2), SP (1)	n/a	0 (0)

EAS emergency abdominal surgery, *IH* incisional hernia, *HRP* hernia repair with polypropylene mesh, *PA* pancreatic abscess, *DD* debridement/drainage, *SI* splenic infarction, *SP* splenectomy, *n/a* not available

Study quality assessment

Based on the NICE guidelines for the quality assessment of case series [9], 6 studies received a score of 7/8 [11–13, 27, 28, 39], 31 studies were graded 6/8 [2, 4, 14–16, 18–23, 25, 26, 29–38, 40–47] and 2 studies 5/8 [17, 24]. Based on the GRADE system [48], 37 studies [2, 4, 11–16, 18–23, 25–47] (94.9 %) were judged as being of low quality, and the remaining 2 studies [17, 24] of very low quality of evidence. Of note, all studies were retrospective, which, by definition, are susceptible of major selection bias as well as misclassification or information bias due to the unknown accuracy of record keeping. NICE guidelines and GRADE system quality assessment are displayed in Fig. 2.

Discussion

The present systematic review is the first to analyze the available literature concerning EAS in transplanted patients. Emergency surgery after transplantation for graft-unrelated acute diseases involved 2.5 % of patients, with the main causes being gallbladder diseases, gastrointestinal perforations, complicated diverticulitis, small bowel obstructions, and appendicitis. Overall, EAS was associated with high morbidity (up to 32.7 %) and mortality (up to 17.5 %) rates, which highlight the particularly challenging surgical management of transplanted patients.

Undoubtedly, one of the most important factors contributing to the high morbidity and mortality in transplanted patients operated for EAS is represented by the use of several immunosuppressive regimens, most frequently consisting in a triple-drug association: calcineurin inhibitors, antiproliferative agents, and corticosteriods [49]. In general, immunosuppressive therapy predisposes transplanted patients to various gastrointestinal diseases [50], lymphoproliferative disorders, infective complications (e.g. Cytomegalovirus, Clostridium difficile), and can mask the presenting signs and symptoms of many disease processes. Moreover, immunosuppression is known to interfere with the patient management for transplant-unrelated surgical procedures in terms of risk for drug interactions, adverse effects, wound healing, and postoperative complications [49].

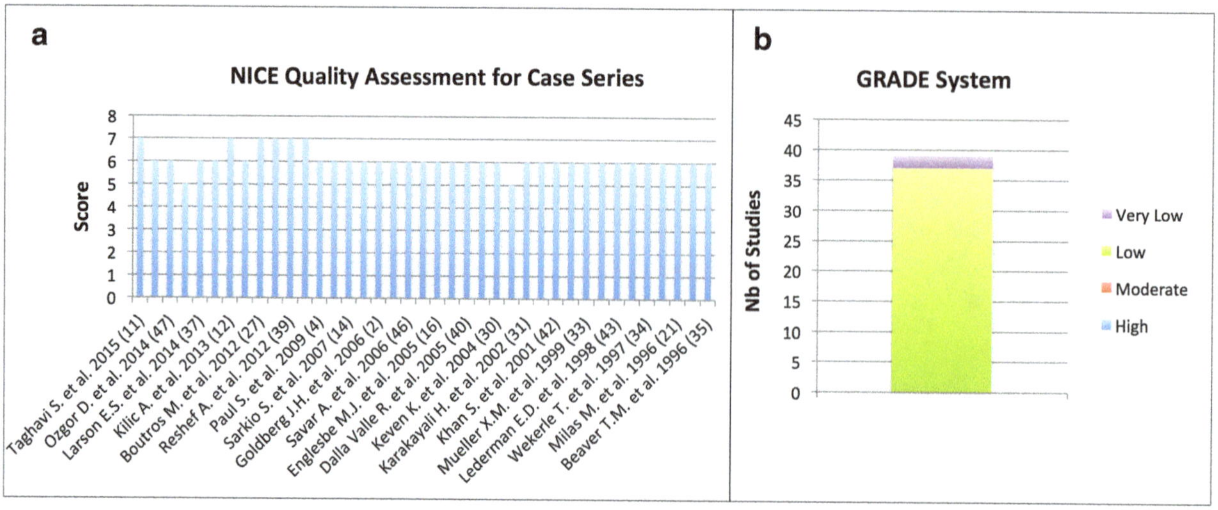

Fig. 2 Study quality assessment by using the NICE (**a**) and GRADE (**b**) systems

Gallbladder diseases were the most frequent reason for EAS after transplantation, which was mainly reported in heart-transplanted patients. Despite actual controversies, the high incidence of biliary tract diseases may be related to cyclosporine-induced perturbation of bile composition resulting in an increased prevalence of biliary stones formation [51, 52]. Other putative explanations include vagotomy and associated biliary stasis, rapid weight loss following transplantation, atherosclerosis, and hemolysis [53]. EAS for gallbladder diseases has been associated with high morbidity (up to 47 %) [17, 20] and mortality rates (up to 29 %) [17, 19], and thus a prophylactic cholecystectomy in asymptomatic patients awaiting transplantation has been proposed as a strategy to avoid symptomatic gallstone diseases later on [54, 55]. This may be particularly indicated before heart and lung transplantation, after which a high incidence of clinical manifestations and increased mortality has been reported [19, 56, 57]. However, this approach remains under debate and it is not routinely performed, also because an emergency cholecystectomy can be highly problematic in patients with end-stage diseases [58]. Both laparoscopy and laparotomy were reported for the surgical management of emergency related to gallbladder diseases. Some evidence suggests that patients undergoing open cholecystectomy develop major post-operative complications (Dindo-Clavien Classification [59] >3) more frequently than patients operated on by laparoscopy [11]. Other studies showed that laparoscopic cholecystectomy can be performed safely in lung-, and kidney-transplanted patients [11, 60], whereas pancreas-transplanted patients may require specific technical modifications in the laparoscopic cholecystectomy procedure, which need to be carefully evaluated preoperatively. In the present systematic review it was not possible to evaluate the rate of post-operative complications and mortality following EAS for gallbladder diseases by specific surgical approach. Nevertheless, the overall morbidity and mortality rates appears to be higher than those found in the literature for non-transplanted patients (estimated at <1 %) [61–64].

Gastrointestinal perforations were the second most frequent cause of EAS after solid organ transplantation. The majority (57.5 %) of the described cases in the literature occurred in kidney-transplanted patients for polycystic kidney disease. Although no precise etiology was found, it seems that transplanted patients for polycystic kidney disease develop more gastrointestinal complications after transplantation than kidney-transplanted patients for other diseases [33], probably due to several biologically active substances that influence the alimentary tract and contribute to the increased incidence of ileus in these patients [65].

In particular, complicated diverticulitis requiring EAS in transplanted patients showed an incidence rate of 0.88 %, which is in accordance with other studies on transplanted patients (1–4 %) [2, 66, 67] and definitely higher than in the general population (estimated incidence of 0.025–0.053 %) [42, 68, 69]. The diagnosis and treatment of diverticulitis after solid organ transplantation are challenging, since immunosuppressive therapies may mask presenting signs and symptoms and impair the ability to contain the infective process [70]. Often, the clinical manifestation and physical examination do not reflect the severity of intra-abdominal disease; signs of infection, such as fever and tachycardia, especially in heart-transplanted patients, could be absent or highly attenuated. Abdominal examination and laboratory testing may be irrelevant, and only the abdominal CT scan appears to be a reliable diagnostic tool to determine the location and severity of the disease. Moreover, morbidity and mortality following emergency colectomy for complicated diverticulitis in transplanted patients are higher (32.7 and 13.6 %, respectively) than those observed in immunocompetent individuals [29, 39].

Another gastrointestinal complication observed in transplanted patients was small bowel obstruction. The most frequent etiologies were post-transplant lymphoproliferative disorders and mechanical obstruction due to adhesions. The first disease is usually diagnosed within the first 2 years after transplantation, and it is strongly associated with high levels of immunosuppressive drugs [71]. The concomitant involvement of both small and large bowels may occur in one third of the patients [72]. These findings stressed the importance of early recognition and systematic referral for endoscopy of any transplanted patient with gastrointestinal symptoms, particularly over the first 2 years after transplantation [26].

Finally, EAS for appendicitis in transplanted patients was described in 0.29 % of cases, mainly in liver-transplanted patients (38.9 %). Appendicitis is one of the most common surgical disease in the general population, with an estimated lifetime risk of 8.6 % in males and 6.7 % in females [73], however only few studies are found in transplanted patients. In all case series, appendectomy was approached by laparotomy. Only a case report in the literature describes laparoscopic appendectomy in two liver and renal transplanted patients with excellent results similar to those in non-transplanted patients [74]. It must be noted that appendicitis in transplanted patients is frequently associated with delayed diagnosis or misdiagnosis, which can lead to complicated appendicitis including rupture and gangrene. As a general rule, appendicitis should be aggressively treated to minimize morbidity in the clinical setting of chronic immunosuppression. Based on the literature findings, surgical morbidity and mortality rates associated with this emergency procedure appear to be much lower than for other gastrointestinal complications [18].

In almost all the included studies, immunosuppressive regimens were maintained unchanged during the post-operative period after EAS. Although the heterogeneity of the literature does not allow pooling data together and analyzing the direct impact of immunosuppressive therapies on post-operative complications, the role of immunosuppression remains crucial since it claims for a more aggressive treatment of acute abdominal diseases. On the other hand, this may contribute to have no cases of graft failure or late rejection following EAS.

Study limitations

The currently available literature on EAS in transplanted patients for graft-unrelated abdominal diseases is based on case series only, which represents a low quality of evidence. However, it may not be feasible to perform randomized controlled trials or even case–control studies in the setting of emergency surgery. Moreover, it was not possible in the present systematic review to perform any quantitative syntheses or risk analysis due to the observational nature of the included studies, the high heterogeneity, and the lack of control groups. Thus, caution should be paid in the interpretation of the results since several biases can be mentioned in the individual studies, such as selection bias, reporting bias, publication bias, and geographical bias. However, we tried to control for search biases by searching the literature on multiple databases, by manual crosscheck of the reference lists, and by performing the critical appraisal by two independent reviewers.

Conclusion

Given the growing number of transplantations per year and the long-term graft survival, EAS for graft-unrelated acute diseases in transplanted patients is not a rare event. The risk of misdiagnosis or delayed diagnosis in chronically immunosuppressed transplanted patients should be minimized by an attentive evaluation of all clinical signs and symptoms. Whenever surgery is indicated, a prompt surgical approach can achieve satisfactory results. However, even common surgical emergencies in transplanted patients are associated with considerable morbidity and mortality. As a general rule, surgeons treating transplanted patients should proceed with caution, apply evidence-based protocols, and expect the unexpected.

Acknowledgements
The authors would like to thank Dr Maria Clotilde Carra for her valuable help in revising the final version of the manuscript.

Funding
Nil.

Authors' contributions
NdeA contributed to concept the study design, literature search, data analysis, data interpretation, and article drafting. FE contributed to literature search, data collection, data analysis, and manuscript drafting. RM contributed to data interpretation, and manuscript critical revision. VL, AMP, FL, PG contributed to literature search, data collection, data analysis, and manuscript revision. FC contributed to concept the study design, data analysis, data interpretation and manuscript critical revision. FB and DA contributed to data interpretation, and manuscript critical revision. All authors read and approved the final version of the manuscript.

Competing interests
The authors declare that they have no competing interests.

Author details
[1]Department of Digestive, Hepatobiliary Surgery and Liver Transplantation, "Henri Mondor" University Hospital, Université Paris Est - UPEC, 51, Avenue du Maréchal de Lattre de Tassigny, 94010 Créteil, France. [2]Department of Hepato-biliary and Pancreatic Surgery, Nouvel Hôpital Civil, Strasbourg, France. [3]Department of Emergency Surgery, University Hospital "Ospedale Maggiore" of Parma, Parma, Italy.

References
1. Mahillo B, Carmona M, Alvarez M, Noel L, Matesanz R. Global database on donation and transplantation: goals, methods and critical issues (http://www.Transplant-observatory.org). Transplant Rev (Orlando). 2013;27:57–60.
2. Goldberg HJ, Hertz MI, Ricciardi R, Madoff RD, Baxter NN, Bullard KM. Colon and rectal complications after heart and lung transplantation. J Am Coll Surg. 2006;202:55–61.
3. Bravo C, Gispert P, Borro JM, de la Torre M, Cifrian Martinez JM, Fernandez Rozas S, Zurbano Goni F, Group MS. Prevalence and management of gastrointestinal complications in lung transplant patients: MITOS study group. Transplant Proc. 2007;39:2409–12.
4. Paul S, Escareno CE, Clancy K, Jaklitsch MT, Bueno R, Lautz DB. Gastrointestinal complications after lung transplantation. J Heart Lung Transplant. 2009;28:475–9.
5. Gautam A, Morrissey PE, Brem AS, Fischer SA, Gohh RY, Yango AF, Monaco AP. Use of an immune function assay to monitor immunosuppression for treatment of post-transplant lymphoproliferative disorder. Pediatr Transplant. 2006;10:613–6.
6. Whiting J. Perioperative concerns for transplant recipients undergoing nontransplant surgery. Surg Clin North Am. 2006;86:1185–94. vi-vii.
7. Moher D, Liberati A, Tetzlaff J, Altman DG, Group P. Preferred reporting items for systematic reviews and meta-analyses: the PRISMA statement. J Clin Epidemiol. 2009;62:1006–12.
8. Abu-Zidan FM, Abbas AK, Hefny AF. Clinical "case series": a concept analysis. Afr Health Sci. 2012;12:557–62.
9. Series NGQAfC: http://www.nice.org.uk/nicemedia/pdf/Appendix_04_qualityofcase_series_form_preop.pdf. Accessed 30 June 2013.
10. Guyatt GH, Oxman AD, Vist GE, Kunz R, Falck-Ytter Y, Alonso-Coello P, Schunemann HJ, Group GW. GRADE: an emerging consensus on rating quality of evidence and strength of recommendations. BMJ. 2008;336:924–6.
11. Taghavi S, Ambur V, Jayarajan SN, Gaughan J, Toyoda Y, Dauer E, Sjoholm LO, Pathak A, Santora T, Goldberg AJ, Rappold J. Postoperative outcomes with cholecystectomy in lung transplant recipients. Surgery. 2015;158:373–8.
12. Kilic A, Sheer A, Shah AS, Russell SD, Gourin CG, Lidor AO. Outcomes of cholecystectomy in US heart transplant recipients. Ann Surg. 2013;258:312–7.
13. Lahon B, Mordant P, Thabut G, Georger JF, Dauriat G, Mal H, Leseche G, Castier Y. Early severe digestive complications after lung transplantation. Eur J Cardiothorac Surg. 2011;40:1419–24.
14. Sarkio S, Salmela K, Kyllonen L, Rosliakova M, Honkanen E, Halme L. Complications of gallstone disease in kidney transplantation patients. Nephrol Dial Transplant. 2007;22:886–90.

15. Takeyama H, Sinanan MN, Fishbein DP, Aldea GS, Verrier ED, Salerno CT. Expectant management is safe for cholelithiasis after heart transplant. J Heart Lung Transplant. 2006;25:539–43.
16. Englesbe MJ, Dubay DA, Wu AH, Pelletier SJ, Punch JD, Franz MG. Gallbladder disease in cardiac transplant patients: a survey study. Arch Surg. 2005;140:399–403. discussion 404.
17. Richardson WS, Surowiec WJ, Carter KM, Howell TP, Mehra MR, Bowen JC. Gallstone disease in heart transplant recipients. Ann Surg. 2003;237:273–6.
18. Hoekstra HJ, Hawkins K, de Boer WJ, Rottier K, van der Bij W. Gastrointestinal complications in lung transplant survivors that require surgical intervention. Br J Surg. 2001;88:433–8.
19. Gupta D, Sakorafas GH, McGregor CG, Harmsen WS, Farnell MB. Management of biliary tract disease in heart and lung transplant patients. Surgery. 2000;128:641–9.
20. Lord RV, Ho S, Coleman MJ, Spratt PM. Cholecystectomy in cardiothoracic organ transplant recipients. Arch Surg. 1998;133:73–9.
21. Bhatia DS, Bowen JC, Money SR, Van Meter Jr CH, McFadden PM, Kot JB, Pridjian AK, Ventura HO, Mehra MR, Smart FW, Ochsner JL. The incidence, morbidity, and mortality of surgical procedures after orthotopic heart transplantation. Ann Surg. 1997;225:686–93. discussion 693–684.
22. Milas M, Ricketts RR, Amerson JR, Kanter K. Management of biliary tract stones in heart transplant patients. Ann Surg. 1996;223:747–53. discussion 753–746.
23. Sharma S, Reddy V, Ott G, Sheppard B, Ratkovec R, Hershberger R, Norman D, Hosenpud J, Cobanoglu A. Gastrointestinal complications after orthotopic cardiac transplantation. Eur J Cardiothorac Surg. 1996;10:616–20.
24. Timrott K, Vondran FW, Kleine M, Warnecke G, Haverich A, Lehner F, Klempnauer J. The impact of abdominal complications on the outcome after thoracic transplantation–a single center experience. Langenbecks Arch Surg. 2014;399:789–93.
25. Lee JT, Dunn TB, Sirany AM, Melton GB, Madoff RD, Kwaan MR. Colorectal surgery after kidney transplantation: characteristics of early vs. late posttransplant interventions. J Gastrointest Surg. 2014;18:1299–305.
26. Cruz Jr RJ, Ramachandra S, Sasatomi E, DiMartini A, de Vera M, Fontes P, Hughes C, Humar A. Surgical management of gastrointestinal posttransplant lymphoproliferative disorders in liver transplant recipients. Transplantation. 2012;94:417–23.
27. Boutros M, Al-Shaibi M, Chan G, Cantarovich M, Rahme E, Paraskevas S, Deschenes M, Ghali P, Wong P, Fernandez M, et al. Clostridium difficile colitis: increasing incidence, risk factors, and outcomes in solid organ transplant recipients. Transplantation. 2012;93:1051–7.
28. Jorgensen KK, Grzyb K, Lundin KE, Clausen OP, Aamodt G, Schrumpf E, Vatn MH, Boberg KM. Inflammatory bowel disease in patients with primary sclerosing cholangitis: clinical characterization in liver transplanted and nontransplanted patients. Inflamm Bowel Dis. 2012;18:536–45.
29. Catena F, Ansaloni L, Gazzotti F, Bertelli R, Severi S, Coccolini F, Fuga G, Nardo B, D'Alessandro L, Faenza A, Pinna AD. Gastrointestinal perforations following kidney transplantation. Transplant Proc. 2008;40:1895–6.
30. Ho GT, Seddon AJ, Therapondos G, Satsangi J, Hayes PC. The clinical course of ulcerative colitis after orthotopic liver transplantation for primary sclerosing cholangitis: further appraisal of immunosuppression post transplantation. Eur J Gastroenterol Hepatol. 2005;17:1379–85.
31. Keven K, Basu A, Re L, Tan H, Marcos A, Fung JJ, Starzl TE, Simmons RL, Shapiro R. Clostridium difficile colitis in patients after kidney and pancreas-kidney transplantation. Transpl Infect Dis. 2004;6:10–4.
32. Karakayalı H, Moray G, Çalişkan K, Başaran Ö, Haberal M. Gastrointestinal complications requiring surgical management in renal transplant recipients. Transplant Proc. 2002;34:2122–3.
33. Andreoni KA, Pelletier RP, Elkhammas EA, Davies EA, Bumgardner GL, Henry ML, Ferguson RM. Increased incidence of gastrointestinal surgical complications in renal transplant recipients with polycystic kidney disease. Transplantation. 1999;67:262–6.
34. Mueller XM, Tevaearai HT, Stumpe F, Hurni M, Ruchat P, Fischer AP, Seydoux C, Goy JJ, von Segesser LK. Gastrointestinal disease following heart transplantation. World J Surg. 1999;23:650–5. discussion 655–656.
35. Wekerle T, Klepetko W, Wisser W, Senbaklavaci O, Artemiou O, Zuckermann A, Wolner E. Incidence and outcome of major non-pulmonary surgical procedures in lung transplant recipients. Eur J Cardiothorac Surg. 1997;12:718–23.
36. Beaver TM, Fullerton DA, Zamora MR, Badesch DB, Weill D, Brown JM, Campbell DN, Grover FL. Colon perforation after lung transplantation. Ann Thorac Surg. 1996;62:839–43.
37. Larson ES, Khalil HA, Lin AY, Russell M, Ardehali A, Ross D, Yoo J. Diverticulitis occurs early after lung transplantation. J Surg Res. 2014;190: 667–71.
38. Scotti A, Santangelo M, Federico S, Carrano R, La Tessa C, Carlomagno N, Palmieri DG, Calogero A, Piantadosi M, Renda A. Complicated diverticulitis in kidney transplanted patients: analysis of 717 cases. Transplant Proc. 2014;46:2247–50.
39. Reshef A, Stocchi L, Kiran RP, Flechner S, Budev M, Quintini C, Remzi FH. Case-matched comparison of perioperative outcomes after surgical treatment of sigmoid diverticulitis in solid organ transplant recipients versus immunocompetent patients. Colorectal Dis. 2012;14:1546–52.
40. Dalla Valle R, Capocasale E, Mazzoni MP, Busi N, Benozzi L, Sivelli R, Sianesi M. Acute diverticulitis with colon perforation in renal transplantation. Transplant Proc. 2005;37:2507–10.
41. Miller CB, Malaisrie SC, Patel J, Garrity E, Vigneswaran WT, Gamelli RL. Intraabdominal complications after lung transplantation. J Am Coll Surg. 2006;203:653–60.
42. Qasabian RA, Meagher AP, Lee R, Dore GJ, Keogh A. Severe diverticulitis after heart, lung, and heart-lung transplantation. J Heart Lung Transplant. 2004;23:845–9.
43. Khan S, Eppstein AC, Anderson GK, Dengal MK, Eggenberger JC, Lee CS, Szilagy EJ, Margolin DA. Acute diverticulitis in heart- and lung transplant patients. Transpl Int. 2001;14:12–5.
44. Lederman ED, Conti DJ, Lempert N, Singh TP, Lee EC. Complicated diverticulitis following renal transplantation. Dis Colon Rectum. 1998;41:613–8.
45. Abt PL, Abdullah I, Korenda K, Frank A, Peterman H, Stephenson GR, Markmann JF, Shaked A, Olthoff KM. Appendicitis among liver transplant recipients. Liver Transpl. 2005;11:1282–4.
46. Savar A, Hiatt JR, Busuttil RW. Acute appendicitis after solid organ transplantation. Clin Transplant. 2006;20:78–80.
47. Ozgor D, Dirican A, Ates M, Yilmaz M, Isik B, Yilmaz S. Incisional hernia in recipients of adult to adult living donor liver transplantation. World J Surg. 2014;38:2122–5.
48. Balshem H, Helfand M, Schunemann HJ, Oxman AD, Kunz R, Brozek J, Vist GE, Falck-Ytter Y, Meerpohl J, Norris S, Guyatt GH. GRADE guidelines: 3. Rating the quality of evidence. J Clin Epidemiol. 2011;64:401–6.
49. Lin S, Cosgrove CJ. Perioperative management of immunosuppression. Surg Clin North Am. 2006;86:1167–83. vi.
50. Popov Z, Ivanovski N, Lekovski L, Stankov O, Dohcev S, Petrovski D, Cakalaroski K, Janculev J, Kolevski P, Abbou CC, Chopin D. [Postoperative complications following kidney transplantation. Ann Urol (Paris). 2000;34:323–9.
51. Hulzebos CV, Bijleveld CM, Stellaard F, Kuipers F, Fidler V, Slooff MJ, Peeters PM, Sauer PJ, Verkade HJ. Cyclosporine A-induced reduction of bile salt synthesis associated with increased plasma lipids in children after liver transplantation. Liver Transpl. 2004;10:872–80.
52. Moran D, De Buitrago JM, Fernandez E, Galan AI, Munoz ME, Jimenez R. Inhibition of biliary glutathione secretion by cyclosporine A in the rat: possible mechanisms and role in the cholestasis induced by the drug. J Hepatol. 1998;29:68–77.
53. Steck TB, Costanzo-Nordin MR, Keshavarzian A. Prevalence and management of cholelithiasis in heart transplant patients. J Heart Lung Transplant. 1991;10:1029–32.
54. Graham SM, Flowers JL, Schweitzer E, Bartlett ST, Imbembo AL. The utility of prophylactic laparoscopic cholecystectomy in transplant candidates. Am J Surg. 1995;169:44–8. discussion 48–49.
55. Kao LS, Kuhr CS, Flum DR. Should cholecystectomy be performed for asymptomatic cholelithiasis in transplant patients? J Am Coll Surg. 2003;197:302–12.
56. Peterseim DS, Pappas TN, Meyers CH, Shaeffer GS, Meyers WC, Van Trigt P. Management of biliary complications after heart transplantation. J Heart Lung Transplant. 1995;14:623–31.
57. Sekela ME, Hutchins DA, Young JB, Noon GP. Biliary surgery after cardiac transplantation. Arch Surg. 1991;126:571–3.
58. Menegaux F, Dorent R, Tabbi D, Pavie A, Chigot JP, Gandjbakhch I. Biliary surgery after heart transplantation. Am J Surg. 1998;175:320–1.
59. Clavien PA, Barkun J, de Oliveira ML, Vauthey JN, Dindo D, Schulick RD, de Santibanes E, Pekolj J, Slankamenac K, Bassi C, et al. The Clavien-Dindo classification of surgical complications: five-year experience. Ann Surg. 2009;250:187–96.
60. Jackson T, Treleaven D, Arlen D, D'Sa A, Lambert K, Birch DW. Management of asymptomatic cholelithiasis for patients awaiting renal transplantation. Surg Endosc. 2005;19:510–3.

61. Dolan JP, Diggs BS, Sheppard BC, Hunter JG. The national mortality burden and significant factors associated with open and laparoscopic cholecystectomy: 1997–2006. J Gastrointest Surg. 2009;13:2292–301.
62. Perissat J. Laparoscopic cholecystectomy: the European experience. Am J Surg. 1993;165:444–9.
63. Stinton LM, Shaffer EA. Epidemiology of gallbladder disease: cholelithiasis and cancer. Gut Liver. 2012;6:172–87.
64. Pulvirenti E, Toro A, Gagner M, Mannino M, Di Carlo I. Increased rate of cholecystectomies performed with doubtful or no indications after laparoscopy introduction: a single center experience. BMC Surg. 2013;13:17.
65. Fleming TW, Barry JM. Bilateral open transperitoneal cyst reduction surgery for autosomal dominant polycystic kidney disease. J Urol. 1998;159:44–7.
66. Hwang SS, Cannom RR, Abbas MA, Etzioni D. Diverticulitis in transplant patients and patients on chronic corticosteroid therapy: a systematic review. Dis Colon Rectum. 2010;53:1699–707.
67. Maurer JR. The spectrum of colonic complications in a lung transplant population. Ann Transplant. 2000;5:54–7.
68. Kang JY, Hoare J, Tinto A, Subramanian S, Ellis C, Majeed A, Melville D, Maxwell JD. Diverticular disease of the colon–on the rise: a study of hospital admissions in England between 1989/1990 and 1999/2000. Aliment Pharmacol Ther. 2003;17:1189–95.
69. Hjern F, Johansson C, Mellgren A, Baxter NN, Hjern A. Diverticular disease and migration–the influence of acculturation to a Western lifestyle on diverticular disease. Aliment Pharmacol Ther. 2006;23:797–805.
70. Detry O, Defraigne JO, Meurisse M, Bertrand O, Demoulin JC, Honore P, Jacquet N, Limet R. Acute diverticulitis in heart transplant recipients. Transpl Int. 1996;9:376–9.
71. Patel H, Vogl DT, Aqui N, Shaked A, Olthoff K, Markmann J, Reddy R, Stadtmauer EA, Schuster S, Tsai DE. Posttransplant lymphoproliferative disorder in adult liver transplant recipients: a report of seventeen cases. Leuk Lymphoma. 2007;48:885–91.
72. Younes BS, Ament ME, McDiarmid SV, Martin MG, Vargas JH. The involvement of the gastrointestinal tract in posttransplant lymphoproliferative disease in pediatric liver transplantation. J Pediatr Gastroenterol Nutr. 1999;28:380–5.
73. Addiss DG, Shaffer N, Fowler BS, Tauxe RV. The epidemiology of appendicitis and appendectomy in the United States. Am J Epidemiol. 1990;132:910–25.
74. Wei CK, Chang CM, Lee CH, Chen JH, Yin WY. Acute appendicitis in organ transplantation patients: a report of two cases and a literature review. Ann Transplant. 2014;19:248–52.

Permissions

All chapters in this book were first published in WJES, by BioMed Central; hereby published with permission under the Creative Commons Attribution License or equivalent. Every chapter published in this book has been scrutinized by our experts. Their significance has been extensively debated. The topics covered herein carry significant findings which will fuel the growth of the discipline. They may even be implemented as practical applications or may be referred to as a beginning point for another development.

The contributors of this book come from diverse backgrounds, making this book a truly international effort. This book will bring forth new frontiers with its revolutionizing research information and detailed analysis of the nascent developments around the world.

We would like to thank all the contributing authors for lending their expertise to make the book truly unique. They have played a crucial role in the development of this book. Without their invaluable contributions this book wouldn't have been possible. They have made vital efforts to compile up to date information on the varied aspects of this subject to make this book a valuable addition to the collection of many professionals and students.

This book was conceptualized with the vision of imparting up-to-date information and advanced data in this field. To ensure the same, a matchless editorial board was set up. Every individual on the board went through rigorous rounds of assessment to prove their worth. After which they invested a large part of their time researching and compiling the most relevant data for our readers.

The editorial board has been involved in producing this book since its inception. They have spent rigorous hours researching and exploring the diverse topics which have resulted in the successful publishing of this book. They have passed on their knowledge of decades through this book. To expedite this challenging task, the publisher supported the team at every step. A small team of assistant editors was also appointed to further simplify the editing procedure and attain best results for the readers.

Apart from the editorial board, the designing team has also invested a significant amount of their time in understanding the subject and creating the most relevant covers. They scrutinized every image to scout for the most suitable representation of the subject and create an appropriate cover for the book.

The publishing team has been an ardent support to the editorial, designing and production team. Their endless efforts to recruit the best for this project, has resulted in the accomplishment of this book. They are a veteran in the field of academics and their pool of knowledge is as vast as their experience in printing. Their expertise and guidance has proved useful at every step. Their uncompromising quality standards have made this book an exceptional effort. Their encouragement from time to time has been an inspiration for everyone.

The publisher and the editorial board hope that this book will prove to be a valuable piece of knowledge for researchers, students, practitioners and scholars across the globe.

List of Contributors

Morihiro Katsura
Department of General Surgery, Okinawa Prefectural Hokubu Hospital, 2-12-3 Onaka, Nago, Okinawa 905-8512, Japan

Hidemitsu Mototake
Department of Cardiovascular Surgery, Okinawa Prefectural Chubu Hospital, Okinawa, Japan

Hiroaki Takara
Department of Radiology, Okinawa Prefectural Chubu Hospital, Okinawa, Japan

Kazuhide Matsushima
Department of Surgery, Penn State Milton S. Hershey Medical Center, PA, USA

Louise S Londero
Department of Cardiothoracic- and Vascular Surgery, University Hospital of Odense, Sdr. Boulevard 29, 5000 Odense C, Denmark

Birgitte Nørgaard
Institute of Public Health, University of Southern Denmark, Sdr. Boulevard 29, 5000 Odense C, Denmark

Kim Houlind
Department of Vascular Surgery, Kolding Hospital, Skovvangen 2, 6000 Kolding, Denmark

Iraklis E Katsoulis, Ioanna Gogoulou, Athanasios Stathoulopoulos and Michael K Digalakis
1st Surgical Department, Asklepieio General Hospital, Voula, Greece

Alexia Balanika and Maria Sakalidou
Computed Tomography Department, Asklepieio General Hospital, Voula, Greece

Hongjin Shim
Department of Surgery, Yonsei University Wonju College of Medicine, Wonju, Korea

Ji Young Jang, Seung Hwan Lee and Jae Gil Lee
Department of Surgery, Yonsei University College of Medicine, 50 Yonsei-ro, Seodaemun-gu, Seoul 120-752, Korea

Markus Udo Wagenhäuser, Tolga Atilla Sagban, Mareike Witte, Mansur Duran, Hubert Schelzig and Alexander Oberhuber
Department of Vascular and Endovascular Surgery, University Hospital Düsseldorf, Moorenstraße.5, 40225 Düsseldorf, Germany

Jonathan C Samuel, Javeria S Qureshi and Gift Mulima
Department of Surgery, Kamuzu Central Hospital, Lilongwe, Malawi

Jonathan C Samuel, Javeria S Qureshi, Bruce A Cairns and Anthony G Charles
Department of Surgery, University of North Carolina, 4001 Burnett Womack Bldg, CB 7050, Chapel Hill, NC, 27599 USA

Carol G Shores
Lineberger Comprehensive Cancer Center, University of North Carolina, CB 7295, Chapel Hill, NC, 27599 USA
Department of Otolaryngology/Head & Neck Surgery, University of North Carolina, 170 Manning Drive, CB 7070, Physician's Office Bldg G-190, Chapel Hill, NC, 27599 USA

Bruce A Cairns
NC Jaycee Burn Center, University of North Carolina, 101 Manning Drive, CB 7600, Chapel Hill, NC, 27599 USA

Fabio Cesare Campanile
Division of Surgery, Ospedale San Giovanni Decollato - Andosilla, Civita Castellana, VT, Italy

Michele Pisano, Federico Coccolini and Luca Ansaloni
General Surgery Department, Papa Giovanni XXIII hospital, Bergamo, Italy

Fausto Catena
Department of Emergency Surgery, Maggiore Parma Hospital, Parma, Italy

Ferdinando Agresta
Department of General Surgery, ULSS19 del Veneto, Adria, RO, Italy

Ali Jawas, Alaa K Abbas and Fikri M Abu-Zidan
Department of Surgery, College of Medicine and Health Sciences, United Arab Emirates University, Al-Ain, United Arab Emirates

Munier Nazzal, Marzoog Albader and Fikri M Abu-Zidan
Department of Surgery, Mubarak Al-Kabeer Teaching Hospital, Jabriya, Kuwait

Munier Nazzal
Division of Vascular and Endovascular Surgery, University of Toledo Medical Center, Toledo, Ohio, USA

Phillipo L Chalya
Department of Surgery, Catholic University of Health and Allied Sciences-Bugando, Mwanza, Tanzania

Anthony N Massinde and Albert Kihunrwa
Department of Obstetrics /Gynecology, Catholic University of Health and Allied Sciences-Bugando, Mwanza, Tanzania

Samson Simbila
Department of Urology, Catholic University of Health and Allied Sciences-Bugando, Mwanza, Tanzania

Flavie Toret-Labeeuw, Cyrille Huchon, Thomas Popowski and Arnaud Fauconnier
Department of Gynecology & Obstetrics, Centre Hospitalier Intercommunal de Poissy - Saint-Germain, University of Versailles Saint-Quentin (UVSQ), 78103 Poissy, France

Cyrille Huchon and Arnaud Fauconnier
EA7285, Risques cliniques et sécurité en santé des femmes et en santé périnatale, University of Versailles Saint-Quentin (UVSQ), Poissy, France

Anne A Chantry
INSERM, UMR S953, 75014 Paris, France

Alexandre Dumont
Institut de recherche pour le développement (Research Institute for Development), UMR IRD 216, 75014 Paris, France

Joao B Rezende-Neto and Fernando A Botoni
sUniversidade Federal de Minas Gerais and Risoleta Tolentino Neves Hospital, Brazil

Argenil J Oliveira and Mario P Neto
Risoleta Tolentino Neves Hospital, Brazil

Sandro B Rizoli
University of Toronto and Sunnybrook Hospital, Canada

Carlos Augusto Gomes
Surgery Department, Therezinha de Jesus University Hospital, Medical and Health Science School, Surgery Unit, Federal University of Juiz de Fora (UFJF), Rua Senador Salgado Filho 510 / 1002, Bairro Bom Pastor, Juiz de Fora, Minas Gerais 36021-660, Brasil

Massimo Sartelli
Department of Surgery, Macerata Hospital, Macerata, Italy

Salomone Di Saverio
Trauma Surgery Unit, Maggiore Hospital, Bologna, Italy

Luca Ansaloni and Federico Coccolini
General Surgery I, Papa Giovanni XXIII Hospital, Bergamo, Italy

Fausto Catena
Emergency Surgery Department, Maggiore Parma Hospital, Parma, Italy

Kenji Inaba and Demetrios Demetriades
University of California, San Francisco, USA

Demetrios Demetriades
Department of Surgery (K.I.), Keck School of Medicine of University of Southern California, Los Angeles, CA, USA

Felipe Couto Gomes
Internal Medicine Departament, Therezinha de Jesus University Hospital, Medical and Health Science School, Juiz de Fora, Brazil

Camila Couto Gomes
Internal Medicine Departament, Monte Sinai Hospital, Juiz de Fora, Minas Gerais, Brazil

Yoram Kluger
Department of Surgery, Rambam Health Care Center, Haifa, Israel

Offir Ben-Ishay and Massimo Sartelli
Department of Surgery, Macerata Hospital, Macerata, Italy

Luca Ansaloni
Department of General Surgery, Ospedali Riuniti, Italy

Tamer El Zalabany
Department of General Surgery, Bahrain Defence Force Military Hospital, West Riffa, Bahrain

Gustavo P Fraga
Department of Surgery, University of Campinas, Campinas, São Paulo, Brazil

Carlos Augusto Gomes
Department of Surgery, Hospital Universitário, Universidade Federal de Juiz de Fora, Juiz de Fora, Minas Gerais, Brazil

Nereo Vettoretto
Department of Surgery, Mellini Hospital, Chiari, Italy

Ernest E Moore
Department of Surgery, Denver Health Medical Center, Denver, Colorado, USA

Japhet M Gilyoma, Darius D Balumuka and Phillipo L Chalya
Department of Surgery, Weill-Bugando University Colleges of Health Sciences, Mwanza, Tanzania

Moritz T Giesecke, Philipp Schwabe, Florian Wichlas, Andrej Trampuz and Christian Kleber
Center for Musculoskeletal Surgery, AG Polytrauma, Charité - Universitätsmedizin, Augustenburger Platz 1, 13353 Berlin, Germany

Sławomir Jabłoński
Department of Thoracic Surgery, General and Oncological Surgery, Medical University of Lodz, 113 Żeromskiego St., 90-547, Łódź, Poland

Marcin Kozakiewicz
Department of Maxillofacial Surgery, Medical University of Lodz, 113 Żeromskiego St., 90- 547, Łódź, Poland

F. Van der Cruyssen
Third year master's student, Faculty of Medicine, Catholic University of Leuven (KU Leuven), Gasthuisberg, Belgium

A. Manzelli
Department of Upper Gastrointestinal Surgery, Royal Devon & Exeter Hospital, Exeter, UK

Massimo Sartelli
Department of Surgery, Macerata Hospital, Via Santa Lucia, 62100 Macerata, Italy

Yoram Kluger
Department of General Surgery, Division of Surgery, Rambam Health Care Campus, Haifa, Israel

Luca Ansaloni
General Surgery Department, "M. Bufalini" Cesena Hospital, Cesena, Italy

Aleksandar Karamarkovic
Clinic for Surgery, University Clinical Center "Zvezdara", Belgrade, Serbia

Jakub Kenig
Third Department of General Surgery, Jagiellonian University Medical College, Krakow, Poland

Vladimir Khokha
Department of Emergency Surgery, City Hospital, Mozyr, Belarus

Francesco M. Labricciosa
Global Alliance for Infections in Surgery, Porto, Portugal

Fausto Catena
Department of Emergency Surgery, Maggiore Hospital, Parma, Italy

Miklosh Bala
Acute Care Surgery and Trauma Unit, General Surgery Department, Hadassah - Hebrew University Medical Center, Kiriat Hadassah, 91120 Jerusalem, Israel

Jeffry Kashuk
Assia Medical Group, Tel Aviv University Sackler School of Medicine, Tel Aviv, Israel

Ernest E. Moore
Department of Surgery, Denver Health Medical Center, University of Colorado, Denver, USA

Nicola de'Angelis
Unit of Digestive, Hepato-Pancreato-Biliary Surgery and Liver Transplantation, Henri Mondor University Hospital, AP-HP, and University of Paris Est, UPEC, 51 Avenue du Maréchal de Lattre de Tassigny, 94010 Créteil, France

Salomone Di Saverio
Department of Surgery, Maggiore Hospital, Bologna, Italy

Osvaldo Chiara
General Surgery and Trauma Team, Niguarda Hospital, Milan, Italy

Pietro Genova
Department of General and Oncological Surgery, University Hospital Paolo Giaccone, Palermo, Italy

Rao Ivatury
Virginia Commonwealth University, Richmond, VA, USA

Jeffry L. Kashuk
Assia Medical Group, Department of Surgery, Sackler School of Medicine, Tel Aviv University, Tel Aviv, Israel

Richard P. ten Broek
Department of Surgery, Radboud University Medical Center, Nijmegen, The Netherlands

Luigi Zorcolo
Department of Surgery, Colorectal Surgery Unit, University of Cagliari, Cagliari, Italy

Maria Clotilde Carra
University Paris Diderot, Rothschild Hospital, AP-HP, Paris, France

Pepijn Krielen
Department of Surgery, Radboud University Medical Center, Nijmegen, The Netherlands

Salomone Di Saverio
Addenbrooke's Hospital, Cambridge, UK

Federico Coccolini
General Emergency and Trauma Surgery, Bufalini hospital, Cesena, Italy

Walter L. Biffl
Acute Care Surgery, The Queen's Medical Center, Honolulu, Hawaii, USA

Zsolt J. Balogh
Department of Traumatology, John Hunter Hospital and University of Newcastle, Newcastle, NSW, Australia

Cino Bendinelli
John Hunter Hospital, New Lambton Heights, New Zealand

Ian Civil
Department of Vascular and Trauma Surgery, Auckland City Hospital, Auckland, New Zealand

Raul Coimbra
Department of Surgery, UC San Diego Health System, San Diego, USA

Nicola De'Angelis
Unit of Digestive Surgery, HPB Surgery and Liver Transplant, Henri Mondor Hospital, Créteil, France

Frank Piscioneri
Canberra Hospital, Canberra, Australia

Joseph M. Galante
Trauma and Acute Care Surgery and Surgical Critical Care Trauma, Department of Surgery, University of California, Davis, USA

Fausto Catena
Emergency and Trauma Surgery, Parma Maggiore hospital, Parma, Italy

Massimo Sartelli
Department of Surgery, Macerata Hospital, Macerata, Italy

Francesco M. Labricciosa and Pamela Barbadoro
Department of Biomedical Sciences and Public Health, Unit of Hygiene, Preventive Medicine and Public Health, Università Politecnica delle Marche, Ancona, Italy

Leonardo Pagani
Infectious Diseases Unit, Bolzano Central Hospital, Bolzano, Italy

Luca Ansaloni
General Surgery Department, Papa Giovanni XXIII Hospital, Bergamo, Italy

Asri Che Jusoh
Department of General Surgery, Kuala Krai Hospital, Kuala Krai, Kelantan, Malaysia

Jill R. Cherry-Bukowiec
Division of Acute Care Surgery, Department of Surgery, University of Michigan, Ann Arbor, MI, USA

Osvaldo Chiara
Niguarda Hospital, Milano, Italy

Elif Colak
Department of General Surgery, Health Sciences University, Samsun Training and Research Hospital, Samsun, Turkey

Tanya L. Zakrison
Division of Trauma and Surgical Critical Care, DeWitt Daughtry Family Department of Surgery, University of Miami, Miami, FL, USA

Brian Zuckerbraun
Department of Surgery, University of Pittsburgh, Pittsburgh, PA, USA

Wietse P. Zuidema
VU University Medical Center, Amsterdam, The Netherlands

Fausto Catena
Department of General Surgery, Maggiore Hospital, Parma, Italy

Ramiro Manzano-Nunez and Claudia P. Orlas
Clinical Research Center, Fundacion Valle del Lili, Cali, Colombia

Ramiro Manzano-Nunez, Juan P. Herrera-Escobar and Justin C. McCarty
Center for Surgery and Public Health - Brigham and Women's Hospital, Harvard Medical School & Harvard T.H. Chan School of Public Health, Boston, MA, USA

Claudia P. Orlas and Carlos A. Ordoñez
Trauma and Acute Care Surgery Division, Department of Surgery, Fundacion Valle del Lili, Cali, Colombia

Samuel M. Galvagno
R. Adams Cowley Shock Trauma Center, Baltimore, MD, USA

Juan J. Melendez and Carlos A. Ordoñez
Trauma Division and Trauma and Emergency Surgery Fellowship, Universidad del Valle, Cali, Colombia

Albaro J. Nieto and Maria F. Escobar-Vidarte
Critical Care Obstetrics, Department of Gynecology and Obstetrics, Fundacion Valle del Lili, Cali, Colombia

Natalia Padilla
School of Medicine, Universidad ICESI, Cali, Colombia

Massimo Sartelli
Department of Surgery, Macerata Hospital, Macerata, Italy

Yoram Kluger
Department of General Surgery, Division of Surgery, Rambam Health Care Campus, Haifa, Israel

Luca Ansaloni
General Surgery Department, Bufalini Hospital, Cesena, Italy

Timothy C. Hardcastle
Trauma Service, Inkosi Albert Luthuli Central Hospital, Durban, South Africa

Kenneth Y. Y. Kok
Department of Surgery, The Brunei Cancer Centre, Jerudong Park, Jerudong, Brunei

Arda Isik
Department of General Surgery, Faculty of Medicine, Erzincan University, Erzincan, Turkey

Francesco M. Labricciosa
Global Alliance for Infections in Surgery, Porto, Portugal

Norio Sato
Department of Aeromedical Services for Emergency and Trauma Care, Graduate School of Medicine, Ehime University, Ehime, Japan

Jay N. Shah
Department of Surgery, Patan Hospital, Patan Academy of Health Sciences Lalitpur, Kathmandu, Nepal

Boonying Siribumrungwong
Department of Surgery, Faculty of Medicine, Thammasat University Hospital, Thammasat University, Rangsit, Pathum Thani, Thailand

Peep Talving
Department of Surgery, North Estonia Medical Center, Tallinn, Estonia

Aidan Lyanzhiang Tan
Preventive Medicine, National University Hospital, Singapore, Singapore

Aidan Lyanzhiang Tan
Health Services Research Unit, Singapore General Hospital, Singapore, Singapore

Yi Chiong
Department of Rehabilitation Medicine, Singapore General Hospital, Singapore, Singapore

Nivedita Nadkarni
Centre for Quantitative Medicine, Duke-NUS Graduate Medical School, Singapore, Singapore

Jolene Yu Xuan Cheng and Ming Terk Chiu
National Trauma Unit, Tan Tock Seng Hospital, Singapore, Singapore

Ming Terk Chiu
Department of General Surgery, Tan Tock Seng Hospital, Singapore, Singapore

Ting Hway Wong
General and Trauma Surgery Singapore General Hospital, Singapore, Singapore
Health Services and Systems Research, Duke-NUS Graduate Medical School, Singapore, Singapore

Emiliano Gamberini, Costanza Martino, Vittorio Albarello, Marco Benni and Vanni Agnoletti
Anesthesia and Intensive Care Department, AUSL Romagna Trauma Center "Maurizio Bufalini" Hospital, Viale Ghirotti 286, 47521 Cesena, Italy

Federico Coccolini and Luca Ansaloni
General and Emergency Surgery Department, ASST Trauma Center "Papa Giovanni XXIII" Hospital, Piazza OMS 1, 24127 Bergamo, Italy

Beatrice Tamagnini
Emergency Medicine, University of Modena and Reggio Emilia, via Università 4, 41121 Modena, Italy

Marcello Bisulli
Interventional Radiology Department, AUSL Romagna Trauma Center "Maurizio Bufalini" Hospital, Viale Ghirotti 286, 47521 Cesena, Italy

Nicola Fabbri
General and Emergency Surgery Department, AUSL Romagna Trauma Center "Maurizio Bufalini" Hospital, Viale Ghirotti 286, 47521 Cesena, Italy

Tal Martin Hörer
Cardiothoracic and Vascular Surgery Department, Örebro University Hospital, Södra Grev Rosengatan, 701 85 Örebro, Sweden

Carlo Coniglio
Anesthesia, Intensive Care and 118 Emergency System Department, AUSL Bologna Trauma Center "Maggiore" Hospital, Largo Nigrisoli 2, 40133 Bologna, Italy

Marco Barozzi
Emergency Medicine Department, AUSL Modena Trauma Center "Sant'Agostino" Hospital, Via Pietro Giardini 1355, 41126 Modena, Italy

Nicola de'Angelis, Francesco Esposito, Vincenzo Lizzi, Aleix Martìnez-Pérez, Filippo Landi, Pietro Genova, Francesco Brunetti and Daniel Azoulay
Department of Digestive, Hepatobiliary Surgery and Liver Transplantation, "Henri Mondor" University Hospital, Université Paris Est - UPEC, 51, Avenue du Maréchal de Lattre de Tassigny, 94010 Créteil, France

Riccardo Memeo
Department of Hepato-biliary and Pancreatic Surgery, Nouvel Hôpital Civil, Strasbourg, France

Fausto Catena
Department of Emergency Surgery, University Hospital "Ospedale Maggiore" of Parma, Parma, Italy

Index

A

Abdominal Hysterectomy, 42, 44, 46, 48

Abdomino-pelvic Surgery, 42-44

Acute Appendicitis, 64-69, 71, 73, 75, 215, 219-220

Acute Cholecystitis, 31-36, 212

Acute Limb Ischemia, 7, 9, 11

Acute Mediastinitis, 91-93, 98

Acute Mesenteric Ischemia, 6, 16, 123, 126-127, 131-133

Acute Pelvic Pain, 50-51, 53-54, 56

Anatomical Polytrauma, 193, 200

Antimicrobial Therapy, 67-68, 82-83, 88-89, 118, 120-121, 143, 152, 177, 192 Aorta, 6, 9, 20, 25, 124, 128, 178-180, 182-183, 201, 203, 206-208

Aortic Balloon Occlusion, 179, 183, 201, 208

Arterial Thrombolysis, 7

Arteriovenous Fistulas, 111-114

B

Balloon Inflation, 201, 207

Blunt Splenic Injury, 103-104, 106-112, 115-116

Bowel Infarction, 20, 23-24, 125, 127-128

Bowel Ischemia, 1, 3-4, 16-17, 20, 123, 125, 127, 129, 161-162

Brachial Arteries, 39

C

C-reactive Protein, 21, 24, 83, 93, 100-102, 140-141, 149, 152

Cardiac Arrest, 13, 15, 204, 207

Cardiopulmonary Resuscitation, 13, 127

Clostridium Difficile Infections, 118

Colonic Necrosis, 13-15

D

Damage Control Surgery, 40-41, 129,

131, 133, 135, 147, 149, 153

Diabetes Mellitus, 21, 24, 71, 137, 166

Diverticulitis, 22, 29, 68, 71, 75, 144-145, 147, 149, 153, 210-212, 214, 216-217, 219-220

E

Edema, 15, 66-67, 89, 125, 158, 190

Endoscopic Submucosal Dissection, 137-139, 148-149, 151-152

Endotracheal Intubation, 76, 78, 81, 101

G

Gastrointestinal Endoscopy, 134, 138-139, 151

Gram Positive Strains, 82

Griggs-portex, 57, 60

H

Hemoperitoneum, 52, 54, 56, 104, 111, 113, 115, 204

Hemorrhagic Shock, 15-16, 132, 183, 201, 207

Hyperemia, 66-67

Hyperlactatemia, 187-188, 190

I

Iatrogenic Colonoscopy Perforation, 134-135, 138-139, 149

Iatrogenic Ureteric Injuries, 42-44, 46, 49

Iliac Arteries, 179-180

Immunosuppressive Therapy, 209, 213-216

Injury Severity Score, 83, 88, 104, 115, 193-196, 198-200

Isolated Dissection, 1-2, 5-6, 20, 24-25

L

L-lactate, 126, 131

Laparoscopic Cholecystectomy, 31-36, 212, 217, 219-220

Logistic Organ Dysfunction Score, 185

M

Magnetic Resonance Imaging, 65, 165

Mesenteric Arterial Occlusion, 123, 125

Meticulous Surgical Technique, 42, 46, 48, 81

Morbidly Adherent Placenta, 178-179, 182-183

Multidetector Computed Tomography, 13, 126, 149

Multiple Organ Dysfunction Score, 17

N

Nasogastric Suction, 20-21, 23, 130

Non-occlusive Ischaemia, 13-14

Nutritional Risk Index, 92, 97-98, 100-101

O

Operative Splenic Salvage, 103-104, 115

Oxygen Radical Activity, 17-19

P
Pathogen Spectrum, 82, 89
Percutaneous Tracheostomy, 57-63
Peritoneal Adhesion Index, 157, 165
Post-partum Hemorrhage, 178-179, 182
Pseudomonas, 82, 85-89

R
Revised Trauma Score, 193-195, 198-199

S
Sepsis, 17-19, 33, 45, 73-74, 91-92, 95, 99-102, 109, 116, 118, 122, 125, 129, 131, 141-144, 146-148, 152, 158, 177, 184-192, 208, 215
Septic Shock, 17-19, 102, 122, 125, 132, 147, 152, 184-192
Small Bowel Perforation, 26-28
Solid Organ Transplantation, 152, 209-210, 212, 215-217
Splenic Artery Embolization, 103, 106-110, 115-116
Sub-/total Traumatic Amputations, 82, 89
Superior Mesenteric Artery, 1, 5-6, 20-21, 24-25, 124, 131-133
Surgical Site Infections, 45, 117, 120
Suture Ligation, 42-44
Systemic Inflammatory Response Syndrome, 15, 143, 184, 187-188, 190, 192

T
Tachycardia, 13, 26-29, 92, 140, 189, 217
Tachypnea, 26-27, 189-190
Thrombocytopenia, 26-28, 63, 190, 206
Thrombocytosis, 26-28
Tissue Plasminogen Activator, 125, 131
Tracheal Breach, 57-58, 60
Tracheostomy Decannulation, 76-77, 79-81
Transvaginal Ultrasonography, 50, 54-55
Transverse Skin Crease Incision, 76-77, 79-80
Tubo-ovarian Abscess, 26-28, 51, 54

U
Ureteroneocystostomy, 42, 45-48

www.ingramcontent.com/pod-product-compliance
Lightning Source LLC
LaVergne TN
LVHW080709210926
848485LV00003B/440

* 9 7 8 1 6 3 9 2 7 4 8 9 5 *